Immunobiology of the Complement System

Immunobiology of the Complement System

Editor: Adah Blair

AMERICAN
MEDICAL PUBLISHERS
www.americanmedicalpublishers.com

AMERICAN
MEDICAL PUBLISHERS
www.americanmedicalpublishers.com

Cataloging-in-Publication Data

Immunobiology of the complement system / edited by Adah Blair.
p. cm.
Includes bibliographical references and index.
ISBN 979-8-88740-203-1
1. Complement (Immunology). 2. Immunology. 3. Complement activation.
4. Immunopathology. 5. Clinical immunology. I. Blair, Adah.
QR185.8.C6 I46 2023
616.079--dc23

American Medical Publishers,
41 Flatbush Avenue,
1st Floor, New York,
NY 11217, USA

ISBN 979-8-88740-203-1 (Hardback)

Contents

Preface

The world is advancing at a fast pace like never before. Therefore, the need is to keep up with the latest developments. This book was an idea that came to fruition when the specialists in the area realized the need to coordinate together and document essential themes in the subject. That's when I was requested to be the editor. Editing this book has been an honour as it brings together diverse authors researching on different streams of the field. The book collates essential materials contributed by veterans in the area which can be utilized by students and researchers alike.

The complement system is a part of the immune system which improves the capability of phagocytic cells and antibodies to take out damaged cells and microbes from the organism's body. Complement control proteins, which are found in a higher concentration in the blood plasma as compared to complement proteins, regulate the complement system. Some of the complement control proteins are found on the membranes of self-cells that protect them from attack by the complement system. This system is considered to be focused on killing bacteria that infect the host organism. Furthermore, it acts as an innate immune surveillance system, which has a significant role to play in host homeostasis, defense against pathogens and inflammation. The dysfunction of the complement system is a major reason of diseases caused in the central nervous system, such as neurodegenerative conditions like spinal cord injuries and Alzheimer's disease. C3 glomerulopathy and atypical hemolytic uremic syndrome have been found linked with mutations in the genes of complement regulators specifically factor H. The readers would gain knowledge that would broaden their perspective about the complement system and its immunobiology through this book. It will help the readers in keeping pace with the rapid changes in this area of study.

Each chapter is a sole-standing publication that reflects each author´s interpretation. Thus, the book displays a multi-facetted picture of our current understanding of application, resources and aspects of the field. I would like to thank the contributors of this book and my family for their endless support.

Editor

1

Complement C3 Produced by Macrophages Promotes Renal Fibrosis via IL-17A Secretion

Yanyan Liu[1†], *Kun Wang*[1†], *Xinjun Liang*[2], *Yueqiang Li*[1], *Ying Zhang*[1], *Chunxiu Zhang*[1], *Haotian Wei*[1], *Ran Luo*[1], *Shuwang Ge*[1] *and Gang Xu*[1*]

[1] *Division of Internal Medicine, Department of Nephrology, Tongji Hospital, Tongji Medical College, Huazhong University of Science and Technology, Wuhan, China,* [2] *Hubei Cancer Hospital, Tongji Medical College, Huazhong University of Science and Technology, Wuhan, China*

***Correspondence:**
Gang Xu
xugang@tjh.tjmu.edu.cn

† These authors have contributed equally to this work

Complement synthesis in cells of origin is strongly linked to the pathogenesis and progression of renal disease. Multiple studies have examined local C3 synthesis in renal disease and elucidated the contribution of local cellular sources, but the contribution of infiltrating inflammatory cells remains unclear. We investigate the relationships among C3, macrophages and Th17 cells, which are involved in interstitial fibrosis. Here, we report that increased local C3 expression, mainly by monocyte/macrophages, was detected in renal biopsy specimens and was correlated with the severity of renal fibrosis (RF) and indexes of renal function. In mouse models of UUO (unilateral ureteral obstruction), we found that local C3 was constitutively expressed throughout the kidney in the interstitium, from which it was released by F4/80^{+}macrophages. After the depletion of macrophages using clodronate, mice lacking macrophages exhibited reductions in C3 expression and renal tubulointerstitial fibrosis. Blocking C3 expression with a C3 and C3aR inhibitor provided similar protection against renal tubulointerstitial fibrosis. These protective effects were associated with reduced pro-inflammatory cytokines, renal recruitment of inflammatory cells, and the Th17 response. *in vitro*, recombinant C3a significantly enhanced T cell proliferation and IL-17A expression, which was mediated through phosphorylation of ERK, STAT3, and STAT5 and activation of NF-kB in T cells. More importantly, blockade of C3a by a C3aR inhibitor drastically suppressed IL-17A expression in C3a-stimulated T cells. We propose that local C3 secretion by macrophages leads to IL-17A-mediated inflammatory cell infiltration into the kidney, which further drives fibrogenic responses. Our findings suggest that inhibition of the C3a/C3aR pathway is a novel therapeutic approach for obstructive nephropathy.

Keywords: complement component 3, macrophage, renal fibrosis (RF), IL-17A, IgAN

INTRODUCTION

Renal fibrosis (RF) has become an important worldwide health problem and represents a major economic burden to society. IgA nephropathy (IgAN) is one of the most common causes of chronic kidney disease (CKD), and the prognosis of IgAN is more closely associated with the severity of interstitial injury and fibrosis than that of glomerular lesions (1). As the common consequence of all forms of CKD, RF is characterized by deposition of extracellular matrix and associated with inflammatory cell recruitment, angiogenesis, lymphangiogenesis, an myofibroblast formation (2–4). Although researchers have confirmed that chronic inflammation, oxidative stress, proteinuria, and abnormal activation of complement are involved in the development and progression of CKD, the pathogenesis of RF remains largely unknown (5–8).

The complement system is a crucial part of the immune system and consists of multiple categories of components. The complement component 3 (C3), a 180 kDa glycoprotein, plays a central role in activation of the complement system. Its activation is required for both classical and alternative complement activation pathways. Circulating C3 is produced by the liver, and its extrahepatic production has been observed in other specialized cells, including mast cells, fibroblasts, smooth muscle cells, and macrophages (9, 10). These cells synthesize C3, presumably through their bioactive products, and have an important role in regulating other aspects of autoimmunity, inflammation, and pathogen host defense. Studies have confirmed that locally synthesized C3 appears to have a stronger influence on rejection than circulating C3 (11). Other reports have demonstrated that the epithelial and vascular tissues at local sites of inflammation could secrete complement components (12). Despite Xavier and Cui have demonstrated that complement C3 activation and macrophage infiltration may play important roles in the progression of interstitial fibrosis in UUO mice and human hypertensive nephropathy, the specific mechanism of local synthesis in renal interstitium by immune cells has not been thoroughly investigated (13, 14).

As early as the 1970s, Pepys first discovered the interactions between complement and adaptive immunity by observing complement-depleted mice that were unable to mount potent antibody responses (15). Previous studies have found that complement C3 deficiency is associated with impaired T cell responses in several disease models, including infections, tumors, autoimmune disease, and renal transplantation (16). More recently, researchers observed that the complement components C3, fB, fD, and C5 were upregulated as regulators of T cell immunity, as well as the C3a receptor and C5a receptor. In some kidney transplant studies, the absence of C3 was correlated with defective T cell priming, reduced T cell proliferation, and cytokine production after donor-specific restimulation (17, 18). Moreover, C3 deficiency or blockade was shown to attenuate the expansion of Ag-specific $CD4^+$ and $CD8^+$ T cell responses to Listeria monocytogenes in mice, and the regulation of T cell functionality by C3 might not involve the C5aR signaling pathway (19).

In this study, we aimed to identify the roles of locally synthesized C3 in the development of RF in a unilateral ureteral obstruction (UUO) model and determine whether this synthesis contributes to M1 cell responses. In addition, we studied the relationships among C3, macrophages and Th17 cells, which are involved in interstitial fibrosis.

MATERIALS AND METHODS

Renal and Blood Samples From Patients With IgAN

Between December 2016 and July 2017, patients aged 18–63 years who underwent kidney biopsy at Tongji Hospital were recruited, and renal biopsy specimens were examined retrospectively. Forty-one patients (20 men and 21 women; mean age = 38.10 ± 12.03 years) with a pathologic diagnosis of IgAN were enrolled. Their renal and/or blood samples were obtained at the time of diagnosis. Patients were excluded from this study if they met the following conditions: <18 years of age, an inability to provide informed consent, presence of active infection, and pregnancy. Our protocol was approved by the institutional review board or ethics committee at each center. Written informed consent was obtained from all patients.

Animal Model

The animals were purchased from Charles river Laboratories (Beijing, China). Unilateral ureteral obstruction (UUO) is a popular experimental model of renal injury. Mice aged 6–8 weeks were anesthetized followed by a lateral incision on the back of the mouse. Subsequently, the left ureter was exposed and tied off with two 4.0 silk suture. Sham-operated mice underwent an identical procedure but without ureteric ligation. The therapeutic experiment was performed with the Compstatin analog Cp40 (dTyr-Ile-[Cys-Val-Trp(Me)-Gln-Asp-Trp-Sar-His-Arg-Cys]-mIle-NH2;1.7kDa) which was produced by solid-phase peptide synthesis (GL Biochem Co., Ltd., Shanghai, China), and SB290157, a C3a receptor antagonist, which was purchased from Sigma-Aldrich. UUO and sham-operated mice were treated with Cp40 (1 mg/kg) via subcutaneous injection every 12 h and SB290157 (30 mg/kg) via intraperitoneal injection daily. After 7 or 14 days, the mice were sacrificed by cervical vertebra dislocation, and then, peripheral blood, spleen, and renal tissues were collected. The mouse kidneys were fixed in 4% formalin for 24 h, processed through dehydration in a graded series of alcohol and embedded in paraffin (Wuhan Goodbio Technology Co., Ltd., Wuhan, China). The remaining sample was frozen in liquid nitrogen for later use. All animal studies were performed in accordance with our university's guidelines for animal care.

IHC and Immunofluorescence

Paraffin-embedded renal sections (3 μm) were subjected to Masson's trichome staining as previously reported (20). Paraffin-embedded renal sections (4 μm) were deparaffinized in xylene and rehydrated in graded alcohol. The endogenous peroxidase activity was blocked with 3% H_2O_2 at room temperature for 15 min, and non-specific proteins were blocked with 10% goat serum for 30 min. Sections were then incubated overnight with antibodies against F4/80, α-SMA (Abcam, Cambridge, MA, USA), C3 (Novus, Littleton, Colorado, USA), iNOS (Santa Cruz, Dallas, Texas, USA), CD68 (Long Island Biotech, Shanghai, China), CD3, CD4, and CD8 (Thermo Scientific, Waltham, MA, USA) at 4°C, followed by incubation with an HRP-conjugated secondary antibody and subsequently visualized with diaminobenzidine substrate and hematoxylin counterstaining. For double-labeling immunofluorescence studies, following incubation with primary antibody, sections were incubated with FITC-conjugated goat anti-rabbit (1:100; Abcam) and Goat anti-rat Alexa Fluor 594 (1:100; Invitrogen Corporation, Carlsbad, CA) for 45 min at 37°C and then counterstained with DAPI

(Vector Laboratories). C3 expression was quantificated by the percentages of positive area at ×400 magnification on 10 fields exclusive of blood vessels and glomerulus per section from six mice in each group. All scorings were carried out by observers blinded to the experimental groups.

Western Blotting

Protein concentrations were quantified by a BCA protein assay kit (Beyotime Institute of Biotechnology, Shanghai, China), and 20 μg of protein was used for gel loading. GAPDH primary antibody (mouse, Santa Cruz, USA) was used at a dilution of 1:3,000, and TGF-β1, collagen I, PDGFR-β, and α-SMA (Abcam, Cambridge, MA, USA) primary antibodies were used at a dilution of 1:2,000. C3 primary antibody (rabbit, Novus, USA), p-ERK, ERK, p-p65, p-STAT3, and p-STAT5 (rabbit, CST, USA) were used at a dilution of 1:1,000. iNOS primary antibody (mouse, Santa, USA) and Arginasel (rabbit, Santa, USA) were used at a dilution of 1:200. C3aR primary antibody (mouse, Abcam, USA) was used at a dilution of 1:1,000. The secondary antibody was used at a dilution of 1:3,000. Western blotting analysis was performed as previously described (21). The signals were detected using enhanced chemiluminescence (ECL) (Amersham Pharmacia Biotech, Piscataway, NJ).

Mouse Cell Preparation

C57BL/6 mice were euthanized by cervical vertebra dislocation, and then, the whole body vasculature was flushed with a 20 ml injection of fresh PBS through a cardiac puncture. Kidneys were harvested and cut into small pieces and placed in RPMI1640 medium containing 2 mg/ml collagenase IV (GIBCO) and 100 mg/ml DNase I (Roche) for 45–60 min at 37°C with intermittent agitation. After tissue disaggregation, cells were filtered through a 40 μm cell strainer (BD Falcon, Franklin Lakes, NJ). Mononuclear cells from kidneys were then washed with cold PBS, counted, and used for flow cytometry.

PBMC Isolation

Patients and normal subjects donated 5 ml of blood collected in heparinized tubes. Blood was diluted 1:1 with PBS and overlaid onto lymphocyte separation medium (TBD sciences, Tianjin, China). After centrifugation, 3 ml of the interface containing the PBMCs was collected and diluted to 6 ml with PBS, then washed twice with cold PBS and counted. The PBMCs were collected for flow cytometric analysis.

CFSE Labeling

A CFSE stock solution (5 mM) was prepared fresh by dissolving lyophilized CFSE (Sigma-Aldrich, USA) in DMSO. Splenocytes were obtained from the spleens of naïve mice, and labeled with CFSE at 5 μM in PBS for 15 min at 37°C. Excess CFSE was quenched by adding three volumes of ice-cold FBS and incubating the cells for 5 min on ice. CFSE labeled cells were then washed three times with PBS and cultured with or without stimulation.

T Cell Activation

The 96-well assay plate precoated with anti-CD3 and anti-CD28 Ab (BD Pharmingen) was incubated at 37°C for 4 h. Splenocytes (1×10^6 cells/well) were obtained from the spleens of naïve mice and were cultured for 3 days in 96-well plates in medium containing IL-2 (10 ng/mL; R&D Systems) as well as IL-12 (10 μg/mL; R&D Systems), or IL-4 (4 ng/mL; BD Pharmingen).

Flow Cytometric Analysis

A single renal cell suspension was prepared and stimulated with PMA/Ionomycin/Golgi-plug for 4 h. The cells were incubated with different primary antibodies or the appropriate isotype control antibodies at 4°C for 30 min. The following antibodies were used PerCP/Cy5.5-conjugated anti-human CD14 (Biolegend), PerCP/Cy5.5-conjugated anti-mouse CD4 (Biolegend), APC-conjugated anti-mouse F4/80 (Biolegend), and PerCP/Cy5.5-conjugated anti-mouse CD11b (Biolegend).After cellular surface staining, cells were fixed and permeabilized with Cytofix/Cytoperm Soln Kit for intracellular staining with Alexa Fluor 488-conjugated anti-human C3 (Abcam) and PE-conjugated anti-mouse IL-17A (eBioscience). All flow cytometric analyses were performed using an LSR II Flow Cytometer (Beckman-Coulter) and Flowjo software.

ELISA

To quantify IL-17A levels in the kidney, samples were analyzed using a mouse IL-17A ELISA (R and D Systems) according to the manufacturer's instructions. All measurements were performed in duplicate.

Real-Time PCR

Real-time PCR was performed as previously described (22). Real-time PCR was carried out using the LightCycler 480 system (Roche, Pleasanton, CA, USA) with the following primers: mouse C3, forward 5′-ACTGTGGACAACAACCTACTGC-3′, reverse 5′-GCATGTTCGTAAAAGGCTCGG-3′; mouse IL-6, forward 5′-TAGTCCTTCCTACCCCAATTTCC-3′, mouse reverse 5′-T TGGTCCTTAGCCACTCCTTC-3′; mouse IL-1β, forward 5′-GAAATGCCACCTTTTGACAGTG-3′, reverse5′-TGGATGCT CTCATCAGGACAG-3′; mouse TNF-α, forward 5′-CCTGTA GCCCACGTCGTA G-3′, reverse 5′-GGGAGTAGACAAGGTA CAACCC-3′; mouse MCP-1, forward 5′-TTAAAAACCTGGA TCGGAACCAA-3′, reverse 5′- GCATTAGCTTCAGATTTAC GGGT-3′; mouse Collagen 1, forward 5′-GTCCTAGTCGAT GGCTGCTC-3′, reverse 5′-CAATGTCCAGAGGTGCAATG-3′; mouse α-SMA, forward 5′-GGAGAAGCCCAGCCAGTCGC-3′, reverse 5′-AGCCGGCCTTACAGAGCCCA-3′; mouse PDGFR-β, forward 5′-GGGTCCGTTCCAGAAAATGT-3′, reverse 5′-GA CAAGGGACCGGGGTCCAA-3′; mouse Arginase, forward 5′-A GCGCCAAGTCCAGAACCATA-3′, reverse 5′-CCATGCAAG TTTCCACTTGT-3′; mouse iNOS, forward 5′-TGGAGCGAGT TGTGGATTGTC-3′, reverse 5′-GTGAGGGCTTGGCTGAGTG A-3′; mouse GAPDH, forward 5′-AGGTCGGTGTGAACGGA TTTG-3′, reverse 5′-GGGGTCGTTGATGGCAACA-3′; mouse C3, forward 5′-ACGGCATCCTCTGTCATCT-3′, reverse 5′-A CGGCATCCTCTGTCATCT-3′; TGF-β1, forward 5′-CGCAAC AACGCCATCTATGA-3′, reverse 5′-ACCAAGGTAACGCCAG GAAT-3′. The relative amounts of mRNA were normalized to GAPDH and were calculated using the $2^{-\Delta\Delta}$Ct approach as previously reported (23).

Statistical Analysis

All statistical analyses were conducted using SPSS 12.0 (SPSS, USA). The values are expressed as the mean ± SEM. Graphpad Prism 5 software (GraphPad Software, La Jolla, CA, USA) was used for the statistical analysis with Student's *t*-test or one-way ANOVA where appropriate. The threshold for statistical significance was set at $P < 0.05$.

RESULTS

Renal Complement C3 Expression Is Elevated and Correlated With Infiltrating CD68^{+} Monocytes/Macrophages in Human IgAN Biopsies

Complement was previously shown to play a key role in IgAN pathogenesis, which involves the aberrant activation of the classic, alternative, and mannose-binding lectin pathways. We recruited IgAN patients whose renal biopsy specimens were reassessed blindly by a single pathologist using the Oxford classification. Notably, in renal biopsy specimens, C3 expression was observed in both renal tubules and the interstitium, and a positive correlation was found between pathologist-assessed Masson's trichrome staining and C3 expression, although the correlation between C3 expression in the interstitium and serum C3 was not statistically significant (**Figures 1A,B**). However, the intensities of C3 in the interstitium were significantly positively correlated to BUN, serum creatinine (SCr), and urine proteinuria/UCr (ACR) and negatively correlated to the eGFR (**Figure 1B**). No correlation was found between the intensities of C3 in the interstitium and ALB. In addition, along with exacerbated RF and enhanced mononuclear leukocyte infiltration, C3 expression increased significantly (**Figure 1C**).

However, evidence of local secretion of complement components by infiltrating cells during IgAN is still absent. To address this, we assessed C3 expression in renal tissues and performed flow cytometric analysis of C3 secretion in peripheral blood of patients with IgAN. C3 secretion was increased significantly in peripheral blood monocytes from IgAN patients (**Figures 1D,E**). Accordingly, C3 expression and monocyte infiltration were examined in paraffin-embedded sections of IgAN tissues by immunofluorescence staining. C3 expression was detected in the interstitium with significant co-staining of macrophages, which was observed as double-positive cells in patients, while healthy individuals showed little or no co-staining (**Figure 1F**). Altogether these results suggest that infiltrating macrophages as well as monocytes are a major source for C3 synthesis in kidney tissue.

Renal Expression of C3 Is Upregulated in the Mouse UUO Model

C3 deposits within the glomerulus have been well-characterized in previous studies. To assess whether expression of C3 in the renal interstitium and kidney tubules is upregulated following UUO-induced renal injury, we performed immunochemical staining, real-time PCR, and Western blot analyses to measure its expression. Extensive stromal fibrosis was detected by Masson's trichrome staining, and increased C3 synthesis, α-SMA expression, and infiltrating macrophages were detected by immunohistochemistry (IHC) in mouse kidneys after the operation compared with those of the sham-operated mice; these parameters peaked on day 14 (**Figures 2A–C, Supplement Figures 1B–E**). Consistent with the histopathological results, C3 mRNA (**Supplement Figure 1A**) and protein (**Figures 2D,E**) levels were significantly increased after 7 and 14 days of UUO. Meanwhile, elevated MCP-1, IL-6, IL-1β, and TNF-α mRNA expression was also observed in UUO mice (**Figure 2F**).

Macrophages Are the Major Source of Complement C3 Production in the Kidney Following Obstructive Injury

Our IHC studies showed C3 overexpression in the interstitium of obstructed kidneys. To further define which cells were the major source of C3 production in UUO kidneys, we performed immunofluorescence staining using CD3, ly6G, F4/80, and α-SMA to identify T cells, PMNs, macrophages, and myofibroblasts, respectively. **Figure 2A** shows macrophages detected in the interstitium with significant C3 co-staining, shown as double-positive cells, in UUO mice, while the sham group showed little or no co-staining. Given that macrophages with different activation phenotypes play distinct roles, we then proceeded to verify which subset of macrophages expressed C3 *in vitro*. Bone marrow-derived macrophages (BMDMs) were assessed after 7 days of culture with L929 supernatant. As previously reported, classically activated macrophages (M1) expressed high levels of iNOS and little Arginase-I, and alternatively activated macrophages (M2) expressed high levels of Arginase-I and little iNOS (**Figure 3A**). We found that C3 was primarily expressed by M1 cells, as shown by immunofluorescence staining and Western blotting (**Figures 3B,C**). Our results show that both tubules and interstitial cells secrete C3. Macrophages in the interstitium are likely to be affected in the microenvironment. As shown in **Figure 3D**, the addition of C3 to the induced differentiated macrophages *in vitro* could stimulate increased iNOS, IL-6, and IL-1β expression and decreased Arginase-I, TGF-β, and TNF-α expression, indicating that C3 could induce macrophage differentiation into M1.

Macrophage Depletion Reduces Complement Expression and Renal Fibrosis

Our above results showed that macrophages, especially M1 macrophages, contribute significantly to C3 secretion. We depleted F4/80^{+} macrophages using clodronate liposomes in UUO mice. As depicted in **Figure 4A**, mice were sacrificed after 7 and 14 days of UUO, and the results showed that macrophages were reduced in UUO mice injected with clodronate compared

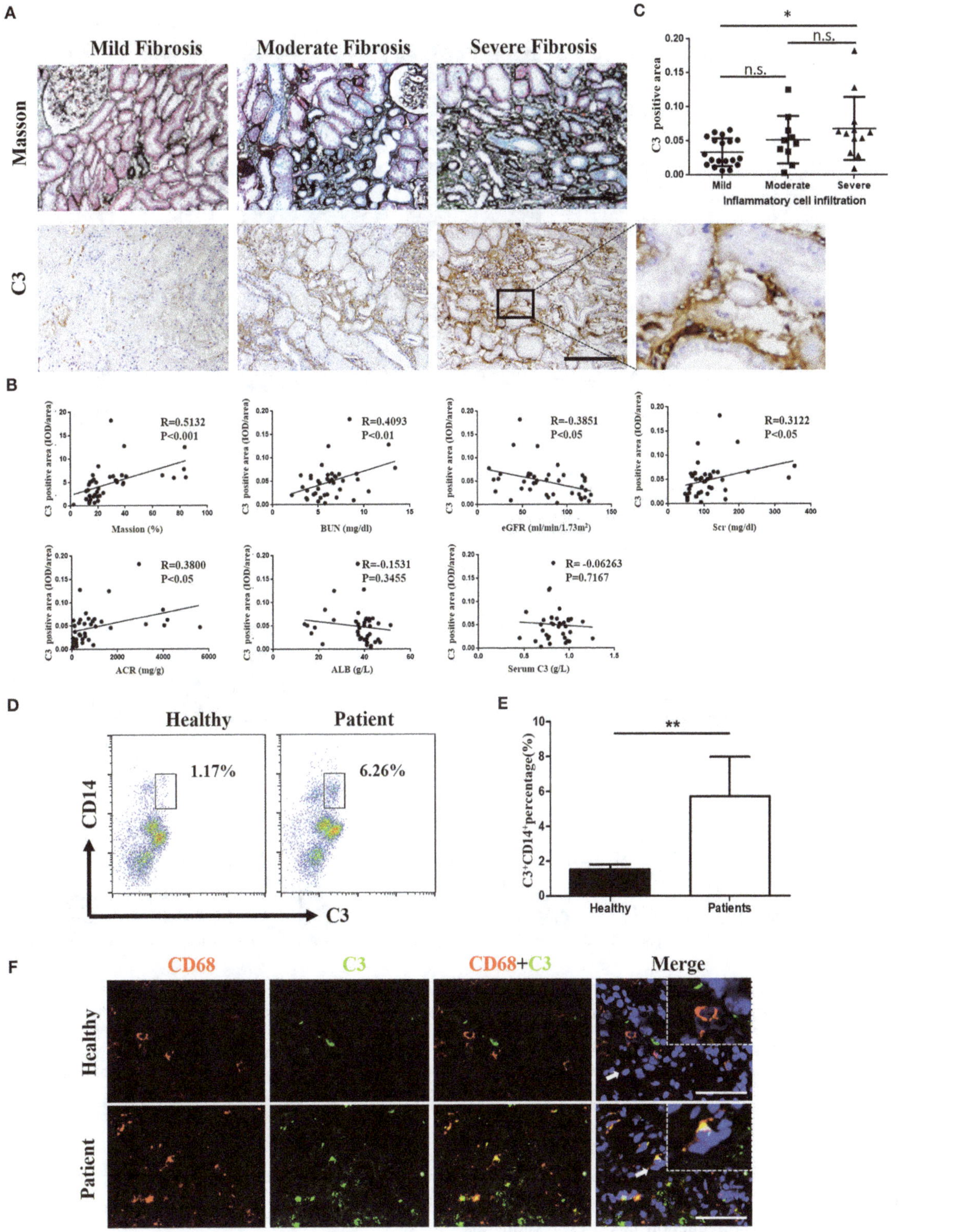

FIGURE 1 | C3 levels were increased in renal tissues and blood samples from patients with IgAN **(A)** Masson's trichome staining showing collagen deposition; IHC analysis of C3 expression in the kidney. $n = 41$ patients with IgAN. **(B)** Relationships between C3 in the interstitium with Masson's trichome staining, BUN, the eGFR, Scr, ACR, ALB, and serum C3. **(C)** Relationships between C3 in the interstitium with the degree of inflammatory cell infiltration. Error bars represent SEM. $^{*}P < 0.05$. **(D)** Flow cytometric analysis showing the percentages of $C3^{+}CD14^{+}$ in PBMC of patients with IgAN. The data shown are representatives of FACS profiles. **(E)** The histograms show the increased the percentages of $C3^{+}CD14^{+}$ in peripheral blood mononuclear in the IgA patients ($n = 41$) compared with the healthy ($n = 37$). The error bars represent the SEM. $^{**}P < 0.01$. **(F)** Immunofluorescence staining of CD68 (red) and C3 (green) in the kidney. Scale bar, 50 μm.

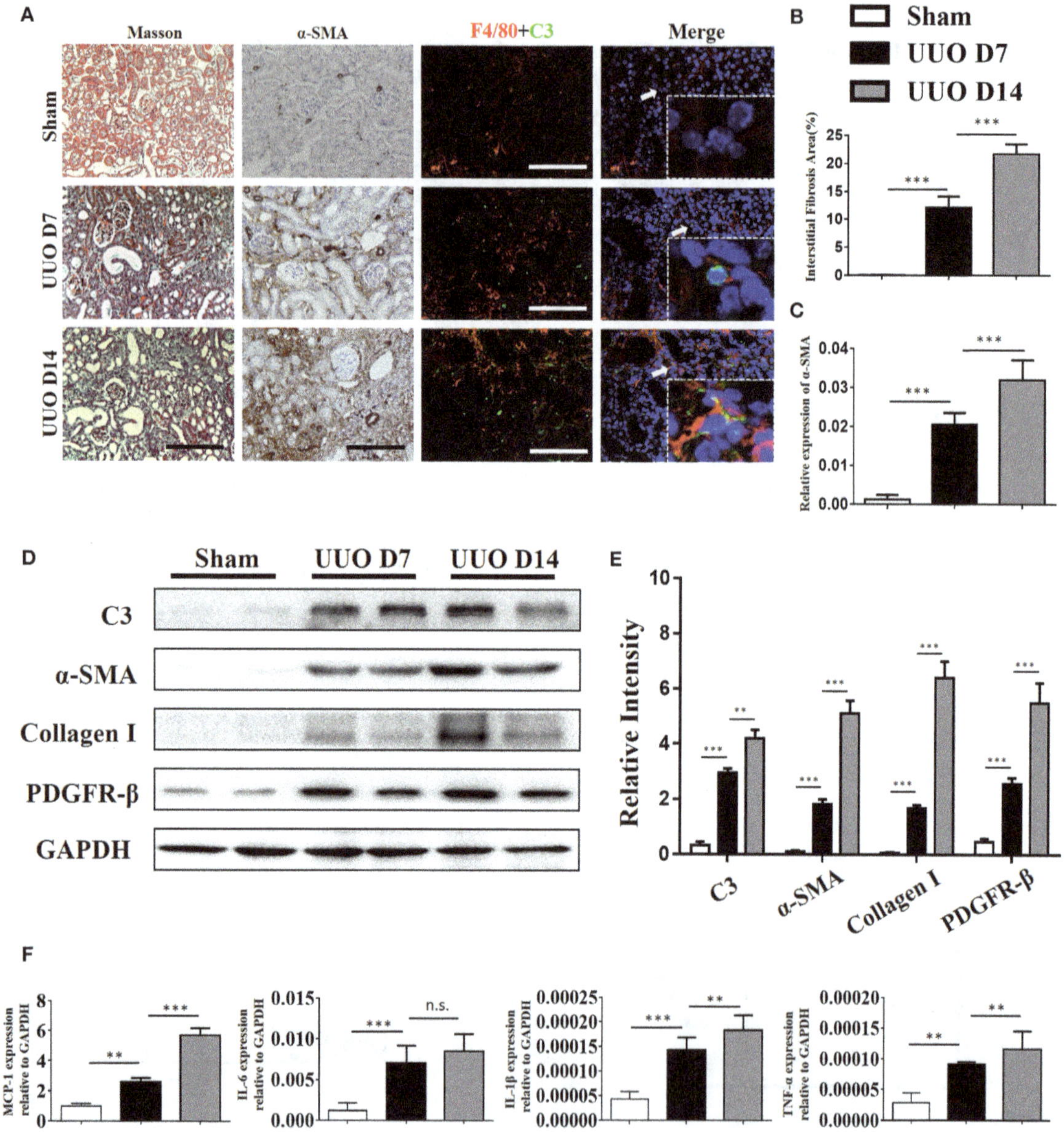

FIGURE 2 | Complement C3 is increased in the obstructed kidney. **(A)** Masson's trichrome staining indicates collagen deposition. IHC staining showing α-SMA expression in the sham control and UUO mice; Immunofluorescence staining showing increased C3 (green) expression in UUO kidneys in the interstitium on days 7 and 14 and colocalization (white arrows) with F4/80 (red) original magnification, ×400. Quantitative positive area of interstitial fibrosis **(B)** and a-SMA **(C)** positive were shown as mean ± SEM. $n = 6$ per group, Scale bar, 50 μm. **(D)** The expression levels of C3 and fibrotic markers (α-SMA, PDGFR-β, and Collagen I) were detected by Western blot, and **(E)** the histogram shows the relative intensity for each marker normalized to GAPDH. $n = 6$ per group. **(F)** Real-time PCR showing relative renal mRNA levels of MCP-1, TNF-α, IL-6, and IL-1β in sham and UUO mice. The error bars represent the SEM. $^{**}P < 0.01$; $^{***}P < 0.001$.

to those injected with control PBS liposomes. Similarly, UUO mice treated with clodronate exhibited significantly decreased C3 expression. The reduction in C3 expression was associated with reduced α-SMA expression and decreased tubulointerstitial fibrosis measured by Masson's trichrome staining (**Figures 4B–F**). In addition, the mRNA and protein levels of C3, α-SMA, and PDGFR-β were reduced in UUO mice receiving clodronate liposomes (**Supplement Figure 2**). These results further support the pathogenic function of macrophage infiltration with increased C3 expression, which leads to RF.

C3 Deficiency Attenuates Fibrosis and Infiltration of Inflammatory Cells in UUO-Induced Renal Fibrosis

To investigate the role of C3 in the pathogenesis of UUO, we used a peptidic C3 inhibitor, Compstatin analog Cp40, to

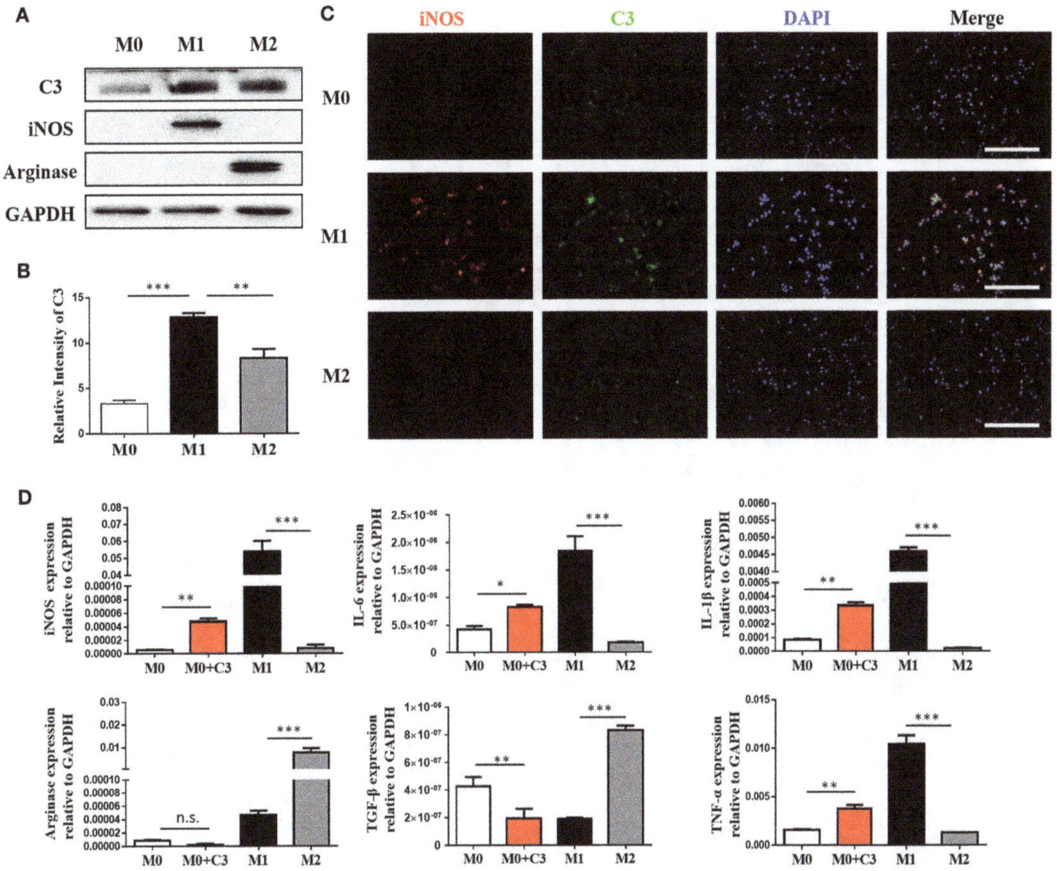

FIGURE 3 | Macrophages are the major source of C3 in the obstructed kidney. **(A)** The protein isolated from BMMs treated for 24 h with either IFN-γ or IL-4 were analyzed by Western blot analyses, and **(B)** the histogram shows the relative intensity for each marker normalized to GAPDH. **(C)** Immunofluorescence staining showing increased C3 (green) primarily expressed in M1 with colocalization with iNOS (red) (original magnification × 400). Scale bar, 50 μm. **(D)** The effect of exogenous C3 on the subtype of macrophage by real-time PCR. The histogram shows the relative mRNA levels of iNOS, IL-6, IL-1β, Arginase, TGF-β, and TNF-α in these groups. $n = 3$. The error bars represent the SEM. $^*P < 0.05$; $^{**}P < 0.01$; $^{***}P < 0.001$. The data were pooled from three independent experiments.

block C3 activation. Masson's staining and α-SMA expression analysis showed that UUO mice injected with 1 mg/kg Cp40 had much less severe interstitial fibrosis than control peptide-injected mice (**Supplement Figures 3A–D**). Western blot analysis also indicated that the α-SMA and PDGFR-β levels were decreased in the Cp40-injected UUO mice (**Supplement Figures 3E,F**). In addition to the attenuated tubulointerstitial fibrosis, renal infiltration of F4/80$^+$ macrophages, CD3$^+$T cells, CD4$^+$T cells, and CD8$^+$T cells was significantly reduced in Cp40-injected UUO mice compared with peptide-injected mice (**Figures 5A–E**). Meanwhile, elevated MCP-1, IL-6, IL-1β, and TNF-α mRNA expression in UUO mice was markedly limited by Cp40 (**Figure 5F**). These data indicate that C3 mediates the infiltration of T cells and macrophages into the kidney in response to obstructive injury.

C3aR Blockade Substantially Attenuates Renal Fibrosis in UUO Mice

C3a is one of the proteins formed by the cleavage of C3 and plays a large role in the immune response. Given that increased generation of C3 was observed in IgAN patients and UUO mice, we proceeded to investigate whether the renal parenchymal loss in UUO mice could be attenuated by C3aR antagonism, SB290157. SB290157 is a selective antagonist of complement anaphylatoxin C3a receptor, a 74 amino acid proinflammatory mediator and chemotactic peptide. It effectively blocks C3aR in humans, rat, guinea pig, and mouse. As shown in **Figures 6A–C**, the progression of renal interstitial fibrosis was dramatically retarded by daily i.p., injection of SB290157, which was initiated on day 7 after the UUO operation. And injection of SB290157 did not affect C3 expression in renal interstitium of UUO mice. Similarly, along with attenuated RF and TGF-β1 release were significantly reduced by treatment with C3aRA (**Figures 6D,E**). In addition, we showed that renal infiltration of F4/80$^+$macrophages, CD3$^+$T cells, CD4$^+$T cells, and CD8$^+$T cells was significantly reduced in SB290157-injected UUO mice compared with that in peptide-injected mice (**Figures 6F–G**). Additionally, elevated MCP-1, IL-6, IL-1β, and TNF-α mRNA expression in UUO mice was markedly limited by SB290157 (**Figure 6H**). Taken together, these data suggest C3-C3aR

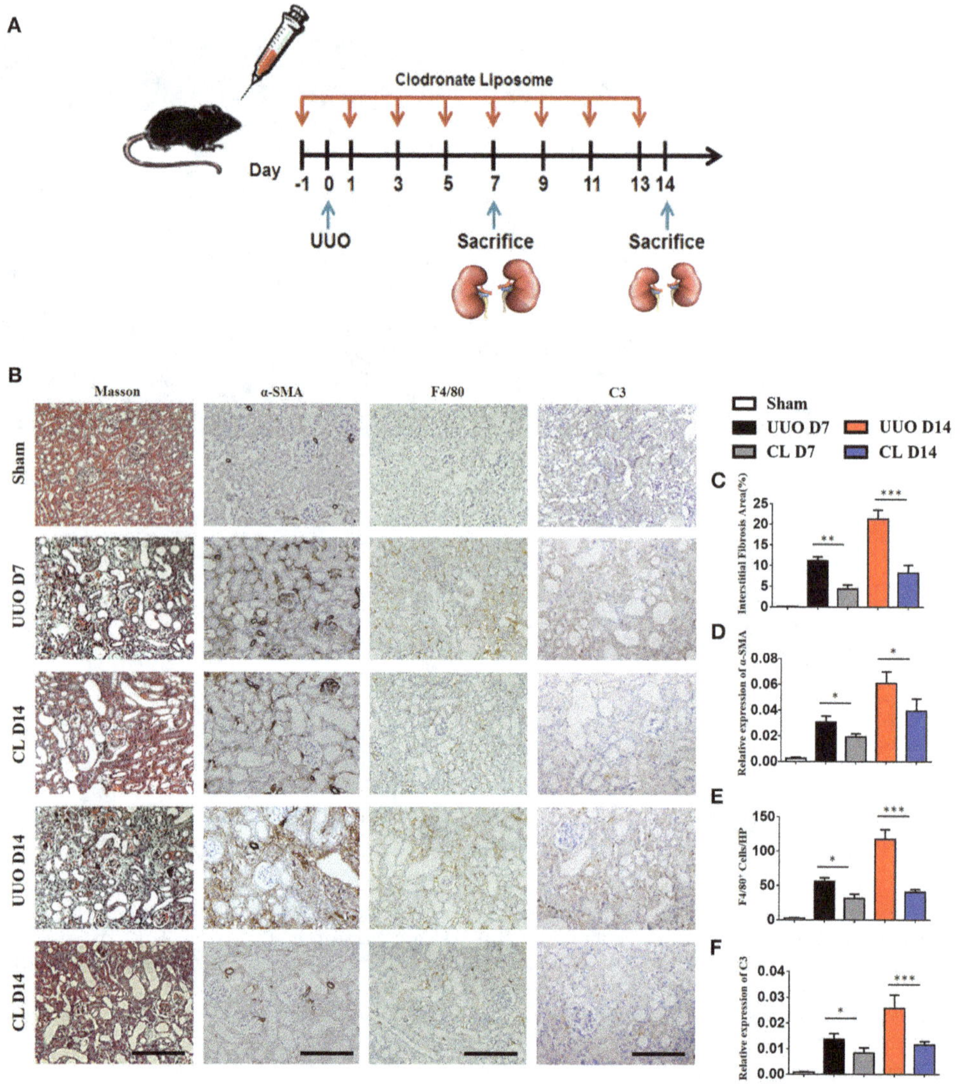

FIGURE 4 | Macrophage depletion protects against renal fibrosis by inhibiting C3 expression. UUO mice were intravenously injected with clodronate liposomes and control liposomes. On days 7 and 14, mice were sacrificed, and the left kidneys were collected. **(A)** Scheme of clodronate liposome-mediated macrophage depletion. **(B)** Masson's trichrome staining indicates collagen deposition. IHC staining showing α-SMA, F4/80, and C3 protein expression in these groups ($n = 6$); original magnification, ×400. Scale bar, 50 μm. Quantitative analysis of interstitial fibrosis**(C)**, a-SMA**(D)**, F4/80 **(E),** and C3 **(F)** positive cells were shown as mean ± SEM. $^*P < 0.05$; $^{**}P < 0.01$; $^{***}P < 0.001$.

signaling promotes RF, and C3aR may be a therapeutic target for renal disease.

Blocking C3-C3aR Signaling Attenuates Renal Fibrosis by Inhibiting IL-17A Production in UUO Mice

As shown in **Figure 7A**, renal mRNA levels of IL-17A were substantially increased in UUO mice compared with sham control mice. In addition, IL-17A levels in the serum of UUO mice were significantly increased in the early and late stages compared with those in the serum of sham control mice (**Figure 7B**). Consistent with the ELISA and mRNA data, the FACS results revealed that 8.48 and 10.9% of $CD4^+$ renal cells in obstructed kidneys expressed IL-17A following UUO, respectively, whereas ≤5.3% were IL-17A$^+$ in sham-operated mice, and this effect was strongly inhibited by Cp40 and SB290157 (**Figures 7C–H**). In addition, we performed analysis of CD11b$^+$F4/80$^+$IL-17$^+$ cells ratio in kidney from C3 blockade UUO mice and UUO mice. The results showed that CD11b$^+$F4/80$^+$IL-17$^+$cells were around 1% in mononuclear cells in two groups, and only slightly changed after blockade C3 with CP40 (**Supplement Figures 4A,B**). Similar results were confirmed in 14 days of UUO mice (**Supplement Figures 4C,D**). Thus, we identified that the main producer of IL-17A in the UUO mice were T cells, which were strikingly increased after unilateral ureteral ligation.

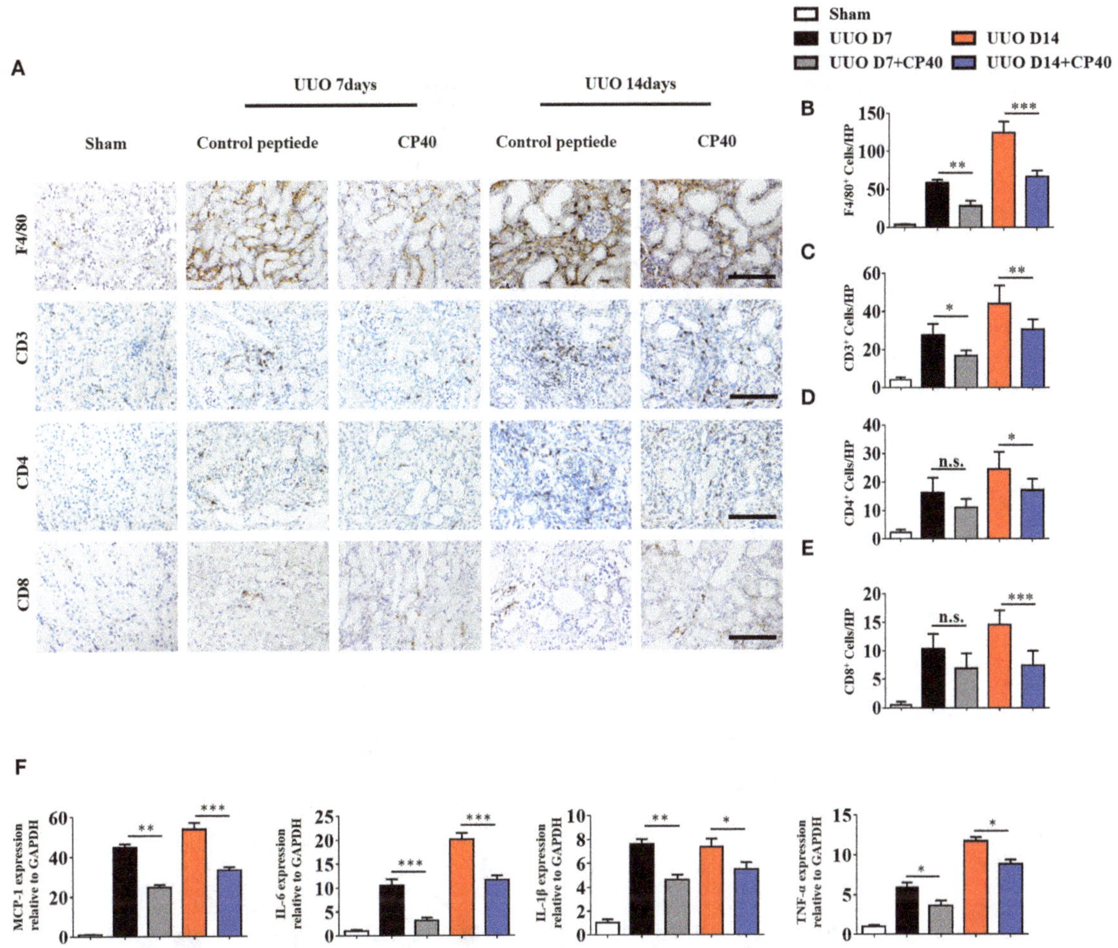

FIGURE 5 | C3 deficiency reduces C3 expression, inflammatory infiltration and fibrosis in kidney during UUO. UUO mice were subcutaneously injected with control peptide and Cp40. On days 7 and 14, mice were sacrificed, and the left kidneys were collected. **(A)** IHC staining showing F4/80 macrophages, CD3$^+$T cells, CD4$^+$T cells, and CD8$^+$T cells in these groups ($n = 6$); original magnification, ×400. Scale bar, 50 μm. Quantitative analysis of F4/80 **(B)**, CD3 **(C)**, CD4 **(D)**, and CD8 **(E)** positive cells were shown as mean ± SEM. **(F)** Real-time PCR showing relative renal levels of MCP-1, IL-6, IL-1β, and TNF-α in these groups ($n = 6$). The error bars represent the SEM. $^*P < 0.05$; $^{**}P < 0.01$; $^{***}P < 0.001$.

To investigate the mechanism by which C3a promotes IL-17A expression, we isolated spleen cells from naïve wild-type mice on anti-CD3/anti-CD28-coated plates *in vitro.* We extended our CFSE dilution assay using splenocytes, and T cells exhibited high levels of proliferation in the presence of mC3a. Inhibition by SB290157 abrogated T cell proliferation; therefore, mC3a is required for T cell proliferation (**Figures 8A,B**). More importantly, blockade of C3a by the C3aR inhibitor drastically suppressed IL-17A expression in C3a-stimulated T cells (**Figures 8C,D**). In this study, we found that C3 deficiency significantly reduced the IL-17A production in obstructed kidneys. Given that IL-17A can stimulate chemokine expression in renal and immune cells, our findings establish C3a as a mediator by which IL-17A initiates infiltration of inflammatory cells during obstructive injury. Thus, complement C3 activation represents a key event for triggering the production of IL-17A during obstructive injury, thereby shaping renal microenvironments.

As the ERK signaling pathway was reported to be indispensable for C3a-mediated effector responses during kidney transplant, we defined the role of ERK signaling in IL-17A release upon C3a stimulation. The results showed that exposure to C3a led to phosphorylation of ERK, STAT3, and STAT5 and activation of NF-kB in T cells (**Figures 9A–D**). To further conformed the impact of C3a on activation of ERK signaling pathway, we knocked down endogenous C3aR in T cells by using specific small-interfering RNAs (siRNAs). As shown in **Supplement Figure 5**, two siRNAs targeting C3aR specifically knocked down endogenous C3aR protein in T cells. siRNA # 2 with higher efficiency was chosen for the subsequent studies. The results showed that T cells depleted in C3aR can inhibit phosphorylation of ERK, STAT3, and STAT5 and activation of NF-kB, which active

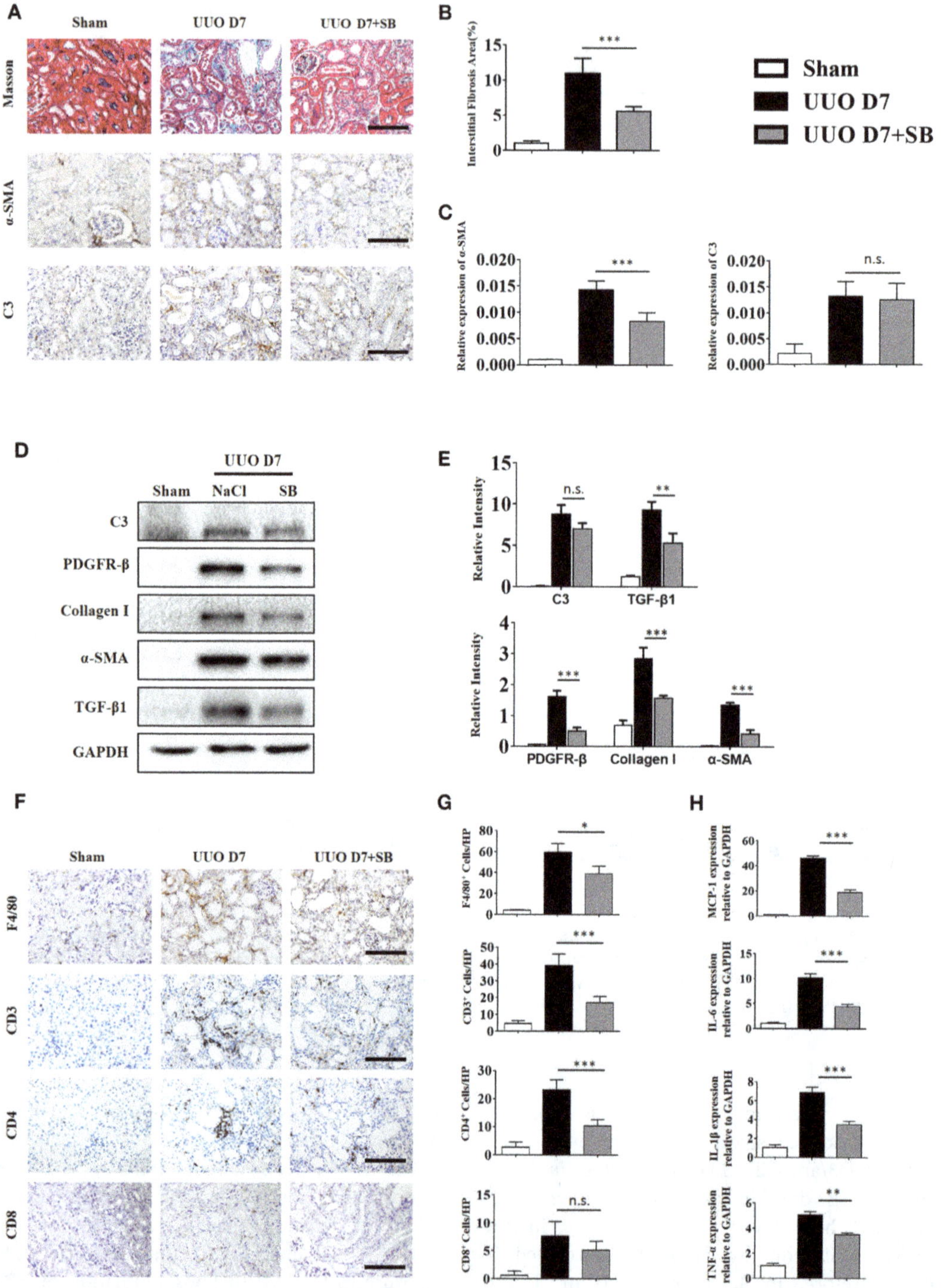

FIGURE 6 | C3aR blockade reduces inflammatory infiltration and fibrosis during UUO. UUO mice were intraperitoneally injected with vehicle and SB290157. On day 7, mice were sacrificed, and the left kidneys were collected. **(A)** Masson's trichrome staining indicates collagen deposition. IHC staining showing α-SMA and C3 protein expression in these groups ($n = 6$); original magnification, ×400. Scale bar, 50 μm. Quantitative analysis of interstitial fibrosis **(B)**, a-SMA **(C),** and C3 positive cells **(C)** were shown as mean ± SEM. **(D)** The expression levels of C3, TGF-β1, and fibrotic markers (α-SMA, PDGFR-β, and Collagen I) were detected by Western blot. **(E)** The histogram shows the relative intensity for each marker normalized to GAPDH. **(F)** IHC staining showing F4/80 macrophages, $CD3^{+}$T cells, $CD4^{+}$T cells, and $CD8^{+}$T cells in these groups ($n = 6$); original magnification, ×400. Scale bar, 50 μm. **(G)** Quantitative analysis of F4/80, CD3, CD4, and CD8 positive cells were shown as mean ± SEM. **(H)** Real-time PCR showing relative renal levels of MCP-1, IL-6, IL-1β, and TNF-α in these groups ($n = 6$). The error bars represent the SEM. $^{*}P<0.05$; $^{**}P<0.01$; $^{***}P<0.001$.

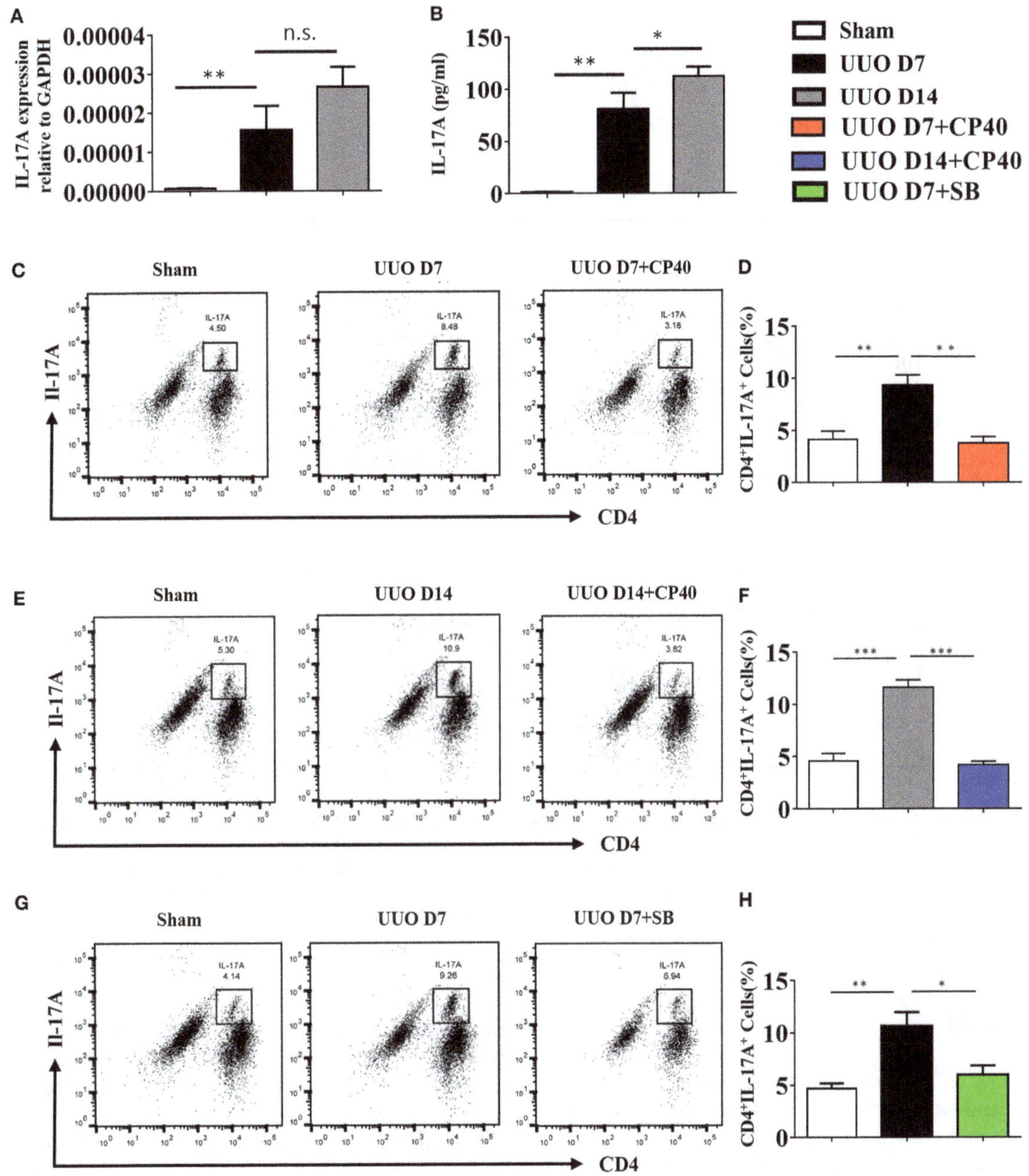

FIGURE 7 | The expression of IL-17A is induced in UUO mice. Mice were subjected to unilateral ureteral obstruction (UUO) by left ureteral ligation for 7 and 14 days ($n = 6$ per group). **(A)** IL-17A mRNA in whole kidneys measured by real-time PCR; $^{**}P < 0.01$ vs. sham operation; $n = 6$. **(B)** Production of IL-17A in obstructed kidneys was determined by CBA and was normalized to total protein content for each sample; $^{**}P < 0.01$, $^{*}P < 0.05$ vs. sham operation; $n = 6$. Flow cytometric analysis **(C,E,G)** and quantification **(D,F,H)** of kidney cell suspensions from the obstructed kidneys injected with or without Cp40/SB290157 during the time course of UUO; $n = 6$. Cells were stimulated *in vitro* with PMA/Ionomycin/Golgi-plug for 4 h. Specific staining of cell markers (anti-CD4) and intracellular staining for IL-17A were performed. Plots are gated for live $CD4^{+}IL\text{-}17A^{+}$ lymphocytes; numbers indicate events in the quadrants as percentages of all gated events. The error bars represent the SEM. $^{*}P < 0.05$; $^{**}P < 0.01$; $^{***}P < 0.001$. The data were pooled from three independent experiments.

by C3a (**Figures 9E–H**). Taken together, our data indicated that C3a could induce ERK and STAT3 signaling pathway activation and promote the IL-17A production in T cells *in vitro*.

Combined with the data obtained from the mouse and cell experiments, the results obtained from IgAN patients further support the notion that local C3 secretion by macrophages leads to renal fibrogenic responses (**Figure 10**).

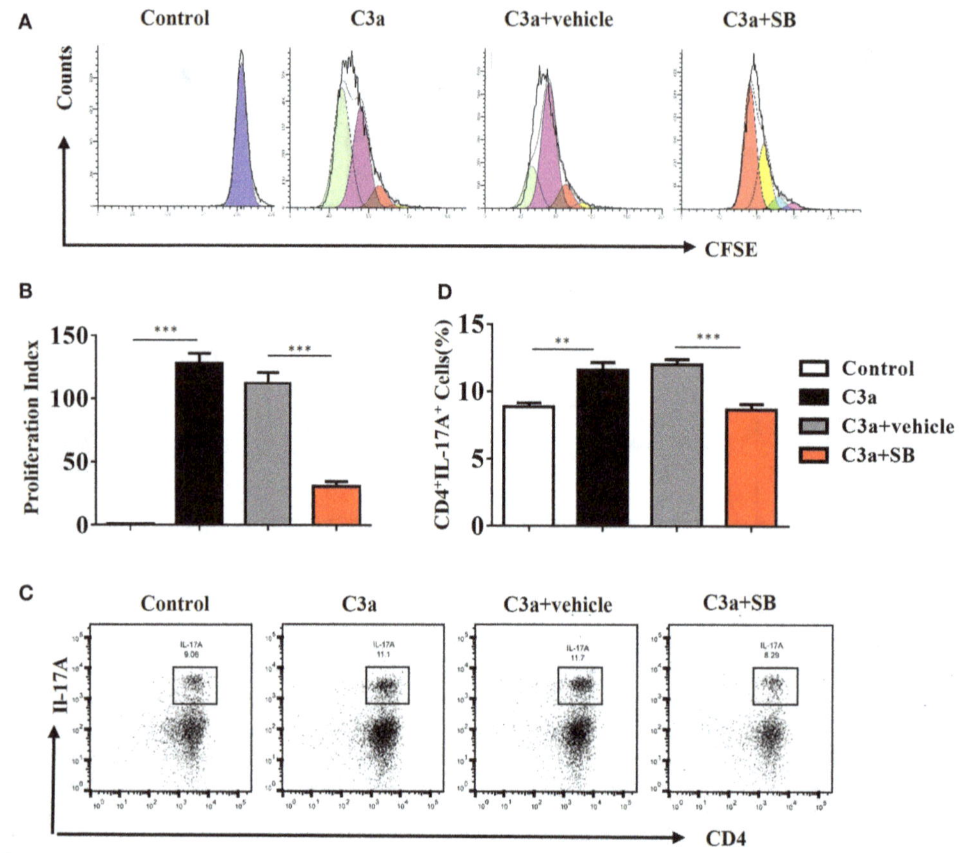

FIGURE 8 | C3a acts as regulator for renal IL-17A. Splenocytes stimulated with recombinant C3a (20 nM) for 72 h in the presence or absence of SB290157. **(A)** Average T cell proliferation increased in response to mC3a, while T cell proliferation decreased in SB290157-treated cultures compared to those containing only mC3a. **(B)**The histograms show the blockade of C3a drastically suppressed T cell proliferation stimulated with C3a. The error bars represent the SEM. ***$P < 0.001$. **(C)** Splenocytes were double-stained for CD4 and IL-17A. Representative dot plots are presented, and the numbers in the quadrants represent the percentage of each population. **(D)** Quantifications of $CD4^{+}IL\text{-}17A^{+}$cells as percentages of splenocytes isolated from the WT mice. The error bars represent the SEM. **$P < 0.01$; ***$P < 0.001$. The data were pooled from three independent experiments.

DISCUSSION

In human samples, we showed that circulating and local C3 was highly expressed in peripheral blood and renal tissues from patients with IgAN. Then, we observed that most of the C3 deposited in the interstitium and its expression were associated with the severity of renal interstitial fibrosis. Previous studies have predominantly investigated C3 glomerulopathy, which is defined as a kidney disease caused by complement dysregulation that results in variable glomerular inflammation (24–26). In most of the cases, C3 deposition in the glomeruli, as shown by immunofluorescence, had no immunoglobulins due to alternative pathway activation. However, further elucidation of C3 deposition in the renal interstitium is needed for a better understanding of its initiation and exacerbation. In our study, the contribution of C3 secretion by macrophages that infiltrated in the kidney appeared to be more important than C3 in the intravascular space as shown by IHC and immunofluorescence in renal tissues. (1) Immunofluorescence of human patients showed that C3 expression was more intense in macrophages than parenchymal cells, and (2) C3 was barely expressed in renal tubules of UUO mice. We further showed that local C3 levels were highly correlated with RF. Consistent with these results, cultured mouse BMDMs under stimulations mimicking the inflammatory microenvironment, M1 and M2 all showed strongly increased secretion of C3. Furthermore, we found that C3 facilitates IL-17A production in T cells, contributing to the development of renal inflammation and fibrosis in UUO mice. In addition, blockage of C3 by Cp40 attenuated RF of UUO mice. Our proposed mechanistic network for the pathogenic role of C3 in the development of RF is also summarized in **Figure 10**.

Renal fibrosis is considered to be a common end point of various types of CKD, and its biological significance depends on the cell types contributing to collagenous and non-collagenous extracellular matrix production (27–33). The associated processes include vascular leakage, leukocyte recruitment, angiogenesis, and the appearance of myofibroblasts. Currently, most data have focused on the precursor cells of renal myofibroblasts, including circulating bone marrow-derived cells, or the transition from epithelial or endothelial cells,

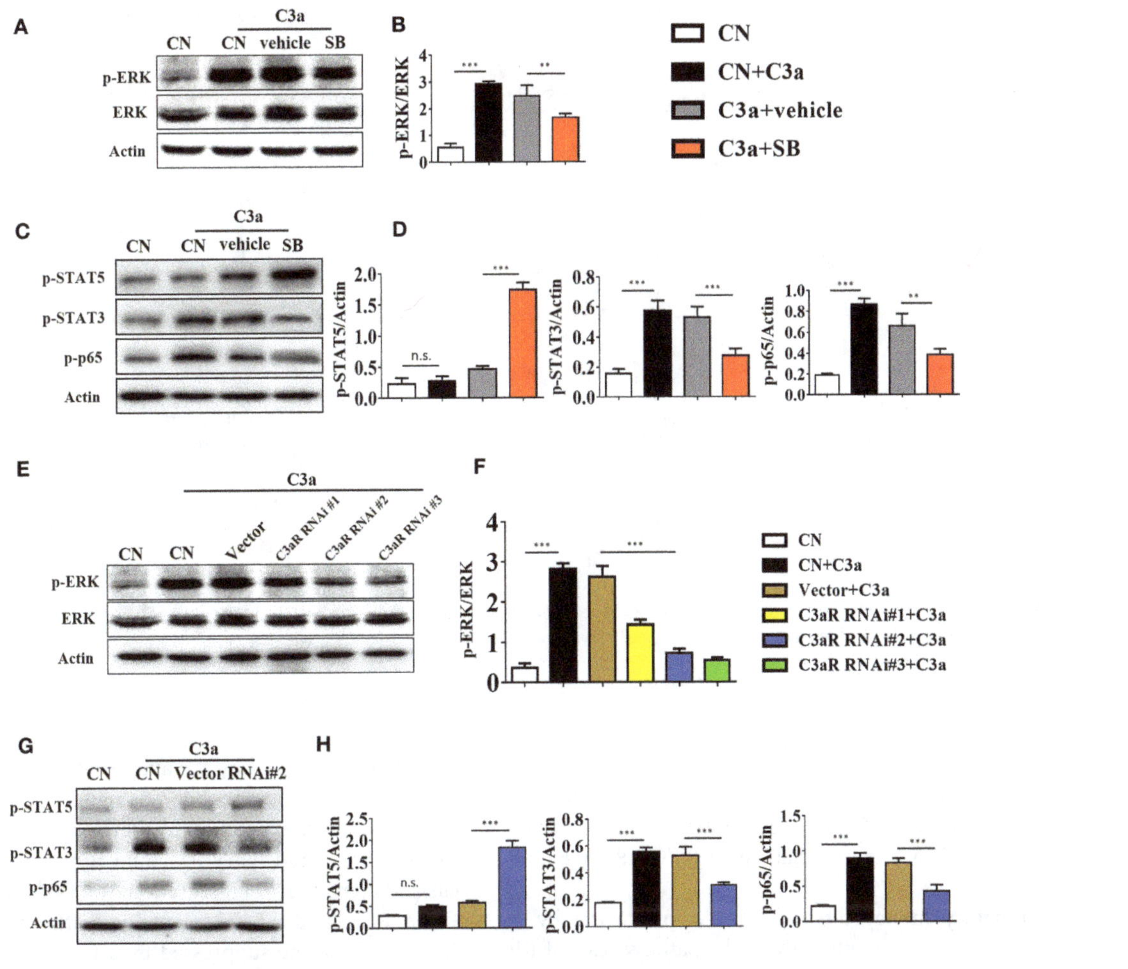

FIGURE 9 | C3a/C3aR signaling promotes the IL-17A production in T cells *in vitro*. **(A,C)** Splenocytes stimulated with C3a (20 nM) for 30 min in the presence or absence of SB290157. Extracellular signal-regulated kinase-1/2 (ERK1/2), signal transducers and activators of transcription-3/5 (STAT3/5), and nuclear factor (NF)-kB p65 subunit phosphorylation were detected by Western blotting. **(B,D)** The histogram shows the relative intensity for each marker normalized to Actin. **(E,G)** T cells were knocked down endogenous C3aR by using siRNAs, and stimulated with C3a (20 nM) for 30 min, p-ERK, p-STAT3, p-STAT5, and p-p65 were detected by Western blotting. **(F,H)** The histogram shows the relative intensity for each marker normalized to Actin. The error bars represent the SEM. $^{**}P < 0.01$; $^{***}P < 0.001$.

pericytes, and resident fibroblasts (34–39). However, these types of transdifferentiation were all triggered by innate and adaptive immune responses through production of proinflammatory and profibrotic molecules. As a model of tubulointerstitial fibrosis, UUO model was thought best for this approach, as it is a rapid and reproducible model of RF in mice, and it mimics the main steps of tubulointerstitial fibrosis in humans (40–42). In this study, we explored the interactions between the innate and adaptive immune systems in the process of promoting RF. In the early stage during the pathogenesis of RF, macrophages are present at the affected areas (43). As an essential component of innate immunity, macrophages also regulate adaptive immune responses by recruiting other immune cells, such as neutrophils, mast cells and lymphocytes (44–49). Our results confirmed that depletion of kidney macrophages by clodronate significantly attenuated RF and function in UUO models, which has been demonstrated by previous reports.

Macrophages are highly heterogeneous cells subdivided according to their distinct functions (50, 51). In CKD, M1 macrophages are increased during early injury and inflammation and persistently surround regions of damaged tissue. Subsequently, macrophages switch to an anti-inflammatory (M2) phenotype and contribute to resolution of inflammation (43). Our evidence showed that resident kidney macrophages can secrete C3, and M1 macrophages secrete higher amounts of C3 than M2 macrophages.

Prominent roles of $CD4^{+}$T cells in chronic diseases have been reported in previous studies (52, 53). Our colleagues showed that massive $CD4^{+}$T lymphocyte infiltration was observed in the fibrotic kidneys of patients and UUO mice (54). After antibodies were used to deplete $CD4^{+}$ T cells, HE and Masson's trichrome staining results showed less inflammatory infiltrates and attenuated interstitial fibrosis in $CD4^{+}$T lymphocyte-depleted mice compared with UUO mice. When we depleted C3 and C3a, the infiltrating inflammatory cells, including

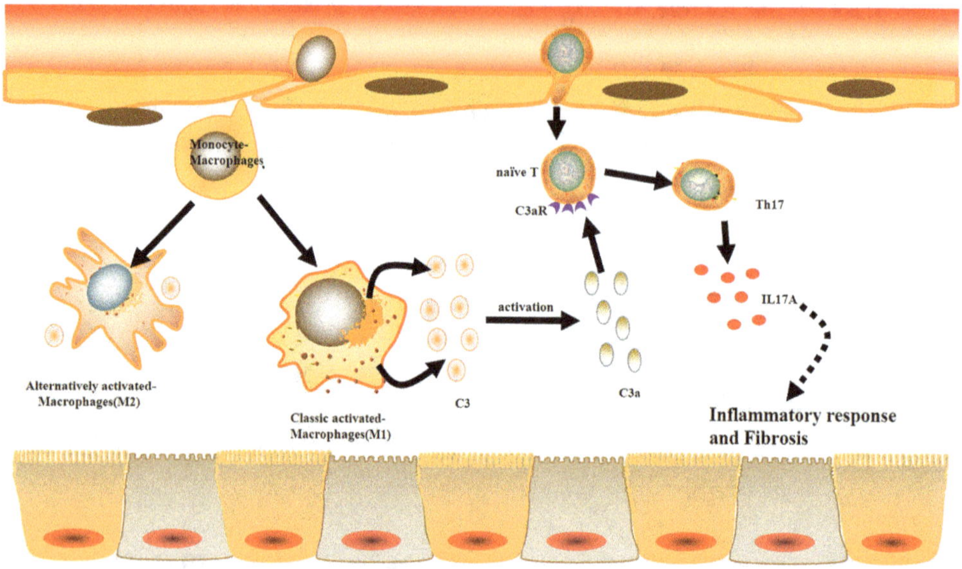

FIGURE 10 | Model summarizing the role of local C3 in the development of renal fibrosis. Local C3 secretion by macrophages may be contributed to the pathogenesis of renal TILs, involving the production of IL-17A and activation of ERK and STAT3 signaling pathway.

macrophages, CD3$^+$T cells, and CD4$^+$T cells, decreased in UUO mice, as demonstrated by IHC and flow cytometric analyses, indicating that CD4$^+$T cell differentiation occurs after UUO. The data suggest that the C3a/C3aR signaling pathway.

In inflammatory kidney diseases, IL-17A producing by T lymphocytes contributes significantly to the pathogenesis of RF (55). A newly-published study has shown that IL-17 acts an inhibitory factor in TGF-β-induced renal fibroblast activation using the UUO model with IL-17$^{-/-}$mice (56). The explanation for this discrepancy might be that the IL-17 cytokine family consists of six members (IL-17A–F), and the potential effect of the other IL-17 family members in renal autoimmunity and inflammation is unknown. Another study has shown that macrophages and neutrophils are major source of IL-17 in different diseases (57–60). But Tamassia noted that the human neutrophils are unable to express and produce IL-17A, IL-17B, or IL-17F *in vitro* (61). Our data show that IL-17A was mainly produced by CD4$^+$Tcell, rather than F4/80$^+$macrophages in UUO mice, which was consistent with previous reports (55, 62).

In addition, IL-17A, which is secreted by CD4$^+$T cells, has been shown to play a major role in post-transplantation allograft rejection and in immune responses in the kidney (63–65). In the presence of TGF-β and IL-6, T cells differentiate into Th17 cells. In this regard, we observed the expression of chemokines (MCP-1, IL-1β, and IL-6) and lymphocyte infiltration in the obstructed kidneys of mice on days 7 and 14 after UUO and IL-17A secretion by CD4$^+$T cells in the UUO mice. The production of IL-17A is negatively regulated by the anaphylatoxins, and C3a signaling elevates Th17 responses, while C5a signaling suppresses Th17 cell differentiation in experimental allergic asthma. As illustrated in **Figure 7**, we found that C3a could promote proliferation of T cells and increase IL-17A secretion by CD4$^+$T cell and activation of the ERK and STAT3 signaling pathways *in vitro*. These phenomena can be suppressed by a C3aR inhibitor, suggesting that the C3a/C3aR pathway participates in the pathogenesis of UUO injury by modulating IL-17A expression, consequently promoting local inflammation and RF.

Combined with the data obtained from patient samples, relevant animal experiments and cell models, our study defines a novel mechanism by which C3 participates in renal inflammation and fibrosis. In response to injury, local C3 secretion by macrophages leads to IL-17A-mediated inflammatory cell infiltration into the kidney, which further drives fibrogenic responses. Our findings suggest that inhibition of the C3a/C3aR pathway could constitute a novel therapeutic approach for obstructive nephropathy.

AUTHOR CONTRIBUTIONS

The experiments were conceived and designed by YyL, XL, and CZ. Experiments were performed by KW, YL, YZ, and HW and data analyzed by KW, RL, and SG. The paper was written by YyL and GX with input from all authors.

FUNDING

This work was partly supported by International (regional) cooperation and exchange projects, (NSFC-DFG, Grant no. 81761138041), the National Natural Science Foundation of China (No.81372244, 81572287, 81772499, and 81470948), Hubei Provincial Health and Family Planning Youth Project of China (no. WJ2015Q007), and the Major Research plan of the National Natural Science Foundation of China (Grant no. 91742204).

ACKNOWLEDGMENTS

The authors thank all of our colleagues working in the Department of Nephrology, Tongji Hospital of Tongji Medical College, Huazhong University of Science and Technology.

SUPPLEMENTARY MATERIAL

Supplement Figure S1 | Complement C3 is increased in the obstructed kidney. **(A)** Real-time PCR showing relative renal mRNA levels of C3, fibrotic markers (α-SMA, PDGFR-β, and Collagen I) in sham control and UUO mice. **(B)** IHC staining showing F4/80 and C3 protein expression in the sham control and UUO mice; original magnification, ×400. Quantitative analysis of F4/80 **(C)** and C3 **(D)** positive cells were shown as mean ± SEM. $n = 6$ per group, Scale bar, 50 μm. **(E)** High magnification of C3 expression in IgA Patient and UUO mouse. The error bars represent the SEM.*$P < 0.05$; **$P < 0.01$; ***$P < 0.001$.

Supplement Figure S2 | Macrophage depletion protects against renal fibrosis by inhibiting C3 expression. UUO mice were intravenously injected with clodronate liposomes and control liposomes. On days 7 and 14, mice were sacrificed, and the left kidneys were collected. The expression levels of C3 and fibrotic markers (α-SMA, PDGFR-β, and Collagen I) were detected by real-time PCR **(A)** and Western blot analyses **(B)**, respectively. **(C)**The histogram shows the relative intensity for each marker normalized to GAPDH. $n = 6$ per group. The error bars represent the SEM. *$P < 0.05$; **$P < 0.01$; ***$P < 0.001$.

Supplement Figure S3 | C3 deficiency reduces C3 expression and fibrosis during UUO. UUO mice were subcutaneously injected with control peptide and Cp40. On days 7 and 14, mice were sacrificed, and the left kidneys were collected. **(A)** Masson's trichrome staining indicates collagen deposition. IHC staining showing α-SMA and C3 protein expression in these groups ($n = 6$); original magnification, ×400. Scale bar, 50 μm. Quantitative analysis of interstitial fibrosis **(B)**, a-SMA**(C)** and C3**(D)** positive cells were shown as mean ± SEM. **(E)** The expression levels of C3, TGF-β1, and fibrotic markers (α-SMA, PDGFR-β, and Collagen I) were detected by Western blot. **(F)** The histogram shows the relative intensity for each marker normalized to GAPDH. $n = 6$ per group. The error bars represent the SEM. *$P < 0.05$; **$P < 0.01$; ***$P < 0.001$.

Supplement Figure S4 | CD11b$^+$F4/80$^+$macrophages are not the main producer of IL-17A in kidney of UUO mice. Flow cytometric analysis of kidney cell suspensions from the obstructed kidneys injected with or without Cp40 at **(A)** 7 days and **(C)** 14 days post UUO; $n = 6$. Cells were stimulated *in vitro* with PMA/Ionomycin/Golgi-plug for 4 h. Specific staining of cell markers (anti-F4/80, anti-CD11b) and intracellular staining for IL-17A were performed. The F4/80$^+$ cells were gated. Among them, the CD11b$^+$IL-17$^+$cells were further gated for the analysis. Plots are gated for live CD11b$^+$F4/80$^+$ IL-17A$^+$ macrophages; numbers indicate events in the quadrants as percentages of all gated events. **(B,D)** Quantifications of CD11b$^+$F4/80$^+$ IL-17A$^+$ cells as percentages of all kidney cells isolated from the C3 blockade UUO mice and UUO mice. The error bars represent the SEM. ***$P < 0.001$. The data were pooled from three independent experiments.

Supplement Figure S5 | T cells were knocked down endogenous C3aR by using three small-interfering RNAs (siRNAs). **(A)** The expression levels of C3aR was detected by Western blot. **(B)** The histogram shows the relative intensity for each marker normalized to Actin. $n = 3$ per group. The error bars represent the SEM. ***$P < 0.001$.

REFERENCES

1. Ai Z, Li M, Liu W, Foo JN, Mansouri O, Yin P, et al. Low α-defensin gene copy number increases the risk for IgA nephropathy and renal dysfunction. *Sci Transl Med.* (2016) 8:345ra88. doi: 10.1126/scitranslmed.aaf2106
2. Humphreys BD. Mechanisms of renal fibrosis. *Annu Rev Physiol.* (2018) 10:309–26. doi: 10.1146/annurev-physiol-022516-034227
3. Liu ZH. Nephrology in China. *Nat Rev Nephrol.* (2013) 9:523–8. doi: 10.1038/nrneph.2013.146
4. Duffield JS. Cellular and molecular mechanisms in kidney fibrosis. *J Clin Invest.* (2014) 6:2299–306. doi: 10.1172/JCI72267
5. Hartupee J, Mann DL. Role of inflammatory cells in fibroblast activation. *J Mol Cell Cardiol.* (2016) 93:143–8. doi: 10.1016/j.yjmcc.2015.11.016
6. Wang P, Yang J, Tong F, Duan Z, Liu X, Xia L, et al. Anti-double-stranded DNA IgG participates in renal fibrosis through suppressing the suppressor of cytokine signaling 1 signals. *Front Immunol.* (2017) 8:610. doi: 10.3389/fimmu.2017.00610
7. Webster AC, Nagler EV, Morton RL, Masson P. Chronic kidney disease. *Lancet* (2017) 389:1238–52. doi: 10.1016/S0140-6736(16)32064-5
8. Barnes JL, Gorin Y. Myofibroblast differentiation during fibrosis: role of NAD(P)H oxidases. *Kidney Int.* (2011) 79:944–56. doi: 10.1038/ki.2010.516
9. Passwell J, Schreiner GF, Nonaka M, Beuscher HU, Colten HR. Local extrahepatic expression of complement genes C3, factor B, C2, and C4 is increased in murine lupus nephritis. *J Clin Invest.* (1988) 82:1676–84. doi: 10.1172/JCI113780
10. Natoli R, Fernando N, Jiao H, Racic T, Madigan M, Barnett NL, et al. Retinal macrophages synthesize C3 and activate complement in AMD and in models of focal retinal degeneration. *Invest Ophthalmol Vis Sci.* (2017) 58:2977–90. doi: 10.1167/iovs.17-21672
11. Tang S, Zhou W, Sheerin S, Vaughan RW, Sacks SH. Contribution of renal secreted complement C3 to the circulating pool in humans. *J Immunol.* (1999) 162:4336–41.
12. Fisher AJ, Cipolla E, Varre A, Gu H, Mickler EA, Vittal R. Potential mechanisms underlying TGF-β-mediated complement activation in lung fibrosis. *Cell Mol Med.* (2017) 3:14.
13. Cui J, Wan J, You D, Zou Z, Chen Y, Li Z, et al. Interstitial complement C3 activation and macrophage infiltration in patients with hypertensive nephropathy. *Clin Nephrol.* (2017) 88:328–37. doi: 10.5414/CN109154
14. Xavier S, Sahu RK, Landes SG, Yu J, Taylor RP, Ayyadevara S, et al. Pericytes and immune cells contribute to complement activation in tubulointerstitial fibrosis. *Am J Physiol Renal Physiol.* (2017) 312:F516–32. doi: 10.1152/ajprenal.00604.2016
15. Pepys MB. Role of complement in the induction of immunological responses. *Transpl Rev.* (1976) 32:93–120.
16. Pratt JR, Basheer SA, Sacks SH. Local synthesis of complement component C3 regulates acute renal transplant rejection. *Nat Med.* (2002) 8:582–7. doi: 10.1038/nm0602-582
17. Heeger PS, Lalli PN, Lin F, Valujskikh A, Liu J, Muqim N, et al. Decay-accelerating factor modulates induction of T cell immunity. *J Exp Med.* (2005) 201:1523–30. doi: 10.1084/jem.20041967
18. Strainic MG, Liu J, Huang D, An F, Lalli PN, Muqim N, et al. Locally produced complement fragments C5a and C3a provide both costimulatory and survival signals to naive CD4+T cells. *Immunity* (2008) 28:425–35. doi: 10.1016/j.immuni.2008.02.001

19. Nakayama Y, Kim SI, Kim EH, Lambris JD, Sandor M, Suresh M. C3 promotes expansion of CD8+ and CD4+ T cells in a *Listeria monocytogenes* infection. *J Immunol.* (2009) 183:2921–31. doi: 10.4049/jimmunol.0801191
20. Zhang J, Zhang Y, Xiao F, Liu Y, Wang J, Gao H, et al. The peroxisome proliferator-activated receptor γ agonist pioglitazone prevents NF-κB activation in cisplatin nephrotoxicity through the reduction of p65 acetylation via the AMPK-SIRT1/p300 pathway. *Biochem Pharmacol.* (2016)101:100–11. doi: 10.1016/j.bcp.2015.11.027
21. Liu YY, Lin SJ, Chen YY, Liu LN, Bao LB, Tang LQ, et al. High-density lipoprotein cholesterol as a predictor of poor survival in patients with nasopharyngeal carcinoma. *Oncotarget* (2016) 7:42978–87. doi: 10.18632/oncotarget.7160
22. Zhan J, Wang K, Zhang C, Zhang C, Li Y, Zhang Y, et al. GSPE inhibits HMGB1 release, attenuating renal IR-induced acute renal injury and chronic renal fibrosis. *Int J Mol Sci.* (2016) 17:E1647. doi: 10.3390/ijms171 01647
23. Zhang S, Lv JW, Yang P, Yu Q, Pang J, Wang Z, et al. Loss of dicer exacerbates cyclophosphamide-induced bladder overactivity by enhancing purinergic signaling. *Am J Pathol.* (2012) 181:937–46. doi: 10.1016/j.ajpath.2012.05.035
24. Fakhouri F, Frémeaux-Bacchi V, Noël LH, Cook HT, Pickering MC. C3 glomerulopathy: a new classification. *Nat Rev Nephrol.* (2010) 6:494–9. doi: 10.1038/nrneph.2010.85
25. Pirozzi N, Stoppacciaro A, Menè P. Dominant C3 glomerulopathy: new roles for an old actor in renal pathology. *J Nephrol.* (2017) 31:503–10. doi: 10.1007/s40620-017-0458-y
26. Hou J, Markowitz GS, Bomback AS, Appel GB, Herlitz LC, Barry Stokes M, et al. Toward a working definition of C3 glomerulopathy by immunofluorescence. *Kidney Int.* (2014) 85:450–6. doi: 10.1038/ki.2013.340
27. Gansevoort RT, Correa-Rotter R, Hemmelgarn BR, Jafar TH, Heerspink HJ, Mann JF, et al. Chronic kidney disease and cardiovascular risk: epidemiology, mechanisms, and prevention. *Lancet* (2013) 382:339–52. doi: 10.1016/S0140-6736(13)60595-4
28. Grgic I, Duffield JS, Humphreys BD. The origin of interstitial myofibroblasts in chronic kidney disease. *Pediatr Nephrol.* (2012) 27:183–93. doi: 10.1007/s00467-011-1772-6
29. Montgomery TA, Xu L, Mason S, Chinnadurai A, Lee CG, Elias JA, et al. Breast regression protein-39/chitinase 3-like 1 promotes renal fibrosis after kidney injury via activation of myofibroblasts. *J Am Soc Nephrol.* (2017) 28:3218–26. doi: 10.1681/ASN.2017010110
30. Kurts C, Panzer U, Anders HJ, Rees AJ. The immune system and kidney disease: basic concepts and clinical implications. *Nat Rev Immunol.* (2013) 13:738–53. doi: 10.1038/nri3523
31. Fogo AB. Causes and pathogenesis of focal segmental glomerulosclerosis. *Nat Rev Nephrol.* (2015) 11:76–87. doi: 10.1038/nrneph.2014.216
32. Pulskens WP, Butter LM, Teske GJ, Claessen N, Dessing MC, Flavell RA, et al. Nlrp3 prevents early renal interstitial edema and vascular permeability in unilateral ureteral obstruction. *PLoS ONE* (2014) 9:e85775. doi: 10.1371/journal.pone.0085775
33. Wang J, Zhuang S. Src family kinases in chronic kidney disease. *Am J Physiol Renal Physiol.* (2017) 313:721–8. doi: 10.1152/ajprenal.00141.2017
34. Wang YY, Jiang H, Pan J, Huang XR, Wang YC, Huang HF, et al. Macrophage-to-Myofibroblast transition contributes to interstitial fibrosis in chronic renal allograft injury. *J Am Soc Nephrol.* (2017) 28:2053–67. doi: 10.1681/ASN.2016050573
35. Liang H, Zhang Z, Yan J, Wang Y, Hu Z, Mitch WE, et al. The IL-4 receptor α has a critical role in bone marrow-derived fibroblast activation and renal fibrosis. *Kidney Int.* (2017) 92:1433–43. doi: 10.1016/j.kint.2017.04.021
36. Djudjaj S, Martin IV, Buhl EM, Nothofer NJ, Leng L, Piecychna M, et al. Macrophage migration inhibitory factor limits renal inflammation and fibrosis by counteracting tubular cell cycle arrest. *J Am Soc Nephrol.* (2017) 28:3590–604. doi: 10.1681/ASN.2017020190
37. Tsukui T, Ueha S, Shichino S, Inagaki Y, Matsushima K. Intratracheal cell transfer demonstrates the profibrotic potential of resident fibroblasts in pulmonary fibrosis. *Am J Pathol.* (2015) 185:2939–48. doi: 10.1016/j.ajpath.2015.07.022
38. Birbrair A, Zhang T, Files DC, Mannava S, Smith T, Wang ZM, et al. Type-1 pericytes accumulate after tissue injury and produce collagen in an organ-dependent manner. *Stem Cell Res Ther.* (2014) 5:122. doi: 10.1186/scrt512
39. LeBleu VS, Taduri G, O'Connell J, Teng Y, Cooke VG, Woda C, et al. Origin and function of myofibroblasts in kidney fibrosis. *Nat Med.* (2013) 19:1047–53. doi: 10.1038/nm.3218
40. Sasaki K, Doi S, Nakashima A, Irifuku T, Yamada K, Kokoroishi K, et al. Inhibition of SET domain-containing lysine methyltransferase 7/9 ameliorates renal fibrosis. *J Am Soc Nephrol.* (2016) 27:203–15. doi: 10.1681/ASN.2014090850
41. Lecru L, Desterke C, Grassin-Delyle S, Chatziantoniou C, Vandermeersch S, Devocelle A, et al. Cannabinoid receptor 1 is a major mediator of renal fibrosis. *Kidney Int.* (2015) 88:72–84. doi: 10.1038/ki.2015.63
42. Iida T, Fujinaka H, Xu B, Zhang Y, Magdeldin S, Nameta M, et al. Decreased urinary calbindin 1 levels in proteinuric rats and humans with distal nephron segment injuries. *Clin Exp Nephrol.* (2014) 18:432–43. doi: 10.1007/s10157-013-0835-3
43. Cao Q, Harris DC, Wang Y. Macrophages in kidney injury, inflammation, and fibrosis. *Physiology* (2015) 30:183–94. doi: 10.1152/physiol.00046.2014
44. Ring NG, Herndler-Brandstetter D, Weiskopf K, Shan L, Volkmer JP, George BM, et al. Anti-SIRPα antibody immunotherapy enhances neutrophil and macrophage antitumor activity. *Proc Natl Acad Sci USA.* (2017) 114:E10578–85. doi: 10.1073/pnas.1710877114
45. Tang Y, Li H, Li J, Liu Y, Li Y, Zhou J, et al. Macrophage scavenger receptor I contributes to pathogenesis of fulminant hepatitis via neutrophil-mediated complement activation. *J Hepatol.* (2017). 68:733–43. doi: 10.1016/j.jhep.2017.11.010
46. Chu YT, Wan SW, Anderson R, Lin YS. Mast cell-macrophage dynamics in modulation of dengue virus infection in skin. *Immunology* (2015) 146:163–72. doi: 10.1111/imm.12492
47. Rodriguez AR, Yu JJ, Navara C, Chambers JP, Guentzel MN, Arulanandam BP. Contribution of FcεRI-associated vesicles to mast cell-macrophage communication following *Francisella tularensis* infection. *Innate Immun.* (2016) 22:567–74. doi: 10.1177/1753425916663639
48. Hams E, Bermingham R, Fallon PG. Macrophage and innate lymphoid cell interplay in the genesis of fibrosis. *Front Immunol.* (2015) 6:597. doi: 10.3389/fimmu.2015.00597
49. Li J, Mo HY, Xiong G, Zhang L, He J, Huang ZF, et al. Tumor microenvironment macrophage inhibitory factor directs the accumulation of interleukin-17-producing tumor-infiltrating lymphocytes and predicts favorable survival in nasopharyngeal carcinoma patients. *J Biol Chem.* (2012) 287:35484–95. doi: 10.1074/jbc.M112.367532
50. Kobori T, Hamasaki S, Kitaura A, Yamazaki Y, Nishinaka T, Niwa A, et al. Interleukin-18 amplifies macrophage polarization and morphological alteration, leading to excessive angiogenesis. *Front Immunol.* (2018) 9:334. doi: 10.3389/fimmu.2018.00334
51. Huen SC, Cantley LG. Macrophages in renal injury and repair. *Annu Rev Physiol.* (2017) 79:449–69. doi: 10.1146/annurev-physiol-022516-034219
52. Ibáñez L, Abou-Ezzi G, Ciucci T, Amiot V, Belaïd N, Obino D, et al. Inflammatory osteoclasts prime TNFα-producing CD4+ T cells and express CX3CR1. *J Bone Miner Res.* (2016) 31:1899–908. doi: 10.1002/jbmr.2868
53. Lim WC, Olding M, Healy E, Millar TM. Human endothelial cells modulate CD4+ T cell populations and enhance regulatory T cell suppressive capacity. *Front Immunol.* (2018) 9:565. doi: 10.3389/fimmu.2018.00565
54. Liu L, Kou P, Zeng Q, Pei G, Li Y, Liang H, et al. CD4+ T Lymphocytes, especially Th2 cells, contribute to the progress of renal fibrosis. *Am J Nephrol.* (2012) 36:386–96. doi: 10.1159/000343283
55. Peng X, Xiao Z, Zhang J, Li Y, Dong Y, Du J. IL-17A produced by both γδ T and Th17 cells promotes renal fibrosis via RANTES-mediated leukocyte infiltration after renal obstruction. *J Pathol.* (2015) 235:79–89. doi: 10.1002/path.4430
56. Sun B, Wang H, Zhang L, Yang X, Zhang M, Zhu X, et al. Role of interleukin 17 in TGF-β signaling-mediated renal interstitial fibrosis. *Cytokine* (2018) 106:80–8. doi: 10.1016/j.cyto.2017.10.015
57. Song C, Luo L, Lei Z, Li B, Liang Z, Liu G, et al. IL-17-producing alveolar macrophages mediate allergic lung inflammation related to asthma. *J Immunol.* (2008) 181:6117–24. doi: 10.4049/jimmunol.181.9.6117
58. Pavlov O, Selutin A, Pavlova O, Selkov S. Macrophages are a source of IL-17 in the human placenta. *Am J Reprod Immunol.* (2018) 29:e13016. doi: 10.1111/aji.13016

59. Li L, Huang L, Vergis AL, Ye H, Bajwa A, Narayan V, et al. IL-17 produced by neutrophils regulates IFN-gamma-mediated neutrophil migration in mouse kidney ischemia-reperfusion injury. *J Clin Invest.* (2010) 120:331–42. doi: 10.1172/JCI38702
60. Hu S, He W, Du X, Yang J, Wen Q, Zhong XP, et al. IL-17 Production of neutrophils enhances antibacteria ability but promotes arthritis development during *Mycobacterium tuberculosis* infection. *EBioMedicine* (2017) 23:88–99. doi: 10.1016/j.ebiom.2017.08.001
61. Tamassia N, Arruda-Silva F, Calzetti F, Lonardi S, Gasperini S, Gardiman E, et al. A reappraisal on the potential ability of human neutrophils to express and produce IL-17 family members *in vitro*: failure to reproducibly detect it. *Front Immunol.* (2018) 9:795. doi: 10.3389/fimmu.2018.00795
62. Wu WP, Tsai YG, Lin TY, Wu MJ, Lin CY. The attenuation of renal fibrosis by histone deacetylase inhibitors is associated with the plasticity of FOXP3+IL-17+ T cells. *BMC Nephrol.* (2017) 18:225. doi: 10.1186/s12882-017-0630-6
63. Liang SC, Long AJ, Bennett F, Whitters MJ, Karim R, Collins M, et al. An IL-17F/A heterodimer protein is produced by mouse Th17 cells and induces airway neutrophil recruitment. *J Immunol.* (2007) 179:7791–9. doi: 10.4049/jimmunol.179.11.7791
64. Kwan T, Chadban SJ, Ma J, Bao S, Alexander SI, Wu H. IL-17 deficiency attenuates allograft injury and prolongs survival in a murine model of fully MHC-mismatched renal allograft transplantation. *Am J Transplant.* (2015) 15:1555–67. doi: 10.1111/ajt.13140
65. Cortvrindt C, Speeckaert R, Moerman A, Delanghe JR, Speeckaert MM. The role of interleukin-17A in the pathogenesis of kidney diseases. *Pathology* (2017) 49:247–58. doi: 10.1016/j.pathol.2017.01.003

2

Development of a Quantitative Assay for the Characterization of Human Collectin-11 (CL-11, CL-K1)

Rafael Bayarri-Olmos [1], Nikolaj Kirketerp-Moller [1], Laura Pérez-Alós [1], Karsten Skjodt [2], Mikkel-Ole Skjoedt [1] and Peter Garred [1]*

[1] Laboratory of Molecular Medicine, Department of Clinical Immunology, Faculty of Health and Medical Sciences, Rigshospitalet, University of Copenhagen, Copenhagen, Denmark, [2] Department of Cancer and Inflammation Research, University of Southern Denmark, Odense, Denmark

Correspondence:
Rafael Bayarri-Olmos
rafael.bayarri.olmos@regionh.dk

Collectin-11 (CL-11) is a pattern recognition molecule of the lectin pathway of complement with diverse functions spanning from host defense to embryonic development. CL-11 is found in the circulation in heterocomplexes with the homologous collectin-10 (CL-10). Abnormal CL-11 plasma levels are associated with the presence of disseminated intravascular coagulation, urinary schistosomiasis, and congenital disorders. Although there has been a marked development in the characterization of CL-11 there is still a scarcity of clinical tools for its analysis. Thus, we generated monoclonal antibodies and developed a quantitative ELISA to measure CL-11 in the circulation. The antibodies were screened against recombinant CL-11 and validated by ELISA and immunoprecipitation of serum and plasma. The best candidates were pairwise compared to develop a quantitative ELISA. The assay was validated regarding its sensitivity, reproducibility, and dilution linearity, demonstrating a satisfactory variability over a working range of 0.29–18.75 ng/ml. The mean plasma concentration of CL-11 in healthy controls was determined to be 289.4 ng/ml (range 143.2–459.4 ng/ml), highly correlated to the levels of CL/10/11 complexes ($r = 0.729$). Plasma CL-11 and CL-10/11 co-migrated in size exclusion chromatography as two major complexes of ~400 and >600 kDa. Furthermore, we observed a significant decrease at admission in CL-11 plasma levels in patients admitted to intensive care with systemic inflammatory response syndrome. By using the in-house antibodies and recombinant CL-11, we found that CL-11 can bind to zymosan independently of calcium by a separate site from the carbohydrate-binding region. Finally, we showed that CL-11/MASP-2 complexes trigger C4b deposition on zymosan. In conclusion, we have developed a specific and sensitive ELISA to investigate the ever-expanding roles of CL-11 in health and disease and shown a novel interaction between CL-11 and zymosan.

Keywords: CL-11, collectin, complement system, lectin pathway, zymosan

INTRODUCTION

CL-11 (alias collectin-11 and CL-K1) is a pattern recognition molecule (PRM) of the lectin pathway of complement with diverse functions such as pathogen recognition, tissue homeostasis, and embryonic development (1–4). It is the most recently discovered member of the collectin family, mammalian C-type lectins involved in the innate immune response of the host.

Collectins recognize conserved pathogen-specific structures and altered-self molecules and mediate their removal by, among others, agglutination, complement activation, and modulation of inflammatory and adaptive immune responses (5). Collectins share a common bouquet-like structure, with monomeric subunits that assemble into oligomers of trimers. Each monomeric subunit is, in turn, composed of a cysteine-rich N-terminal region, a collagen-like domain, an α-helical neck domain, and a C-terminal carbohydrate recognition domain (CRD). The biological functions of the collectins rely on the high-avidity binding resulting from the oligomerization and clustering of the CRDs.

CL-11 is a secreted collectin found in the circulation (6–8). Elevated CL-11 plasma levels are associated with a decreased risk of contracting urinary schistosomiasis (9) and the presence of disseminated intravascular coagulation (8), characterized by simultaneous clotting and bleeding that frequently leads to multiple organ failure and death. CL-11 deficiency is one of the causes of the 3MC (Malpuech, Michels, Mingarelli, and Carnevale) syndrome (3, 10), a congenital disorder associated with craniofacial dysmorphism, mental retardation, growth deficiency, and physical abnormalities. CL-11 is expressed ubiquitously in the body and it appears to play an important role in maintaining homeostasis in the tissue of expression (1, 11). During embryonic development, CL-11 is highly expressed in the craniofacial cartilage and vertebral bodies, where together with MASP-3 and CL-10, may act as a guidance cue for neural crest cell migration (12). In the mature kidney, locally-produced CL-11 appears to be critical for the development of renal injury after hypoxic and hypothermic stress (13), while in the retina local CL-11 facilitates phagocytosis of photoreceptor outer segments and modulates cytokine production in the retina (4).

Recently, CL-11 has been observed to circulate in complex with another member of the collectin family, CL-10 (collectin-10, CL-L1), forming high molecular weight heterocomplexes (i.e., CL-10/11) that interact strongly with the MASPs (14). Upon binding of CL-11 or CL-10/11 heterocomplexes to carbohydrate structures on the surface of microorganisms, the MASPs activate complement by cleaving C4 and C2 and generating the lectin pathway C3 convertase (C4b2a) (2, 15). Besides their role as the central lectin pathway enzymes, the MASPs are also involved in a variety of biological processes (16–18). MASP-1 has a particularly broad substrate-specificity and it is known to participate in the coagulation cascade, inflammatory reactions, and cell activation; MASP-2 is associated with the development of renal ischemia/reperfusion injury; while MASP-3 might be involved in the modulation of the alternative pathway by activating pro-FD in resting blood.

The multiplicity of biological functions attributed to CL-11 results from its ability to both associate with the MASPs and to interact with a broad range of self and non-self structures, such as yeast, bacteria, viruses, and apoptotic cells (1, 6, 19). Glycan array studies revealed that CL-11 has a preference toward high-mannose oligosaccharides and a subset of fucosylated glycans (10). This unusual binding specificity, different from the other collectins, can be explained by the presence of an extended binding site on the CRD that recognizes both the terminal and the penultimate sugar. Moreover, CL-11 has been observed to bind to certain ligands—e.g., nucleic acids (19), Aspergillus (2), and 9-O-acetylneuraminic acid (10)—in the absence of calcium via a binding site distinct from the carbohydrate-binding region.

Though the biological importance of CL-11 is evident, there is still a scarcity of clinical tools for its analysis. In this study, we generated monoclonal antibodies (mAbs) for the study of human CL-11. The mAbs were screened against serum and plasma using different immunological methods. Furthermore, we developed a quantitative ELISA based on two mAbs to measure the concentration of CL-11 in the circulation. The assay was thoroughly validated and used to determine the levels of CL-11 in plasma from healthy individuals. Our measurements of CL-11 are in good agreement with the literature and are tightly associated with those of CL-10/11. By size exclusion chromatography of plasma, we show that CL-11 forms complexes of 300–400 kDa and >600 kDa with a distinct composition of CL-10 glycosylation states and CL-11 isoforms. Finally, we demonstrate that CL-11 recognizes zymosan in a calcium-independent manner, and triggers C4b deposition in the presence of MASP-2.

MATERIALS AND METHODS

Buffers

The following buffers were used: PBS (10.1 mM disodium phosphate, 1.5 mM monopotassium phosphate, 137 mM NaCl, 2.7 mM KCl), PBS-Tw (PBS, 0.5% Tween-20), TBS-Tw ± Ca/EDTA/Mg-EGTA (10 mM Tris, 150 mM NaCl, 0.05% Tween-20, ±2.5 mM $CaCl_2$/10 mM EDTA/2 mM $MgCl_2$, 10 mM EGTA), sample buffer (TBS-Tw-EDTA, 0.1% v/v bovine serum), barbital-Tw ± EDTA (4 mM sodium barbitone, 145 mM NaCl, 2.6 mM $CaCl_2$, 2.1 mM $MgCl_2$, with 0.05% Tween-20, ± 5 mM EDTA).

Generation of Anti-CL-11 Monoclonal Antibodies (mAbs)

Two outbred NMRI mice were immunized subcutaneously three times with 25 μg of purified recombinant CL-11 (rCL-11) (R&D, USA) adsorbed to $Al(OH)_3$ and diluted 1:1 with Freund's incomplete adjuvant (Sigma-Aldrich, USA). Three days prior to the fusion, the mice received a final intravenous injection of 25 μg of antigen and adrenalin. The fusion and subsequent selection were done according to the principles of the hybridoma technology (20). Positive clones were screened in MaxiSorp microtiter plates (Thermo Fisher Scientific, USA) coated with 0.6 μg/ml of polyclonal antibody (pAb) rabbit anti-CL-11 (15269-1-AP, Proteintech, USA) and in-house rCL-11 as antigen. Selected mAbs were purified using a HiTrap Protein G column in an Äkta Pure system (both from GE Healthcare, UK). Briefly, clarified hybridoma supernatant was applied onto the column and washed until a stable UV reading was observed. Bound antibodies were eluted with 0.5% citric acid and neutralized with 0.1 M Tris pH 9. Elution fractions were pooled and dialyzed against PBS. MAbs were biotinylated with 20% w/w (+)-Biotin N-hydroxysuccinimide ester (Sigma, USA) for 3 h at room temperature (RT), followed by dialysis against PBS to remove unreacted biotin.

Production of Recombinant Proteins

Recombinant CL-11 (rCL-11) and CL-10 (rCL-10) were produced in Flp-In^{TM}-CHO cells (Invitrogen, USA). The coding sequences (NM_024027.4 and NM_006438.4, respectively) were retrieved from the RefSeq NCBI nucleotide database and cloned into pcDNA^{TM}5/FRT vectors flanked by two Flp recombinase target (FRT) sites. Stable transfectants were generated by co-transfecting the coding vectors with a pOG44 plasmid encoding the Flp recombinase. Positive clones were selected for Hygromycin resistance and grown in Ham's F-12 Nutrient Mix supplemented with 0.5% FBS, 0.1 mg/ml of Penicillin/Streptomycin (Sigma) and 2 mM of L-Glutamine (all from Gibco, Thermo Fisher Scientific unless otherwise stated) according to the manufacturer's recommendations. The concentration of rCL-11 in the supernatant was calculated using commercially-available rCL-11 (R&D) as calibrator.

Immunoprecipitation

Anti-CL-11 mAbs Hyb-15 and Hyb-17 (described in section Generation of Anti-CL-11 Monoclonal Antibodies and Development of a CL-11 Specific Sandwich ELISA), or mouse IgG1κ isotype control (BD Biosciences, USA) (2 μg each) were coupled to 25 μl of sheep anti-mouse IgG Dynabeads (Invitrogen) end-over-end for 30 min at RT. The conjugated beads were washed with PBS-Tw and incubated end-over-end 1 h at RT with serum diluted 1:1 in TBS-Tw-EDTA. After washing with PBS-Tw, bound CL-11 was eluted with 0.5% citric acid and subjected to SDS-PAGE as described below.

SDS-Page and Western Blot

Denatured samples were separated by electrophoresis in NuPAGE® Tris-Acetate 3–8% gels (Invitrogen, USA) according to the manufacturer's recommendation. Proteins were blotted onto a PVDF membrane (Amersham Bioscience, UK). Membranes were blocked with 5% skim milk (Merck Millipore, USA) and incubated overnight with 0.2 μg/ml of pAb rabbit anti-CL-11 (15269-1-AP, Proteintech) followed by 1 h incubation with pAb swine anti-rabbit-HRP (P0399, Dako, Denmark) in a 1:5000 dilution. After thorough washing, the membranes were developed with SuperSignal^{TM} West Femto Maximum Sensitivity Substrate (Thermo Fisher Scientific) and imaged with Microchemi (Bio-imaging systems, Israel).

CL-11 Specific Sandwich ELISA

MaxiSorp microtiter plates were coated overnight at 4°C with 2 μg/ml mAb Hyb-17 in PBS. Serial dilutions of the calibrator, serum and plasma samples in sample buffer were applied to the plate and incubated for 2 h, followed a 2 h incubation with 2 μg/ml of biotinylated mAb Hyb-15 in PBS-Tw. Streptavidin-HRP conjugate (RPN1231V, Sigma) was added to the wells for 1 h in a 1:2000 dilution in PBS-Tw. TMB One (KemEnTec Diagnostics, Denmark) was used as substrate. The reaction was stopped with 0.2 M H_2SO_4 and the optical density (OD) was recorded at 450 nm using an ELx80 absorbance reader (BioTek, USA). Plates were washed with PBS-Tw between steps and unless otherwise stated all incubations took place at RT. The optimal combination and concentration of mAbs was determined using a two-dimensional of capture and detection antibodies against serial dilutions of serum and plasma and rated according to their signal intensity and signal-to-noise ratio. The optimal incubation times and sample buffer composition were determined based on the same criteria.

Assay Validation: Parallelism, Precision, Limit of Detection, Working Range, and Variation

Supernatant from Flp-In CHO cells expressing rCL-11 was used as calibrator. The calibrator was applied in a two-fold dilution to generate an eight-point curve with a concentration ranging from 37.5 to 0.29 ng/ml. OD values from serial dilutions of the calibrator, commercial rCL-11 (R&D), serum and EDTA plasma pools (25 and 10 donors, respectively) were logistically-transformed and a log(agonist) vs. response equation was applied to evaluate the parallelism between the best-fit hill slopes. The calibrator was stored at −20°C in single-use aliquots. The limit of detection of the assay was expressed as the background absorbance plus two times the standard deviation (SD). The precision of the assay was evaluated by calculating the ratio between the OD and the mean OD of the triplicates of five donors over a 10-point dilution curve. The dilution linearity was calculated as the ratio between the interpolated concentration for each dilution and the mean concentration calculated from the linear part of the curve. The working range was determined as the concentrations for which both the ratio OD/mean OD and ratio concentration/mean concentration had a coefficient of variation (CV) <20%. Intra-assay variation was calculated as the CV of a plasma pool in 40 wells of a single microtiter plate. To calculate the inter-assay variation, serum and plasma pools were run in triplicates on four separate plates over six different days.

Stability of CL-11 in Serum and Plasma Samples

Serum and plasma samples from three healthy individuals were stored at 4°C, RT, or 37°C for up to 72 h. To study the effect of repeated freeze-thaw cycles, serum and plasma samples from a healthy donor were frozen at −80°C and thawed at RT five times. The levels of CL-11 were compared to a control sample subjected to a single freeze-thaw cycle.

Measurement of CL-10/11 Complexes in Plasma

MaxiSorp microtiter plates were coated overnight at 4°C with 2 μg/ml mAb anti-CL-10 (HM2356, Hycult) in PBS. Serial dilutions of the calibrator and EDTA plasma 1:40 in sample buffer were incubated for 2 h. Detection and development were performed as described in section CL-11 Specific Sandwich ELISA.

Serum and Plasma Samples

The concentration of CL-11 and CL-10/11 complexes in the circulation was determined from blood of Danish healthy volunteers ($n = 126$). In addition, CL-11 levels were measured in plasma from patients at admission to an Intensive Care Unit at Rigshospitalet diagnosed with systemic inflammatory syndrome ($n = 65$). The patients have been described elsewhere (21). Informed consent was obtained from the patients or their relatives in accordance with the Helsinki Protocol. The study was approved by the local ethics committee for Copenhagen County (record no. KA 96097). Serum and plasma were processed within 1 h of blood collection and stored at −80°C. Plasma was obtained by incubating fresh blood with EDTA, citrate, or hirudin—a naturally occurring anticoagulant that binds to and inhibits activated thrombin while maintaining complement activity in blood.

Size Exclusion Chromatography

Serum (100 µl) from a pool of blood donors was applied into a Superdex 200 HR 10/30 column (GE Healthcare) at a flow rate of 0.5 ml/min at RT with PBS 2 mM EDTA. The relative molecular weight of CL-11 and CL-10/11 complexes was estimated using a gel filtration marker kit (29–700 kDa, Sigma). CL-11 and CL-10/CL-11 levels in the elution fractions were measured by ELISA as described previously. Results were confirmed by western blotting following Trichloroacetic acid (TCA, Sigma) precipitation. Briefly, elution fractions (500 µl) were incubated 30 min on ice with 10% v/v TCA and centrifuged at 13,000 × g for 30 min at 4°C. Supernatants were discarded and the pellet was washed with ice-cold acetone (Sigma) at 13,000 × g for another 30 min at 4°C. Dry precipitates were resuspended in SDS loading buffer and separated by SDS-PAGE as described above. Anti-CL-10 (0.05 µg/ml, HM2356, Hycult) and pAb rabbit anti-CL-11 (0.05 µg/ml, 15269-1-AP, Proteintech) were used as detection antibodies with rCL-10 and rCL-11 (in-house) as controls.

Binding of rCL-11 to Ligands

Ligand interaction studies were performed in the fluid and solid phase. Unless otherwise stated, all reagents were purchased from Sigma. Fluid phase binding was analyzed by incubating 100 µl of zymosan particles (100 µg, Z4250), mannan-agarose (M9917), D-mannose-agarose (M6400), and Sepharose CL-2B (CL2B300) with 2.75 µg of rCL-11 in 500 µl of TBS-Tw-Ca or TBS-Tw-EDTA for 1.5 h at RT in an end-over-end shaker. Samples were washed thrice with their respective buffer and centrifuged at 3000 × g for 30 min. Pellets were resuspended in SDS loading buffer and subjected to SDS-PAGE using anti-CL-11 Hyb-6 (2 µg/ml) and pAb anti-CL-11 (15269-1-AP, Proteintech) as detection antibodies under non-reducing and reducing conditions, respectively.

Solid-phase binding was determined on microtiter plates coated with zymosan (Z4250), mannan (M7504), BSA (A2153), and D-mannose-BSA (NGP1108, Dextra, UK) in two-fold dilutions starting at 10 µg/ml in PBS overnight at 4°C. The plates washed between steps with TBS-Tw, and unless otherwise stated all incubations took place at RT. rCL-11 (1 µg/ml) was diluted in TBS-Tw-Ca, TBS-Tw-EDTA or TBS-Tw-Mg-EGTA and incubated for 2 h. Hyb-15 (2 µg/ml) in matching buffer was used as detection antibody for 2 h, followed by 1 h incubation with Streptavidin-HRP conjugate (RPN1231V) in a 1:2000 dilution. Development was performed as described previously.

To study the effect of soluble inhibitors on the binding to zymosan and mannan, rCL-11 was incubated with two-fold dilutions of L-fucose (F2252), N-acetyl-glucosamine (A3286), or human genomic DNA (isolated in-house) in TBS-Tw-Ca or TBS-Tw-EDTA for 1 h. Protein/ligand mixes were applied to Maxisorp plates pre-coated with zymosan or mannan (10 µg/ml) and were allowed to bind for 2 h. Quantification of bound rCL-11 was carried out as described before.

CL-11 Mediated C4 Deposition on Zymosan

Microtiter plates were coated as for the solid-phase binding studies. rCL-11 (2 µg/ml) in barbital-Tw or barbital-Tw-EDTA was applied to the wells and incubated for 2 h at RT, followed by rMASP-2 produced in CHO DG44 cells (0.5 µg/ml, in-house) in barbital-Tw or barbital-Tw-EDTA for 4 h at 37°C. Subsequently, purified C4 (0.5 µg/ml, CompTech, USA) in barbital-Tw was added to the plate for 1 h 37°C. Polyclonal rabbit anti-C4c (2 µg/ml, Dako) was used as a detection antibody for 1.5 h at RT, followed by swine anti-rabbit-HRP (0.15 µg/ml, P0399, Dako). The plates were washed between steps with barbital-Tw. Development and data recoding were carried out as before.

Statistical Analyses

Statistical analyses were performed using GraphPad Prism version 7.02 (GraphPad Software, USA). Measurements of samples and the calibrator were performed in duplicates unless otherwise stated. The concentration of CL-11 in serum and plasma was interpolated by regression analysis using a four-parameter logistic curve fitting. Effect of storage of CL-11 concentration and differences between measured CL-11 in serum and plasma samples was analyzed using two-way ANOVA with Dunnett's multiple comparisons tests. Two-tailed person correlation coefficient was used to determine the correlation between CL-11 and CL-10/CL-11 levels. Differences between CL-11 levels in controls and SIRS patients were analyzed with the Mann-Whitney test. The half maximal inhibitory concentration (IC50) was calculated using the inhibitor concentration vs. response equation on a nonlinear curve fitting constraining the top and bottom parameter to equal 100 and 0, respectively. The significance of observed differences on C4 deposition on zymosan was assessed via one-way ANOVA with Tukey's corrections for multiple comparisons. Data are represented as mean ± SEM of three independent experiments.

RESULTS

Generation of Anti-CL-11 Monoclonal Antibodies and Development of A CL-11 Specific Sandwich ELISA

Stable monoclonal hybridoma populations were generated by several rounds of cloning by limiting dilution. Each cloning round, culture supernatants were screened by indirect ELISA with rCL-11. Selected positive clones were characterized further by immunoprecipitation of native CL-11 from serum followed by western blotting. As seen in **Figure 1**, under reducing conditions both mAbs Hyb-15 and Hyb-17 precipitated a protein with an apparent molecular mass of ~34 kDa corresponding to the CL-11 monomer. Under non-reducing conditions, a characteristic

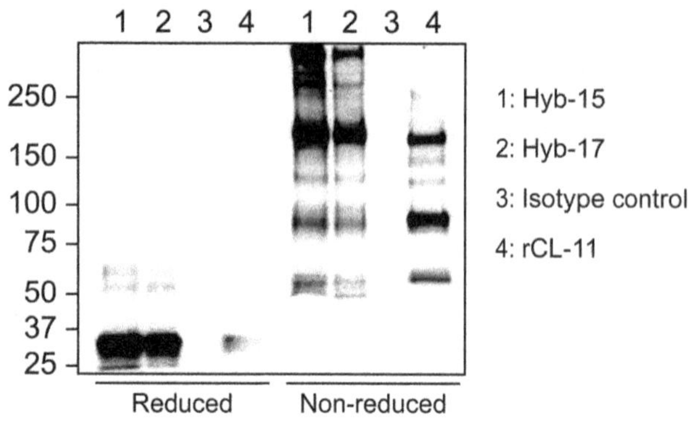

FIGURE 1 | Western blot of serum after immunoprecipitation using CL-11 specific mAbs Hyb-17 and Hyb-15 or a mouse IgG1κ isotype control antibody under reducing and non-reducing conditions. Supernatant from CHO cells expressing rCL-11 was used as positive control. The blots were developed with pAb rabbit anti-CL-11.

ladder-like banding pattern is visible with a major protein band around 180 kDa and several others larger than 250 kDa indicating that CL-11 assembles into high molecular weight oligomers held together by interchain disulfide bridges. rCL-11 used as positive control appeared to form predominantly lower oligomeric forms. An equivalent banding pattern was also seen with the other tested mAbs (data not shown). No bands were apparent when using a mouse IgG1κ control as precipitating antibody.

The best candidates were pairwise screened by sandwich ELISA against a serum and plasma pool. The optimal combination and concentration of mAbs was determined using a two-dimensional of capture and detection antibodies and rated according to their signal intensity and signal-to-noise ratio. Based on their properties, Hyb-17 and Hyb-15 were selected as capture and detection antibody, respectively. No signals were obtained when an irrelevant mouse antibody was used as capture or detection antibody (data not shown).

Assay Validation

Supernatant from CHO cells expressing rCL-11 was used as calibrator. A four-parameter fit model using the equation log(agonist) vs. response was applied to estimate the concentration of rCL-11 in the supernatant ($R^2 > 0.996$ for all curves). Parallelism was observed between the slopes of the calibrator and two batches of commercial rCL-11 (**Figure 2A**). Log-transformed values fitted a linear regression with $R^2 > 0.98$ and the slopes (ranging from 0.56 to 0.58) did not differ significantly ($p > 0.05$). Parallelism was also observed between the slopes of serial dilutions of the calibrator and serum and plasma pools in the range 0.29–37.5 ng/ml, with slopes between −0.7 and −0.77 that were not significantly different ($p > 0.05$) (**Figure 2B**). The limit of detection, defined as the mean background absorbance plus two times the SD, was 0.17 and 0.19 ng/ml in serum and plasma respectively. The precision of the assay, evaluated using the ratio between individual OD values and the mean OD values of triplicate measurements for five different donors (**Figure 2C**), was found to be acceptable (CV < 20%) for concentrations above 0.29 ng/ml. To determine the dilution linearity the ratio between the interpolated concentrations and the mean concentration of a plasma pool was calculated for each dilution of a 10-point dilution curve (**Figure 2D**). The dilution linearity was satisfactory in the range 0.15–18.75 ng/ml with a deviation under 20% from the mean concentration. The working range of the assay—defined based on the parallelism, limit of detection, precision, and dilution linearity—was 0.29–18.75 ng/ml.

Intra- and inter-assay variation were calculated to estimate the variation of the assay. The intra-assay CV, calculated by measuring one sample forty times on the same plate, was 3.96 % (**Table 1**). The inter-assay CV was 10.5%, measured in triplicates on four plates analyzed on six different occasions.

Effect of Storage and Freeze-Thawing

The effect of temperature on the stability of CL-11 in blood samples was evaluated on matched serum and plasma from three different donors stored at 4°C, RT, or 37°C for up to three days, whereas the effect of freezing and thawing was studied on serum and plasma samples from a single donor over five consecutive cycles. No significant trend on CL-11 levels was observed when the samples were stored at 4°C (**Figure 3A**) or at RT (**Figure 3B**), nor after repeated freeze-thawing cycles (**Figure 3D**). On the other hand, storage at 37°C degrees caused a highly significant drop in CL-11 concentration in citrate and EDTA plasma (**Figure 3C**). CL-11 levels in serum and plasma did not differ significantly.

CL-11 Levels in Plasma

CL-11 concentration in plasma was calculated from EDTA plasma samples of 126 Danish blood donors (mean 289.4 ng/ml, range 143.2–459.4 ng/ml) using rCL-11 as calibrator (**Figure 4A**). Since it has been reported that a major fraction of CL-11 exists in complex with the homologous CL-10, we measured the same samples by sandwich ELISA using an anti-CL-10 as capture antibody and anti-CL-11 Hyb-15 as detection. The estimated mean concentration of CL-10/11 complexes in plasma was 256.2 μg/ml (range 37.89–622.7) and there was a strong correlation between CL-11 and CL-10/11 levels ($r = 0.729$, **Figure 4B**. A pool of EDTA plasma from 10 healthy individuals was subjected to size exclusion chromatography followed by sandwich ELISA in order to define the relationship of CL-11 and CL-10/11 across their molecular weight distribution (**Figure 4C**). CL-11 and CL-10/11 migrated as two major oligomerization forms of approximately 400 and >600 kDa. ELISA results were confirmed by western blot using anti-CL-11 (**Figure 4D** above) and anti-CL-10 antibodies (**Figure 4D** below), where most of the protein is observed in fractions 7–8 and 13–14. Under reducing conditions, CL-10 migrates as a triple band of ~40 kDa. CL-11 present in the high molecular weight complexes migrates as a single band of ~34 kDa, whereas in the lower oligomers it appears as a double band—hinting at the occurrence of two different isoforms.

In light of the tight association between CL-11 and CL-10, we conclude that the ELISA developed in the current work is

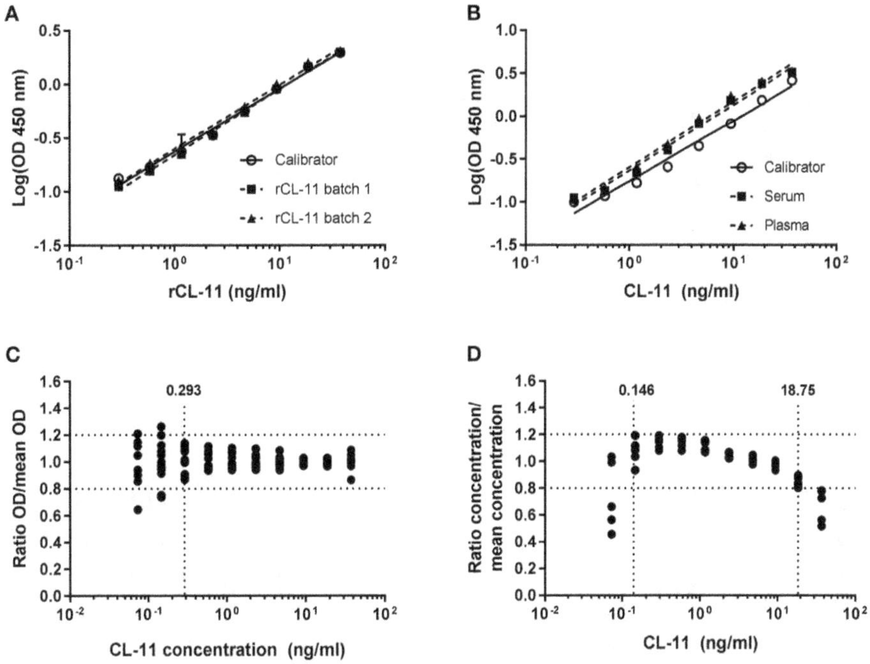

FIGURE 2 | Sandwich ELISA validation. Parallelism between serial dilutions of rCL-11 produced in CHO cells, used as calibrator, and two different batches of purified rCL-11 **(A)** and a serum and plasma pool **(B)** over a 10-point serial dilution series using a log(agonist) vs. response equation (R^2 > 0.99 for all curves). Error bars indicate the standard deviation of the mean of duplicate measurements. **(C)** Precision of the assay on plasma from five donors calculated as the range of concentrations for which the variation of the ratio OD/mean OD of the triplicates is <20% (i.e., > 0.293 ng/ml). **(D)** Dilution linearity on plasma from five donors calculated as the range of concentrations for which the variation of the interpolated concentration/mean concentration of the triplicates is <20% (i.e., 0.146–18.75 ng/ml).

TABLE 1 | Intra- and inter-assay variation of ELISA.

Sample	*n*	CL-11(ng/ml)		SD	CV(%)
		Mean	Range		
INTRA-ASSAY VARIATION					
Plasma	40	282.6	250.2–299.1	11.2	3.96
INTER-ASSAY VARIATION					
Plasma	6	286.7	257–335.2	30.1	10.5
Serum	6	247.1	187.8–331.7	49.47	20.02

The intra-assay variation was calculated by measuring a plasma pool sample on the same microtiter plate. The inter-assay variation was determined by comparing the mean of triplicates of a serum and plasma pool on four microtiter plates on six different days.

accurate and relevant to describe the natural situation of CL-11 in the circulation.

CL-11 Levels in Patients With Systemic Inflammatory Response Syndrome (SIRS)

Since CL-11 is expected to participate in the response against invading pathogens by activating the lectin pathway of complement, we measured the levels of CL-11 in 65 randomly selected plasma samples from patients admitted to the intensive care unit with SIRS [reported elsewhere(21)] (**Figure 5A**). Compared to healthy controls ($n = 69$), CL-11 was significantly decreased in patients with SIRS and spanned a wider range of concentrations (mean 276.4 ng/ml, range 136.2–511.7 vs. 240 ng/ml, range 73.76–876.4 ng/ml for controls and SIRS patients, respectively). As observed in healthy individuals, the concentration of CL-11 in SIRS plasma was strongly correlated with that of CL-10/11 complexes ($r = 0.915$, **Figure 5B**).

Ligand Characterization

Using our validated antibodies, we studied the ligand binding characteristics of CL-11 to identify a suitable ligand for *in vitro* complement activation assays. Binding was performed in the presence of calcium or EDTA (as cationic chelator) in the fluid phase using zymosan particles, mannan-agarose, D-mannose-agarose, and Sepharose as negative control. CL-11 displayed a characteristic C-type lectin activity and bound to D-mannose and mannan in the presence of calcium (1, 6) (**Figures 6A,B**). Remarkably, CL-11 was also able to bind to zymosan in a calcium-independent manner, suggesting an alternative ligand recognition mechanism. We confirmed the results by coating two-fold dilutions of mannan, zymosan, D-mannose-BSA, and BSA as negative control (**Figures 6C–F**). Binding of rCL-11 (1 μg/ml) was performed in the presence of calcium, EDTA, and magnesium-EGTA (a commonly used buffer for alternative pathway activation). As seen in the fluid-phase assay, calcium was required for binding to mannan and D-mannose (**Figures 6C,E**) but not to zymosan (**Figure 6D**). No binding to BSA was observed regardless of the buffer (**Figure 6F**).

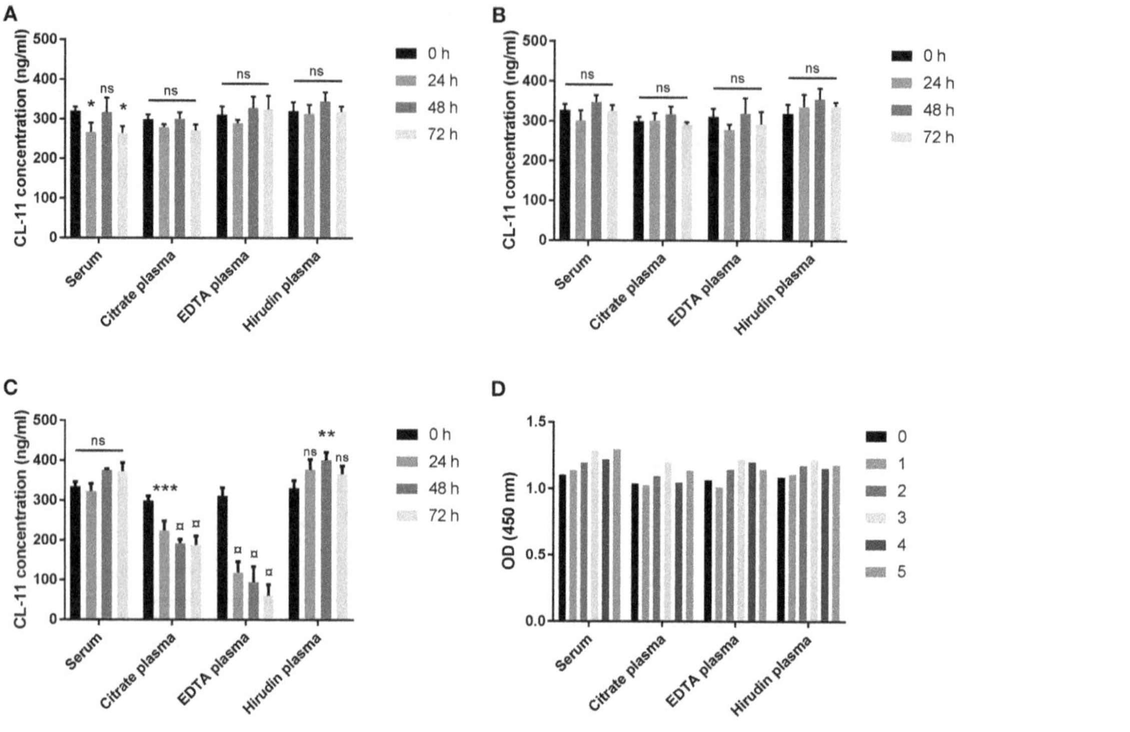

FIGURE 3 | Sample stability. Effect of temperature on CL-11 concentration in serum and plasma from three donors after storage at 4°C **(A)**, RT **(B)**, or 37°C **(C)** for three days. **(D)** Effect of freeze-thawing cycles on CL-11 measurements serum and plasma from the same donor. $^{*}p < 0.05$, $^{**}p < 0.01$; $^{***}p < 0.001$; ¤, $p = 0.0001$.

In order to determine whether the observed binding profiles are a result of the involvement of different binding sites for mannan and zymosan, we compared the effect of L-fucose (a strong ligand), N-Acetyl glucosamine (GlcNAc, a weak ligand), and genomic DNA (a calcium-independent ligand) on the binding to mannan and zymosan (**Figure 7**). Briefly, CL-11 was co-incubated with serial dilutions of L-fucose or GlcNAc starting in a 125 mM, or human genomic DNA starting at 30 μg/ml prior to addition to coated plates. L-fucose was an effective inhibitor of the binding to mannan in the presence of calcium with an IC50 of 36.48 mM, whereas N-acetyl-glucosamine had just a minor effect (IC50 > 125 mM) (**Figure 7A**). On zymosan, L-fucose was only a moderate inhibitor in the presence of calcium, forming an apparent plateau around 50% inhibition, while GlcNAc had no effect (**Figure 7B**). The limited effect of L-fucose suggests the presence of two separate binding sites for zymosan and carbohydrates.

CL-11 has been reported to bind to DNA in a calcium-independent fashion via an alternative binding-site. Co-incubation with DNA in the presence of calcium increased the binding to mannan, suggesting a cooperative effect between both molecules (see Discussion) (**Figure 7C**). DNA did not affect zymosan binding under calcium conditions, whereas in EDTA it showed a pronounced inhibition with an IC50 of 2.3 μg/ml (**Figure 7D**). These results indicate the presence of a shared binding site for nucleic acids and zymosan. Bearing all of the above in mind, we have identified a novel interaction with zymosan independent of divalent cations that we hypothesize may be relevant in environments where the binding to calcium is impaired, such as the gastrointestinal tract.

CL-11-Mediated C4 Deposition on Zymosan

To investigate if CL-11 bound to zymosan could trigger the lectin complement pathway, we developed an *in vitro* assay using rMASP-2 and purified C4 (**Figure 8**). CL-11/MASP-2 complexes on zymosan caused a significant C4b deposition under calcium conditions in a level comparable to mannan. In the presence of EDTA, C4 activation was only seen on the zymosan ligand. No C4b deposition was observed on BSA, nor in the absence of CL-11 and MASP-2.

DISCUSSION

We have generated mAbs against human CL-11 and established a quantitative sandwich ELISA. The antibody-producing hybridomas underwent successive selection rounds using first rCL-11, and later serum and plasma by ELISA and western immunoblotting. While all clones readily bound rCL-11, just a few reacted strongly with native CL-11. This is probably due to the existence of complexes in the circulation that hide epitopes otherwise exposed in the homomeric rCL-11 used as immunogen. In fact, immunoprecipitation of serum demonstrates that native CL-11 has a different oligomeric distribution than our recombinant protein (**Figure 1**). The best candidates were pairwise compared to develop a sandwich

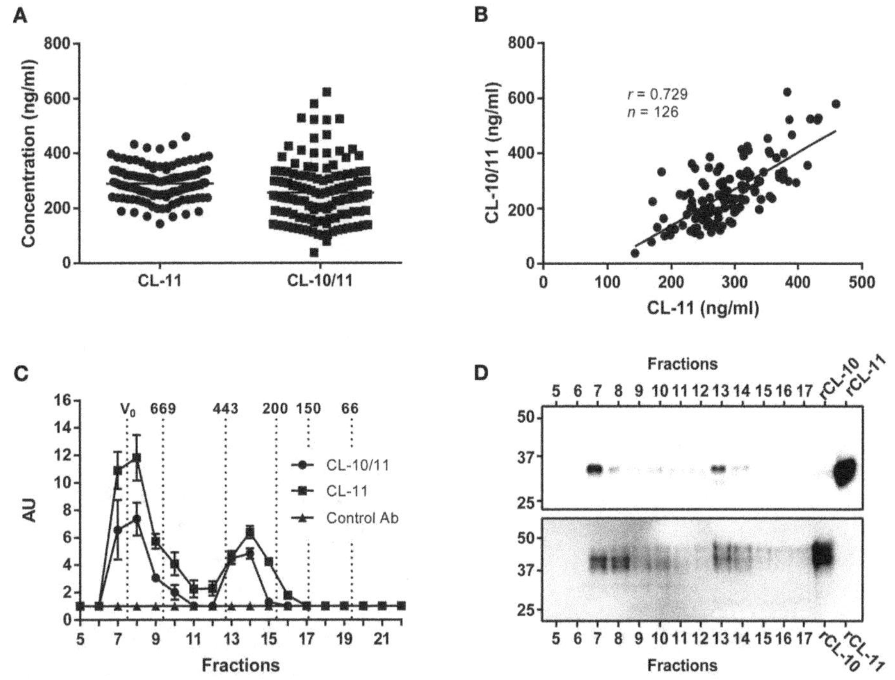

FIGURE 4 | Concentration and molecular weight distribution of CL-11 and CL-10/11 complexes in plasma. **(A)** CL-11 and CL-10/11 concentration in plasma of 126 Danish blood donors using the validated assay described here and a semi quantitative CL-10/CL-11 sandwich ELISA. Horizontal lines represent mean. **(B)** Spearman's rank correlation between measured CL-11 and CL-10/11 levels. **(C)** Detection of CL-11 and CL-10/11 complexes in the elution fractions of size exclusion chromatography of plasma by sandwich ELISA. Relative levels of CL-11 and CL-10/11 complexes in the elution fractions are reported as arbitrary units (AU). Vertical dotted lines indicate the molecular masses of thyroglobulin (669 kDa), apoferritin (443 kDa), β-amylase (200 kDa), alcohol dehydrogenase (150 kDa), BSA (66 kDA), carbonic anhydrase (29 kDa). Western blot of elution fractions from size exclusion chromatography using Hyb-6 anti-CL-11 (**D above**) or anti-CL-10 (**D below**). rCL-11 and rCL-10 produced in CHO cells were used as positive controls.

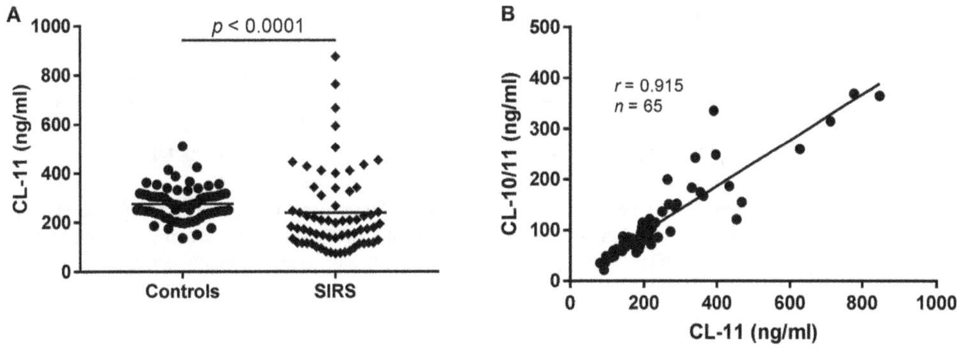

FIGURE 5 | CL-11 levels in plasma from patients with SIRS and controls. **(A)** CL-11 concentration was measured in 65 SIRS plasma samples and 69 controls using the quantitative ELISA described here. Horizontal lines represent mean. **(B)** Spearman's rank correlation between CL-11 and CL-10/11 concentration in SIRS plasma samples.

ELISA. Two antibodies were selected as capture and detection antibody in the basis of their signal-to-noise ratio. The assay was validated in terms of linearity, variability, and precision, demonstrating a satisfactory variability, and parallelism between calibrator and serum and plasma across a working range of 0.29–18.75 ng/ml (**Figure 2**). We observed no significant differences between CL-11 concentration in serum and four different widely used plasma preparations (**Figure 3**). Similarly, common storage conditions and freeze-thawing procedures did not affect the measurements of CL-11, highlighting the suitability of this assay for routine measurements in the clinic. Of interest, some of the mAbs cross-reacted with CL-11 from other species, granting the possibility of forthcoming studies into CL-11 in animal models of disease.

When optimizing the sandwich ELISA we noticed that EDTA was required to detect native CL-11 in serum and plasma (but not

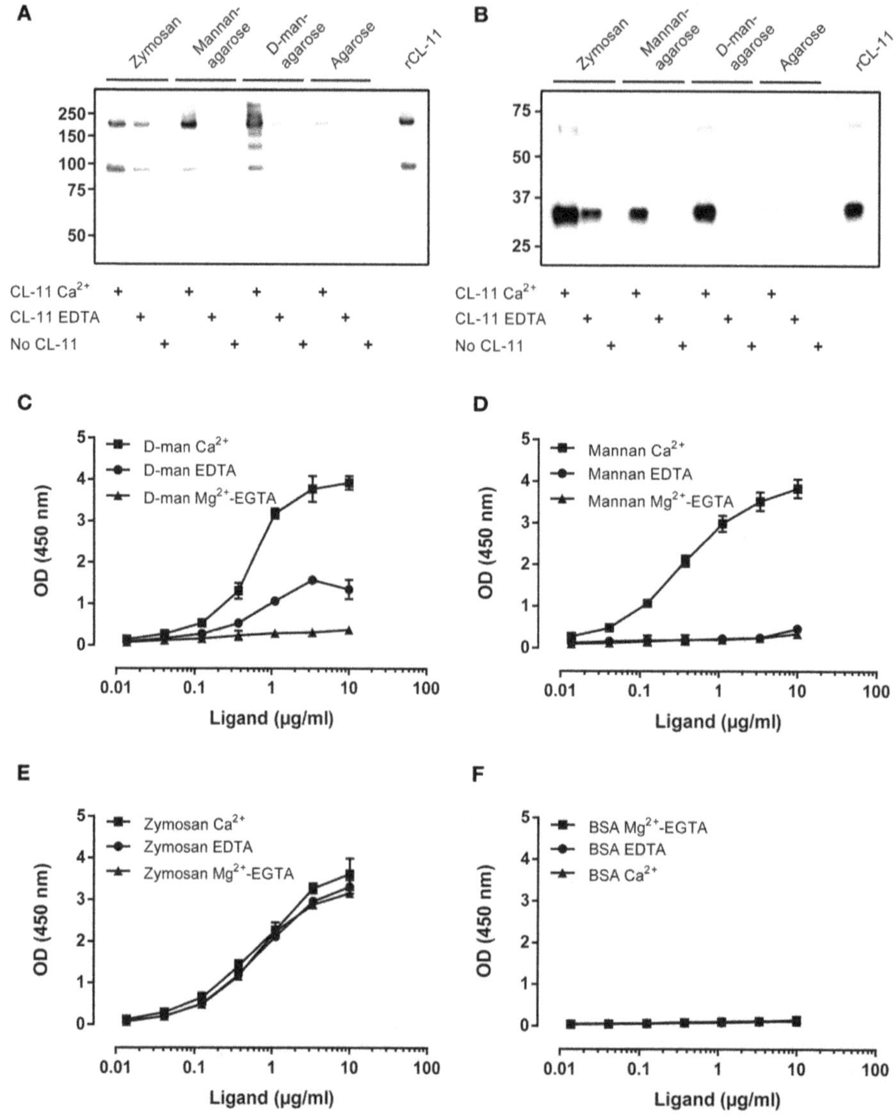

FIGURE 6 | Characterization of CL-11 ligand binding. Western blot of rCL-11 co-precipitated with zymosan particles, mannan-agarose, D-mannose-agarose, or Sepharose in the presence of Ca^{2+} or EDTA under non-reducing **(A)** and reducing conditions **(B)**. Binding of rCL-11 (1 μg/ml) to serial dilutions of coated D-mannose-BSA **(C)**, mannan **(D)**, zymosan **(E)**, and BSA **(F)** in the presence of Ca^{2+}, EDTA, and Mg^{2+}-EGTA. Data is reported as mean ± SEM of three independent experiments.

rCL-11) (**Supplementary Figures 1A–C**). Moreover, Western blot results following immunoprecipitation of serum CL-11 in a calcium-containing buffer vs. EDTA buffer resulted in a different banding pattern (**Supplementary Figure 1D**). Calcium stabilizes the tertiary structure of the CRD of CL-11 (10), and is required for the association of the MASPs with the collagen stalks of the PRMs (22, 23). To determine whether the EDTA-dependent detection of native CL-11 was due to a change in its three-dimensional structure or masking of the epitope by bound MASPs, we incubated rCL-11 in the presence of calcium, EDTA, and MASP-3. Calcium and MASP-3 had no effect on the detection of rCL-11. It has been frequently observed that serum can inhibit the binding of spiked collectins and ficolins to their ligands (14). This inhibition is greatly reduced when using EDTA in the dilution buffer. At the same time others have reported the use of a calcium-dependent antibody for the purification of native CL-10/11 complexes (24). Our hypothesis is that CL-11 (or CL-10) exists in a calcium-dependent complex with a hitherto unknown protein that both interferes with detection of native CL-10/11 complexes at low serum dilutions and inhibits the binding of spiked CL-11.

Since it appears that CL-11 is found in the circulation associated with the homologous CL-10 (14), we used our assay and a semiquantitative ELISA to compare the levels of CL-11 and CL-10/11 complexes in plasma from Danish blood donors (**Figure 4**). The mean plasma concentration of CL-11

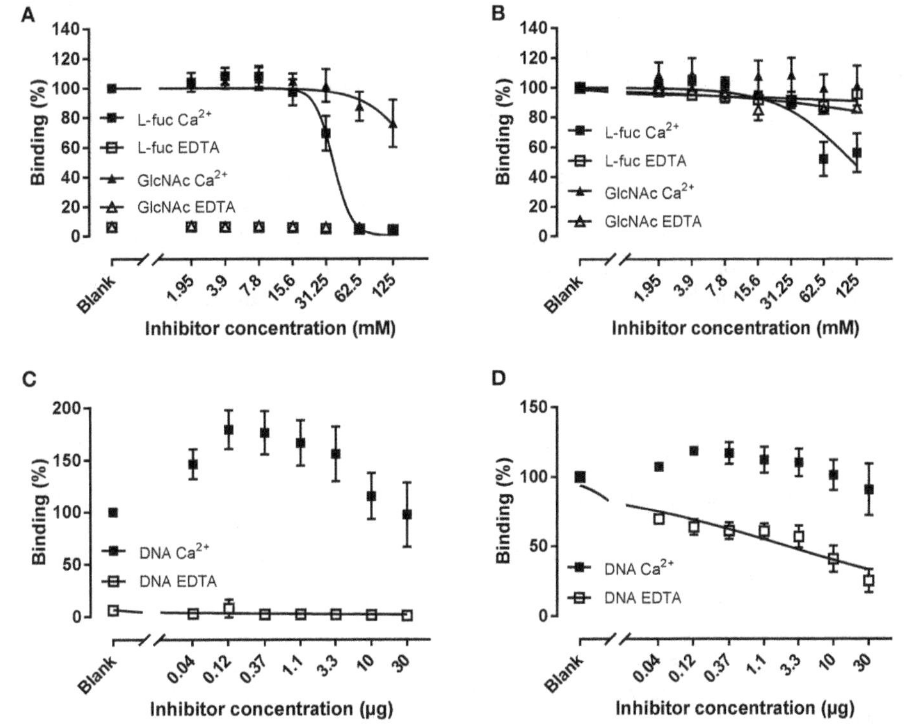

FIGURE 7 | Inhibition of binding of rCL-11 to coated mannan **(A,C)** or zymosan **(B,D)**. Serial dilutions of L-fucose (L-fuc), N-acetyl-glucosamine (GlcNAc), or genomic DNA were incubated with rCL-11 (1 µg/ml) in the presence of Ca^{2+} or EDTA. Data is reported as percent binding compared to the well without inhibitor. Bound rCL-11 was measured with biotinylated mAb anti-CL-11 Hyb-15. Connecting lines represent nonlinear regression fits using the equation inhibitor concentration vs. response with variable slope. Data is reported as mean ± SEM of three independent experiments.

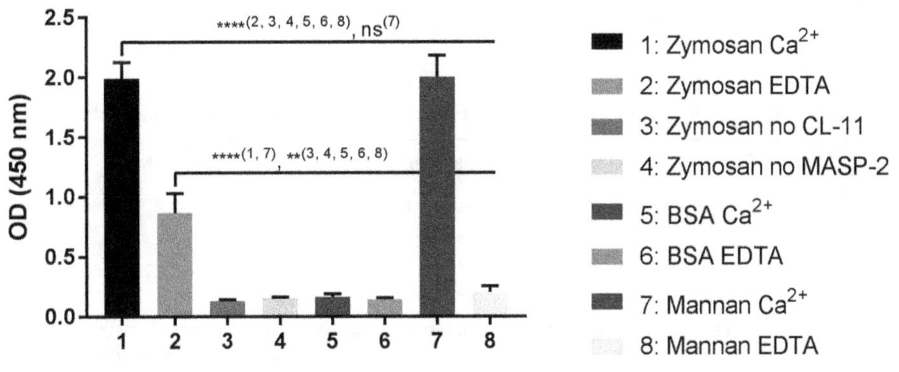

FIGURE 8 | C4 deposition on zymosan. CL-11 (2 µg/ml) was allowed to bind to zymosan or mannan-coated plates (10 µ/ml) for 2 h in the presence of calcium or EDTA, followed by incubation with rMASP-2 (0.5 µg/ml) and purified C4 (0.5 µg/ml) for 4 h and 1 h respectively at 37°C. C4b deposition was measured using a pAb anti-C4c. Data is reported as mean ± SEM of three independent experiments. Numbers between parentheses are columns compared by ANOVA. $^{**}p < 0.01$; $^{****}p < 0.0001$.

was 289.4 ng/ml, range 143.2–459.4 ng/ml, in agreement with two previously published Danish and Japanese cohorts (284 ng/ml and 340 ng/ml, respectively) (7, 25), and equivalent to the estimated concentration of CL-10/11 (256.2 ng/ml, range 37.89–622.7 ng/ml). However, we want to remark that lacking a carefully validated ELISA for CL-10/11, the later concentration is merely an educated guess. There was a strong correlation between CL-11 and CL-10/11 levels in plasma ($r = 0.729$) apparent across a wide range of molecular masses after subjecting plasma to size exclusion chromatography and measuring the levels of CL-11 and CL-10/11 in the elution fractions by ELISA and western blot. This tight association previously reported for CL-11 and CL-10 (26–28), conforms with quantitative mass spectrometry estimates suggesting that the CL-10/11 subunit is composed of one CL-11 and two CL-10 polypeptide chains (14). Plasma CL-11 and CL-10/11 eluted as two distinct peaks at 300–400 kDa and >600 kDa that may correspond with tetramers of trimeric subunits and higher forms, respectively. Although direct area-under-the-curve comparisons suggest that most of CL-10 and CL-11 exist as high molecular weight complexes in the circulation, the lack of resolution beyond 700 kDa makes it impossible to differentiate hexamers of trimers from higher oligomeric forms, that could otherwise elute in distinct peaks with a similar area-under-the-curve as the ~400 kDa peak. Western blot of the elution fractions under-reducing conditions revealed multiple monomer bands for CL-10 and CL-11 in agreement with the observations of Henriksen et al. that CL-10 is found in the circulation as three glycosylated states and CL-11 as two differentially-spliced isoforms (14). Detection of CL-11 demonstrated the presence of a second band in the low molecular weight complexes, possibly corresponding to the shorter isoform D. Of the five isoforms predicted to be secreted by *in silico* analyses (29), only isoform A and D have been detected in blood (1, 14, 25). Isoform D has a shorter collagen-like domain (48 amino acids as opposed to 72 in isoform A) and lacks the putative MASP-binding motif HGKIGP (**Figure 9**). Though shorter, isoform D maintains intact the Gly-X-Y repeats of the collagen-like domain required for the formation of interchain

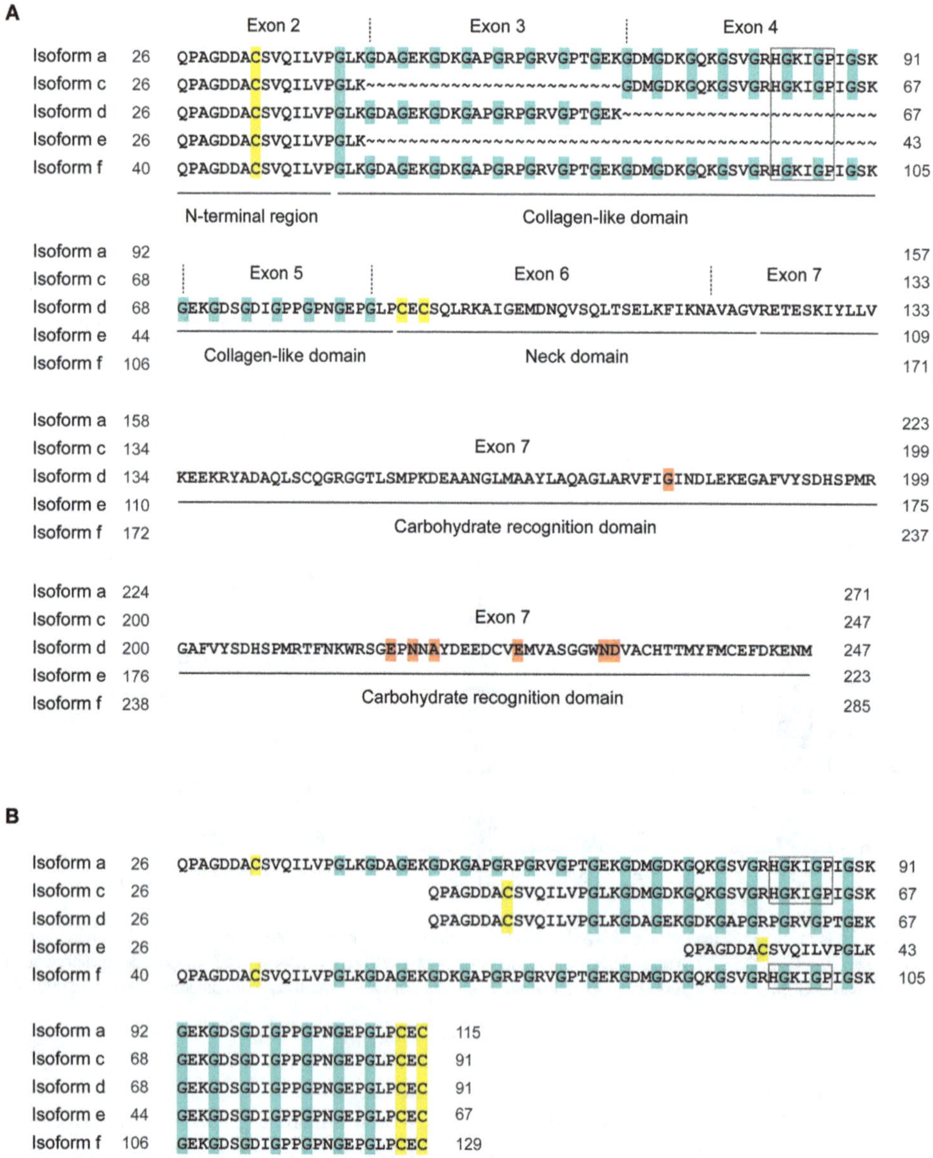

FIGURE 9 | Exon and domain organization of CL-11 isoforms. The five isoforms predicted to be secreted are aligned from the N-terminus **(A)** with the missing amino acids represented by tildes (~), or from the cysteine pair in the neck domain **(B)**. Exons 5 to 7, numbered according to isoform a, are shown once for they are conserved between isoforms. Cysteines are highlighted in yellow, glycines in Gly-X-Y collagen repeats in blue, amino acids involved in carbohydrate binding in red. Grey box, putative MASP-binding motif. Isoform a, NM_024027.4; isoform c, NM_001255982.1; isoform d, NM_001255983; isoform e, NM_001255984.1; isoform f, NM_001255985.1.

hydrogen bonds and stabilization of the collagen triple helix (30, 31). Because the C-terminus of isoforms A and D are identical, we hypothesize that the neck domain could direct the assembly of a trimer with a ragged N-terminal region with cysteines incapable of stabilizing high order oligomeric structures (32). Detection of CL-10 in the elution fractions revealed that non- or singly-glycosylated CL-10 was more abundant in the ~600 kDa oligomers, while the doubly-glycosylated form was more abundant in the ~400 kDa complexes. It has been suggested that CL-11 stabilizes and facilitates secretion of CL-10 (14), in part due to the difficulties of expressing the CL-10 recombinantly (33, 34). In the current work we describe the production of rCL-10 using stable transfected CHO cells. The protein was secreted into the supernatant and appeared to form oligomers of trimers (data not shown). Further studies in the characterization of homomeric CL-10 and the influence of alternative spliced variants and glycosylation states in the oligomerization of CL-10/11 are guaranteed, as are studies on the effect (if any) of the isoform D lacking the MASP binding motif in the weak interaction of low molecular weight CL-10/11 with the MASPs.

Based on the putative role of CL-11 in the modulation of the immune response against pathogens (2, 9), we performed a pilot study on randomly-selected plasma samples from patients diagnosed with SIRS (**Figure 5**). Notably, the mean CL-11 plasma concentration was significantly decreased in SIRS patients upon admission compared to healthy controls ($p < 0.0001$). Nonetheless, we choose to remain cautious and refrain from any biological interpretation until a thorough analysis of new ongoing projects can be performed. The levels of homomeric and heteromeric CL-11 were strongly associated in SIRS patients ($r = 0.915$), as seen for healthy controls, reinforcing the current opinion that CL-10 and CL-11 are co-regulated and exist as a hybrid molecule.

CL-11 has been shown to bind to several microorganisms (6), with a preference for complex sugars as opposed to other collectins (10). Using the developed mAbs we confirmed that our in-house recombinant protein displays the characteristics of native CL-11 and binds to mannan and D-mannose in a calcium-dependent manner (**Figure 6**). As expected, L-fucose—but not GlcNAc—was an effective inhibitor of the binding to mannan (IC50 = 36.48 mM). Interestingly, rCL-11 also bound to zymosan in a calcium-independent manner that could be only partially inhibited by L-fucose in the presence of calcium. Zymosan is a major constituent of the cell wall of the yeast *Saccharomyces cerevisiae*. It is composed mainly of cross-linked β-glucan and α-mannan, and has been widely used to elicit immune and inflammatory responses (35–38). Several calcium-independent ligands, such as nucleic acids, have been reported for CL-11 reflecting complex interactions beyond its lectin activity (2, 10, 19). Thus, we incubated rCL-11 with DNA and measured the amount of bound CL-11 to coated mannan and zymosan (**Figure 7**). On mannan DNA appeared to increase the binding to the coated ligand. The same phenomenon has been reported by Henriksen et al., where the authors concluded that DNA may increase the avidity or align the CRDs in a more favorable conformation (19). On zymosan, DNA had a minor effect in calcium, while in EDTA buffer it was a moderately effective inhibitor (IC50 = 2.3 μg/ml). We propose that CL-11 recognizes zymosan via two distinct mechanisms: a classical calcium-dependent lectin activity, and an alternative calcium-independent interaction shared with nucleic acids. Other C-type lectins, such as dectin-1 and Reg family proteins III and IV, are also capable of recognizing fungal and bacterial ligands in a metal ion-independent fashion (39–41). Interestingly, it has been proposed that the Reg family proteins evolved to bind sugars without calcium to carry their antimicrobial function in the gastrointestinal tract, where the low pH may impair the ability of classical C-type lectins to bind to carbohydrates. Similar low pH, low calcium conditions result from infection-induced local inflammation (42). Immunohistochemical analyses have revealed that CL-11 is expressed (among others) in the stomach and the intestines (11). At this stage we can only conjecture whether the calcium-independent zymosan interaction may be of biological relevance in acidic environments with low calcium availability.

Finally, we measured the ability of rCL-11 to trigger lectin pathway activation on zymosan (**Figure 8**). It has been reported that serum inhibits the binding of purified and recombinant collectins and ficolins to their ligands (14). At the same time, the relatively low concentration of CL-11 in circulation requires using serum dilutions that would trigger complement activation via the alternative pathway. To circumvent these limitations, we employed a step-wise activation assay using recombinant and purified proteins in a buffer that allows the cleavage of C4 by MASP-2—the first step of the activation of the lectin pathway. Binding of rCL-11 followed by incubation with rMASP-2 and purified C4 resulted in the deposition of C4b on coated zymosan, comparable to that on mannan. Calcium was not necessary for the binding of rCL-11 to zymosan, but for the complex formation with rMASP-2. We consider that not requiring calcium is an asset when designing a specific assay to discriminate the contribution of CL-11 from the other PRMs of the lectin pathway.

In conclusion, we have developed monoclonal antibodies and a robust and sensitive sandwich ELISA for the quantification of CL-11 in the circulation and used them to study native CL-11 in plasma and the binding characteristics of rCL-11 to different ligands.

AUTHOR CONTRIBUTIONS

RB-O, NK-M, LP-A, and KS performed the experiments. RB-O, KS, M-OS, and PG designed the study. RB-O, PG wrote the manuscript. All authors critically reviewed the manuscript.

FUNDING

The Danish Research Foundation of Independent Research (DFF-6110-00489), the Sven Andersen Research Foundation, and Novo Nordisk Research Foundation.

ACKNOWLEDGMENTS

The authors would like to thank Ms Jytte Bryde Clausen, Mr Lars Vitved, and Mr Jesper Andresen for their excellent technical assistance.

SUPPLEMENTARY MATERIAL

Supplementary Figure 1 | Effect of calcium in the detection of native CL-11. The concentration of CL-11 was measured in three different donors in a three-fold dilution of serum **(A)** and plasma **(B)** or supernatant from CHO cells **(C)** with and without EDTA the sample buffer. **(D)** Western blot of immunoprecipitation (IP) of CL-11 from serum in a calcium or EDTA-containing buffer under non-reducing conditions. Lanes 1 and 2, purified rCL-11 and supernatant from CHO cells expressing rCL-11. Lane 3, serum before IP. Lanes 4 to 9, serum after IP using CL-11 specific mAbs Hyb-15 and Hyb-17 or a mouse IgG1κ isotype control antibody. The blots were developed with pAb rabbit anti-CL-11. ELISA, IP and Western blotting were performed according to sections CL-11 Specific Sandwich ELISA, Immunoprecipitation, SDS-page and western blot, respectively.

REFERENCES

1. Keshi H, Sakamoto T, Kawai T, Ohtani K, Katoh T, Jang S, et al. Identification and characterization of a novel human collectin CL-K1. *Microbiol Immunol.* (2006) 50:1001–13. doi: 10.1111/j.1348-0421.2006.tb03868.x
2. Ma YJ,Skjoedt MO, Garred P. Collectin-11/MASP complex formation triggers activation of the lectin complement pathway-The fifth lectin pathway initiation complex. *J Innate Immun.* (2013) 5:242–50. doi: 10.1159/000345356
3. Rooryck C, Diaz-Font A, Osborn DPS,Chabchoub E, Hernandez-Hernandez V, Shamseldin H, et al. Mutations in lectin complement pathway genes COLEC11 and MASP1 cause 3MC syndrome. *Nat Genet.* (2011) 43:197–203. doi: 10.1038/ng.757
4. Dong X, Wu W, Ma L, Liu C, Bhuckory MB,Wang L, et al. Collectin-11 is an important modulator of retinal pigment epithelial cell phagocytosis and cytokine production. *J Innate Immun.* (2017) 9:529–45. doi: 10.1159/000478042
5. Van De Wetering JK, Van Golde LMG, Batenburg JJ. Collectins: players of the innate immune system. *Eur J Biochem.* (2004) 271:1229–49. doi: 10.1111/j.1432-1033.2004.04040.x
6. Hansen S, Selman L, Palaniyar N, Ziegler K, Brandt J, Kliem A, et al. Collectin 11 (CL-11, CL-K1) is a MASP-1/3-associated plasma collectin with microbial-binding activity. *J Immunol.* (2010) 185:6096–104. doi: 10.4049/jimmunol.1002185
7. Yoshizaki T, Ohtani K, Motomura W, Jang SJ,Mori KI, Kitamoto N, et al. Comparison of human blood concentrations of collectin kidney 1 and mannan-binding lectin. *J Biochem.* (2012) 151:57–64. doi: 10.1093/jb/mvr114
8. Takahashi K, Ohtani K, Larvie M, Moyo P, Chigweshe L, Van Cott EM,et al. Elevated plasma CL-K1 level is associated with a risk of developing disseminated intravascular coagulation (DIC). *J Thromb Thrombolysis* (2014) 38:331–8. doi: 10.1007/s11239-013-1042-5
9. Antony JS,Ojurongbe O, Kremsner PG, Velavan TP. Lectin complement protein collectin 11 (CL-K1) and susceptibility to urinary schistosomiasis. *PLoS Negl Trop Dis.* (2015) 9:e0003647. doi: 10.1371/journal.pntd.0003647
10. Venkatraman Girija U, Furze CM,Gingras AR,Yoshizaki T, Ohtani K, Marshall JE, et al. Molecular basis of sugar recognition by collectin-K1 and the effects of mutations associated with 3MC syndrome. *BMC Biol.* (2015) 13:27. doi: 10.1186/s12915-015-0136-2
11. Hansen SWK,Aagaard JB,Bjerrum KB,Hejbøl EK,Nielsen O, Schrøder HD, et al. CL-L1 and CL-K1 exhibit widespread tissue distribution with high and co-localized expression in secretory epithelia and mucosa. *Front. Immunol.* (2018) 9:1757. doi: 10.3389/fimmu.2018.01757
12. Munye MM, Diaz-Font A, Ocaka L, Henriksen ML, Lees M, Brady A, et al. COLEC10 is mutated in 3MC patients and regulates early craniofacial development. *PLoS Genet.* (2017) 13:e1006679. doi: 10.1371/journal.pgen.1006679
13. Farrar CA,Tran D, Li K, Wu W, Peng Q, Schwaeble W, et al. Collectin-11 detects stress-induced L-fucose pattern to trigger renal epithelial injury. *J Clin Invest.* (2016) 126:1911–25. doi: 10.1172/JCI83000
14. Henriksen ML,Brandt J, Andrieu J-P, Nielsen C, Jensen PH,Holmskov U, et al. Heteromeric complexes of native collectin kidney 1 and collectin liver 1 are found in the circulation with MASPs and activate the complement system. *J Immunol.* (2013) 191:6117–27. doi: 10.4049/jimmunol.1302121
15. Garred P, Genster N, Pilely K, Bayarri-Olmos R, Rosbjerg A, Ma YJ, et al. A journey through the lectin pathway of complement—MBL and beyond. *Immunol Rev.* (2016) 274:74–97. doi: 10.1111/imr.12468
16. Dobó J, Pál G, Cervenak L, Gál P. The emerging roles of mannose-binding lectin-associated serine proteases (MASPs) in the lectin pathway of complement and beyond. *Immunol Rev.* (2016) 274:98–111. doi: 10.1111/imr.12460.
17. Asgari E, Farrar CA,Lynch N, Ali YM,Roscher S, Stover C, et al. Mannan-binding lectin-associated serine protease 2 is critical for the development of renal ischemia reperfusion injury and mediates tissue injury in the absence of complement C4. *FASEB J.* (2014) 28:3996–4003. doi: 10.1096/fj.13-246306
18. Dobó J, Szakács D, Oroszlán G, Kortvely E, Kiss B, Boros E, et al. MASP-3 is the exclusive pro-factor D activator in resting blood: the lectin and the alternative complement pathways are fundamentally linked. *Sci Rep.* (2016) 6:31877. doi: 10.1038/srep31877
19. Henriksen ML,Brandt J, Iyer SSC,Thielens NM, Hansen S. Characterization of the interaction between collectin 11 (CL-11, CL-K1) and nucleic acids. *Mol Immunol.* (2013) 56:757–67. doi: 10.1016/j.molimm.2013.07.011
20. Kohler G, Milstein C. Continuous cultures of fused cells secreting antibody of predefined specificity. *Nature* (1975) 256:495–7. doi: 10.1038/256495a0
21. Garred P, Strøm JJ,Quist L, Taaning E, Madsen HO. Association of mannose-binding lectin polymorphisms with sepsis and fatal outcome, in patients with systemic inflammatory response syndrome. *J Infect Dis.* (2003) 188:1394–403. doi: 10.1086/379044
22. Wallis R, Dodd RB. Interaction of mannose-binding protein with associated serine proteases. Effects of naturally occurring mutations. *J Biol Chem.* (2000) 275:30962–9. doi: 10.1074/jbc.M004030200
23. Thielens NM,Cseh S, Thiel S, Vorup-Jensen T, Rossi V, Jensenius JC, et al. Interaction properties of human mannan-binding lectin (MBL)-associated serine proteases-1 and−2, MBL-associated protein 19, and MBL. *J Immunol.* (2001) 166:5068–77. doi: 10.4049/jimmunol.166.8.5068
24. Henriksen ML,Madsen KL,Skjoedt K, Hansen S. Calcium-sensitive immunoaffinity chromatography: gentle and highly specific retrieval of a scarce plasma antigen, collectin-LK (CL-LK). *J Immunol Methods* (2014) 413:25–31. doi: 10.1016/j.jim.2014.07.006
25. Selman L, Henriksen ML,Brandt J, Palarasah Y, Waters A, Beales PL, et al. An enzyme-linked immunosorbent assay (ELISA) for quantification of human collectin 11 (CL-11, CL-K1). *J Immunol Methods* (2012) 375:182–8. doi: 10.1016/j.jim.2011.10.010
26. Bayarri-Olmos R, Hansen S, Henriksen ML,Storm L, Thiel S, Garred P, et al. Genetic variation of COLEC10 and COLEC11 and association with serum levels of collectin liver 1 (CL-L1) and collectin kidney 1 (CL-K1). *PLoS ONE* (2015) 10:e0114883. doi: 10.1371/journal.pone.0114883
27. Troldborg A, Thiel S, Jensen L, Hansen S, Laska MJ,Deleuran B, et al. Collectin liver 1 and collectin kidney 1 and other complement-associated pattern recognition molecules in systemic lupus erythematosus. *Clin Exp Immunol.* (2015) 182:132–8. doi: 10.1111/cei.12678
28. Smedbr J, Fagerland MW,Hansen SWK,Smedbråten J, Sagedal S, Åsberg A, et al. Collectin liver 1 and collectin kidney 1 of the lectin complement pathway are associated with mortality after kidney transplantation. *Am Transplant J.* (2016) 17:265–71. doi: 10.1111/ajt.13933
29. Petersen TN,Brunak S, von Heijne G, Nielsen H. SignalP 4.0: discriminating signal peptides from transmembrane regions. *Nat Methods* (2011) 8:785–6. doi: 10.1038/nmeth.1701
30. Beck K, Brodsky B. Supercoiled protein motifs: the collagen triple-helix and the α-helical coiled coil. *J Struct Biol.* (1998) 122:17–29. doi: 10.1006/jsbi.1998.3965

31. Boudko SP,Engel J, Bachinger HP. The crucial role of trimerization domains in collagen folding. *Int J Biochem Cell Biol.* (2012) 44:21–32. doi: 10.1016/j.biocel.2011.09.009
32. Hoppe H-J, Barlow PN, Reid KBM. A parallel three stranded α-helical bundle at the nucleation site of collagen triple-helix formation. *FEBS Lett.* (1994) 344:191–5.
33. Ohtani K, Suzuki Y, Eda S, Kawai T, Kase T, Yamazaki H, et al. Molecular cloning of a novel human collectin from liver (CL-L1). *J Biol Chem.* (1999) 274:13681–9. doi: 10.1074/jbc.274.19.13681
34. Axelgaard E, Jensen L, Dyrlund TF,Nielsen HJ,Enghild JJ,Thiel S, et al. Investigations on collectin liver 1. *J Biol Chem.* (2013) 288:23407–20. doi: 10.1074/jbc.M113.492603
35. Di Carlo FJ, Fiore JV. On the composition of zymosan. *Science* (1958) 127:756LP–7LP.
36. Ikeda Y, Adachi Y, Ishibashi K, Miura N, Ohno N. Activation of toll-like receptor-mediated NF-κβ by zymosan-derived water-soluble fraction: possible contribution of endotoxin-like substances. *Immunopharmacol Immunotoxicol.* (2005) 27:285–98. doi: 10.1081/IPH-200067943
37. Sato M, Sano H, Iwaki D, Kudo K, Konishi M, Takahashi H, et al. Direct binding of toll-like receptor 2 to zymosan, and zymosan-induced NF-κB activation and TNF-α secretion are down-regulated by lung collectin surfactant protein A. *J Immunol.* (2003) 171:417LP–25LP. doi: 10.4049/jimmunol.171.1.417
38. V Sanguedolce M, Capo C, Bongrand P, Mege JL. Zymosan-stimulated tumor necrosis factor-alpha production by human monocytes. Down-modulation by phorbol ester. *J Immunol.* (1992) 148:2229–36.
39. Brown GD. Dectin-1: a signalling non-TLR pattern-recognition receptor. *Nat Rev Immunol.* (2006) 6:33. doi: 10.1038/nri1745
40. Lehotzky RE, Partch CL, Mukherjee S, Cash HL, Goldman WE, Gardner KH, et al. Molecular basis for peptidoglycan recognition by a bactericidal lectin. *Proc Natl Acad Sci USA.* (2010) 107:7722–7. doi: 10.1073/pnas.0909 449107
41. Ho M-R, Lou YC, Wei S-Y, Luo S-C, Lin W-C, Lyu P-C, et al. Human RegIV protein adopts a typical C-type lectin fold but binds mannan with two calcium-independent sites. *J Mol Biol.* (2010) 402:682–95. doi: 10.1016/j.jmb.2010.07.061
42. Zhang J, Koh J, Lu J, Thiel S, Leong BSH,Sethi S, et al. Local inflammation induces complement crosstalk which amplifies the antimicrobial response. *PLOS Pathog.* (2009) 5:e1000282. doi: 10.1371/journal.ppat. 1000282

3

Ficolin-1 and Ficolin-3 Plasma Levels are Altered in HIV and HIV/HCV Coinfected Patients from Southern Brazil

Maria Regina Tizzot[1], Kárita Cláudia Freitas Lidani[1], Fabiana Antunes Andrade[1], Hellen Weinschutz Mendes[1], Marcia Holsbach Beltrame[1], Edna Reiche[2], Steffen Thiel[3], Jens C. Jensenius[3] and Iara J. de Messias-Reason[1]*

[1] *Laboratory of Molecular Immunopathology, Department of Medical Pathology, Federal University of Paraná, Curitiba, Brazil,* [2] *Clinic Hospital, Estate University of Londrina, Londrina, Brazil,* [3] *Department of Biomedicine, Aarhus University, Aarhus, Denmark*

***Correspondence:**
Maria Regina Tizzot
retizzot@gmail.com

The complement system is a key component of the innate immune system, participating in the surveillance against infectious agents. Once activated by one of the three different pathways, complement mediates cell lysis, opsonization, signalizes pathogens for phagocytosis and induces the adaptive immune response. The lectin pathway is constituted by several soluble and membrane bound proteins, called pattern recognition molecules (PRM), including mannose binding lectin (MBL), Ficolins-1, -2, and -3, and Collectin 11. These PRMs act on complement activation as recognition molecules of pathogen-associated molecular patterns (PAMPs) such as N-acetylated, found in glycoproteins of viral envelopes. In this study, Ficolin-1 and Ficolin-3 plasma levels were evaluated in 178 HIV patients (93 HIV; 85 HIV/HCV) and 85 controls from southern Brazil. Demographic and clinical-laboratory findings were obtained during medical interview and from medical records. All parameters were assessed by logistic regression, adjusted for age, ancestry, and sex. Significantly lower levels of Ficolin-1 were observed in HIV/HCV coinfected when compared to HIV patients ($p = 0.005$, median = 516 vs. 667 ng/ul, respectively) and to controls ($p < 0.0001$, 1186 ng/ul). Ficolin-1 levels were lower in males than in females among HIV patients ($p = 0.03$) and controls ($p = 0.0003$), but no association of Ficolin-1 levels with AIDS was observed. On the other hand, Ficolin-3 levels were significantly lower in controls when compared to HIV ($p < 0.0001$, medians 18,240 vs. 44,030 ng/ml, respectively) and HIV/HCV coinfected ($p < 0.0001$, 40,351 ng/ml) patients. There was no correlation between Ficolin-1 and Ficolin-3 levels and age, HIV viral load or opportunistic infections. However, Ficolin-3 showed a positive correlation with T CD4 cell counts in HIV monoinfected patients ($p = 0.007$). We provide here the first assessment of Ficolin-1 and–3 levels in HIV and HIV/HCV coinfected patients, which indicates a distinct role for these pattern recognition molecules in both viral infections.

Keywords: Ficolin-1, Ficolin-3, complement system, HIV infection, hepatitis C virus

INTRODUCTION

Infection by the Human Immunodeficiency Virus (HIV) leads to a chronic disease and, when not treated, to Acquired Immune Deficiency Syndrome (AIDS). HIV/AIDS currently affects 36.9 million people worldwide, with a high rate of mortality and morbidity (1–3). The number of HIV cases has increased despite the decrease in the number of new infection cases, which was estimated to be 3.3 million in 2002 and 2.3 million people in 2012 (1, 2). The implementation of strategies which includes prevention campaigns, increased access to treatment, and the use of less toxic and more efficient anti-retroviral therapies (*highly active antiretroviral therapy-* HAART), have all contributed to increase the survival and decrease the infection rates in risk groups, thereby changing the HIV infection epidemiologic profile in the last decade (1, 2).

Coinfection with other pathogens such as hepatitis B virus (HBV) and hepatitis C virus (HCV), and related diseases are known to be aggravating factors in the clinical condition of HIV patients (4–6). In addition, mortality related to chronic liver diseases has increased significantly in the last decade in HIV patients, with about 24% of AIDS mortality being due to end-stage liver diseases (ESLD), where 66% were attributed to HCV and 17% to HBV coinfection (7–11). It is important to note that these viruses share the same transmission routes, including sexual and blood, both contributing to the high prevalence of HIV/HCV and HIV/HBV coinfection worldwide (6).

The complement system is a key element of innate immunity which plays a crucial role in the host surveillance against pathogens, including HIV and HCV (12–19). Complement comprises a variety of membrane associated and soluble recognition molecules, known as pattern recognition molecules (PRM), and they include Ficolins (Ficolin-1, Ficolin-2, and Ficolin-3), mannose-binding lectin (MBL) and Collectin 11 (CL-K1) (14). These PRMs are able to recognize a variety of pathogen-associated molecular patterns (PAMPs), such as carbohydrates, N-glycan, LPS and sialic acid residues at the microorganism surface as well as endogenous altered cells and double strand RNAs (12, 14), leading to complement activation. This activation may occur through three different pathways: the classic, the alternative and the lectin pathways, which result in a proteolytic cascade that culminates in multiple biological processes including opsonization and phagocytosis of pathogenic agents and altered cells, production of cytokines, inflammation, and induction of adaptive immune response and homeostasis (14–16).

Ficolin-1 is a non-serum type Ficolin that is found as a membrane-associated protein expressed mainly by monocytes and granulocytes, being the less abundant Ficolin in plasma (average of 1.07 µg/mL) (12, 14, 20). On the other hand, Ficolin-3 being the most abundant Ficolin in circulation (average of 26 µg/mL) is a serum type protein expressed in alveolar macrophages type II, bronchial epithelial cells and hepatocytes (12, 21). Several studies showed that Ficolins have an important role in viral infections (17–19, 22–31). Denner et al. (31) reported that incubation of mononuclear cells with HIV-1 immunosuppressive gp41 peptides resulted in low Ficolin-1 mRNA concentrations. The authors suggested that Ficolin-1 may be downregulated by the isu domain of gp41 thereby preventing early local innate response, allowing infection and virus replication (31). A possible role for Ficolin-1 in the protection against HCV infection was proposed in a clinical study by Urban et al. (30), who observed the upregulated expression of Ficolin-1 in chronic HCV patients with *IL28B* rs12979860 CC genotype, which was associated to a favorable response to pegylated interferon-α and ribavirin treatment (30). In addition, Verma et al. (29), demonstrated in an experimental study the binding of Ficolin-3 to influenza A virus which inhibited viral infectivity thereby contributing to host defense against the virus (29). However, there are no prior studies evaluating the role of Ficolin- 1 and -3 in patients with HIV infection, with this now being the first study.

MATERIALS AND METHODS

Subjects and Samples

This study was approved by the Human Research Ethic Committee of the Clinical Hospital of the Federal University of Parana (1409.074/2007-04). All patients gave written informed consent in accordance with the Declaration of Helsinki. A total of 178 HIV-1 patients (positive for anti-HIV-1, negative for anti-HIV-2 according to Brazilian Ministry of Health guideline) (32) were attending at the Ambulatory of Infectious and Parasitic Diseases at the Clinical Hospital of the Federal University of Parana, in Curitiba, and the Infectology Ambulatory at the Clinical Hospital of the Londrina State University. Among the patients 85 presented coinfection with HCV (Anti-HCV antibody determination by immunoenzimatic micro assay with chemiluminescence QMA Architect—Abbott, USA). As control group, 85 HIV/HCV negative individuals without any clinical complaints were included. The clinical epidemiology data was obtained during the appointments with a questionnaire referring to HIV risk factors and by retrospective analyses of medical records. The following variables were analyzed: age, sex, date of first HIV positive result, possible forms of virus transmission. Same risk factors was also analyzed such as, injected drugs usage, sexual activity, and blood transfusion history as well as clinical progression, T CD4 counts, anti-retroviral treatments and opportunistic diseases (**Table 1**).

FICOLIN-1 AND FICOLIN-3 PLASMA LEVELS

Ficolin-1 plasma concentration was determined by the in-house monoclonal antibody-based method of *time-resolved immunofluorometric assay* (TRIFMA) and were carried out at the Institute of Medical Microbiology and Immunology at University of Aarhus, Denmark (20) on 178 patients (93 HIV and 85 HIV/HCV) and 85 controls. Ficolin-3 plasma levels were determined by the enzyme-linked immune-sorbent (ELISA) assay HK 340 (Hycult Biotechnology, Uden, The Netherlands) in 79 patients (59 HIV and 20 HIV/HCV) and 85 controls. A total of 10 ml of peripheral whole blood was drawn and separated by

TABLE 1 | Clinical and demographic characteristics of controls, HIV and HIV/HCV patients.

Parameters	Patients (n = 178)		Controls (n = 85)
	HIV (n = 93)	HIV/HCV (n = 85)	
Median age (years) [min–max]	47 [20–76]	44 [22–71]	38 [18–57]
SEX			
Female % (n)	43.5 (40/92)	36.9 (31/84)	41.2 (35/85)
Male % (n)	56.5 (52/92)	63.1 (53/84)	58.8 (50/85)
ANCESTRY			
Euro-Brazilians % (n)	81.1 (73/90)	76.2 (64/84)	71.4 (60/85)
Afro-Brazilians % (n)	18.9 (17/90)	23.8 (20/84)	28.6 (24/85)
T CD4 cell Counts	193.5 (n = 82)	129.5 (n = 30)	N/A
HIV Viral load	106500 (n = 64)	51100 (n = 23)	N/A
AIDS % (n)	69.6 (62/89)	75.0 (24/32)	N/A
Progression to AIDS (years) median [min–max]	8.8 [2.7–24]	9.41 [3.0–18.2]	N/A
Opportunistic infection % (n)	59.0% (49/83)	61.5% (16/26)	N/A
Bacterial % (n)	19.1 (9/49)	12.5 (2/16)	N/A
Viral % (n)	8.2 (4/49)	0	N/A
Parasitic/fungal % (n)	53.1 (26/49)	66.8 (11/16)	N/A

centrifugation for 10 min at 1,000–2,000 × g in plasma samples using vacutainer plastic blood collection tubes with K2EDTA (BD Vacutainer® Blood Collection Tubes, Curitiba, Brazil).

Data Analyses

Clinical and demographic data was analyzed with GraphPad Prism 3.0 Software (GraphPad Software, Inc., Califórnia, EUA). The distribution of all quantitative variables was evaluated with Kolmogorov-Smirnov and Shapiro-Wilk tests. When normal hypothesis was rejected, medians were compared using non-parametric Mann-Whitney and Kruskal-Wallis and Spearman correlation tests. The associations of Ficolin-1 and -3 levels with HIV and HIV/HCV infection were corrected by multiple logistic regression analysis using STATA 9.2 (StataCorp, Texas, USA). The age, sex, T CD4-cell count and viral load were included as variables in the regression model when the univariate analyses resulted in $p < 0.2$. Ficolin-1 and -3 levels descriptive statistics were presented with medians and percentiles. P-values lower than 0.05 were considered statistically significant.

RESULTS

Ficolin-1 plasma levels were significantly lower in HIV/HCV coinfected when compared to HIV patients (medians of 516 ng/ml vs. 667 ng/ml, respectively; $p = 0.005$) and to controls (medians of 516 ng/ml vs. 1,186 ng/ml, respectively; $p < 0.0001$). HIV infected patients also presented lower levels of Ficolin-1 when compared to controls (medians of 667 ng/ml vs. 1186 ng/ml, respectively; $p < 0.0001$) (**Figure 1A**). These values were corrected for age and sex with logistic regression and were still significant for the findings above.

The presence of AIDS, opportunistic infection and both T CD4 counts and viral load did not alter Ficolin-1 levels in HIV infected or coinfected patients (**Figures 1B–E**). There was also no significant correlation between Ficolin-1 levels and AIDS progression time, which was similar for both groups (medians of 8.8 years for HIV and 9.1 years for HIV/HCV patients; $p = 0.4$).

Lower Ficolin-1 levels were observed in males compared to females both in controls (medians of 1,079 vs. 1,457 ng/ml, respectively; $p = 0.0003$) and in HIV patients (medians of 500 vs. 859 ng/ml respectively; $p = 0.03$), but not in HIV/HCV coinfected subjects ($p = 0.6$) (**Figure 1F**).

Ficolin-3 levels were significantly increased in HIV patients (medians of 44030 vs. 18240 ng/ml, respectively; $p < 0.0001$) and HIV/HCV coinfected patients (40351 ng/ml; $p < 0.0001$) when compared to controls, with no difference between HIV and HIV/HCV coinfected patients (medians of 44,030 vs. 40,351 ng/ml, respectively; $p = 0.6$) (**Figure 2A**).

The presence of AIDS was associated with lower Ficolin-3 levels in HIV patients (medians of 20,658 vs. 28,306 ng/ml, respectively; $p = 0.02$) (**Figure 2B**). A statistically significant correlation was observed between Ficolin-3 levels and CD4 cell counts in HIV patients ($p = 0.007$, $r = 0.33$) (**Figure 2D**). There was no difference, however, for the presence of opportunistic diseases in HIV or in HIV/HCV patients (**Figure 2C**), HIV viral load (**Figure 2E**), and AIDS progression time in both patient groups.

Male HIV/HCV patients presented higher Ficolin-3 plasma levels compared to female (medians of 47,095 vs. 28,693 ng/ml, respectively; $p = 0.01$), with the same trend in HIV (medians of 39,110 vs. 28,784 ng/ml, respectively; $p = 0.06$) but no difference within the control group ($p = 0.1$) (**Figure 2F**). Ficolin-3 but not Ficolin-1 plasma levels correlated with the age in both groups of patients ($p = 0.02$, $r = -0.27$; HIV $p = 0.009$ $r = -0.37$, e HIV/HCV $p = 0.65$ $r = -0.04$).

DISCUSSION

We presented here novel evidence that both Ficolin-1 and -3 plasma levels are altered in HIV and HIV/HCV coinfection. Whereas Ficolin-1 levels were found lower in HIV and HIV/HCV coinfected patients, Ficolin-3 were higher in these patients in comparison to controls. Our results indicate that Ficolin-1 and Ficolin-3 may operate as a PRM in a distinct manner facing HIV infection and HIV/HCV coinfection.

These findings are in fact in accordance with the notion that Ficolins—although presenting high structural and molecular homology and specification overlap to PAMPs binding—exhibit differences in functional activities and in the pattern of tissue expression, with consequences in the potential to activate complement as well having other roles in the immune response (14). Ficolins can interact with viral glycoproteins which are constituted of N-Acetylglucosamine (GlcNAc), such as gp120 and gp41, which are essential for cell binding and infection onset, but is also a target for Ficolin-1 and Ficolin-3 (17–19). Considering

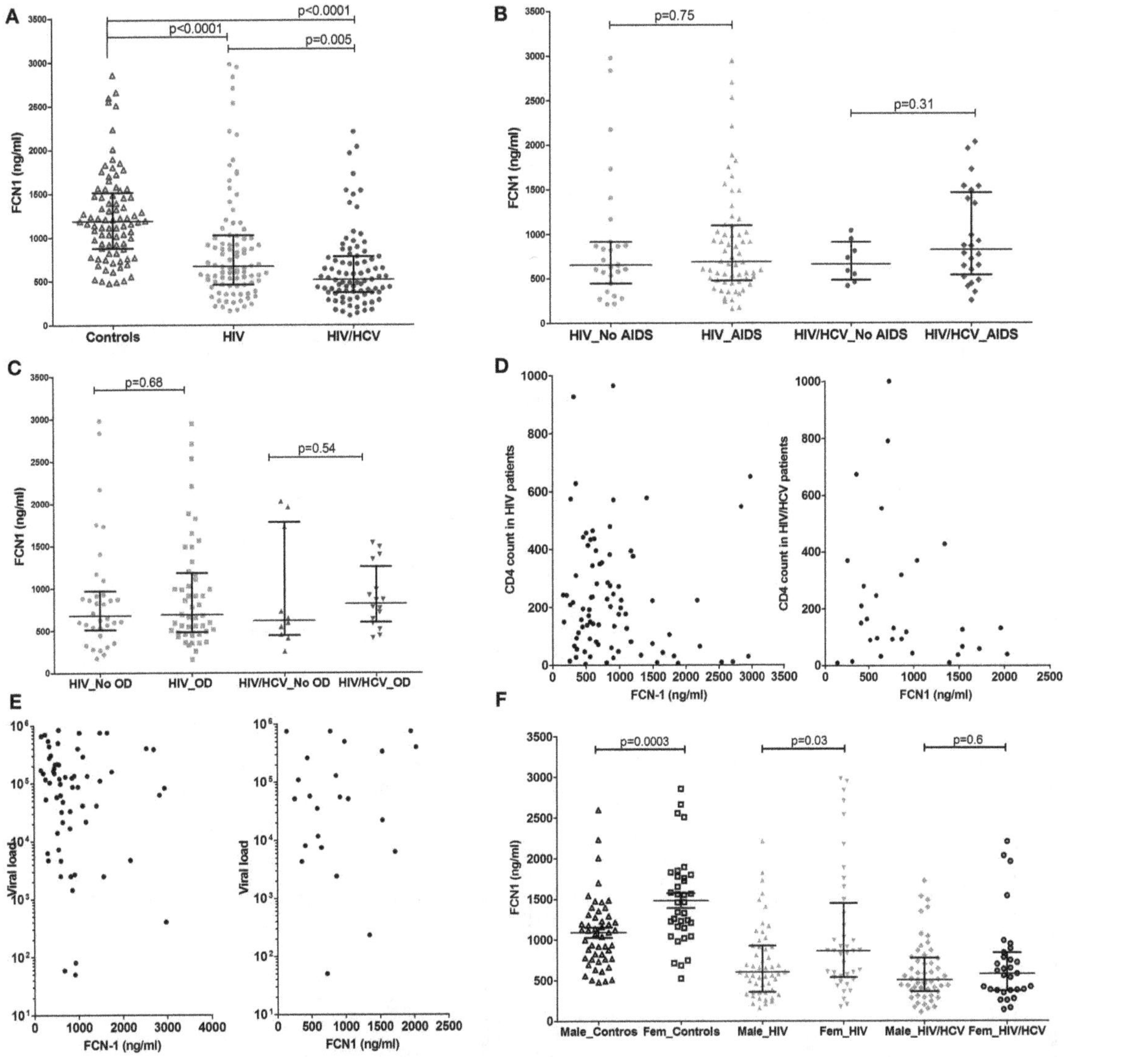

FIGURE 1 | Ficolin-1 plasma levels in controls and HIV infected and HIV/HCV coinfected patients **(A)**, considering the presence of AIDS **(B)** or opportunistic diseases **(C)**. Correlation between Ficolin-1 and T CD4 cell counts **(D)**, Ficolin-1 and HIV viral load **(E)** (Values are in Log10 scale) in patients of HIV and HIV/HCV. Ficolin-1 levels in male and female controls and patients **(F)**.

that PRMs bind to these viral surface glycoproteins, they may have a role in the process of HIV infection. In fact, complement may play different activities in HIV pathogenesis, such as blocking virus entrance into the cell, signalizing phagocytosis, inflammation, as well as forming the lytic complex at the infected cell membranes (17–19, 22–31). On the other hand, viruses may bind to complement proteins impairing an effective adaptive immune response thereby facilitating its entrance into target cells through complement receptors (CR) (17–19, 22).

Studies relating the role of Ficolin-1 and -3 in viral infections are scarce (29–31) and to our knowledge, this is the first study evaluating the levels of Ficolin-1 and -3 in HIV and HIV/HCV coinfected patients. The low Ficolin-1 levels observed in HIV and HIV/HCV patients suggests possible protein consumption due to viral infection. It is known that neutrophil autocrine Ficolin-1 can bind to CD43 (a neutrophil membrane sialoprotein) inducing neutrophil adhesion at the beginning of an inflammatory response (14, 33). On the other hand, in the late phase Ficolin-1 was shown to have strong affinity to C-reactive protein resulting in downregulation of pro-inflammatory cytokines (34, 35). In addition, Ficolin-1 levels could be reduced due to downregulation effect of the viruses as described for HIV gp41 immunosuppressive (isu) domain (31). Interestingly, Ficolin-1 levels were even lower in HIV/HCV patients when compared to HIV. It is known that HCV coinfection is an aggravating factor in the clinical condition of HIV patient exacerbating the existing inflammatory process (4–6), and that complement can interact with glycoproteins of

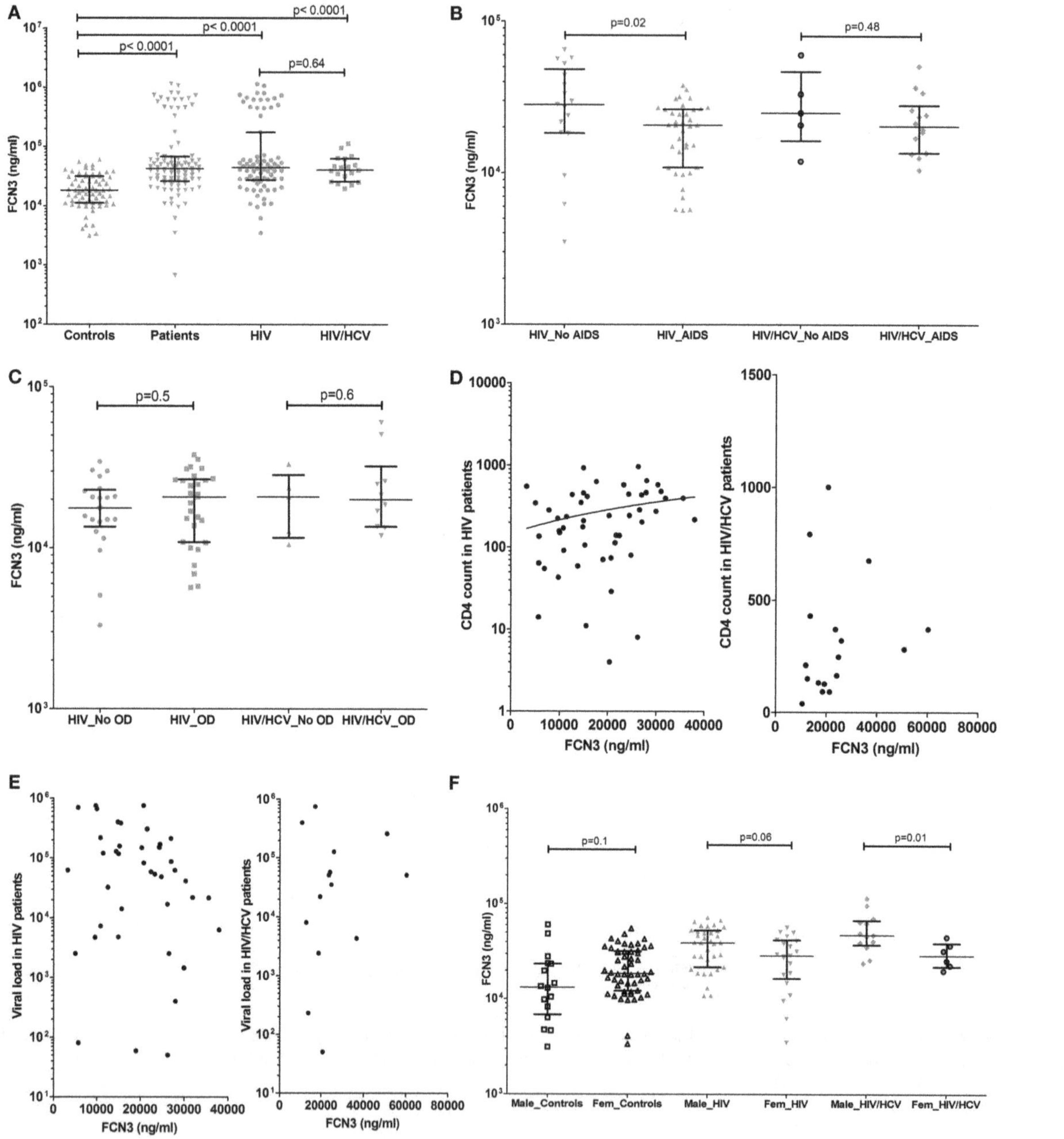

FIGURE 2 | Ficolin-3 plasma levels in controls, HIV patients and HIV/HCV coinfected patients **(A)**, considering the presence of AIDS **(B)** and opportunistic diseases **(C)**. Correlation between Ficolin-3 and T CD4 cell counts **(D)**, Ficolin-1 and HIV viral load **(E)** (Values are in Log10 scale) in HIV and HIV/HCV patients. Ficolin-3 levels in male and female controls and patients **(F)**.

both virus (17, 19, 25). Thus, our results suggest that low Ficolin-1 levels might be a consequence of the interaction with both HCV and HIV in addition to an immunomodulatory effect due to chronic inflammatory process.

Meanwhile, the elevated Ficolin-3 levels found in HIV and HIV/HCV patients compared to controls may derive from compensatory mechanisms of upregulation of this protein due to its interaction with viral glycoproteins as well as complement activation. Ficolin-3 binding to HIV or HCV has not yet been reported, however, it is known that HIV gp120 is rich in fucose, which is a particular ligand of Ficolin-3 (36). Still, high expression of Ficolin-3 found in both viral infections could be related to the inflammatory status seen in co-infected patients, contributing to the chronic process of these conditions. Elevated Ficolin-3 levels were also observed in ovarian tumor patients (37), related to shorter graft survival after kidney transplantation (38), in patients with Leprosy (39) and Systemic Lupus Erythematosus (40, 41), all conditions associated with inflammatory process.

Higher Ficolin-1 levels in female HIV patients and controls corroborates previous findings (42), but, such difference was not observed in HCV coinfected patients, what could be due to the higher male frequency in this group. Ficolin-3 levels were higher in males only in the co-infected group, a sex difference previously observed in healthy subjects (42).

This study has some limitations. First, polymorphisms shown association to Ficolin-1 (rs7857015, rs10120023, rs10117466) (43, 44) and Ficolin-3 (rs532781899, rs28362807, and rs4494157) (39) concentrations, that could have contributed to the variation of protein concentration in HIV and HIV/HCV patients, were not assessed. Future studies in this cohort of patients should include the investigation of these variants. Second, although Ficolins concentration showed significant results among the groups the relevance of these findings should be confirmed in a larger sample of patients, and, in experimental studies showing Ficolins 1 and 3 interaction with both HIV and HCV. Third, the status of HCV co-infection was based only on anti-HCV test, which is an evidence for prior exposure to HCV. Since all patients were attending the HIV ambulatory whose routine for HCV is based on serology, molecular tests were not available at the time of the study. In order to established direct evidence of current infection both the presence of HCV RNA and a longitudinal follow-up in HIV/HCV patients should be considered.

Nevertheless, our data represent a pioneer study on the role of Ficolin-1 and -3 in HIV/HCV infections. This novel finding suggests that these proteins contribute in a different manner to host defense against these viruses and may be helpful for future studies in understanding the function of Ficolins in HIV/HCV infection as well as in the development of new therapeutic targets.

AUTHOR CONTRIBUTIONS

IM-R, ST, JJ, and MT contributed with conception and design of the study. MT, HM, MB, and FA executed laboratory procedures. KL performed the statistical analysis. MT, KL, FA, and MB wrote the original draft of the manuscript. ER performed the recruitment of patients. All authors contributed to manuscript revision, read, and approved the submitted version.

ACKNOWLEDGMENTS

We gratefully acknowledge the subjects of this investigation for their consent in participating in the study, and to the staff of the Laboratório de Imunopatologia Molecular in Curitiba for DNA extraction. We also thank the Institute of Medical Microbiology and Immunology at University of Aarhus, Denmark for collaboration in plasma Ficolin-1 quantification. This work was supported by grants and scholarships from Conselho Nacional de Desenvolvimento Científico e Tecnológico (CNPq).

REFERENCES

1. Nakagawa F, May M, Phillips A. Life expectancy living with HIV. *Curr Opin Infect Dis.* (2013) 26:17–25. doi: 10.1097/QCO.0b013e32835ba6b1
2. Katz IT, Maughan-Brown B. Improved life expectancy of people living with HIV: who is left behind? *Lancet HIV.* (2017) 4:e324–6. doi: 10.1016/S2352-3018(17)30086-3
3. *UNAIDS -JOINT UNITED NATIONS PROGRAMME ON HIV/AIDS.* Available online at: http://unaids.org.br/tag/atualizacao-sobre-a-aids-no-mundo-2016/
4. Laskus T, Kibler KV, Chmielewski M, Wilkinson J, Adair D, Horban A, et al. Effect of hepatitis C infection on HIV-induced apoptosis. *PLoS ONE.* (2013) 8:e75921. doi: 10.1371/journal.pone.0075921
5. Zeremski M, Martinez AD, Talal AH. Editorial commentary: management of hepatitis C virus in HIV-infected patients in the era of direct-acting antivirals. *Clin Infect Dis.* (2014) 58:880–2. doi: 10.1093/cid/cit804
6. Sulkowski MS. Viral hepatitis and HIV coinfection. *J Hepatol.* (2008) 48:353–67. doi: 10.1016/j.jhep.2007.11.009
7. Joshi D, O'Grady J, Dieterich D, Gazzard B, Agarwal K. Increasing burden of liver disease in patients with HIV infection. *Lancet* (2011) 377:1198–209. doi: 10.1016/S0140-6736(10)62001-6
8. Soriano V, Vispo E, Labarga P, Medrano J, Barreiro P. Viral hepatitis and HIV co-infection. *Antiviral Res.* (2010) 85:303–15. doi: 10.1016/j.antiviral.2009.10.021
9. Weber R, Ruppik M, Rickenbach M, Spoerri A, Furrer H, Battegay M, et al. Decreasing mortality and changing patterns of causes of death in the Swiss HIV Cohort Study. *HIV Med.* (2013) 14:195–207. doi: 10.1111/j.1468-1293.2012.01051.x
10. Kim AY, Onofrey S, Church DR. An epidemiologic update on hepatitis C infection in persons living with or at risk of HIV infection. *J Infect Dis.* (2013) 207(Suppl. 1):S1–6. doi: 10.1093/infdis/jis927
11. Soriano V, Vispo E, Fernandez-Montero JV, Labarga P, Barreiro P. Update on HIV/HCV Coinfection. *Curr HIV/AIDS Rep.* (2013) 10:226–34. doi: 10.1007/s11904-013-0169-5
12. Garred P, Genster N, Pilely K, Bayarri-Olmos R, Rosbjerg A, Ma YJ, et al. A journey through the lectin pathway of complement-MBL and beyond. *Immunol Rev.* (2016) 274:74–97. doi: 10.1111/imr.12468
13. Fabiana Antunes Andrade, Kárita CF. Lidani, Sandra J. Catarino IJMR. *Proteases in Physiology and Pathology.* In: Chakraborti S, Dhalla NS, editors. Singapore: Springer Singapore (2017). p. 397–420.
14. Endo Y, Matsushita M, Fujita T. New insights into the role of ficolins in the lectin pathway of innate immunity. *Int Rev Cell Mol Biol.* (2015)316:49–110. doi: 10.1016/bs.ircmb.2015.01.003
15. Ricklin D, Hajishengallis G, Yang K, Lambris JD. Complement: a key system for immune surveillance and homeostasis. *Nat Immunol.* (2010) 11:785–97. doi: 10.1038/ni.1923
16. Dunkelberger JR, Song WC. Complement and its role in innate and adaptive immune responses. *Cell Res.* (2010) 20:34–50. doi: 10.1038/cr.2009.139
17. Mason C, Tarr A. Human lectins and their roles in viral infections. *Molecules* (2015) 20:2229–71. doi: 10.3390/molecules20022229
18. Datta PK, Rappaport J. HIV and complement: hijacking an immune defense. *Biomed Pharmacother.* (2006) 60:561–8. doi: 10.1016/j.biopha.2006.07.087
19. Ballegaard V, Haugaard AK, Garred P, Nielsen SD, Munthe-Fog L. The lectin pathway of complement: advantage or disadvantage in HIV pathogenesis? *Clin Immunol.* (2014) 154:13–25. doi: 10.1016/j.clim.2014.06.002
20. Wittenborn T, Thiel S, Jensen L, Nielsen HJ, Jensenius JC. Characteristics and biological variations of M-Ficolin, a pattern recognition molecule, in Plasma. *J Innate Immun.* (2010) 2:167–80. doi: 10.1159/000218324
21. Schlapbach LJ, Aebi C, Hansen AG, Hirt A, Jensenius JC, Ammann RA. H-ficolin serum concentration and susceptibility to fever and neutropenia in paediatric cancer patients. *Clin Exp Immunol.* (2009) 157:83–9. doi: 10.1111/j.1365-2249.2009.03957.x
22. Frank MM, Hester C, Jiang H. Complement and the control of HIV infection. *Curr Opin HIV AIDS* (2014) 9:278–90. doi: 10.1097/COH.0000000000000058

23. Luo F, Chen T, Liu J, Shen X, Zhao Y, Yang R, et al. Ficolin-2 binds to HIV-1 gp120 and blocks viral infection. *Virol Sin.* (2016) 31:406–14. doi: 10.1007/s12250-016-3808-3
24. Zhao Y, Ren Y, Zhang X, Zhao P, Tao W, Zhong J, et al. Ficolin-2 inhibits hepatitis C virus infection, whereas apolipoprotein E3 mediates viral immune escape. *J Immunol.* (2014) 193:783–96. doi: 10.4049/jimmunol.1302563
25. Liu J, Ali MA, Shi Y, Zhao Y, Luo F, Yu J, et al. Specifically binding of L-ficolin to N-glycans of HCV envelope glycoproteins E1 and E2 leads to complement activation. *Cell Mol Immunol.* (2009) 6(4): 235–44. doi: 10.1038/cmi.2009.32
26. Hu YL, Luo FL, Fu JL, Chen TL, Wu SM, Zhou YD, et al. Early increased ficolin-2 concentrations are associated with severity of liver inflammation and efficacy of anti-viral therapy in chronic hepatitis C patients. *Scand J Immunol.* (2013) 77:144–50. doi: 10.1111/sji.12014
27. Tong HV, Toan NL, Song LH, Ouf EA, Bock CT, Kremsner PG, et al. Ficolin-2 levels and FCN2 haplotypes influence hepatitis b infection outcome in vietnamese patients. *PLoS ONE* (2011) 6:e28113. doi: 10.1371/journal.pone.0028113
28. Pan Q, Chen H, Wang F, Jeza VT, Hou W, Zhao Y, et al. L-Ficolin binds to the glycoproteins hemagglutinin and neuraminidase and inhibits influenza A virus infection both *in vitro* and *in vivo*. *J Innate Immun.* (2012) 4:312–24. doi: 10.1159/000335670
29. Verma A, White M, Vathipadiekal V, Tripathi S, Mbianda J, Ieong M, et al. Human H-ficolin inhibits replication of seasonal and pandemic influenza A viruses. *J Immunol.* (2012) 189:2478–87. doi: 10.4049/jimmunol.1103786
30. Urban TJ, Thompson AJ, Bradrick SS, Fellay J, Schuppan D, Cronin KD, et al. IL28B genotype is associated with differential expression of intrahepatic interferon-stimulated genes in patients with chronic hepatitis C. *Hepatology* (2010) 52:1888–96. doi: 10.1002/hep.23912
31. Denner J, Eschricht M, Lauck M, Semaan M, Schlaermann P, Ryu H, et al. Modulation of cytokine release and gene expression by the immunosuppressive domain of gp41 of HIV-1. *PLoS ONE* (2013) 8:e55199. doi: 10.1371/journal.pone.0055199
32. *Manual Técnico Para o Diagnóstico Da Infecção Pelo HIV.* 2nd ed. Brasília : Ministério da Saúde, Ministério da Saúde, Secretaria de Vigilância em Saúde, Departamento de Vigilância, Prevenção e Controle das Doenças Sexualmente Transmissíveis, Aids e Hepatites Virais (2015).
33. Moreno-Amaral AN, Gout E, Danella-Polli C, Tabarin F, Lesavre P, Pereira-da-Silva G, et al. M-ficolin and leukosialin (CD43): new partners in neutrophil adhesion. *J Leukoc Biol.* (2012) 91:469–74. doi: 10.1189/jlb.0911460
34. Tanio M, Wakamatsu K, Kohno T. Binding site of C-reactive protein on M-ficolin. *Mol Immunol.* (2009) 47:215–21. doi: 10.1016/j.molimm.2009.09.032
35. Zhang J, Yang L, Ang Z, Yoong SL, Tran TT, Anand GS, et al. Secreted M-ficolin anchors onto monocyte transmembrane G protein-coupled receptor 43 and cross talks with plasma C-reactive protein to mediate immune signaling and regulate host defense. *J Immunol.* (2010) 185:6899–910. doi: 10.4049/jimmunol.1001225
36. Sugimoto R, Yae Y, Akaiwa M, Kitajima S, Shibata Y, Sato H, et al. Cloning and characterization of the hakata antigen, a member of the ficolin/opsonin p35 lectin family. *J Biol Chem.* (1998) 273:20721–7. doi: 10.1074/jbc.273.33.20721
37. Szala A, Sawicki S, Swierzko AS, Szemraj J, Sniadecki M, Michalski M, et al. Ficolin-2 and ficolin-3 in women with malignant and benign ovarian tumours. *Cancer Immunol Immunother.* (2013) 62:1411–9. doi: 10.1007/s00262-013-1445-3
38. Smedbråten YV, Sagedal S, Mjøen G, Hartmann A, Fagerland MW, Rollag H, et al. High ficolin-3 level at the time of transplantation is an independent risk factor for graft loss in kidney transplant recipients. *Transplantation* (2015) 99:791–6. doi: 10.1097/TP.0000000000000422
39. Andrade FA, Beltrame MH, Bini VB, Gonçalves LB, Boldt AB, Messias-Reason IJ. Association of a new FCN3 haplotype with high ficolin-3 levels in leprosy. *PLoS Negl Trop Dis.* (2017) 11:e0005409. doi: 10.1371/journal.pntd.0005409
40. Andersen T, Munthe-Fog L, Garred P, Jacobsen S. Serum levels of ficolin-3 (Hakata Antigen) in patients with systemic lupus erythematosus. *J Rheumatol.* (2009) 36:757–9. doi: 10.3899/jrheum.080361
41. Hein E, Nielsen LA, Nielsen CT, Munthe-Fog L, Skjoedt MO, Jacobsen S, et al. Ficolins and the lectin pathway of complement in patients with systemic lupus erythematosus. *Mol Immunol.* (2015) 63:209–14. doi: 10.1016/j.molimm.2014.07.003
42. Troldborg A, Hansen A, Hansen SWK, Jensenius JC, Stengaard-Pedersen K, Thiel S. Lectin complement pathway proteins in healthy individuals. *Clin Exp Immunol.* (2017) 188:138–47. doi: 10.1111/cei.12909
43. Ammitzbøll CG, Kjær TR, Steffensen R, Stengaard-Pedersen K, Nielsen HJ, Thiel S, et al. Non-synonymous polymorphisms in the FCN1 gene determine ligand-binding ability and serum levels of M-ficolin. *PLoS ONE* (2012) 7:e50585. doi: 10.1371/journal.pone.0050585
44. Munthe-Fog L, Hummelshoj T, Honoré C, Moller ME, Skjoedt MO, Palsgaard I, et al. Variation in FCN1 affects biosynthesis of ficolin-1 and is associated with outcome of systemic inflammation. *Genes Immun.* (2012) 13:515–22. doi: 10.1038/gene.2012.27

4

Alternative Pathway is Essential for Glomerular Complement Activation and Proteinuria in a Mouse Model of Membranous Nephropathy

Wentian Luo[1,2], Florina Olaru[1†], Jeffrey H. Miner[3], Laurence H. Beck Jr[4], Johan van der Vlag[5], Joshua M. Thurman[6] and Dorin-Bogdan Borza[2,7]*

[1] Division of Nephrology, Department of Medicine, Vanderbilt Medical Center, Nashville, TN, United States, [2] Vanderbilt Center for Kidney Disease, Vanderbilt Division of Nephrology, Nashville, TN, United States, [3] Renal Division, Washington University School of Medicine, St. Louis, MO, United States, [4] Division of Nephrology, Boston University Medical Center, Boston, MA, United States, [5] Department of Nephrology, Radboud University Medical Center, Nijmegen, Netherlands, [6] Department of Medicine, University of Colorado School of Medicine, Aurora, CO, United States, [7] Department of Microbiology, Immunology and Physiology, Meharry Medical College, Nashville, TN, United States

***Correspondence:**
Dorin-Bogdan Borza
dborza@mmc.edu

†Present address:
Department of Dermatology, Heidelberg University Hospital, Heidelberg, Germany

Membranous nephropathy is an immune kidney disease caused by IgG antibodies that form glomerular subepithelial immune complexes. Proteinuria is mediated by complement activation, as a result of podocyte injury by C5b-9, but the role of specific complement pathways is not known. Autoantibodies-mediating primary membranous nephropathy are predominantly of IgG4 subclass, which cannot activate the classical pathway. Histologic evidence from kidney biopsies suggests that the lectin and the alternative pathways may be activated in membranous nephropathy, but the pathogenic relevance of these pathways remains unclear. In this study, we evaluated the role of the alternative pathway in a mouse model of membranous nephropathy. After inducing the formation of subepithelial immune complexes, we found similar glomerular IgG deposition in wild-type mice and in factor B-null mice, which lack a functional alternative pathway. Unlike wild-type mice, mice lacking factor B did not develop albuminuria nor exhibit glomerular deposition of C3c and C5b-9. Albuminuria was also reduced but not completely abolished in C5-deficient mice. Our results provide the first direct evidence that the alternative pathway is necessary for pathogenic complement activation by glomerular subepithelial immune complexes and is, therefore, a key mediator of proteinuria in experimental membranous nephropathy. This knowledge is important for the rational design of new therapies for membranous nephropathy.

Keywords: membranous nephropathy, glomerulonephritis, albuminuria, alternative pathway, membrane attack complex, factor B, complement C5, mouse models

INTRODUCTION

Membranous nephropathy (MN), one of the leading causes of nephrotic syndrome in adults, is an antibody-mediated kidney disease clinically characterized by proteinuria, often heavy and persistent. MN is a disease of heterogeneous etiology, defined histologically by immune complexes deposited on the subepithelial side of glomerular basement membrane (GBM), together with GBM thickening

---

Abbreviations: AP, alternative pathway; GBM, glomerular basement membrane; MN, membranous nephropathy; PLA2R, phospholipase A2 receptor; THSD7A, thrombospondin type-1 domain-containing 7A.

and podocyte foot process effacement, but little glomerular inflammation. The most prevalent form is primary MN, now understood as an autoimmune disease in which IgG autoantibodies (predominantly of IgG4 subclass) form subepithelial immune complexes with autoantigens expressed on podocyte cell surface (1, 2). About 70% of patients with primary MN have autoantibodies targeting phospholipase A2 receptor (PLA2R), and an additional 3–5% have autoantibodies targeting thrombospondin type-1 domain-containing 7A (THSD7A) (3, 4). Secondary MN can occur when circulating antibodies bind to antigens planted in the subepithelial space, such as cationic bovine serum albumin of dietary origin (5).

In the current paradigm for the pathogenesis of MN, complement activation is a major effector mechanism of subepithelial immune complexes (1, 6). Complement activation is initiated by three canonical pathways. The classical pathway is triggered by immune complexes and the lectin pathway—by certain danger patterns, while the alternative pathway (AP) is constitutively active and self-amplifies on foreign surfaces. The AP also amplifies activation that is initiated through the other two pathways. All three pathways converge toward the assembly of C3 and C5 convertases, which generate pro-inflammatory anaphylatoxins (C3a, C5a), opsonins that mediate immune adhesion (C3b, iC3b), and the membrane attack complex (C5b-9), which lyses cells. In human MN, C3 fragments and C5b-9 are present alongside IgG in subepithelial deposits, while urinary excretion of sC5b-9 associates with immune disease activity (7–9). Studies in passive Heymann nephritis, a faithful rat model of MN, have specifically implicated C5b-9 as a key mediator of podocyte injury and proteinuria (10, 11). However, the role of different complement pathways upstream of C5 activation in human and experimental MN remains largely unknown.

How immune complexes activate complement in MN remains a conundrum because the autoantibodies implicated in primary MN are predominantly of IgG4 subclass (6, 12–14). Although immune complexes typically bind C1q and activate the classical pathway, IgG4 does not bind C1q and is considered unable to activate complement—at least not *via* the classical pathway (15–17). In kidney biopsies from patients with primary MN, glomerular staining for C1q is almost always weak or absent, while staining for mannan-binding lectin (MBL) and C4d is usually positive (except in patients with MBL deficiency), consistent with the activation of the lectin pathway (18–20). Beck and Salant proposed that the lectin pathway may be activated by IgG4 glycoforms that lack terminal galactose and sialic acid, and, therefore, can bind MBL (1, 6). However, the occurrence of primary MN in patients with MBL deficiency shows that the lectin pathway is not absolutely required (21). Glomerular deposition of properdin and factor B—which is indicative of the AP activation—is also common in MN (18, 21), but the pathogenic relevance of this pathway is not known.

The goal of this study was to determine the contribution of the AP to glomerular injury and proteinuria mediated by subepithelial immune complexes. For this purpose, we used a mouse model that recapitulates clinical and morphologic features of human MN (22–25) and which was found to exhibit proteinuria exacerbated by C5 activation. Using $Cfb^{-/-}$ mice, which lack factor B (an essential component of the AP), we found that the absence of a functional AP prevented complement activation by subepithelial immune complexes (as assessed from the glomerular deposition of C3c and C5b-9) and abolished proteinuria. These findings provide the first direct evidence implicating the AP activation in the pathogenesis of MN. This knowledge may provide a framework for developing new therapeutic strategies for MN.

MATERIALS AND METHODS

Materials

The recombinant non-collagenous (NC1) domain of human α3(IV) collagen (rh-α3NC1) was expressed in HEK293 cells and purified as described (26).

Animal Experiments

DBA/1J (D1), DBA/2J (D2), and C57Bl/6J (B6) mice were purchased from The Jackson Laboratory (Bar Harbor, ME, USA). Breeding pairs of $Cfb^{-/-}$ mice backcrossed on the B6 background for more than nine generations (B6.$Cfb^{-/-}$) were obtained from Dr. Joshua Thurman and maintained by homozygous breeding. D1.$Cfb^{-/-}$ mice were generated by backcrossing onto the D1 background for four generations and then intercrossing F4 heterozygous mice. Mice were housed in a specific pathogen-free facility with free access to food and water. The study was carried out in accordance with the recommendations of the National Institutes of Health Guide for Care and Use of Laboratory Animals and the protocol was approved by the local Institutional Animal Care and Use Committee.

To induce experimental membranous nephropathy, mice (6–10 weeks old, both male and female) were immunized subcutaneously at two sites on the back with rh-α3NC1 antigen (30 μg in 50 μL sterile phosphate-buffered saline) emulsified in an equal volume of Complete Freund's Adjuvant (Sigma, St. Louis, MO, USA). D1 and D2 mice received one booster immunization with the rh-α3NC1 antigen in Incomplete Freund's Adjuvant (Sigma, St. Louis, MO, USA) on day 21 after the first immunization. B6 mice were boosted four times with rh-α3NC1 in Incomplete Freund's Adjuvant, at 10 days interval starting on day 14 after the first immunization. As negative controls, some mice were immunized with adjuvant alone in each experiment. Unless otherwise indicated, mice were euthanized at 8 weeks (for D1 and D2 mice) or 12 weeks (for B6 mice) after the initial immunization, and tissues and blood were collected for further evaluations.

Evaluation of Kidney Function

Spontaneously voided spot urine samples were collected by placing mice over 96-well microtiter plates and then analyzed as follows. Urinary albumin was measured by capture ELISA using a mouse albumin quantitation kit (Bethyl, Montgomery, TX, USA). Urine creatinine and blood urea nitrogen levels were measured using Infinity creatinine and urea liquid stable reagents (Thermo Fisher Scientific, Middletown, VA, USA), according to the manufacturer's protocols. To account for urine tonicity, albuminuria was expressed as urinary albumin-to-creatinine ratio (ACR).

Evaluation of Mouse IgG Autoantibody Production

Sera were assayed for the presence of IgG antibodies to rh-α3NC1 by ELISA. Briefly, 96-well microtiter plates (Nunc MaxiSorp) were coated overnight with rh-α3NC1 (100 ng per well) in carbonate-bicarbonate buffer, pH 9.6. After blocking with 1% bovine serum albumin, the wells were incubated for 1 h with mouse sera diluted 1/5,000 for detection of total IgG, 1/2,000 for detection of IgG1, or 1/500 for detection of IgG2a and IgG2b. Secondary antibodies were alkaline phosphatase-conjugated goat anti-mouse IgG (Rockland Immunochemicals, Gilbertsville, PA, USA) and horseradish peroxidase-conjugated goat anti-mouse IgG1, IgG2a, IgG2b, or IgG2c (Bethyl, Montgomery, TX, USA). Plates were developed with p-nitrophenol phosphate or tetramethylbenzidine (Sigma, St. Louis, MO, USA) as substrate, and absorbance was read at 405 nm with a SpectraMax ELISA plate reader (Molecular Devices, Sunnyvale, CA, USA).

Renal Histopathology and Immunofluorescence Microscopy

For light microscopy, portions of mouse kidneys were fixed in 10% buffered formalin, dehydrated through a graded ethanol series, and embedded in paraffin. Paraffin sections (2 μm thick) were stained with periodic-acid Schiff reagent. Transmission electron microscopy was performed as described (27). For immunofluorescence, portions of mouse kidneys embedded in OCT were snap-frozen in isopentane and stored at −70°C. Cryosections cut at a thickness of 5 μm were fixed in cold acetone for 10 min. Mouse IgG was visualized using FITC-conjugated goat anti-mouse IgG (BD Bioscience Pharmingen, San Jose, CA, USA). Complement C3 was visualized using FITC-conjugated goat anti-mouse C3c (Nordic Immunology, Tilburg, Netherlands). Kidney deposition of rh-α3NC1 was visualized with rat IgG mAb RH34 (a gift from Dr. Yoshikazu Sado, Shigei Medical Research Institute, Japan), which is specific for human but not mouse α3NC1 (28). Mouse C5b-9, properdin, factor H, and C4 were visualized using rabbit anti-C5b9 (Abcam; Cambridge, MA, USA), rabbit anti-properdin (Santa Cruz, CA, USA), rat IgG anti-mouse C4d mAb (HyCult, Netherlands), and rat IgG anti-mouse factor H mAb (MAB4999, R&D Systems, Minneapolis, MN, USA). Nephrin was visualized using guinea pig anti-nephrin (Progen, Germany). Heparan sulfate chains were visualized with mouse IgM mAb JM403 (29). Agrin was visualized using a rabbit anti-agrin polyclonal antibody (kindly provided by Dr. Takako Sasaki, Oita University, Japan), as previously described (27). Secondary antibodies were Alexa Fluor 488-conjugated goat anti-rabbit IgG, goat anti-rat IgG, donkey anti-guinea pig IgG, goat anti-mouse IgM (Invitrogen, Carlsbad, CA, USA), and FITC-goat anti-rat IgG (BD Bioscience Pharmingen, San Jose, CA, USA). Sections were mounted with anti-fade reagent (Invitrogen, Carlsbad, CA, USA), then cover-slipped and observed using a fluorescence microscope (Nikon Eclipse E800). Photomicrographs were captured with a digital camera attached to the microscope, using the same exposure settings for each primary antibody. For quantitative analyses, images were analyzed with Image J software, as described (30). All sections from one experiment were stained and analyzed at the same time.

In Vitro Complement Activation

Fresh frozen normal mouse serum, collected from DBA/1 mice, and stored in aliquots at −70°C, was used as a source of complement. Cryosections of mouse kidneys fixed in cold acetone were incubated overnight at 37°C with normal mouse serum diluted 1:3 in veronal buffered saline (Sigma, St. Louis, MO, USA) containing 0.1% Tween 20 and supplemented with: (a) 2.5 mM calcium chloride and 0.7 mM magnesium chloride; or (b) 2.5 mM magnesium chloride and 6.2 mM EGTA; or (c) 25 mM EDTA. Complement activation was visualized by staining with FITC-conjugated goat anti-mouse C3c, as described above.

Statistical Analyses

Analyses were performed using GraphPad Prism 7.00 software (San Diego, CA, USA). ACRs were log transformed. The significance of differences was determined by unpaired *t* test or by one-way analysis of variance (ANOVA) with Dunnett's correction for multiple comparisons. A value of $P < 0.05$ was considered statistically significant. Values are presented as means ± SEM.

RESULTS

Complement C5 Deficiency Ameliorates Albuminuria Induced by Subepithelial Immune Complexes in Mice Immunized With α3NC1

DBA/1 (D1) mice immunized with α3NC1 develop kidney disease recapitulating clinical and morphologic features of human MN (22–25). This model exhibits proteinuria associated with subepithelial immune complexes and glomerular deposition of IgG, C3, and C5b-9, but the role of complement activation in proteinuria is not known. We reasoned that if C5b-9 is pathogenic in this mouse model (analogous to the rat Heymann nephritis model), then, proteinuria would be ameliorated by the genetic deficiency of complement C5, which occurs naturally in several inbred strains of mice (31). To test this conjecture, we induced experimental MN in C5-deficient DBA/2 (D2) mice, which are nearly 95% genetically identical to C5-sufficient D1 mice (32).

Compared to D1 mice, D2 mice immunized with α3NC1 developed much milder albuminuria (**Figure 1A**). At week 8 after the first immunization, the endpoint for this experiment, the urine ACR in α3NC1-immunized D2 mice (2.4 ± 0.96) was significantly lower ($P < 0.001$) than that in α3NC1-immunized D1 mice (77.1 ± 20.8), albeit greater than in control D2 mice immunized with adjuvant alone (ACR 0.16 ± 0.07) (**Figure 1B**). Blood urea nitrogen levels did not increase over the baseline (mean values at week 0 and at week 8 were 23.1 and 20.3 mg/dL for D1 mice, 27.8 and 25.4 mg/dL for D2 mice), indicating that the renal function did not decline during the duration of the experiment. Serum levels of mouse IgG anti-α3NC1 antibodies were similar in D1 and D2 mice (data not shown). Kidneys were collected at 8 weeks post-immunization for morphologic evaluation. By light microscopy, kidneys from α3NC1-immunized mice

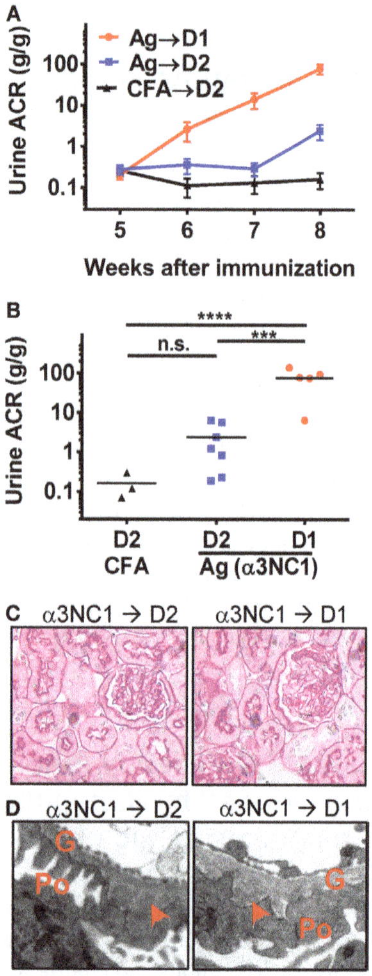

FIGURE 1 | C5 deficiency protects against albuminuria in experimental MN. **(A)** Time course of urinary albumin-to-creatinine ratio (ACR) in D1 mice (circles) and D2 mice (squares) immunized with α3NC1 (N = 5–7 per group). Control D2 mice (triangles) were immunized with adjuvant alone (N = 3). Shown are means and SEM. **(B)** Scatterplot depicting the final ACR values (at week 8). The significance of differences among groups was analyzed by one-way ANOVA with Dunnett's correction for multiple comparisons. ***P < 0.001, ****P < 0.0001. n.s., not significant. **(C)** Light microscopy shows normal appearance of glomeruli and tubules in α3NC1-immunized D2 and D1 mice (periodic acid–Schiff staining; original magnification 400x). **(D)** Transmission electron microscopy shows subepithelial electron dense deposits (arrowhead), areas of glomerular basement membrane (G) thickening, and effacement of podocyte (Po) foot processes. Original magnification 7,500x.

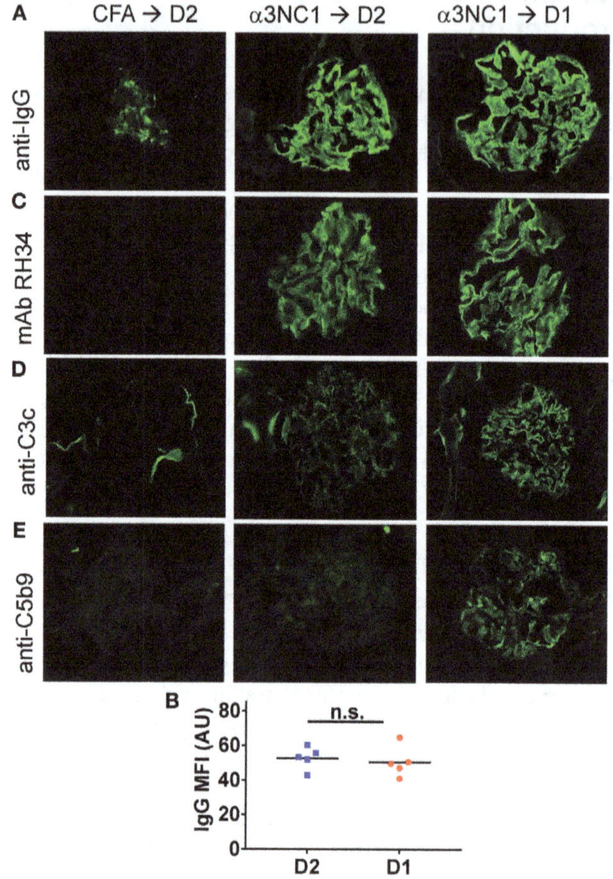

FIGURE 2 | Analysis of glomerular immune complexes and complement deposition in D1 and D2 mice immunized with α3NC1. Kidneys were collected at week 8 post-immunization from adjuvant immunized D2 mice (left), α3NC1-immunized D2 mice (middle), and α3NC1-immunized D1 mice (right). **(A)** Direct immunofluorescence staining shows mouse IgG binding along the glomerular basement membrane (GBM) in α3NC1-immunized D1 and D2 mice. Control mice show non-specific mesangial deposition of mouse IgG. **(B)** Mean fluorescence intensity (MFI) of IgG staining, expressed in arbitrary units (AU), was compared in α3NC1-immunized D2 and D1 mice. The difference was not significant (n.s.) by t test. **(C)** Indirect immunofluorescence staining with mAb RH34 shows GBM deposition of exogenous antigen in all α3NC1-immunized mice, which is absent in adjuvant-immunized mice. **(D)** Direct immunofluorescence staining reveals C3c deposition along the capillary loops in α3NC1-immunized D1 and D2 mice. In control mice, C3c staining is positive in the Bowman's capsule and kidney tubules. **(E)** Indirect immunofluorescence shows capillary loop staining for C5b-9 in α3NC1-immunized D1 mice. A weak background of non-specific immunofluorescence is observed in adjuvant-immunized and α3NC1-immunized D2 mice. Original magnification 400x.

appeared relatively normal, with little glomerular inflammation (**Figure 1C**); however, electron microscopy revealed areas of thickened GBM surrounding subepithelial deposits and podocyte foot process effacement (**Figure 1D**).

Immunofluorescence microscopy showed mouse IgG staining along the GBM in all α3NC1-immunized mice (**Figure 2A**). The IgG staining intensity was similar in D1 and D2 mice (**Figure 2B**). Staining with an antibody that binds to human but not mouse α3NC1 (mAb RH34) showed capillary loop deposition of exogenous antigen in α3NC1-immunized but not control mice (**Figure 2C**). GBM staining for C3c, which indicates recent complement activation, was also found in all α3NC1-immunized mice (**Figure 2D**). However, glomerular deposition of C5b-9 was only found in α3NC1-immunized D1 mice (**Figure 2E**), as expected based on the C5 deficiency in D2 mice. A decrease in nephrin staining in α3NC1-immunized D1 mice compared to D2 mice confirmed an injured podocyte phenotype (not shown). These results imply that C5 activation exacerbates proteinuria induced by subepithelial immune complexes in α3NC1-immunized mice, presumably as a result of podocyte injury by C5b-9.

Evidence of the AP Activation by Subepithelial Immune Complexes

To determine which complement pathways may be activated by subepithelial immune complexes, we assessed glomerular deposition of properdin, factor H, and C4d. Properdin and factor H are positive and negative regulators of the AP, respectively, while C4d is a marker of the classical and lectin pathway activation. Capillary loop staining for both properdin (**Figure 3A**) and factor H (**Figure 3B**) was found in α3NC1-immunized D1 mice but not in control mice. All mice had staining for C4d in a non-specific mesangial pattern (**Figure 3C**), also commonly seen in normal human glomeruli (33). In addition, α3NC1-immunized mice also had segmental staining for C4d along the capillary loops, suggesting that subepithelial immune complexes formed in these mice activate multiple complement pathways, similar to what is observed in human MN (18). While these results are indicative of the AP activation, the pathogenic relevance of the AP cannot be inferred from morphologic findings alone.

B6.Cfb$^{-/-}$ Mice Immunized With α3NC1 Develop Subepithelial Immune Complexes but Are Protected Against Albuminuria and Do Not Exhibit Glomerular Complement Deposition

The absence of a functional AP in Cfb$^{-/-}$ mice afforded a strategy to investigate the role of the AP in experimental MN. We initially obtained Cfb$^{-/-}$ mice backcrossed on the B6 background for nine generations (B6.Cfb$^{-/-}$), which allowed us to compare the course of albuminuria induced by α3NC1 immunization in B6.Cfb$^{-/-}$ mice to congenic wild-type B6 mice (B6.Cfb$^{+/+}$) (**Figure 4A**). At the endpoint in this experiment (i.e., at 12 weeks after the initial immunization), the urinary ACR in α3NC1-immunized B6.Cfb$^{-/-}$ mice (0.11 ± 0.05) was similar to that in adjuvant-immunized B6 mice (0.057 ± 0.011); both were significantly lower ($P < 0.0001$) than the urine ACR in α3NC1-immunized B6.Cfb$^{+/+}$ mice (10.6 ± 5.9) (**Figure 4B**). Two mice from each group were observed for an additional 4 weeks; albuminuria further increased in Cfb$^{+/+}$ mice but not in Cfb$^{-/-}$ mice. In both groups of α3NC1-immunized B6 mice, kidney morphology mice appeared relatively normal by light microscopy (**Figure 4C**).

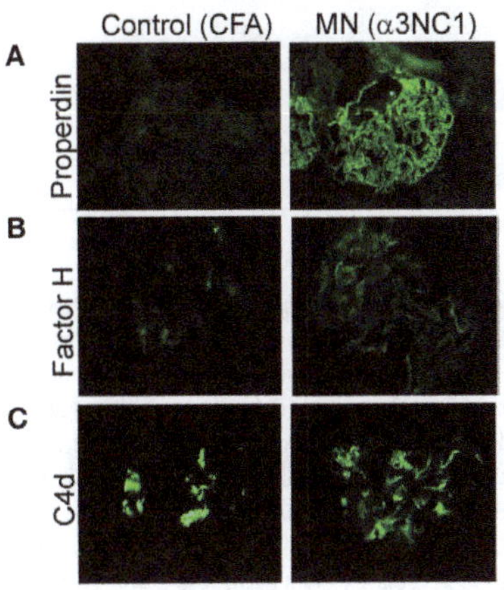

FIGURE 3 | Histologic evidence of AP activation in experimental MN. Glomerular deposition of properdin **(A)**, factor H **(B)**, and C4d **(C)** was evaluated by indirect immunofluorescence staining of frozen kidney sections from α3NC1-immunized D1 mice and adjuvant-immunized control mice. Properdin and factor H staining along the capillary loops was found in α3NC1-immunized D1 mice, but not in adjuvant-immunized mice. Mesangial C4d staining was found in all mice, while weaker segmental staining for C4d along capillary loops was also present in α3NC1-immunized mice.

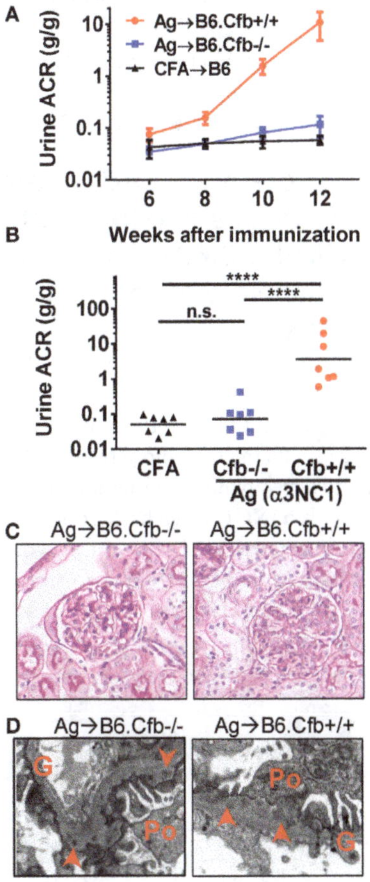

FIGURE 4 | B6.Cfb$^{-/-}$ mice immunized with α3NC1 are protected against albuminuria despite developing subepithelial immune complexes. **(A)** Time course of urinary albumin-to-creatinine ratio (ACR) in B6.Cfb$^{+/+}$ mice (circles) and B6.Cfb$^{-/-}$ mice (squares) immunized with α3NC1 ($N = 7$ per group). Control B6 mice (triangles), including both genotypes, were immunized with adjuvant alone ($N = 7$). Shown are means and SEM. **(B)** Scatterplot depicts the ACR values at the endpoint of this experiment (week 12). The significance of differences among groups was analyzed by one-way ANOVA with Dunnett's correction for multiple comparisons. ***$P < 0.001$, ****$P < 0.0001$. n.s., not significant. **(C)** Morphology of kidneys from α3NC1-immunized B6.Cfb$^{-/-}$ and B6.Cfb$^{+/+}$ mice appears normal by light microscopy (periodic acid–Schiff staining, original magnification 400×). **(D)** Transmission electron microscopy shows subepithelial electron dense deposits (arrowhead), expansion of the glomerular basement membrane (G), and podocyte (Po) foot process effacement. Original magnification 7,500×.

Electron microscopy showed features of MN including subepithelial deposits, GBM expansion, and foot process effacement (**Figure 4D**).

Humoral immune responses to α3NC1 were comparable in immunized B6.Cfb$^{-/-}$ and B6.Cfb$^{+/+}$ mice, as shown by similar levels of circulating mouse IgG, IgG1, IgG2b, and IgG2c anti-α3NC1 antibodies (**Figure 5**). Immune complexes and complement deposition were evaluated by immunofluorescence microscopy (**Figure 6**). GBM staining for mouse IgG was found in all α3NC1-immunized mice (**Figure 6A**), with similar intensity in B6.Cfb$^{-/-}$ and B6.Cfb$^{+/+}$ mice (**Figure 6B**). GBM deposition of exogenous antigen in α3NC1-immunized mice was indicated by positive staining with mAb RH34 (**Figure 6C**). Deposition of C3c along the GBM was found in α3NC1-immunized Cfb$^{+/+}$ mice but was completely absent in immunized Cfb$^{-/-}$ mice (**Figure 6D**); as also found for C5b-9 (**Figure 6E**). These results indicate that the absence of factor B does not affect the formation of subepithelial immune complexes but prevents glomerular complement activation and abolishes proteinuria induced by immunization with α3NC1.

Absence of Proteinuria and Glomerular Complement Deposition in D1.Cfb$^{-/-}$ Mice Immunized With α3NC1 Corroborates the Pathogenic Role of the AP in Experimental MN

We sought to verify whether the ablation of the AP also prevents albuminuria in D1 mice, which are more susceptible to MN. Results in B6 mice cannot be directly compared to those in D1 and D2 mice because B6 mice are more resistant to experimental kidney disease and develop milder proteinuria requiring repeated immunizations with α3NC1. After backcrossing to D1 for four generations, we generated D1.Cfb$^{-/-}$ mice, which had about 94% D1 genetic background (comparable to almost 95% genetic similarity between D1 and D2 mice).

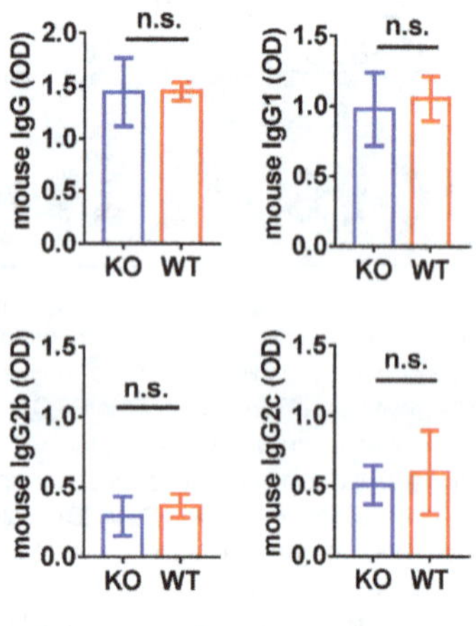

FIGURE 5 | Analysis of circulating anti-α3NC1 mouse IgG antibodies. The levels of circulating mouse IgG, IgG1, IgG2b, and IgG2c antibodies binding to rh-α3NC1 were measured by indirect ELISA. Mouse sera were diluted 1/5,000 for total IgG, 1/2,000 for IgG1, and 1/500 for IgG2b and IgG2c. The significance of differences between Cfb$^{-/-}$ (KO) and Cfb$^{+/+}$ (WT) mice was evaluated by *t*-test (n.s., not significant).

D1.Cfb$^{-/-}$ mice were resistant to development of albuminuria induced by α3NC1 immunization (**Figure 7A**). At the final time point (at week 8 post-immunization), urine ACR in α3NC1-immunized D1.Cfb$^{-/-}$ mice (0.36 ± 0.12) was similar to that in adjuvant-immunized D1 mice (0.078 ± 0.023); both were significantly lower ($P < 0.0001$) than urine ACR in α3NC1-immunized D1.Cfb$^{+/+}$ mice (78.8 ± 18.1) (**Figure 7B**). Morphologic analyses of the kidneys collected at week 8 largely recapitulated the findings from B6 mice. Light microscopy did not show major glomerular abnormalities (**Figure 7C**), while electron microscopy showed subepithelial deposits with GBM thickening and effaced podocyte foot processes (**Figure 7D**). GBM staining for mouse IgG was found in all α3NC1-immunized but not control mice (**Figure 8A**). The IgG

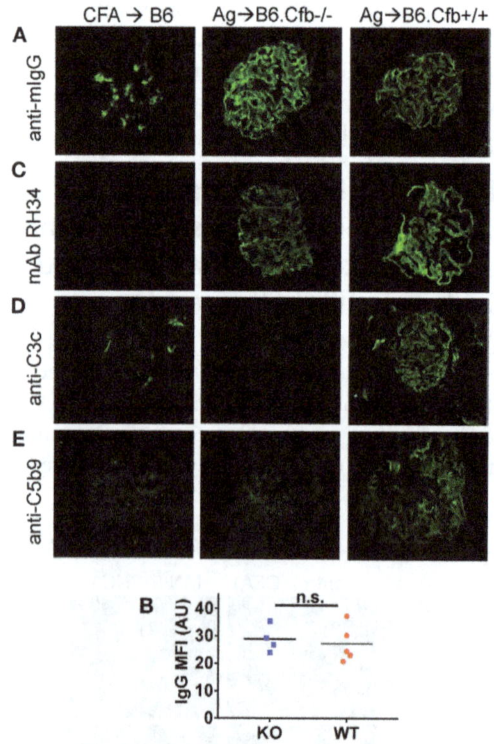

FIGURE 6 | Analysis of glomerular immune complexes and complement deposition in B6 mice immunized with α3NC1. Kidneys from adjuvant-immunized B6 mice (left), α3NC1-immunized B6.Cfb$^{-/-}$ mice (middle), and α3NC1-immunized B6.Cfb$^{-/-}$ mice (right) were collected at week 12 after the initial immunization. **(A)** Immunofluorescence staining for mouse IgG shows glomerular basement membrane (GBM) staining in α3NC1-immunized B6.Cfb$^{-/-}$ and B6.Cfb$^{+/+}$ mice. Adjuvant-immunized mice show non-specific mesangial IgG deposition. **(B)** Mean fluorescence intensity (MFI) of IgG staining, expressed in arbitrary units (AU), was compared in α3NC1-immunized B6.Cfb$^{-/-}$ and B6.Cfb$^{+/+}$ mice. Significance was evaluated by *t* test (n.s., not significant). **(C)** Staining with mAb RH34 shows GBM deposition of exogenous antigen in α3NC1 immunized B6.Cfb$^{-/-}$ and B6. Cfb$^{+/+}$ mice, which is absent in control mice. **(D)** Direct immunofluorescence staining reveals C3c deposition in a capillary loop pattern in α3NC1-immunized B6.Cfb$^{+/+}$ mice. C3c staining is absent in B6.Cfb$^{-/-}$ mice. **(E)** Indirect immunofluorescence shows C5b-9 deposition along the GBM in α3NC1-immunized B6.Cfb$^{+/+}$ mice, but not B6.Cfb$^{-/-}$ mice. Original magnification 400x.

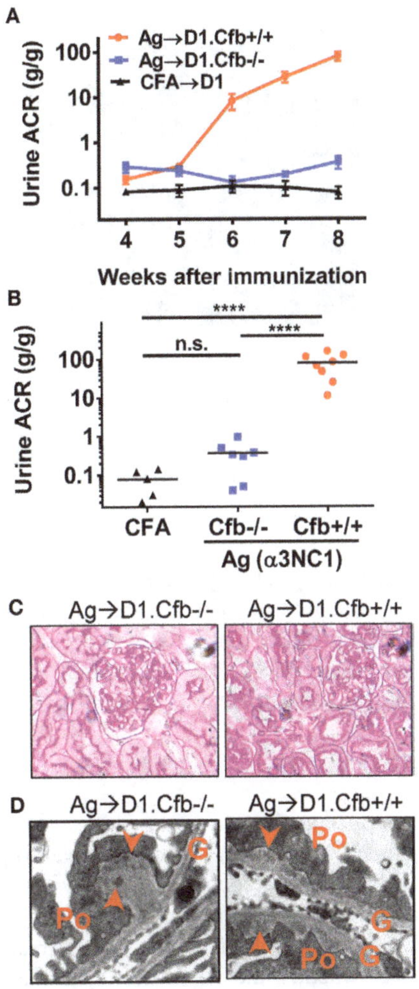

FIGURE 7 | D1.Cfb$^{-/-}$ mice immunized with α3NC1 are protected against albuminuria despite developing subepithelial immune complexes. **(A)** Time course of urinary albumin-to-creatinine ratio (ACR) in D1.Cfb$^{+/+}$ mice (circles) and D1.Cfb$^{-/-}$ mice (squares) immunized with α3NC1 (N = 7–8 per group). Control D1 mice (triangles), including both genotypes, were immunized with adjuvant alone (N = 5). Shown are means and SEM. **(B)** Scatterplot depicts the ACR values at the last time point (week 8). The significance of differences among groups was analyzed by one-way ANOVA with Dunnett's correction multiple comparisons. ***P < 0.001, ****P < 0.0001, n.s., not significant. **(C)** Morphology of kidneys from α3NC1-immunized D1.Cfb$^{-/-}$ (left) and D1.Cfb$^{+/+}$ mice (right) appeared normal by light microscopy (periodic acid–Schiff staining, original magnification 400×). **(D)** Transmission electron microscopy shows subepithelial electron dense deposits (arrowhead), thickening of the glomerular basement membrane (G), and podocyte (Po) foot process effacement. Original magnification 15,000×.

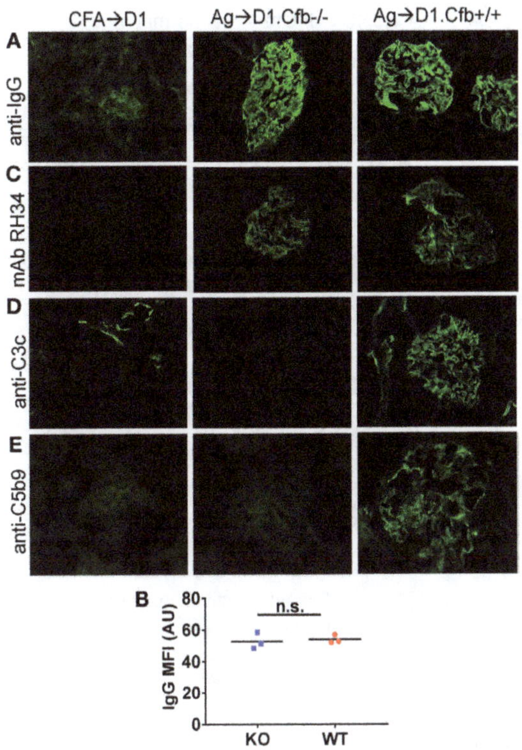

FIGURE 8 | Analysis of glomerular immune complexes and complement deposition in D1 mice immunized with α3NC1. Kidneys were collected from adjuvant immunized D1 mice (left), α3NC1-immunized D1.Cfb$^{-/-}$ mice (middle), and α3NC1-immunized D1.Cfb$^{-/-}$ mice (right) at week 8 after the initial immunization. **(A)** Immunofluorescence staining for mouse IgG shows glomerular basement membrane (GBM) staining in α3NC1-immunized D1.Cfb$^{-/-}$ and D1.Cfb$^{+/+}$ mice. Adjuvant-immunized control mice show non-specific mesangial IgG deposition. **(B)** Mean fluorescence intensity (MFI) of IgG staining, expressed in arbitrary units (AU), was compared in α3NC1-immunized D1.Cfb$^{-/-}$ and D2.Cfb$^{+/+}$ mice. The difference was not significant (n.s.) by t test. **(C)** Staining with mAb RH34 shows the GBM deposition of exogenous antigen in both groups of α3NC1-immunized mice, which is absent in control mice. **(D)** Direct immunofluorescence staining reveals capillary loop deposition of C3c in α3NC1-immunized D1.Cfb$^{+/+}$ mice, while C3c staining is absent in D1.Cfb$^{-/-}$ mice. **(E)** Indirect immunofluorescence shows C5b-9 deposition along the GBM in α3NC1-immunized D1.Cfb$^{+/+}$ mice but not D1.Cfb$^{-/-}$ mice. Original magnification 400×.

staining intensity was similar in D1.Cfb$^{-/-}$ and D1.Cfb$^{+/+}$ mice (**Figure 8B**). Staining with mAb RH34 showed GBM deposition of exogenous antigen in these mice (**Figure 8C**). Capillary loop deposition of C3c (**Figure 8D**) and C5b-9 staining (**Figure 8E**) was observed in α3NC1-immunized D1.Cfb$^{+/+}$ mice but was absent from α3NC1 immunized D1.Cfb$^{-/-}$ mice. These results confirm that the AP is essential for pathogenic complement activation by subepithelial immune complexes and further show that the ablation of the AP abolishes proteinuria to a greater extent than C5 deficiency under comparable experimental conditions.

Subepithelial Immune Complexes Activate Complement *In Vitro via* the AP

Since α3NC1-immunized Cfb$^{-/-}$ mice had glomerular IgG but not C3c deposition, we investigated whether immune complexes formed in these mice can activate complement *in vitro*. To this end, kidney cryosections from D1.Cfb$^{-/-}$ mice were incubated with normal mouse serum as a source of complement. As shown in **Figure 9**, glomerular capillary loops deposition of C3c was found after incubation with normal mouse serum in the presence of Ca^{2+} and Mg^{2+} (in which all three pathways are active), and also in the presence of Mg^{2+} and EGTA (conditions under which the

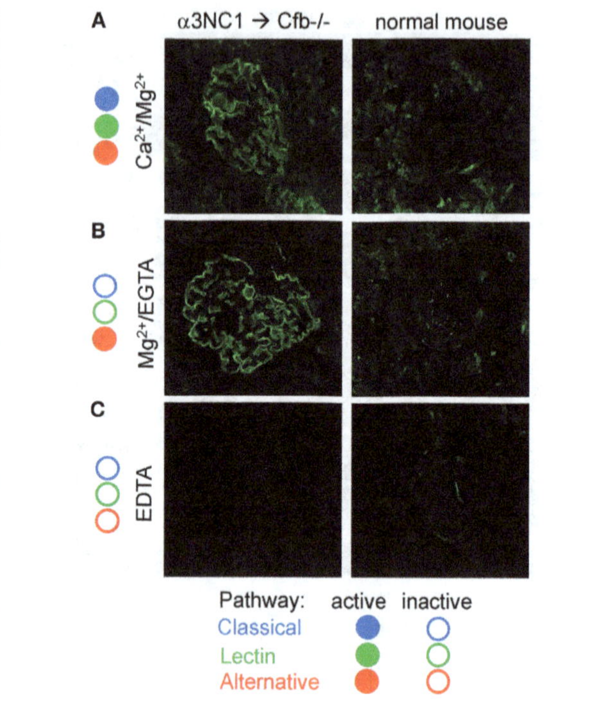

FIGURE 9 | *In vitro* complement activation by glomerular immune complexes from α3NC1-immunized $Cfb^{-/-}$ mice. Immunofluorescence analysis of C3c deposition onto kidneys cryosections from α3NC1-immunized D1.$Cfb^{-/-}$ mice (left) and control non-immunized wild-type DBA/1 mice (right), after incubation with 33% normal mouse serum in buffer containing Ca^{2+} and Mg^{2+} **(A)**, Mg^{2+} and EGTA **(B)**, or EDTA **(C)**. Complement pathways active in each buffer are indicated on the left, according to the key shown at the bottom.

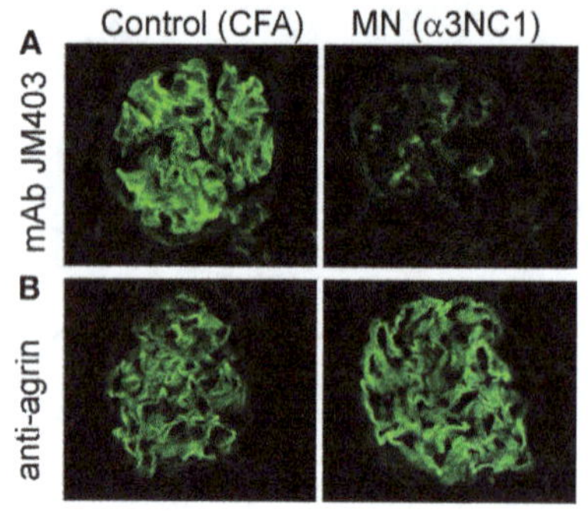

FIGURE 10 | Decreased glomerular basement membrane (GBM) staining by anti-heparan sulfate mAb JM403 in experimental MN. **(A)** Immunofluorescence staining with anti-heparan sulfate mAb JM403 revealed intense staining in the GBM of control mice, which was markedly decreased in α3NC1-immunized B6.$Cfb^{+/+}$ mice. **(B)** GBM staining for agrin core protein was similar in both groups.

alternative pathway is active, but the classical and lectin pathways are inhibited), but not in the presence EDTA (which inhibits all thee pathways). In control experiments using kidney cryosections from a non-immunized wild-type mouse (i.e., without glomerular IgG deposits), no C3c deposition along the capillary loops was observed under any conditions. Similar results were obtained using human serum as complement source (not shown). These results indicate that glomerular immune complexes formed *in vivo* in α3NC1-immunized $Cfb^{-/-}$ mice have the intrinsic ability to activate complement *via* the AP.

The Loss of GBM Heparan Sulfate in Experimental MN May Affect the Local AP Regulation

Activation of the AP on extracellular matrices, which are not protected by intrinsic complement regulators, is largely controlled by factor H. Factor H selectively inhibits the AP on host surfaces by recognizing polyanions such as heparan sulfate as markers of self. The normal GBM contains heparan sulfate chains attached to the agrin core protein, but the GBM staining for heparan sulfate epitopes is markedly decreased in human MN and rat Heymann nephritis (34–36). We investigated whether similar changes occur after the induction of experimental MN in mice. Compared to adjuvant-immunized control mice, α3NC1-immunized B6 (**Figure 10**) and D1 mice (not shown) with proteinuria had almost complete loss of GBM staining by anti-heparan sulfate mAb JM403, while staining for agrin core protein was not changed. These results demonstrate the loss of heparan sulfate epitopes from the GBM of α3NC1-immunized mice, which may locally dysregulate the AP by reducing the recruitment of factor H (37).

DISCUSSION

Whereas podocyte injury by C5b-9 is a major effector mechanism of the subepithelial immune complexes that lead to proteinuria in MN, the role of specific complement pathways upstream of C5 activation remains poorly understood. Glomerular deposition of complement components specific to the AP in human MN raises the question of whether the AP activation is pathogenically relevant or just an epiphenomenon. We addressed this question by evaluating how the absence of a functional AP affects kidney disease in a mouse model of MN. We found that $Cfb^{-/-}$ and $Cfb^{+/+}$ mice immunized with α3NC1 developed subepithelial immune complexes, with similar IgG deposition. However, $Cfb^{-/-}$ mice were protected against proteinuria and did not exhibit glomerular deposition of C3c and C5b-9. These results imply that the AP is required for glomerular complement activation by subepithelial immune complexes, which in turn is necessary for proteinuria. We thus provide the first direct evidence implicating the AP in the pathogenesis of experimental MN.

Complement activation can contribute to kidney disease at several levels, by causing direct injury at the glomerular filtration barrier, and also by augmenting the production of pathogenic antibodies (38). The latter appears unlikely in our model, as the levels of circulating anti-α3NC1 antibodies and kidney-bound IgG were similar in $Cfb^{-/-}$ and wild-type mice. Hence, the more likely mechanism by which the absence of factor B protects against proteinuria is *via* the reduced complement activation at the level of C3 and C5, as implied by the absence of glomerular C3c and C5b-9 staining in $Cfb^{-/-}$ mice despite the presence of subepithelial immune deposits. While immune complexes typically activate complement *via* the classical pathway, the AP is secondarily activated and forms an amplification loop. In a quantitative assay of complement activation initiated *via* the classical pathway (by IgM or aggregated IgG), the AP accounted for more than 80% of the C5 activation products (C5a, sC5b-9) generated in the assay (39). This amplification explains the pathogenic role of the AP in various animal models of immune complex-mediated diseases, including lupus nephritis (40–42). An increased generation of C3b would exacerbate the formation of C5b-9, which is pathogenic in MN, because C5 binding to C3b is a prerequisite for C5 activation, and very high affinity C5 convertases only form at high surface density of C3b (43, 44).

How glomerular immune complexes activate complement depends on several factors, including their ultrastructural localization and immunoglobulin composition. In human anti-GBM disease, IgG1 auto-antibodies that bind to α345(IV) collagen in the human GBM (usually specific for α3NC1) cause severe glomerulonephritis, often featuring C3 deposition along the GBM (45). By contrast, in wild-type mice, human or murine IgG antibodies that bind to α345(IV) collagen in the mouse GBM are insufficient to cause local complement activation or glomerular injury (46, 47). It is, therefore, remarkable that subepithelial immune complexes formed by mouse IgG anti-α3NC1 antibodies with exogenous rh-α3NC1 antigen (*via* a planted antigen mechanism) are able to activate complement *in vivo* and *in vitro*, even though anti-α3NC1 antibodies are predominantly of mouse IgG1 subclass. Mouse IgG1 functionally resembles human IgG4 (the predominant IgG subclass in human primary MN), in that neither binds C1q to activate the classical pathway (48). However, mouse IgG1 can activate the AP (49), as do human IgG2 and IgA (50). Whether human IgG4 can activate the AP remains an important question yet to be solved. In preliminary studies, we found that the AP amplifies *in vitro* complement activation by immune complexes formed by human anti-PLA2R IgG autoantibodies (Dorin-Bogdan Borza and Laurence H. Beck, unpublished observations).

The extent to which the AP is activated is also modulated by the local microenvironment. Although the AP is constitutively active and self-amplifies on foreign surfaces, its activation on self-surfaces is normally restricted by host complement regulatory proteins that inactivate C3 and C5 convertases. In glomeruli, podocytes are protected by membrane-bound regulators such as CR1, while plasma factor H is recruited to inhibit the AP in the GBM (51). Studies in the nephrotoxic nephritis model, in which the AP contributes to chronic but not acute kidney injury, suggest that the mechanisms controlling the AP may be impaired over time by the persistence of antibodies or by glomerular injury (52). One mechanism that could locally dysregulate the AP is the loss of heparan sulfate chains, which factor H normally recognizes as markers of self (37). Decreased GBM staining by anti-heparan sulfate mAb JM403 occurs in α3NC1-immunized mice (this study) and also in human MN (53) and a rat model of MN, active Heymann nephritis (36). The loss of GBM heparan sulfate may be the result of enzymatic cleavage by heparanase, which is often upregulated in glomerular disease (54), including in Heymann nephritis (55). It may also be due to other mechanisms (56). An apparent loss of heparan sulfate occurs in lupus nephritis due to masking by immune complexes (57). Besides factor H, heparan sulfate can also bind properdin, thus serving as a platform for AP activation on some surfaces, such as the apical surface of kidney tubules or apoptotic T cells (58, 59). In our model, given the loss of GBM heparan sulfate, glomerular deposition of properdin is more likely due to properdin binding to C3b and stabilization of the C3bBb convertase (60). Elucidating the relationships among the loss of GBM heparan sulfate, local complement regulation and proteinuria is an area for future investigations.

The role of C5b-9 in proteinuria induced by subepithelial immune complexes has been demonstrated in passive Heymann nephritis (11), but not validated in other models of MN to date. In this study, we found that C5-deficient DBA/2 mice developed significantly less proteinuria than C5-sufficient DBA/1 mice, which further supports the paradigm that C5 activation mediates glomerular injury by subepithelial immune complexes. Cleavage of C5 generates C5b, a precursor for C5b-9, and also C5a, a pro-inflammatory anaphylatoxin. Although our results cannot formally exclude a pathogenic role for C5a in the MN model used in this study, there is currently no evidence to implicate C5a as meditator of glomerular injury in MN, and inflammatory cells are usually not detected in glomeruli in MN.

An unexpected finding in this study was that the absence of factor B abolished proteinuria to a greater extent than the absence of complement C5. Under similar experimental conditions, albuminuria in C5-deficient D2 mice (ACR 2.38 ± 0.96) was reduced by a factor of about 30 compared to C5-sufficient D1 mice (ACR 77.1 ± 20.8), while albuminuria in D1.Cfb$^{-/-}$ mice (ACR 0.36 ± 0.12) was reduced by a factor of about 200 compared to D1.Cfb$^{+/+}$ mice (ACR 78.8 ± 18.1)—a sixfold difference. This difference may be explained by the fact the absence of C5 only prevents events downstream of C5 activation (such as C5b-9 formation), while the absence of factor B also inhibits complement activation at the level of C3. Indeed, glomerular C3c deposition was absent in Cfb$^{-/-}$ mice but present in C5-null mice. These results suggest that complement activation at the level of C3 may also contribute to proteinuria in MN, independently of C5b-9-mediated glomerular injury.

Our study has some limitations. The role of the AP in experimental MN was only investigated using genetic approaches. Further corroboration by pharmacologic inhibition of the AP in a clinically relevant setting is desirable. This is evaluated in ongoing studies. Another potential caveat is that subepithelial immune complexes induced by immunization with α3NC1 are formed by a planted antigen mechanism, recapitulating secondary MN rather than primary MN. Nonetheless, glomerular deposition of factor B occurs not only in primary but also secondary MN (6), suggesting that the AP is involved regardless of how subepithelial immune complexes form. We expect that future studies will address the pathogenic role of the AP in emerging animal models of MN, which target autoantigens implicated in human disease. Of interest in this regard, mice injected with human anti-THSD7A antibodies develop mild proteinuria with histologic features of MN (61). However, efforts to develop models of MN targeting PLA2R have been hampered by the fact that rodents (unlike humans) do not express PLA2R on podocytes.

A better understanding of the complement-mediated mechanisms of injury in MN may help develop novel therapies for MN. MN is a common cause of nephrotic syndrome in adults, and up to 40% of patients eventually develop end-stage renal disease (62). Current therapies use non-specific immunosuppressive drugs, which have significant toxic side effects and are ineffective in about 25–30% of patients (2, 63, 64). Therapeutic inhibition of complement may be a viable approach for treating MN (65), especially in patients who do not respond to conventional therapy or have rapid deterioration of renal function. One anti-complement agent already in clinical use is eculizumab, a humanized IgG2/IgG4 anti-C5 monoclonal antibody that blocks C5 activation. An early, unpublished clinical trial of eculizumab in primary MN did not find a significant remission of proteinuria after 16 weeks of treatment, which may be explained by the insufficient dosage of the drug. Indeed, a recent study has found that C5 inhibition by eculizumab is incomplete at high C3b density (44), a setting relevant to MN. Compared to eculizumab, which does not prevent potentially harmful C3 activation, agents that inhibit complement at the level of both C3 and C5 may offer additional therapeutic benefit. The results of this study identify the AP as a novel target for therapy in MN. Inhibition of the AP has the advantage of leaving the classical and lectin pathways intact for defense against pathogens and other homeostatic functions.

In summary, our results suggest that the AP is necessary for sustained complement activation by subepithelial immune complexes, leading to glomerular deposition of C3c and C5b-9. Furthermore, the activation of the AP is essential for the devel¯opment of proteinuria in experimental MN. These findings may provide a framework for the rational design of new therapies for MN.

AUTHOR CONTRIBUTIONS

D-BB conceived the idea, designed the experiments, performed data analysis, and wrote the manuscript. WL and FO performed experiments and collected, assembled, and interpreted data. JM performed experiments. JV provided reagents. JT provided mice and reagents and interpreted data. LB analyzed and interpreted data. All authors contributed to editing, reviewed and approved the final manuscript.

ACKNOWLEDGMENTS

We thank Linna Ge for excellent technical assistance. Polyclonal anti-agrin antibody was a gift from Dr. Takako Sasaki (Oita University, Japan). Rat mAb RH34 was a generous gift from Dr. Yoshikazu Sado (Shigei Medical Research Institute, Okayama, Japan).

FUNDING

This work was supported by Paul Teschan Research Fund grant from the Dialysis Clinic Inc. (DB-B), by Meharry Translational Research Center grant U54 MD007593 from the National Institute on Minority Health and Health Disparities of the National Institutes of Health, by the Norman S. Coplon Extramural Grant Program from Satellite Healthcare (DB-B), and by internal funds from the Meharry Medical College (DB-B). Support was also received from the National Institutes of Health grants DK113586 and DK076690 (JMT) and R01DK078314 (JM). Electron microscopy was performed by the Washington University O'Brien Center for Kidney Disease Research, supported by grant P30 DK079333.

REFERENCES

1. Beck LH Jr, Salant DJ. Membranous nephropathy: from models to man. *J Clin Invest* (2014) 124(6):2307–14. doi:10.1172/JCI72270
2. Cattran DC, Brenchley PE. Membranous nephropathy: integrating basic science into improved clinical management. *Kidney Int* (2017) 91(3):566–74. doi:10.1016/j.kint.2016.09.048
3. Beck LH Jr, Bonegio RG, Lambeau G, Beck DM, Powell DW, Cummins TD, et al. M-type phospholipase A2 receptor as target antigen in idiopathic membranous nephropathy. *N Engl J Med* (2009) 361(1):11–21. doi:10.1056/NEJMoa0810457
4. Tomas NM, Beck LH Jr, Meyer-Schwesinger C, Seitz-Polski B, Ma H, Zahner G, et al. Thrombospondin type-1 domain-containing 7A in idiopathic membranous nephropathy. *N Engl J Med* (2014) 371(24):2277–87. doi:10.1056/NEJMoa1409354
5. Debiec H, Lefeu F, Kemper MJ, Niaudet P, Deschenes G, Remuzzi G, et al. Early-childhood membranous nephropathy due to cationic bovine serum albumin. *N Engl J Med* (2011) 364(22):2101–10. doi:10.1056/NEJMoa1013792
6. Ma H, Sandor DG, Beck LH Jr. The role of complement in membranous nephropathy. *Semin Nephrol* (2013) 33(6):531–42. doi:10.1016/j.semnephrol.2013.08.004
7. Brenchley PE, Coupes B, Short CD, O'Donoghue DJ, Ballardie FW, Mallick NP. Urinary C3dg and C5b-9 indicate active immune disease in human membranous nephropathy. *Kidney Int* (1992) 41(4):933–7. doi:10.1038/ki.1992.143
8. Zhang R, Zheng ZY, Lin JS, Qu LJ, Zheng F. The continual presence of C3d but not IgG glomerular capillary deposition in stage I idiopathic membranous nephropathy in patients receiving corticosteroid treatment. *Diagn Pathol* (2012) 7:109. doi:10.1186/1746-1596-7-109
9. Papagianni AA, Alexopoulos E, Leontsini M, Papadimitriou M. C5b-9 and adhesion molecules in human idiopathic membranous nephropathy. *Nephrol Dial Transplant* (2002) 17(1):57–63. doi:10.1093/ndt/17.1.57
10. Cybulsky AV, Rennke HG, Feintzeig ID, Salant DJ. Complement-induced glomerular epithelial cell injury. Role of the membrane attack complex in rat membranous nephropathy. *J Clin Invest* (1986) 77(4):1096–107. doi:10.1172/JCI112408
11. Baker PJ, Ochi RF, Schulze M, Johnson RJ, Campbell C, Couser WG. Depletion of C6 prevents development of proteinuria in experimental membranous nephropathy in rats. *Am J Pathol* (1989) 135(1):185–94.
12. Doi T, Mayumi M, Kanatsu K, Suehiro F, Hamashima Y. Distribution of IgG subclasses in membranous nephropathy. *Clin Exp Immunol* (1984) 58(1):57–62.
13. Kanigicherla D, Gummadova J, McKenzie EA, Roberts SA, Harris S, Nikam M, et al. Anti-PLA2R antibodies measured by ELISA predict long-term outcome in a prevalent population of patients with idiopathic membranous nephropathy. *Kidney Int* (2013) 83(5):940–8. doi:10.1038/ki.2012.486
14. Larsen CP, Messias NC, Silva FG, Messias E, Walker PD. Determination of primary versus secondary membranous glomerulopathy utilizing phospholipase A2 receptor staining in renal biopsies. *Mod Pathol* (2013) 26(5):709–15. doi:10.1038/modpathol.2012.207

15. van der Zee JS, van Swieten P, Aalberse RC. Inhibition of complement activation by IgG4 antibodies. *Clin Exp Immunol* (1986) 64(2):415–22.
16. Vidarsson G, Dekkers G, Rispens T. IgG subclasses and allotypes: from structure to effector functions. *Front Immunol* (2014) 5:520. doi:10.3389/fimmu.2014.00520
17. Tao MH, Canfield SM, Morrison SL. The differential ability of human IgG1 and IgG4 to activate complement is determined by the COOH-terminal sequence of the CH2 domain. *J Exp Med* (1991) 173(4):1025–8. doi:10.1084/jem.173.4.1025
18. Segawa Y, Hisano S, Matsushita M, Fujita T, Hirose S, Takeshita M, et al. IgG subclasses and complement pathway in segmental and global membranous nephropathy. *Pediatr Nephrol* (2010) 25(6):1091–9. doi:10.1007/s00467-009-1439-8
19. Kusunoki Y, Itami N, Tochimaru H, Takekoshi Y, Nagasawa S, Yoshiki T. Glomerular deposition of C4 cleavage fragment (C4d) and C4-binding protein in idiopathic membranous glomerulonephritis. *Nephron* (1989) 51(1):17–9. doi:10.1159/000185234
20. Val-Bernal JF, Garijo MF, Val D, Rodrigo E, Arias M. C4d immunohistochemical staining is a sensitive method to confirm immunoreactant deposition in formalin-fixed paraffin-embedded tissue in membranous glomerulonephritis. *Histol Histopathol* (2011) 26(11):1391–7. doi:10.14670/HH-26.1391
21. Bally S, Debiec H, Ponard D, Dijoud F, Rendu J, Faure J, et al. Phospholipase A2 receptor-related membranous nephropathy and mannan-binding lectin deficiency. *J Am Soc Nephrol* (2016) 27(12):3539–44. doi:10.1681/ASN.2015101155
22. Zhang JJ, Malekpour M, Luo W, Ge L, Olaru F, Wang XP, et al. Murine membranous nephropathy: immunization with alpha3(IV) collagen fragment induces subepithelial immune complexes and FcgammaR-independent nephrotic syndrome. *J Immunol* (2012) 188(7):3268–77. doi:10.4049/jimmunol.1103368
23. Borza DB, Zhang JJ, Beck LH Jr, Meyer-Schwesinger C, Luo W. Mouse models of membranous nephropathy: the road less travelled by. *Am J Clin Exp Immunol* (2013) 2(2):135–45.
24. Hopfer H, Holzer J, Hunemorder S, Paust HJ, Sachs M, Meyer-Schwesinger C, et al. Characterization of the renal CD4(+) T-cell response in experimental autoimmune glomerulonephritis. *Kidney Int* (2012) 82(1):60–71. doi:10.1038/ki.2012.73
25. Hopfer H, Hunemorder S, Treder J, Turner JE, Paust HJ, Meyer-Schwesinger C, et al. Glomerulopathy induced by immunization with a peptide derived from the goodpasture antigen alpha3IV-NC1. *J Immunol* (2015) 194(8):3646–55. doi:10.4049/jimmunol.1401267
26. Boutaud A, Borza DB, Bondar O, Gunwar S, Netzer KO, Singh N, et al. Type IV collagen of the glomerular basement membrane: evidence that the chain specificity of network assembly is encoded by the noncollagenous NC1 domains. *J Biol Chem* (2000) 275:30716–24. doi:10.1074/jbc.M004569200
27. Harvey SJ, Jarad G, Cunningham J, Rops AL, van der Vlag J, Berden JH, et al. Disruption of glomerular basement membrane charge through podocyte-specific mutation of agrin does not alter glomerular permselectivity. *Am J Pathol* (2007) 171(1):139–52. doi:10.2353/ajpath.2007.061116
28. Heidet L, Borza DB, Jouin M, Sich M, Mattei MG, Sado Y, et al. A human-mouse chimera of the alpha3alpha4alpha5(IV) collagen protomer rescues the renal phenotype in Col4a3(-/-) Alport mice. *Am J Pathol* (2003) 163(4):1633–44. doi:10.1016/S0002-9440(10)63520-1
29. van den Born J, van den Heuvel LP, Bakker MA, Veerkamp JH, Assmann KJ, Berden JH. A monoclonal antibody against GBM heparan sulfate induces an acute selective proteinuria in rats. *Kidney Int* (1992) 41(1):115–23. doi:10.1038/ki.1992.15
30. Olaru F, Luo W, Suleiman H, St John PL, Ge L, Mezo AR, et al. Neonatal fc receptor promotes immune complex-mediated glomerular disease. *J Am Soc Nephrol* (2014) 25(5):918–25. doi:10.1681/ASN.2013050498
31. Wetsel RA, Fleischer DT, Haviland DL. Deficiency of the murine fifth complement component (C5). A 2-base pair gene deletion in a 5'-exon. *J Biol Chem* (1990) 265(5):2435–40.
32. Wade CM, Daly MJ. Genetic variation in laboratory mice. *Nat Genet* (2005) 37(11):1175–80. doi:10.1038/ng1666
33. Zwirner J, Felber E, Herzog V, Riethmuller G, Feucht HE. Classical pathway of complement activation in normal and diseased human glomeruli. *Kidney Int* (1989) 36(6):1069–77. doi:10.1038/ki.1989.302
34. van den Born J, van den Heuvel LP, Bakker MA, Veerkamp JH, Assmann KJ, Weening JJ, et al. Distribution of GBM heparan sulfate proteoglycan core protein and side chains in human glomerular diseases. *Kidney Int* (1993) 43(2):454–63. doi:10.1038/ki.1993.67
35. Levidiotis V, Freeman C, Punler M, Martinello P, Creese B, Ferro V, et al. A synthetic heparanase inhibitor reduces proteinuria in passive Heymann nephritis. *J Am Soc Nephrol* (2004) 15(11):2882–92. doi:10.1097/01.ASN.0000142426.55612.6D
36. Raats CJ, Luca ME, Bakker MA, Van Der Wal A, Heeringa P, Van Goor H, et al. Reduction in glomerular heparan sulfate correlates with complement deposition and albuminuria in active Heymann nephritis. *J Am Soc Nephrol* (1999) 10(8):1689–99.
37. Borza DB. Glomerular basement membrane heparan sulfate in health and disease: a regulator of local complement activation. *Matrix Biol* (2017) 57-58:299–310. doi:10.1016/j.matbio.2016.09.002
38. Carroll MC, Isenman DE. Regulation of humoral immunity by complement. *Immunity* (2012) 37(2):199–207. doi:10.1016/j.immuni.2012.08.002
39. Harboe M, Ulvund G, Vien L, Fung M, Mollnes TE. The quantitative role of alternative pathway amplification in classical pathway induced terminal complement activation. *Clin Exp Immunol* (2004) 138(3):439–46. doi:10.1111/j.1365-2249.2004.02627.x
40. Banda NK, Thurman JM, Kraus D, Wood A, Carroll MC, Arend WP, et al. Alternative complement pathway activation is essential for inflammation and joint destruction in the passive transfer model of collagen-induced arthritis. *J Immunol* (2006) 177(3):1904–12. doi:10.4049/jimmunol.177.3.1904
41. Mihai S, Chiriac MT, Takahashi K, Thurman JM, Holers VM, Zillikens D, et al. The alternative pathway of complement activation is critical for blister induction in experimental epidermolysis bullosa acquisita. *J Immunol* (2007) 178(10):6514–21. doi:10.4049/jimmunol.178.10.6514
42. Watanabe H, Garnier G, Circolo A, Wetsel RA, Ruiz P, Holers VM, et al. Modulation of renal disease in MRL/lpr mice genetically deficient in the alternative complement pathway factor B. *J Immunol* (2000) 164(2):786–94. doi:10.4049/jimmunol.164.2.786
43. Rawal N, Pangburn M. Formation of high-affinity C5 convertases of the alternative pathway of complement. *J Immunol* (2001) 166(4):2635–42. doi:10.4049/jimmunol.166.4.2635
44. Harder MJ, Kuhn N, Schrezenmeier H, Hochsmann B, von Zabern I, Weinstock C, et al. Incomplete inhibition by eculizumab: mechanistic evidence for residual C5 activity during strong complement activation. *Blood* (2017) 129(8):970–80. doi:10.1182/blood-2016-08-732800
45. Borza DB. Autoepitopes and alloepitopes of type IV collagen: role in the molecular pathogenesis of anti-GBM antibody glomerulonephritis. *Nephron Exp Nephrol* (2007) 106(2):e37–43. doi:10.1159/000101791
46. Olaru F, Wang XP, Luo W, Ge L, Miner JH, Kleinau S, et al. Proteolysis breaks tolerance toward intact alpha345(IV) collagen, eliciting novel anti-glomerular basement membrane autoantibodies specific for alpha345NC1 hexamers. *J Immunol* (2013) 190(4):1424–32. doi:10.4049/jimmunol.1202204
47. Luo W, Wang XP, Kashtan CE, Borza DB. Alport alloantibodies but not Goodpasture autoantibodies induce murine glomerulonephritis: protection by quinary crosslinks locking cryptic alpha3(IV) collagen autoepitopes in vivo. *J Immunol* (2010) 185(6):3520–8. doi:10.4049/jimmunol.1001152
48. Lilienthal G-M, Rahmöller J, Petry J, Bartsch YC, Leliavski A, Ehlers M. Potential of murine IgG1 and human IgG4 to inhibit the classical complement and Fcγ receptor activation pathways. *Front Immunol* (2018) 9:958. doi:10.3389/fimmu.2018.00958
49. Seino J, Eveleigh P, Warnaar S, van Haarlem LJ, van Es LA, Daha MR. Activation of human complement by mouse and mouse/human chimeric monoclonal antibodies. *Clin Exp Immunol* (1993) 94(2):291–6. doi:10.1111/j.1365-2249.1993.tb03446.x
50. Lucisano Valim YM, Lachmann PJ. The effect of antibody isotype and antigenic epitope density on the complement-fixing activity of immune complexes: a systematic study using chimaeric anti-NIP antibodies with human Fc regions. *Clin Exp Immunol* (1991) 84(1):1–8. doi:10.1111/j.1365-2249.1991.tb08115.x
51. Laskowski J, Renner B, Le Quintrec M, Panzer S, Hannan JP, Ljubanovic D, et al. Distinct roles for the complement regulators factor H and Crry in protection of the kidney from injury. *Kidney Int* (2016) 90(1):109–22. doi:10.1016/j.kint.2016.02.036
52. Thurman JM, Tchepeleva SN, Haas M, Panzer S, Boackle SA, Glogowska MJ, et al. Complement alternative pathway activation in the autologous phase of nephrotoxic serum nephritis. *Am J Physiol Renal Physiol* (2012) 302(12):F1529–36. doi:10.1152/ajprenal.00422.2011

53. Borza DB. Alternative pathway dysregulation and the conundrum of complement activation by IgG4 immune complexes in membranous nephropathy. *Front Immunol* (2016) 7:157. doi:10.3389/fimmu.2016.00157
54. van den Hoven MJ, Rops AL, Vlodavsky I, Levidiotis V, Berden JH, van der Vlag J. Heparanase in glomerular diseases. *Kidney Int* (2007) 72(5):543–8. doi:10.1038/sj.ki.5002337
55. Levidiotis V, Freeman C, Tikellis C, Cooper ME, Power DA. Heparanase is involved in the pathogenesis of proteinuria as a result of glomerulonephritis. *J Am Soc Nephrol* (2004) 15(1):68–78. doi:10.1097/01.ASN.0000103229.25389.40
56. Raats CJ, Van Den Born J, Berden JH. Glomerular heparan sulfate alterations: mechanisms and relevance for proteinuria. *Kidney Int* (2000) 57(2):385–400. doi:10.1046/j.1523-1755.2000.00858.x
57. van Bruggen MC, Kramers K, Hylkema MN, van den Born J, Bakker MA, Assmann KJ, et al. Decrease of heparan sulfate staining in the glomerular basement membrane in murine lupus nephritis. *Am J Pathol* (1995) 146(3):753–63.
58. Kemper C, Mitchell LM, Zhang L, Hourcade DE. The complement protein properdin binds apoptotic T cells and promotes complement activation and phagocytosis. *Proc Natl Acad Sci U S A* (2008) 105(26):9023–8. doi:10.1073/pnas.0801015105
59. Zaferani A, Vives RR, van der Pol P, Hakvoort JJ, Navis GJ, van Goor H, et al. Identification of tubular heparan sulfate as a docking platform for the alternative complement component properdin in proteinuric renal disease. *J Biol Chem* (2011) 286(7):5359–67. doi:10.1074/jbc.M110.167825
60. Harboe M, Johnson C, Nymo S, Ekholt K, Schjalm C, Lindstad JK, et al. Properdin binding to complement activating surfaces depends on initial C3b deposition. *Proc Natl Acad Sci U S A* (2017) 114(4):E534–9. doi:10.1073/pnas.1612385114
61. Tomas NM, Hoxha E, Reinicke AT, Fester L, Helmchen U, Gerth J, et al. Autoantibodies against thrombospondin type 1 domain-containing 7A induce membranous nephropathy. *J Clin Invest* (2016) 126(7):2519–32. doi:10.1172/JCI85265
62. Fervenza FC, Sethi S, Specks U. Idiopathic membranous nephropathy: diagnosis and treatment. *Clin J Am Soc Nephrol* (2008) 3(3):905–19. doi:10.2215/CJN.04321007
63. Glassock RJ. The treatment of idiopathic membranous nephropathy: a dilemma or a conundrum? *Am J Kidney Dis* (2004) 44(3):562–6. doi:10.1016/S0272-6386(04)00868-6
64. Ruggenenti P, Fervenza FC, Remuzzi G. Treatment of membranous nephropathy: time for a paradigm shift. *Nat Rev Nephrol* (2017) 13(9):563–79. doi:10.1038/nrneph.2017.92
65. Wiggins RC, Alpers CE, Holzman LB, He JC, Salant DJ, Chugh SS, et al. Glomerular disease: looking beyond pathology. *Clin J Am Soc Nephrol* (2014) 9(6):1138–40. doi:10.2215/CJN.01450214

5

Analysis of C3 Gene Variants in Patients with Idiopathic Recurrent Spontaneous Pregnancy Loss

*Frida C. Mohlin[1], Piet Gros[2], Eric Mercier[3], Jean-Christophe Raymond Gris[3] and Anna M. Blom[1]**

[1] Department of Translational Medicine, Lund University, Malmö, Sweden, [2] Crystal and Structural Chemistry, Bijvoet Center for Biomolecular Research, Department of Chemistry, Utrecht University, Utrecht, Netherlands, [3] Laboratory of Hematology, University Hospital, Nimes, France

***Correspondence:**
Anna M. Blom
anna.blom@med.lu.se

Miscarriage is the most common complication of pregnancy. Approximately 1% of couples trying to conceive will experience recurrent miscarriages, defined as three or more consecutive pregnancy losses and many of these cases remain idiopathic. Complement is implicated both in the physiology and pathology of pregnancy. Therefore, we hypothesized that alterations in the C3 gene could potentially predispose to this disorder. We performed full Sanger sequencing of all exons of C3, in 192 childless women, with at least two miscarriages and without any known risk factors. All exons carrying non-synonymous alterations found in the patients were then sequenced in a control group of 192 women. None of the identified alterations were significantly associated with the disorder. Thirteen identified non-synonymous alterations (R102G, K155Q, L302P, P314L, Y325H, V326A, S327P, V330I, K633R, R735W, R1591G, G1606D, and S1619R) were expressed recombinantly, upon which C3 expression and secretion were determined. The L302P and S327P were not secreted from the cells, likely due to misfolding and intracellular degradation. Y325H, V326A, V3301I, R1591G, and G1606D yielded approximately half C3 concentration in the cell media compared with wild type (WT). We analyzed the hemolytic activity of the secreted C3 variants by reconstituting C3-depleted serum. In this assay, R1591G had impaired hemolytic activity while majority of remaining mutants instead had increased activity. R1591G also yielded more factor B activation in solution compared with WT. R1591G and G1606D showed impaired degradation by factor I, irrespectively if factor H, CD46, or C4b-binding protein were used as cofactors. These two C3 mutants showed impaired binding of the cofactors and/or factor I. Taken together, several alterations in C3 were identified and some of these affected the secretion and/or the function of the protein, which might contribute to the disorder but the degree of association must be evaluated in larger cohorts.

Keywords: reproductive immunology, miscarriage, complement system, C3, mutation

INTRODUCTION

Spontaneous pregnancy loss, or miscarriage, is the most common complication of pregnancy and includes all pregnancy losses from conception until 24 weeks of gestation. It is believed that as many as 50% of all conceptions and 15% of clinically recognized pregnancies end up in miscarriage (1). The definition of recurrent spontaneous pregnancy loss (RSPL) differs among international societies.

Abbreviations: AMD, age-related macular degeneration; C4BP, C4b-binding protein; HEK, human embryonic kidney; RSPL, recurrent spontaneous pregnancy loss; WT, wild type.

The American Society for Reproductive Medicine defines RSPL as two or more pregnancy losses (2), affecting around 5% of couples trying to conceive, while The European Society for Human Reproduction and Embryology defines it as three or more consecutive losses (3), affecting around 1% of couples trying to conceive. Over the years, various etiologies have been identified, such as genetic, structural, autoimmune, endocrine, thrombophilic abnormalities, together with infections. However, approximately 40–50% of the cases still remain idiopathic (1).

Pregnancy is a complex process, where on the one hand significant adaptations of the immune system is needed to tolerate the semiallogenic fetus but on the other hand, an active immune system is needed to defend the mother and fetus from infections. The complement system, which is a pivotal part of our innate immunity, has been shown to play an important role for a successful pregnancy. Studies have shown that too little or too much complement at the wrong time during pregnancy can have devastating consequences for the pregnancy outcome. Too much complement activation in the placenta may lead to placental damage, with a potential risk of fetal loss and therefore complement inhibition in the placenta is of great importance. Complement inhibitors, such as CD46, CD55, and CD59, are expressed in the placenta and on the surface of the trophoblast (4–6), and the critical role of these inhibitors is demonstrated by the embryonic lethality in mice deficient in Crry (7), an important mouse complement inhibitor that resembles human CD46. Previously, we hypothesized that alterations in the complement inhibitors C4b-binding protein (C4BP), CD46, and CD55 might be associated with an increased complement activation, at the trophoblastic maternal interface, leading to pregnancy loss. Several alterations in C4BP and CD46 were identified and some of these caused altered expression and/or function of the proteins (8). However, complement is not only needed for fighting infections during pregnancy but also for proper placental and fetal development. Despite the complement inhibitors presence in the placenta, some degree of complement activation is seen during normal pregnancy. One example of this importance is that mice deficient in C1q, had abnormal development of the placenta, reduced litter size and fetal weight (9). These mice demonstrated a preeclamptic-like phenotype with proteinuria and increased blood pressure, which indicates that C1q plays an important role for a successful pregnancy. Furthermore, C1q in human placenta has also been implicated in preeclampsia (6).

Complement component C3 is the key protein of the complement system and composed of two polypeptide chains, α- and β-chain. The importance of C3 is demonstrated by the high plasma concentration of 1–1.5 mg/ml (10). The cleavage of C3 by C3-convertases is the central reaction of all three complement pathways and results in the biologically active components C3a, an anaphylatoxin and C3b, a potent opsonin. C3b has an exposed thioester bond, allowing C3b to rapidly bind covalently to cell surfaces and promote further complement activation. C3b will participate to form the C5-convertase and in the final step of the complement cascade, the membrane-attack complex is formed, which has the ability to lyse some target cells, e.g., Gram-negative bacteria (11). Activation of complement can be limited by degradation and inactivation of C3b by factor I, in the presence of different cofactors, such as factor H, CD46, and C4BP (12). C3, along with C3b and most importantly iC3b (the inactivated form of C3b), has been shown to be embryotrophic factors. These factors are mainly derived from the uterus and promote embryonic growth prior to the development of the placenta. In humans, the most abundant embryotrophic factor is embryotrophic factor 3 and this was later found to contain mainly C3, C3b, and iC3b (13). It has also been demonstrated that rat C3 on the visceral yolk sac is important for early embryonic development and in explant rat embryo culture, adding intact C3 significantly favors development, without the requirement of C3 activation (14). C3 knockout mice also demonstrate smaller blastocysts, higher resorption rates, and smaller sizes of the placenta (15). In humans, C3 levels was shown to be higher in patients suffering three consecutive miscarriages, compared with women who went on having a live birth after two miscarriages (16). *In vitro* data also suggest that mutations in *FOXD1*, a transcription factor that directly seems to target C3, leading to both decreased and increased C3 expression, were deleterious (17). Genetic variants in the *C3* gene have also been reported to be associated with severe preeclampsia (18). Thus, C3 appears to have an important physiological role in the early phase of pregnancy and in placental development and a subtle fine-tuning of the C3 level is necessary for optimal function.

Due to the role of C3 in the physiology and pathology of pregnancy, we hypothesized that maternal mutations and polymorphisms in C3 might be associated with pregnancy loss. Herein, we performed full Sanger sequencing of all coding exons of *C3* in women experiencing idiopathic RSPL and we found several heterozygous non-synonymous alterations. The C3 mutants were expressed recombinantly and some of the alterations affected the secretion and/or the function of the protein, which might contribute to the disorder.

MATERIALS AND METHODS

Patients and Controls

Our cohort was previously described in detail (8). Briefly, patients with recurrent pregnancy losses were referred to the Department of Gynecology and Obstetrics or the Hematology Laboratory, University Hospital of Nîmes, France. In total, 1,359 women were pre-selected but the focus was on the 962 most severe cases, defined by at least three consecutive embryonic losses before the 10th gestational week, or two consecutive fetal losses at and beyond the 10th gestational week, all occurring in childless women. These women were screened for classical risk factors for pregnancy loss, such as abnormal parental karyotypes, infectious diseases during pregnancy, uterine anatomical abnormalities, diabetes mellitus, thyroid dysfunction, hyperprolactinaemia prior to luteal phase defects, erythroblastosis fetalis, immune thrombocytopenic purpura, feto-maternal alloimmune thrombocytopenia, and antiphospholipid antibodies. Women were excluded from the study if they had any of the above classical risk factors, previous occurrence of superficial or deep vein thrombosis, were positive for constitutional thrombophilia, preeclampsia, or were of non-Caucasian origin, since this might have introduced consistent confounding heterogeneities in the local frequencies of the polymorphisms and mutations under focus. In the end, 453 women fulfilled all of the criteria and after informed consent was obtained, 429 patients were finally recruited. DNA samples from controls were obtained from women referred to the Department of Gynecology and Obstetrics for a systematic medical exam such as implementation of a new contraception or evaluation of the pelvic floor after pregnancy. Women with no previous pregnancy loss but with at least two uneventful pregnancies were selected ($n = 261$) and similar to cases, these controls were also screened for classical risk factors for pregnancy loss. In total, 224 controls were finally recruited, after informed consent was obtained.

DNA Sequencing

All exons of C3 were sequenced in 192 patients by Polymorphic DNA Technologies (Alameda, CA, USA). A nested PCR amplification of the specific exons preceded the Sanger dideoxy sequencing. The primers used are listed in **Table 1**. The identified non-synonymous alterations found in the patients were then analyzed in a control group of 192 women. All patients and controls were randomly chosen from the cohort defined above. There were no statistical differences in baseline characteristics (age, BMI, ethnicity, and risk factors for vascular diseases) between the patients and controls (**Table 2**). The NHLBI Exome Sequencing Project database[1] was used for investigating the frequencies of the identified C3 non-synonymous alterations in the general population. The PolyPhen software[2] was used for determining the potential effect on the protein function. The sequencing data have been deposited at DDBJ/EMBL/GenBank Targeted Locus Study project under the accession KCDD00000000. The version described in this paper is the first version, KCDD0100000.

Proteins

Factor B, factor D, factor H, C3, and properdin were purchased from Complement Technology. Factor I (19), C4BP (20), CD55 (21), and CD46 (21) were expressed recombinantly and purified, as described previously.

Expression of C3 Variants

The non-synonymous C3 variants of interest (**Table 3**) were expressed recombinantly. cDNA coding for human C3 was used as template and the mutations were introduced by site directed mutagenesis, according to the manufacturer's instruction (QuikChange Lightning, Agilent Technologies). The primers used for mutagenesis are listed in **Table 4**. Automated DNA sequencing confirmed the correct mutations and the constructs were cloned into the mammalian expression vector pCEP4 (Thermo Fisher Scientific). The constructs were transiently transfected into either human embryonic kidney-293 adherent cells (ATCC) using Lipofectamine 2000 (Thermo Fisher Scientific) or Freestyle 293-F cells (Thermo Fisher Scientific) using FreeStyle MAX reagent (Thermo Fisher Scientific). To evaluate the expression and secretion levels of the mutants, the C3 concentration in the supernatants and cell lysates after transient transfection in adherent cells, were determined by ELISA (described below). The same volume (5 µl) of these cell supernatants was also analyzed by Western Blotting, both under non-reducing and reducing (25 mM DTT) conditions. A polyclonal goat anti-human C3 antibody (Quidel), followed by a HRP-conjugated rabbit anti-goat antibody (Dako), were used for detection. The blots were developed using enhanced chemiluminescence (Merck-Millipore). The supernatants from the Freestyle 293-F cells were collected, concentrated, C3 concentration determined by the same ELISA and used in the functional assays. Supernatant from cells transfected with empty pCEP vector were treated in the same manner and used as negative control in all assays. For some functional assays, C3b-like molecules were needed, and this was achieved by treatment of the C3 cell media with 0.1 M methylamine hydrochloride pH 8.0, for 1 h at 37°C, followed by a buffer exchange to TBS (Zeba Spin desalting columns, Thermo Fisher Scientific). Methylamine will create C3met, a C3b-like molecule, by breaking the labile thioester bond in C3 and inducing a conformational change.

C3 Concentration Determination by ELISA

To determine the C3 concentration after protein expression, an ELISA was performed. Two polyclonal antibodies were used, to eliminate the risk that a monoclonal antibody will recognize the mutants differently. Microtiter plates were coated with rabbit anti-human C3c antibody (Dako), diluted in 75 mM sodium carbonate, pH 9.6. The wells were washed with washing buffer (50 mM Tris–HCl, pH 8.0, 0.15 M NaCl, 0.1% Tween) and blocked with 3% fish gelatin (Norland Products) in washing buffer. The samples were diluted in blocking buffer, supplemented with 10 mM EDTA, and incubated on the plate for 1 h at 37°C. Purified C3 from Complement Technology was used as a standard. C3 was then detected using a goat anti-human C3 antibody (Quidel), followed by a HRP-conjugated rabbit anti-goat antibody (Dako). After 1 h incubation at RT for each of the antibodies, the plates were developed using OPD-tablets (Kem-En-Tec). The absorbance at 490 nm was measured spectrophotometrically.

Hemolytic Assay

To assess the hemolytic activity of the C3 variants, a hemolytic assay using C3-depleted serum was performed, essentially as described previously (22). Briefly, antibody-sensitized sheep erythrocytes (Håtunalab AB) was incubated in a V-bottom microtiter plate with 1% C3-depleted serum (Quidel) and four different concentrations (0–2 µg/ml) of either wild type (WT) or mutant C3, in DGVB++ buffer (2.5 mM veronal buffer pH 7.3, containing 70 mM NaCl, 140 mM dextrose, 0.1% porcine gelatin, 1 mM $MgCl_2$, and 0.25 mM $CaCl_2$). The plate was incubated for 1 h at 37°C, during shaking, followed by centrifugation to pellet unlysed erythrocytes. The hemolytic activity was then evaluated by measuring the absorbance, i.e., amount of released hemoglobin, in the supernatant at 405 nm.

Degradation of C3 by Factor I

C3b can be degraded by factor I, in the presence of cofactors such as factor H, CD46, and C4BP. C3 cell media treated with methylamine (C3met) were used. In a total volume of 15 µl, 20 ng of C3met, 25 ng factor I, and either 200 ng factor H or 100 ng CD46 were added in TBS. For C4BP, 20 ng C3met, 50 ng

[1] http://evs.gs.washington.edu/EVS (Accessed: 20 February, 2018).
[2] http://genetics.bwh.harvard.edu/pph2/ (Accessed: 20 February, 2018).

TABLE 1 | Primers used for sequencing of all C3 exons.[a]

Exon no.	Outer primers 5′	Outer primers 3′	Inner primers 5′	Inner primers 3′
1	TGCTGGGGAACATGC	ACAGGCAGCCCAAATAT	GGACTGAAAAGCTTAGGA	ATCATTCCCAACCTGCTAA
2	CCAGAGAAGATAATGGCAT	AAGGAGAGGCGACTC	CGGCAGTCACTGGAT	GGCTTAGAAAGGGAGAA
3–4 (a)	CTCGCACCTCCTTCA	TGACCATGACCGTCC	TCCCTCCCCAAAACG	GTGAAGATCCGATAGAGAA
3–4 (b)	AGGGAGTTCAAGTCAGA	CTGTGTCTCTGCCACT	GTTCGTGACCGTGCA	GCCTCTCCTAAGCCT
5–7 (a)	CTGGGTCCCTGTTCTTA	TCGAAACTGGGCAGC	CTTAACCACAGTAGACACT	GAGATGGCGTTGGTG
5–7 (b)	ACCAGCTTGGCGTCT	CCCACCTGGTCTTCA	CTTGTCTTGGGACATTC	CCTCACCTGGCTCTT
8–9 (a)	TGGGAGTGGGGCAA	GGTGGCAGACACGTA	AGAGGCCAGCAGTG	CAGGTCTTCTGCTCG
8–9 (b)	TCCCGTAGGTTCCTC	CCATCTTCATACTCGGC	GAGGGAACTGCCTTTG	GAACCCCACTTTCACTC
10–11 (a)	CAAGGCCAGTATAAAGGT	TTGGCCACGCCATCT	GTATGAAAGTGGACTCTACT	GACTGCACAGTGTCCT
10–11 (b)	AGATCCACTTCACCAAG	CGCAGGAGAGAACCT	AAGACACCCAAGTACTTC	CTATGCAGATGAGAATATCTGT
12	ATCTCCAGATCCCTAACT	TCCCGCCTTCAACAG	CTAACTTAATCCCATCTGCAA	ACAGGCTGGCATCAG
13	CGCTACTACACCTACC	ACAGTTGAGAGACAGAGA	CCACCTGGAAACCTC	GAGAGAGGAGTAGGGA
14	CTCCCCCCAACCTT	GTCCAACCTCATTCCCA	TTCTGTCTTTCCACTCTAG	CAGCTTCAACCATCCCT
15	ACAGAGCAAGACTCCAT	GTGTTCCTGCTCCCAT	AGGAAGGGCAGAAGC	TGATGGAAGAGCAAACTGA
16	ATGCTGGGAGCAGAG	CAGCACTTGCGCAG	GCCTGGGTTCAAGC	TACTTGCCGACTGCG
17	CGTGCAGGAGCCA	GGCCTCCTCCAGC	AGGGAGGAGGGGA	CCACCCCCACCAG
18	GTCCTGACCTCAAGC	GACAGGCTGGAAGG	CACCCACCTCAGC	GCCTCCATGTAGGTC
19	CATGCACCTGCTATCTC	TGACTCTTGGCTGAATTCT	TCTGGAATCACAGTGCA	AGGAACTAAGGATTCCCA
20	TCATTTGTCGCCATTGAC	GCACGATGACATATGGA	TTCACAGGCTTCAGCAA	CTGGTGACGCCTCTT
21	CCGAGCCGTTCTCTA	ACTTTACCCCAATCCTG	GGCAGAACCAAGAGCT	CAAATTTCCTAAGCTGGACA
22–23	CTCCCAAAGTGCTAGGA	GTAAAAGAGGGAAAACAGATC	GCCCGGCAATGCTA	GGGCTGTTCTAGCTGAA
24	CCGCAGTCACATCC	GGCCTCAAATGAGGG	CTCGCCTGTCCCTA	GGCTAGGAGAGAAGGT
25	CCCTTGTCCTCTTGAGA	CTGGTTTGCCTTCCCA	TCCACCTCCTCGTTC	GTGCTTAAGGATGCTTAATG
26	GCATCCTTAAGCACGGA	ATGCTGGAGTGACGC	CAACAGCTGGGTCCT	CCCAATCTTTGCAAAGG
27	CATTGACATTTGCAGAAGGA	CATGTGAAACTATTAGAGGG	CAAATTGTTGCATGAATTAATACTA	TGTATTAGATGAGTTAAGTGCT
28	GCTAAAATATCTGGGAAATTCT	ACCTGCGAAAACTTAGAG	GAAATTCTCAAAAATGGACAAATCT	CCAGCTTGATACCTTAG
29	AAACAAGAGAGGTAAGGCA	AACCTATAGATGGGTTTGC	CAAGTAATTGAGAGCCTC	TTCTCAACTCCACTGCAAT
30	CCTCAGAGTCCAGTGA	TGGGTTTCTGTTCCTTAC	CCCTGCACTCTCTAG	AACCCTCATTTTCCTTGGT
31–32	GGTACAGTCACCCAG	GGTGACCTAGCTTCTTA	GCTGTCTCCCCCTA	CCTGAGGCCTCTTTTCT
33	GCTGACATTGTGTCTCC	GTGTACTTTCCTCCATTGAT	CCAAAGATCAACTCACC	TTACGTGGTCATTGCTG
34–35	CTTTGGGGAAATGTTTCCTAAA	ATAGAAGATGCTGGGTTGA	CCTCTGTGCTGCTATG	CCTTATTTTACAAGCTCCTTC
36	GCCACACCTAATTGAAAGA	AGAACCTCAGAACCTCAA	AGAAAGGTAGTCTCACTG	CGTGGGACCTTCATAC
37–38 (a)	CCAAAGATCAGAAAGTAGAG	TGGCTCACAGGCCTT	GAGGGGTTGAAGACCTA	CTTCCAGGGTGACCTT
37–38 (b)	GGAGGATGGAAAGCTGA	GCCCCTCACAATACATG	CTCTGCCGTGATGAAC	CACACACCACAGTCAC
39–40	GGCCATAGTGTGACTG	CTTCCCGATGATGTAGC	GCTGTGATTCTGCAACTT	GAATGGCAGGTCAGGAA
41	TTCATCAGCCCCATCAA	CACTAGCAGGCGAAC	CTCATGTGGGGTCTC	ATGCGGTGGGAACAG

[a]The specific exons were first amplified from genomic DNA using nested PCR. The nested PCR product was subsequently sequenced, using Sanger dideoxy method and the inner primer pairs.

TABLE 2 | Baseline characteristics of the sequenced patients and controls.[a]

	Patient group	Control group
N	192	192
Age, years[b]	29 (4) [18–44]	30 (5) [17–44]
Age >35 years[c]	8 (4.2%)	10 (5.2%)
BMI, kg/m²[b]	25.9 (4.2) [13.5–34.1]	25.6 (4.5) [15.3–36.1]
BMI >30[c]	21 (10.9%)	19 (9.9%)
BMI <18.5[c]	2 (1.1%)	3 (1.6%)
Ethnicity[c]		
Caucasian-European	158 (82.3%)	155 (80.7%)
Caucasian-North African	24 (12.5%)	26 (13.5%)
Black African	7 (3.6%)	9 (4.7%)
Asian	3 (1.6%)	2 (1.1%)
Risk factors for vascular diseases[c]		
Current smokers	22 (11.5%)	20 (10.4%)
Hypertension	7 (3.6%)	5 (2.6%)
Hypercholesterolemia	9 (4.7%)	10 (5.2%)
Hypertriglyceridemia	7 (3.6%)	8 (4.2%)
Diabetes mellitus	2 (1.9%)	3 (1.6%)

[a]No statistical differences were detected between the two groups, for either of the parameters. The significance was assessed with Mann-Whitney test for the quantitative data and Chi-Square test for the qualitative data.

[b]Quantitative data: median, interquartile range, and range values.

[c]Qualitative data: numbers and percentages.

factor I, and 4 μg C4BP were mixed. The samples were then incubated for 60 and 90 min, and the reaction was terminated by addition of SDS-PAGE sample buffer, containing 25 mM DTT. The samples were heated at 95°C for 5 min, applied on a 10% SDS-PAGE, and transferred to a PVDF-membrane for Western Blotting. The C3 Western Blot procedure is described above. The intensity of the intact α′-chain of C3met and the 46 kDa degradation product were analyzed, and the results are shown as a ratio of the two.

Direct Binding Assays

Binding of C3 to the different ligands factor H, CD46, C4BP, factor I, CD55, factor B, and properdin was assessed in plate assays. The ligands were immobilized on microtiter plates at 5 μg/ml (except factor B which was coated at 10 μg/ml) in PBS and the plates were washed and blocked as described above for the C3 ELISA. The different C3 cell media (mock cell medium was used as negative control), treated with methylamine, were then diluted to four different concentrations in a low salt buffer (10 mM Tris, pH 7.2, 25 mM NaCl, 0.05% Tween 20, 4% BSA) and incubated on the plate for 2 h at 37°C. For binding to factor H and CD46,

TABLE 3 | Mutations and polymorphisms found in *C3*.[a]

Amino acid[b]	cDNA ATG+1	SNP no.	Exon	Domain	Polyphen[c]	MAF, %[d]	Frequency in patients, % (no.)	Frequency in controls, % (no.)
p.R102G	c.304 C>G	rs2230199	3	β-chain/MG1	Benign	15.5	40.1 (77)	32.8 (63)
p.K155Q	c.463A>C	rs147859257	4	β-chain/MG2	Benign	0.3	0.5 (1)	
p.S297SfsX5	c.891delG	Novel	9	β-chain/MG3	–	0	1 (2)	
p.L302P	c.905 T>C	Novel	9	β-chain/MG3	Probably damaging	0	0.5 (1)	
p.P314L	c.941 C>T	rs1047286	9	β-chain/MG3	Benign	14.9	34.4 (66)	25.5 (49)
p.Y325H	c.973 T>C	Novel	9	β-chain/MG3	Possibly damaging	0	0.5 (1)	
p.V326A	c.977 T>C	Novel	9	β-chain/MG3	Possibly damaging	0		0.5 (1)
p.S327P	c. 979T>C	Novel	9	β-chain/MG3	Probably damaging	0		0.5 (1)
p.V330I	c. 988G>A	Novel	9	β-chain/MG3	Probably damaging	0		0.5 (1)
p.K633R	c.1898 A>G	rs140655115	15	β-chain/LNK	Benign	0.07	1 (2)	
p.R735W	c.2203 C>T	rs117793540	17	α-chain/ANA/C3a	Probably damaging	0.3	0.5 (1)	0.5 (1)
p.R1591G	c.4771 A>G	Novel	40	α-chain/C345C	Probably damaging	0	0.5 (1)	
p.G1606D	c.4817 G>A	Novel	40	α-chain/C345C	Probably damaging	0	0.5 (1)	
p.S1619R	c.4855 A>C	rs2230210	41	α-chain/C345C	Possibly damaging	0.2	0.5 (1)	0.5 (1)

[a]*All mutations were found in heterozygous form. None of the found alterations were significantly associated with the disorder, as determined by Fisher's exact test.*
[b]*Numbering including signal peptide, Met = 1.*
[c]*Polyphen predication of the protein function: http://genetics.bwh.harvard.edu/pph2/.*
[d]*MAF, minor allelle frequency in NHLBI Exome Sequencing Project database.*

TABLE 4 | Primer sequences (5′–3′) used to introduce site directed mutations in *C3*.

C3 mutation	Primer sequence (5′–3′)[a]
R102G	GTCAGAAAAGGGGGGCAACAAGTTCGTG
K155Q	CACCGTCAACCACCAGCTGCTACCC
L302P	GGGAGGTTGTGCCGAGCCGGAAGGTAC
P314L	GGTGCAGAACCTCCGAGCAGAAGAC
Y325H	GGGAAGTCTTTGCACGTGTCTGCCAC
V326A	GGAAGTCTTTGTACGCGTCTGCCACCGTC
S327P	GTCTTTGTACGTGCCTGCCACCGTCATC
V330I	CGTGTCTGCCACCATCATCTTGCACTC
K633R	CGGGCAGTGGGAGGGATTACGCCGG
R735W	CATCACAGAGCTGTGGCGGCAGCACGC
R1591G	CCCATCAAGTGCGGAGAAGCCCTGAAGC
G1606D	CTACCTCATGTGGGATCTCTCCTCCG
S1619R	GAGAAGCCCAACCTCCGCTACATCATCGG

[a]*Nucleotides corresponding to the changed amino acid residue are underlined.*

C3 variants were tested at 250, 125, 62, and 31 ng/ml; for C4BP, properdin and CD55 at 500, 250, 125, and 62 ng/ml; for factor I at 1,000, 500, 250, and 125 ng/ml; and for factor B at 2,000, 1,000, 500, and 250 ng/ml. The amount of bound C3met was then detected using a rabbit anti-human C3c antibody (Dako), followed by a HRP-conjugated goat anti-rabbit antibody (Dako). Both antibodies were incubated for 1 h at 37°C and developed as described above.

Factor B Cleavage

The cleavage of factor B by factor D was determined in solution, in the presence of methylamine-treated C3 WT, R1591G, or mock cell medium as negative control. A mixture of 2 μg/ml factor B, 2 μg/ml C3, and 0.1 μg/ml factor D was prepared in Mg^{2+} EGTA buffer (2.5 mM veronal buffer, pH 7.3, 70 mM NaCl, 140 mM glucose, 0.1% gelatin, 7 mM $MgCl_2$, and 10 mM EGTA) and incubated for 0.5, 1, 2, and 4 h at 37°C. At each time point, 10 μl was removed from the mixture, and the reaction stopped by addition of SDS-PAGE sample buffer. The samples were heated at 95°C for 5 min, subjected to SDS-PAGE (10% gel, non-reduced), and transferred to a PVDF-membrane for Western Blotting. Intact factor B, together with the cleavage products Bb (60 kDa) and Ba (33 kDa), were then detected using a polyclonal goat anti-human factor B antibody (Complement Technologies), followed by a HRP-conjugated rabbit anti-goat antibody (Dako). Both antibodies were diluted 1:10,000 and developed using enhanced chemiluminescence (Merck-Millipore). The intensity of the intact factor B band and Bb degradation product were analyzed, and the results are shown as a ratio of the two.

Structural Analysis

Structure files were downloaded from the Protein Data Bank (23) and visualized using the molecular graphics program PyMOL.[3]

Statistical Analysis

Fisher's exact test was used to assess statistical association between the found C3 alterations and the disorder. The statistical differences in baseline characteristics between the patient and the control group were assessed with Mann–Whitney test for the quantitative data and Chi-square test for the qualitative data. For all experimental data in the figures, statistical significance was determined using either one-way or two-way ANOVA with Dunnett's multiple comparison test. The results are shown as the mean + SD of at least three independent experiments and values of $p < 0.05$ were considered significant ($^{*}p < 0.05$, $^{**}p < 0.01$, and $^{***}p < 0.001$).

RESULTS

Alterations Identified in *C3*

All exons of *C3* were sequenced in 192 patients with RSPL. The exons carrying identified non-synonymous alterations found in

[3]https://pymol.org/2/ (Accessed: 2 March, 2018).

the patient group were then analyzed in a control group of 192 women. Altogether, 13 heterozygous, non-synonymous alterations were found both in patient and control groups (**Table 3**). Seven novel alterations in C3 were found in total, four in the patient group (L302P, Y325H, R1591G, and G1606D) and three in the control group (V326A, S327P, and V330I). The remaining alterations have been identified previously in other patient cohorts or are common polymorphisms (R102G and P314L). We also identified a novel heterozygous deletion (p.S297SfsX5) in two patients, which results in a frame shift and an introduction of a premature stop codon. This mutant was not expressed recombinantly as it could only yield a 30-kDa truncated fragment of C3 without function. None of the found alterations in the patient group were statistically significantly associated with RPSL, as determined by Fisher's exact test. With the available sample size we had a power of at least 0.80 to detect an association for alleles with risk allele frequencies >0.07, assuming a population prevalence of 0.05, an alpha of 0.05, and a genotype relative risk of 2. Power was calculated using the Genetic Power Calculator (24).

Expression, Secretion, and Characterization of C3 Variants

To be able to elucidate whether the found C3 variants altered the expression, secretion, or function of the protein, all 13 identified alterations were expressed recombinantly. Transient transfections revealed that two of the mutants (L302P, identified in one patient and S327P, identified in one control) were expressed but not secreted from the cells into the supernatant (**Figure 1A**). Five other alterations (Y325H, V326A, V330I, R1591G, and G1606D) yielded approximately half C3 concentration in the supernatant compared with WT. The supernatants from the transient transfections were also subjected to Western Blotting under both non-reducing (**Figure 1B**) and reducing (**Figure 1C**) conditions. All mutants migrated with the same apparent velocity to 185 kDa for non-reduced C3 and to 110 and 75 kDa for the α- and β-chain, respectively, under reducing conditions.

Hemolytic Activity

To assess the hemolytic activity of the C3 variants, C3-depleted serum was reconstituted with C3 WT or variants (or

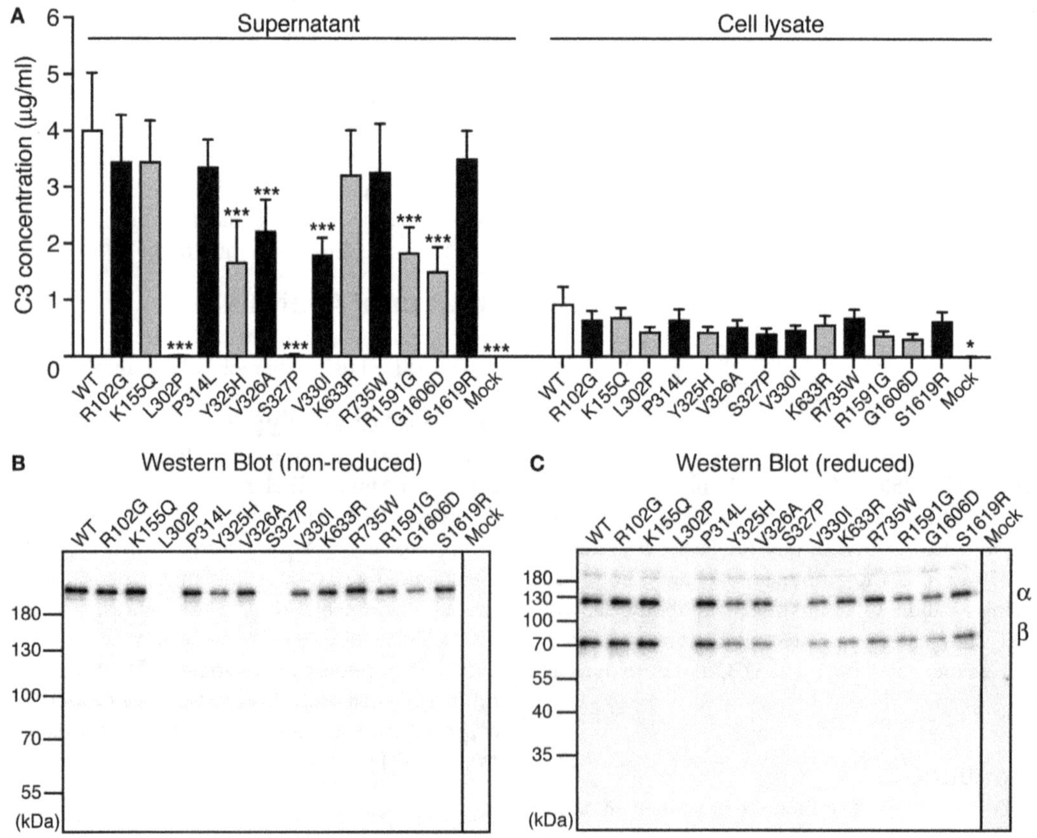

FIGURE 1 | Expression of C3 variants. **(A)** C3 variants, together with wild type (WT) and negative control (mock = empty vector), were transiently transfected into adherent human embryonic kidney (HEK) 293 cells. After four independent transfections, the C3 concentration was measured both in the conditioned cell media (supernatant) and the cell lysate using ELISA. The results are shown as mean + SD and the statistical significance of the differences between WT and mutants was determined using two-way ANOVA with Dunnett's multiple comparisons test, *$p < 0.05$, ***$p < 0.001$. The C3 alterations identified only in patients are marked in gray. **(B,C)** After transient transfections, the same volume of each cell supernatant was also subjected to SDS-PAGE under both **(B)** non-reducing and **(C)** reducing conditions, followed by Western blotting. C3 was detected using a polyclonal anti-C3 antibody.

corresponding volumes of mock medium as negative control), added to antibody-sensitized sheep erythrocytes and the amount of hemoglobin released from lysed erythrocytes was measured spectrophotometrically. Four concentrations of C3 were tested (2, 1, 0.5, and 0.25 μg/ml) in the hemolytic assay but for clarity only the result for 2 μg/ml is shown in **Figure 2**. Several variants showed increased hemolytic activity compared with WT while K633R and R1591G showed instead impaired activity. However, for the K633R mutant, the impaired activity was only clearly observed for the one shown concentration. The other three tested concentrations showed the same hemolytic activity as for WT. The rest of the mutants displayed the same activity for all tested concentrations (data not shown).

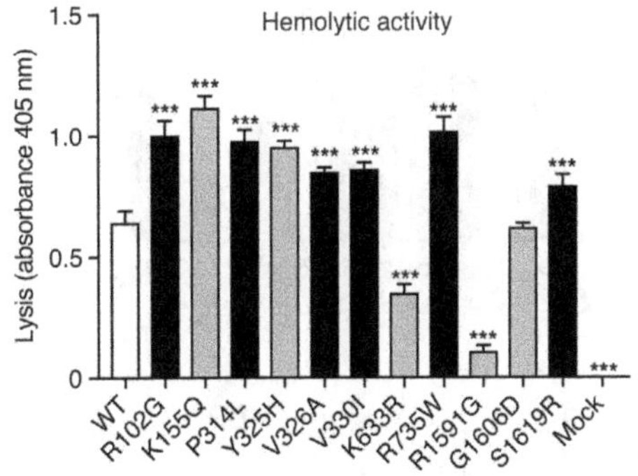

FIGURE 2 | Hemolytic activity. C3-depleted serum was reconstituted with either C3 wild type (WT), the different C3 variants or the negative control (corresponding volumes of cell media from mock-transfected cells). This was added to antibody-sensitized sheep erythrocytes and the hemolytic activity, i.e., lysis of the erythrocytes, was determined by measuring the absorbance of the supernatant at 405 nm (free hemoglobin). C3 was added in different concentrations but for clarity only one concentration (2 μg/ml) is shown in the figure. The experiment was performed three independent times in duplicates, and the results are shown as mean + SD. Statistical significance of the differences between WT and mutants was determined using one-way ANOVA with Dunnett's multiple comparisons test, $^{***}p < 0.001$. The C3 alterations identified only in patients are marked in gray.

Factor B Cleavage in Solution for R1591G

Since R1591G showed decreased hemolytic activity, we hypothesized that this mutant might cause more cleavage of factor B by factor D in solution and thereby less C3 will be available for the cell surface. Indeed, in the presence of R1591G, an increased cleavage of factor B in solution was observed, compared with C3 WT (**Figure 3**). This was statistically significant after 4 h cleavage but the trend was visible at all tested time points.

Degradation of C3 by Factor I

Degradation assays in fluid phase were performed to study if the different C3 variants could be degraded by factor I, in the presence of the cofactors factor H, CD46, and C4BP. C3 cell media were treated with methylamine to create C3met, a C3b-like molecule, and this was incubated for either 30 min (data not shown) or 90 min (**Figure 4**) with factor I and the different cofactors. Two of the mutants (R1591G and G1606D) showed statistically significantly impaired degradation compared with WT, regardless of which cofactor used. Degradation assays using factor H (**Figures 4A,B**), CD46 (**Figures 4C,D**), and C4BP (**Figures 4E,F**) all displayed the same result. The same trend was also seen at 30 min cleavage (data not shown).

Binding Assays

Direct binding assays were performed to elucidate if the C3 variants showed altered binding to factor H, CD46, C4BP, factor I, CD55, factor, and properdin. Corresponding volumes of mock medium was used as negative control. Four different concentrations of C3 were tested in each binding assay but for clarity only one concentration is shown in **Figure 5**. Small differences in binding could be observed. R1591G, that showed both impaired hemolytic activity and impaired degradation by factor I, also showed a somewhat decreased binding to factor H, CD46, and properdin. The other mutant, G1606D, that also showed impaired degradation by factor I, also displayed somewhat impaired binding to factor H, CD46, C4BP, factor I, CD55, and properdin.

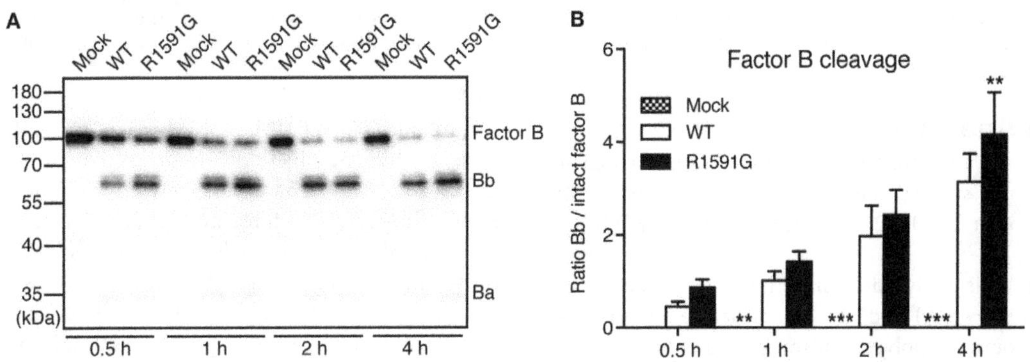

FIGURE 3 | Factor B cleavage in solution. Methylamine-treated C3 wild type (WT) or R1591G (or mock medium as negative control) was incubated with factor B and factor D for indicated time points, before being subjected to Western Blotting and factor B detection. A representative blot is shown in panel **(A)**. The bands corresponding to intact factor B as well as the Bb degradation product were quantified by densitometry. Data in panel **(B)** show the ratio between the intensity of these two bands. Each sample was analyzed in a single replicate, and the data are shown as mean + SD from four independent experiments. Two-way ANOVA with Dunnett's multiple comparisons test was used to calculate statistical significance of the difference between WT and R1591G, $^{**}p < 0.01$ and $^{***}p < 0.001$.

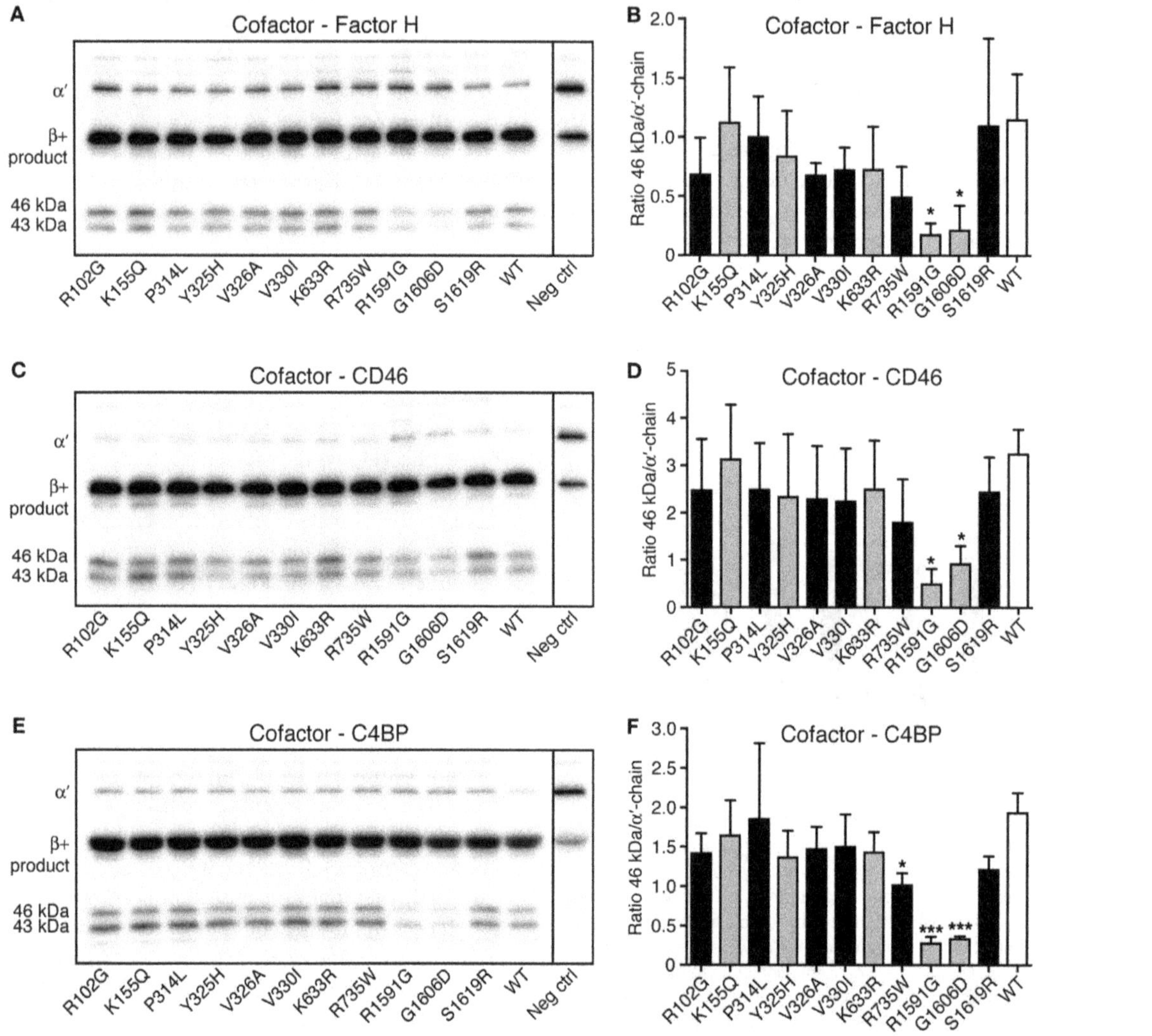

FIGURE 4 | Degradation of C3met by factor I, in the presence of different cofactors. The ability of the C3 variants to be degraded by factor I, in the presence of the different cofactors **(A,B)** factor H, **(C,D)** CD46, and **(E,F)** C4b-binding protein (C4BP) was determined. C3met, either wild type (WT) or variants, was incubated with factor I, together with the cofactor for 90 min. The degradation of C3met was evaluated by Western Blotting [representative blots can be seen in panels **(A,C,E)**] and the bands corresponding to intact α′-band of C3met as well as the 46 kDa degradation product were quantified by densitometry. Data in panels **(B,D,F)** show the ratio between the intensity of these two bands. The negative control shown in the blots is C3 WT at 0 min. Each sample was analyzed in a single replicate, and the data are shown as mean + SD from at least three independent experiments. Statistical significance of the differences between WT and mutants was determined using one-way ANOVA with Dunnett's multiple comparisons test, *$p < 0.05$ and ***$p < 0.001$. The C3 alterations identified only in patients are marked in gray.

Structural Analysis

Next, we tried to rationalize the functional consequences of the identified and studied alterations in the context of the known C3 (pdb-id: 2A73) (25) and C3b (pdb-id: 5FO7) (26) structures.

All C3 alterations analyzed in this study were mapped onto both the C3 (**Figure 6A**) and the C3b structure (**Figure 6B**). R102G is the common polymorphism also known as C3 S/F (slow/fast) and located in the macroglobulin (MG) 1 domain. Mutants K155Q, located in the MG2 domain; K633R in the LNK domain; R735W in ANA/C3a domain and S1619R in the C345C (CTC) domain, all showed normal expression and normal or only slightly altered function.

Mutants L302P, P314L, Y325H, V326A, S327P, and V330I are all located in the MG3 domain of C3. For two of the mutants, L302P and S327P, C3 was not secreted from the cells after transient transfections. In these mutants, leucine 302 and serine 327 are changed to proline residues, which most probably will cause misfolding and degradation of the protein intracellularly. The others are relatively structurally subtle mutations, changing a proline into leucine, a tyrosine into histidine, a valine into an alanine, and a valine into a leucine in MG3. Structurally, MG3 plays a critical role in the conversion from C3 to C3b and its contacts with MG7 and MG8 are changed drastically when converting C3 into C3b by removal of the anaphylatoxin (ANA/C3a) domain. Apparently, the minor alterations in the MG3 domain affected the secretion

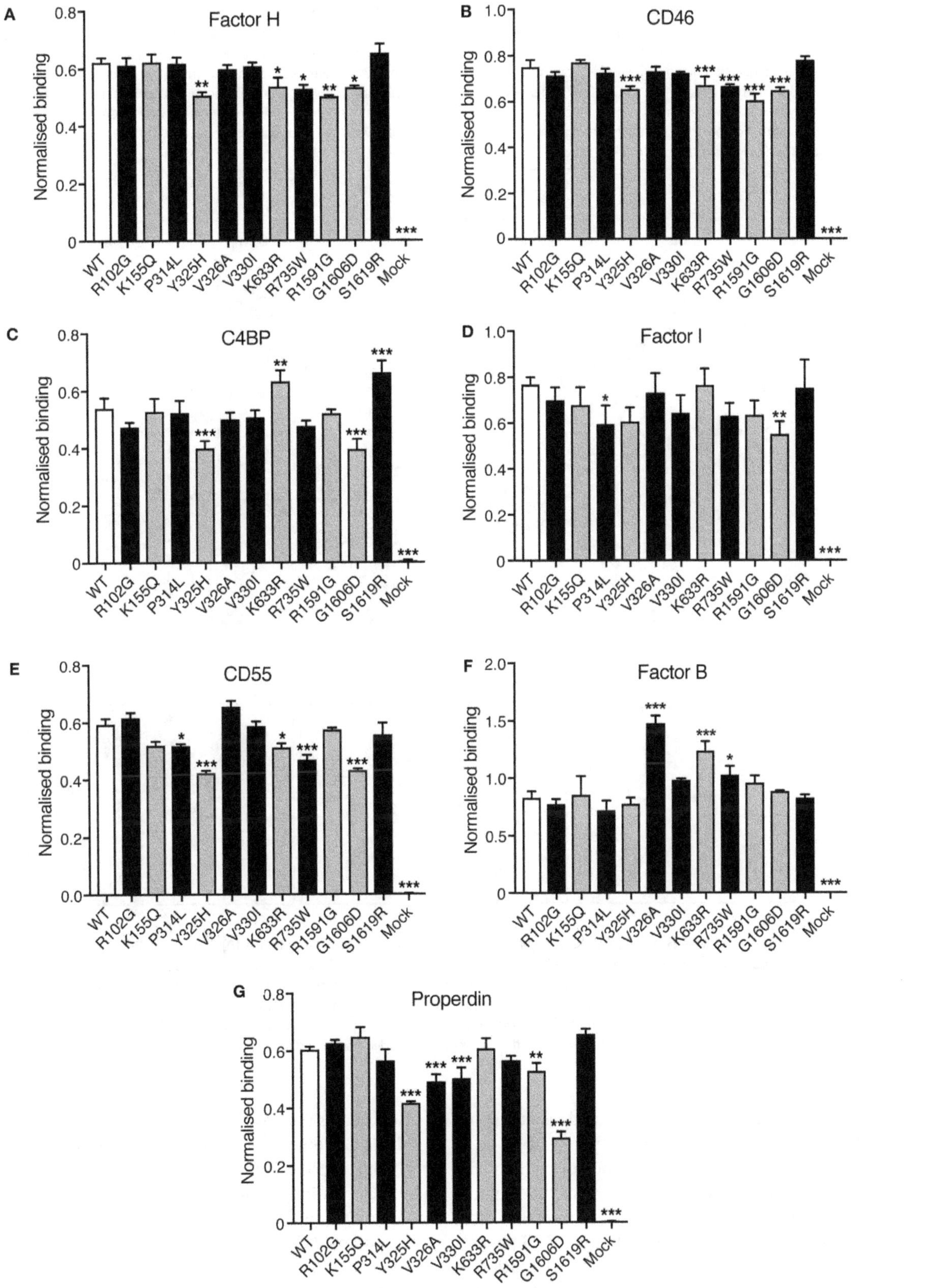

FIGURE 5 | Continued

FIGURE 5 | Binding of factor H, CD46, C4b-binding protein (C4BP), factor I, CD55, factor B, and properdin to C3met. Microtiter plates were coated with the different ligands for C3b: **(A)** factor H, **(B)** CD46, **(C)** C4BP, **(D)** factor I, **(E)** CD55, **(F)** factor B, and **(G)** properdin. C3met, either WT, variants or corresponding volumes of cell media from mock-transfected cells as a negative control, was added to the coated plates and the ability of the variants to bind the different ligands was detected using a polyclonal anti-human C3 antibody. Four different concentrations of C3met were tested but for clarity only one concentration for each ligand is shown in the figure (125 ng/ml for factor H and CD46; 250 ng/ml for C4BP, properdin, and CD55; 1 µg/ml for factor B; and 500 ng/ml for factor I). Each concentration was analyzed in duplicates, and the data are shown as mean + SD from three independent experiments. One-way ANOVA with Dunnett's multiple comparisons test was used for determining the statistical significance of the differences between WT and mutants, *$p < 0.05$, **$p < 0.01$, and ***$p < 0.001$. The C3 alterations identified only in patients are marked in gray.

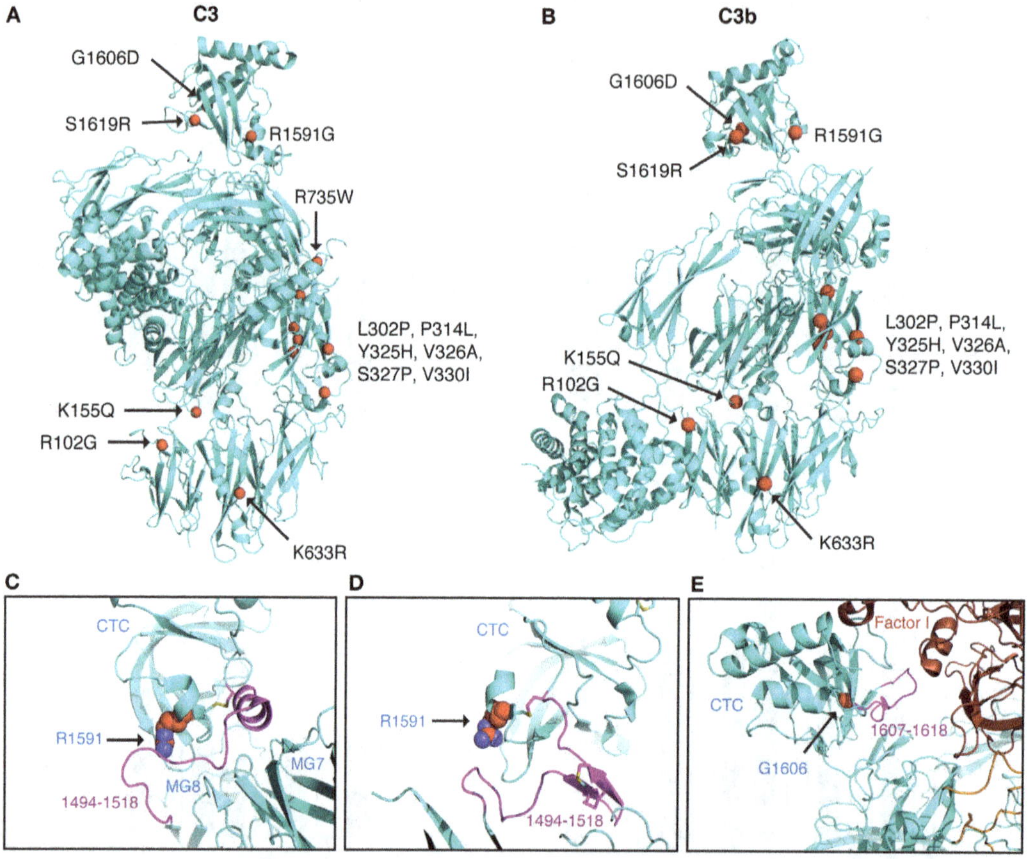

FIGURE 6 | Structural analysis of C3 alterations. The C3 alterations analyzed in this study were mapped onto the **(A)** C3 (pdb-id: 2A73) and **(B)** C3b (pdb-id: 5FO7) structures, using the molecular graphics program PyMOL. R735W is located in C3a and therefore absent in the C3b molecule. For R1591G; structures are shown of **(C)** C3 (pdb-id: 2A73) and **(D)** C3b (pdb-id: 5FO7). Both C3 and C3b are colored in cyan with indicated in purple the neck region (res. 1494–1518), connecting the CTC domains to the C3 and C3b body. R1591 is indicated by spheres and disulfide bridge Cys1518–Cys1590 shown in sticks. **(E)** For G1606D; the structure of C3b—mini-factor H—factor I (pdb-id: 5O32) is shown. The glycine C[alpha] atom is indicated by a red sphere. Mutation G1606D likely induces local rearrangement affecting its subsequent loop (res. 1617–1618, highlighted in purple) that is directly involved in contacting factor I.

of the protein (all except P314L showed decreased secretion) and also resulted in an increased hemolytic activity.

Mutant R1591G showed impaired hemolytic activity but instead yielded increased cleavage of factor B in the solution. In C3, R1591 is involved in interactions with residues of the "neck" region (res. 1494–1517) in native C3. Mutation R1591G possibly destabilizes these interactions and thereby alters or destabilizes the MG7-MG8 domain arrangement (**Figures 6C,D**). Destabilization of the MG7-MG8 arrangement in C3 is likely to induce generation of C3(H_2O) more readily, leaving less native C3 available for hemolytic activity. Moreover, enhanced generation of C3(H_2O) also explains the observed increased cleavage of factor B, due to soluble C3 convertase, i.e., C3(H_2O)Bb, generation.

Both R1591G and G1606D showed impaired degradation by factor I, independently of which cofactor that was used. Both mutations R1591 and G1606 are located in the C-terminal CTC domain. Interactions between the C3b-CTC domain and the heavy chain of factor I (pdb-id: 5O32) are needed to bind factor I and activate its catalytic serine-protease domain for cleaving C3b (26). Mutation G1606D possibly induces local rearrangements that disturb neighboring contact sites required for factor I binding (**Figure 6E**). R1591G, however, is positioned opposite of the factor I binding interface on the CTC domain. Putatively, a distortion of the "neck" conformation mis-orients the CTC domain for proper factor I binding needed for inducing catalytic activity.

DISCUSSION

Miscarriage is unfortunately a common complication of pregnancy and RSPL affects around 1–5% of couples trying to conceive. Evidence-based treatments, e.g., aspirin and heparin treatment for antiphospholipid syndrome and surgical corrections for uterine abnormalities, have improved the outcome for couples over the years but 40–50% of the cases still remain idiopathic. The complement system has been shown to be involved both in the physiology and the pathology of pregnancy. Furthermore, C3—the central protein of the complement cascade—appears to have an important role in the early phase of pregnancy and in the development of the placenta. In this study, we therefore set out to determine whether maternal variations in C3 are associated with idiopathic RSPL.

We performed full Sanger sequencing of all exons of the *C3* gene, in 192 patients with RSPL. The exons carrying identified alterations were then analyzed in a control group of 192 women and a total of 13 heterozygous non-synonymous alterations were found in both groups. Four of these (L302P, Y325H, R1591G, and G1606D) were novel mutations only found in the patient group and three (V326A, S327P, and V330I) were novel ones only found in the control group. We found the two common C3 polymorphisms in many of both the patients and controls; R102G (27) and P314L (28), which both have been associated with age-related macular degeneration (AMD) in many studies (29–31). R102G is also known as the C3S/F (slow/fast) allele and has been associated not only with AMD but also other immune-mediated disorders, such as IgA nephropathy, systemic vasculitis, partial lipodystrophy, and membranoproliferative glomerulonephritis type II (32). K155Q is a rare mutation, found previously in AMD patients (33) and we found this mutation in one RSPL patient as well. We also identified K633R in two RSPL patients, which has previously been identified to be a rare variant in atypical hemolytic uremic syndrome patients (34). Both R735W and S1619R were each found in one patient and one control and the former has previously been reported before in atypical hemolytic uremic syndrome (35) and the latter in AMD (36). None of the C3 alterations identified in the patients were associated with RSPL. However, we used a relatively small cohort and several of the found mutations are rare variants, which makes it difficult to appropriately statistically analyze the association between rare variants and disease. To be able to conclude a significant association, replication in larger cohorts is needed.

We decided to recombinantly express and analyze all our found alterations, also those only found in the control group. The women in the control group were selected on the basis of no previous pregnancy loss, at least two uneventful pregnancies and no known classical risk factors for pregnancy loss. However, they could potentially have other, unknown medical conditions, not related to pregnancy loss. Transient transfections of all C3 variants revealed that two mutants, L302P (identified in one patient) and S327P (identified in one control), were not secreted from the cells. These proline substitutions will most probably misfold the protein, leading to intracellular degradation. However, it should be noted that all identified C3 alterations in this study were in heterozygous form, which means that the individuals with the L302P and S327P alterations could theoretically have C3 concentration in blood decreased by 50%. We could unfortunately not confirm this, due to lack of blood samples from these individuals. Functional testing of the mutants that were secreted revealed that several of the alterations had increased hemolytic activity compared with C3 WT, e.g., R102G and P314L, which is in accordance with previous reports (37, 38). However, in that previous report, the authors also observed a 1.3-fold lower binding affinity for R102G to factor H, something we did not observe. The reason for this could be the use of different methods; we detected factor H binding using a microtiter plate assay and the former report used surface plasmon resonance. The K155Q mutant was previously reported in AMD (39) with impaired degradation of this mutant by factor I, in the presence of factor H as a cofactor. When using CD46 as a cofactor, the activity was normal. However, in our degradation assay, this mutant showed normal activity, for both the cofactors factor H and CD46. Furthermore, we did not see any altered binding for K155Q to factor H in our microtiter plate assay, which is in accordance with Seddon et al. However, Seddon et al. did see a decreased binding of K155Q to factor H using surface plasmon resonance. The only difference we observed for this mutant was an increased hemolytic activity. R735W was previously tested functionally, for its binding to CD46, factor H, factor B, and soluble CR1, together with its degradation by factor I, using CD46 as the cofactor (35). In that report, no functional changes were observed. In our report, we could see a slightly impaired degradation by factor I, when using C4BP as a cofactor but in accordance with the previous report, the activity was normal when using CD46 as the cofactor. We could also see a somewhat decreased binding to factor H and CD46, together with an increased binding to factor B. However, these changes were only minor.

Two novel mutations, importantly only found in the patient group, displayed the most functional impairment and also decreased secretion of the protein into the cell media after transient transfection: R1591G and G1606D. Both of these mutations showed impaired degradation by factor I, independently of which cofactor that was used (factor H, CD46, or C4BP). Binding of R1591G to factor H and CD46 was slightly impaired but we could not observe any impaired binding to factor I in a microtiter plate assay. However, to become active, factor I needs to bind to C3b in a way that it stabilizes the conformation of its catalytic domain. R1591G is positioned opposite of the factor I binding interface on the CTC domain. A distortion of the "neck" conformation could mis-orient the CTC domain for proper factor I binding needed for inducing catalytic activity. R1591G also displayed a decreased hemolytic activity but instead an increased cleavage of factor B in the solution. This might lead to consumption of C3 in the solution, resulting in less activity on the cell surface. Structural analysis of this mutant indicated that R1591G is involved in interactions with the neck region of native C3 and could possibly destabilize that region. This could also lead to more C3(H_2O) generation and subsequently less native C3 available for hemolytic activity. The other mutant, G1606D, also showed impaired degradation by factor I. Structural analysis of this mutant revealed that this amino acid change could induce a significant local rearrangement, which might affect the residues that are involved in binding to factor I. We did indeed observe a slightly impaired binding of this mutant to factor I, together with impaired binding to factor H, CD46 and C4BP, which could all together result in the impaired degradation we see by factor I.

Taken together, several C3 alterations were identified both in patients and controls. Since we used a relatively small cohort, none of the found alterations in the patient group were associated with RSPL in a statistically significant manner. To be able to determine an association with the disease, larger cohorts need to be analyzed. Two mutants (L302P, found in one patient and S327P, found in one control) were not secreted from the cells, probably due to misfolding and two others (R1591G and G1606D), found in patients, showed both decreased secretion and functional impairment. Some of the identified C3 alterations might result in *in vivo* consequences and contribute to RPSL.

AUTHOR CONTRIBUTIONS

AB and J-CG designed the study. J-CG and EM provided the patient and control samples, together with the clinical data. FM performed the functional experiments. PG performed the structural analysis. FM, AB, PG, and J-CG wrote the manuscript, and all authors approved it.

ACKNOWLEDGMENTS

We would like to thank all the patients and controls for their contribution to this study. We would also like to thank Emma Ahlqvist at Lund University for her kind help with power calculations. This work was supported by the Swedish Research Council (2016-01142) and a grant for clinical research (ALF).

REFERENCES

1. Rai R, Regan L. Recurrent miscarriage. *Lancet* (2006) 368(9535):601–11. doi:10.1016/S0140-6736(06)69204-0
2. Practice Committee of the American Society for Reproductive Medicine. Evaluation and treatment of recurrent pregnancy loss: a committee opinion. *Fertil Steril* (2012) 98(5):1103–11. doi:10.1016/j.fertnstert.2012.06.048
3. Jauniaux E, Farquharson RG, Christiansen OB, Exalto N. Evidence-based guidelines for the investigation and medical treatment of recurrent miscarriage. *Hum Reprod* (2006) 21(9):2216–22. doi:10.1093/humrep/del150
4. Holmes CH, Simpson KL, Okada H, Okada N, Wainwright SD, Purcell DF, et al. Complement regulatory proteins at the feto-maternal interface during human placental development: distribution of CD59 by comparison with membrane cofactor protein (CD46) and decay accelerating factor (CD55). *Eur J Immunol* (1992) 22(6):1579–85. doi:10.1002/eji.1830220635
5. Buurma A, Cohen D, Veraar K, Schonkeren D, Claas FH, Bruijn JA, et al. Preeclampsia is characterized by placental complement dysregulation. *Hypertension* (2012) 60(5):1332–7. doi:10.1161/HYPERTENSIONAHA.112.194324
6. Lokki AI, Heikkinen-Eloranta J, Jarva H, Saisto T, Lokki ML, Laivuori H, et al. Complement activation and regulation in preeclamptic placenta. *Front Immunol* (2014) 5:312. doi:10.3389/fimmu.2014.00312
7. Xu C, Mao D, Holers VM, Palanca B, Cheng AM, Molina H. A critical role for murine complement regulator Crry in fetomaternal tolerance. *Science* (2000) 287(5452):498–501. doi:10.1126/science.287.5452.498
8. Mohlin FC, Mercier E, Fremeaux-Bacchi V, Liszewski MK, Atkinson JP, Gris JC, et al. Analysis of genes coding for CD46, CD55 and C4b-binding protein in patients with idiopathic, recurrent, spontaneous pregnancy loss. *Eur J Immunol* (2013) 43(6):1617–29. doi:10.1002/eji.201243196
9. Agostinis C, Bulla R, Tripodo C, Gismondi A, Stabile H, Bossi F, et al. An alternative role of C1q in cell migration and tissue remodeling: contribution to trophoblast invasion and placental development. *J Immunol* (2010) 185(7):4420–9. doi:10.4049/jimmunol.0903215
10. Ricklin D, Reis ES, Mastellos DC, Gros P, Lambris JD. Complement component C3 – the "Swiss Army Knife" of innate immunity and host defense. *Immunol Rev* (2016) 274(1):33–58. doi:10.1111/imr.12500
11. Kolev M, Le Friec G, Kemper C. Complement – tapping into new sites and effector systems. *Nat Rev Immunol* (2014) 14(12):811–20. doi:10.1038/nri3761
12. Blom AM. The role of complement inhibitors beyond controlling inflammation. *J Intern Med* (2017) 282(2):116–28. doi:10.1111/joim.12606
13. Lee YL, Lee KF, Xu JS, He QY, Chiu JF, Lee WM, et al. The embryotrophic activity of oviductal cell-derived complement C3b and iC3b, a novel function of complement protein in reproduction. *J Biol Chem* (2004) 279(13):12763–8. doi:10.1074/jbc.M311160200
14. Usami M, Mitsunaga K, Miyajima A, Sunouchi M, Doi O. Complement component C3 functions as an embryotrophic factor in early postimplantation rat embryos. *Int J Dev Biol* (2010) 54(8–9):1277–85. doi:10.1387/ijdb.092993mu
15. Chow WN, Lee YL, Wong PC, Chung MK, Lee KF, Yeung WS. Complement 3 deficiency impairs early pregnancy in mice. *Mol Reprod Dev* (2009) 76(7):647–55. doi:10.1002/mrd.21013
16. Sugiura-Ogasawara M, Nozawa K, Nakanishi T, Hattori Y, Ozaki Y. Complement as a predictor of further miscarriage in couples with recurrent miscarriages. *Hum Reprod* (2006) 21(10):2711–4. doi:10.1093/humrep/del229
17. Laissue P, Lakhal B, Vatin M, Batista F, Burgio G, Mercier E, et al. Association of FOXD1 variants with adverse pregnancy outcomes in mice and humans. *Open Biol* (2016) 6(10):160109. doi:10.1098/rsob.160109
18. Lokki AI, Kaartokallio T, Holmberg V, Onkamo P, Koskinen LLE, Saavalainen P, et al. Analysis of complement C3 gene reveals susceptibility to severe preeclampsia. *Front Immunol* (2017) 8:589. doi:10.3389/fimmu.2017.00589
19. Nilsson SC, Karpman D, Vaziri-Sani F, Kristoffersson AC, Salomon R, Provot F, et al. A mutation in factor I that is associated with atypical hemolytic uremic syndrome does not affect the function of factor I in complement regulation. *Mol Immunol* (2007) 44(8):1845–54. doi:10.1016/j.molimm.2006.10.005
20. Blom AM, Kask L, Dahlbäck B. Structural requirements for the complement regulatory activities of C4BP. *J Biol Chem* (2001) 276(29):27136–44. doi:10.1074/jbc.M102445200
21. Harris CL, Spiller OB, Morgan BP. Human and rodent decay-accelerating factors (CD55) are not species restricted in their complement-inhibiting activities. *Immunology* (2000) 100(4):462–70. doi:10.1046/j.1365-2567.2000.00066.x
22. Ruseva MM, Heurich M. Purification and characterization of human and mouse complement C3. In: Gadjeva M, editor. *The Complement System: Methods and Protocols*. Totowa, NJ: Humana Press (2014). p. 75–91.
23. Berman HM, Westbrook J, Feng Z, Gilliland G, Bhat TN, Weissig H, et al. The protein data bank. *Nucleic Acids Res* (2000) 28(1):235–42. doi:10.1093/nar/28.1.235

24. Purcell S, Cherny SS, Sham PC. Genetic power calculator: design of linkage and association genetic mapping studies of complex traits. *Bioinformatics* (2003) 19(1):149–50. doi:10.1093/bioinformatics/19.1.149
25. Janssen BJ, Huizinga EG, Raaijmakers HC, Roos A, Daha MR, Nilsson-Ekdahl K, et al. Structures of complement component C3 provide insights into the function and evolution of immunity. *Nature* (2005) 437(7058):505–11. doi:10.1038/nature04005
26. Xue X, Wu J, Ricklin D, Forneris F, Di Crescenzio P, Schmidt CQ, et al. Regulator-dependent mechanisms of C3b processing by factor I allow differentiation of immune responses. *Nat Struct Mol Biol* (2017) 24(8):643–51. doi:10.1038/nsmb.3427
27. Alper CA, Propp RP. Genetic polymorphism of the third component of human complement (C'3). *J Clin Invest* (1968) 47(9):2181–91. doi:10.1172/JCI105904
28. Botto M, Fong KY, So AK, Koch C, Walp MJ. Molecular basis of polymorphisms of human complement component C3. *J Exp Med* (1990) 172(4):1011–7. doi:10.1084/jem.172.4.1011
29. Maller JB, Fagerness JA, Reynolds RC, Neale BM, Daly MJ, Seddon JM. Variation in complement factor 3 is associated with risk of age-related macular degeneration. *Nat Genet* (2007) 39(10):1200–1. doi:10.1038/ng2131
30. Yates JR, Sepp T, Matharu BK, Khan JC, Thurlby DA, Shahid H, et al. Complement C3 variant and the risk of age-related macular degeneration. *N Engl J Med* (2007) 357(6):553–61. doi:10.1056/NEJMoa072618
31. Park KH, Fridley BL, Ryu E, Tosakulwong N, Edwards AO. Complement component 3 (C3) haplotypes and risk of advanced age-related macular degeneration. *Invest Ophthalmol Vis Sci* (2009) 50(7):3386–93. doi:10.1167/iovs.08-3231
32. Peruzzi B, Serra M, Pescucci C, Sica M, Lastraioli S, Rondelli T, et al. Easy genotyping of complement C3 'slow' and 'fast' allotypes by tetra-primer amplification refractory mutation system PCR. *Mol Cell Probes* (2010) 24(6):401–2. doi:10.1016/j.mcp.2010.07.002
33. Zhan X, Larson DE, Wang C, Koboldt DC, Sergeev YV, Fulton RS, et al. Identification of a rare coding variant in complement 3 associated with age-related macular degeneration. *Nat Genet* (2013) 45(11):1375–9. doi:10.1038/ng.2758
34. Noris M, Galbusera M, Gastoldi S, Macor P, Banterla F, Bresin E, et al. Dynamics of complement activation in aHUS and how to monitor eculizumab therapy. *Blood* (2014) 124(11):1715–26. doi:10.1182/blood-2014-02-558296
35. Fremeaux-Bacchi V, Miller EC, Liszewski MK, Strain L, Blouin J, Brown AL, et al. Mutations in complement C3 predispose to development of atypical hemolytic uremic syndrome. *Blood* (2008) 112(13):4948–52. doi:10.1182/blood-2008-01-133702
36. Duvvari MR, Paun CC, Buitendijk GH, Saksens NT, Volokhina EB, Ristau T, et al. Analysis of rare variants in the C3 gene in patients with age-related macular degeneration. *PLoS One* (2014) 9(4):e94165. doi:10.1371/journal.pone.0094165
37. Heurich M, Martinez-Barricarte R, Francis NJ, Roberts DL, Rodriguez de Cordoba S, Morgan BP, et al. Common polymorphisms in C3, factor B, and factor H collaborate to determine systemic complement activity and disease risk. *Proc Natl Acad Sci U S A* (2011) 108(21):8761–6. doi:10.1073/pnas.1019338108
38. Abrera-Abeleda MA, Nishimura C, Frees K, Jones M, Maga T, Katz LM, et al. Allelic variants of complement genes associated with dense deposit disease. *J Am Soc Nephrol* (2011) 22(8):1551–9. doi:10.1681/ASN.2010080795
39. Seddon JM, Yu Y, Miller EC, Reynolds R, Tan PL, Gowrisankar S, et al. Rare variants in CFI, C3 and C9 are associated with high risk of advanced age-related macular degeneration. *Nat Genet* (2013) 45(11):1366–70. doi:10.1038/ng.2741

6

MASP-1 and MASP-2 Serum Levels are Associated with Worse Prognostic in Cervical Cancer Progression

Carlos Afonso Maestri[1,2], Renato Nisihara[2,3], Hellen Weinschutz Mendes[3], Jens Jensenius[4], Stephen Thiel[4], Iara Messias-Reason[3] and Newton Sérgio de Carvalho[5]*

[1] Liga Paranaense de Combate ao Câncer, Erasto Gaertner Hospital, Curitiba, Brazil, [2] Department of Medicine, Positivo University, Curitiba, Brazil, [3] Immunopathology Laboratory, Department of Clinical Pathology, Federal University of Parana, Curitiba, Brazil, [4] Department of Biomedicine, Aarhus University, Aarhus, Denmark, [5] Department of Gynecology, Clinical Hospital, Federal University of Parana, Curitiba, Brazil

***Correspondence:**
Renato Nisihara
renatonisihara@up.edu.br;
renatonisihara@gmail.com

Background: MBL-associated serine proteases (MASP-1, MASP-2, MASP-3, MAp-44, and MAp-19) are key factors in the activation of the lectin pathway of complement. Serum levels of these components have been associated with recurrence and poor survival of some types of cancer, such as colorectal and ovarian cancer. In this investigation, we determined the serum levels of MASP-1, MASP-2, MASP-3, MAp-44, and MAp-19 in patients with cervical cancer and cervical intraepithelial neoplasia (CIN).

Methods: A total of 351 women who underwent screening for cervical cancer or treatment at the Erasto Gaertner Cancer Hospital in Curitiba-Brazil, were enrolled in the study. Based on their latest cervical colposcopy-guided biopsy results, they were divided into four groups: CIN-I: $n = 52$; CIN-II: $n = 73$; CIN-III: $n = 141$; and invasive cancer: $n = 78$. All the serum protein levels were determined by time-resolved immunofluorometric assay (TRIFMA).

Results: Patients with invasive cancer presented significantly higher MASP-2, MASP-1, and MAp-19 serum levels than other groups ($p < 0.0001$; $p = 0.012$; $p = 0.025$ respectively). No statistically significant differences in MASP-3 and MAp-44 serum levels were found between the four studied groups. In addition, high MASP-2, MASP-1, and MAp-19 serum levels were significantly associated with poor survival in patients with invasive cancer and relapse ($p = 0.002$, $p = 0.0035$ and $p = 0.025$, respectively).

Conclusion: High MASP-2, MASP-1, and MAp-19 serum levels were associated with cervical cancer progression and worse disease prognosis. These novel findings demonstrate the involvement of the serine proteases of the lectin pathway in the pathogenesis of cervical cancer and future investigations should clarify their role in the disease process.

Keywords: complement, lectin pathway, HPV, cervical intraepithelial neoplasia, cervical cancer

INTRODUCTION

Human papilloma virus (HPV) is amongst the most common worldwide viral infection transmitted sexually. And although most HPV infections generally clear up on its own, a small percentage of these infections caused by specific HPV types can persist and evolve to cancer. The highest prevalence rate of HPV is observed in women younger than 25 years and decreases at later ages, but in many populations, there is a secondary peak in peri-menopause (1, 2). Young infected patients can usually eliminate the virus without presenting clear clinical evidence, due to an effective cell-mediated immune response causing the lesions to regress. The inability to develop an effective immune response to clear or control infection results in persistent infection that, in the case of oncogenic HPVs, creates a greater likelihood of progression to high-grade cervical intraepithelial neoplasia (CIN-2, CIN-3) and carcinoma. On the other hand, about 50% of HPV infections in women with normal cytology will resolve in less than 1 year, and approximately 90% of women with either normal cytology or CIN-1 diagnoses will ultimately resolve on their own (2).

It is known that HPV has a variety of strategies to evade the immune response, and when this occurs, HPV replication continues leading to persistent infection (1, 2). Among the approaches used by HPV to evade the host immune response are suppression of important inflammatory/immunological pathways that enable virus escaping from host immune surveillance (3). Due to suppression of some danger signals, HPV infection does not produce cytolysis, cytopathic cell death or interferon (IFN) release, leading to lower grade inflammation (1, 4, 5).

Chronic inflammation in the tumor microenvironment and evasion of the antitumor effector immune response are two of the hallmarks required for oncogenesis and cancer progression. The innate immune system not only plays a critical role in perpetuating these tumor-promoting hallmarks but also in developing antitumor adaptive immune responses (6). Thus, understanding the dual role of the innate system in cancer immunology is required for the design of combined immunotherapy strategies able to tackle established tumors (6). The lectin pathway of the complement system is part of innate response, being triggered when pattern recognition molecules (PRMs), including the two collectins [mannan-binding lectin (MBL) and collectin-LK] and three ficolins (ficolin-1,-2, and-3) initiate the complement activation upon binding to carbohydrates present on the surfaces of microbes or altered tissues. When this occurs, three MBL-associated proteases (MASP-1,-2, and-3) provide activation of the complement system, and two MBL-associated proteins (MAp44 and MAp19) serve as natural endogenous competitive inhibitors (7). The proteins MASP-1, MASP-3, and Map44 arise from the *MASP1* gene by mutually exclusive splicing (8). In a similar mode, MASP-2 and MAp19 arise from the *MASP2* gene (7). All these components are key factors in the activation of the lectin pathway of complement. Serum levels of these components were associated with recurrence and poor survival of some types of cancer such as colorectal or ovarian cancer (9, 10). Increased serum levels of MBL and MASP-2 were found in patients with colorectal cancer, which were not explained by genetic profiles (9, 10). So far, no study has addressed the serine proteases of the lectin pathway proteins in relation to cervical intraepithelial neoplasia and carcinoma. Our research group had previously reported on the MBL concentrations in women presenting with HPV-associated cervical lesions, showing there was no statistically significant difference between the median serum MBL concentrations in women presenting with CIN-1, CIN-2, CIN-3 lesions or invasive cervical cancer (11).

The aim of the present study was to investigate whether MASP-1, MASP-2, MASP-3, MAp-44, and MAp-19 serum levels are involved in the pathogenesis and progression of cervical intraepithelial neoplasia by measuring their concentrations in women presenting moderate grade of cervical intraepithelial neoplasia and cervical invasive cancer.

SUBJECTS AND METHODS

This cross-sectional study was carried out at the Erasto Gaertner Cancer Hospital (HEG) in Curitiba, southern Brazil, which is a reference center for the treatment of gynecological malignancies. The Institutional Ethics Committee approved the study.

All subjects were followed at the out-patient clinic of the HEG and were consecutively included from January 2011 to March 2012. Inclusion criteria were cervical cancer screening and treatment at HEG. We also collected historical data on disease progression from patients' medical records. Exclusion criteria were pregnancy, HIV-positivity, systemic infection, autoimmune disease, and blood transfusion within the last 60 days. Written informed consent was obtained from all patients.

A group of 344 women was included in this study. Based on their latest cervical colposcopy-guided biopsy, the subjects were divided into four groups: low grade CIN-1: $n = 52$ (control group); moderate CIN-2: $n = 73$; CIN-3: $n = 141$; and invasive cancer (Ca): $n = 78$. The loop electrical excision procedure or cold-knife cone excision was used to confirm the previous biopsy results. A 3-ml sample of venous blood was collected from each subject and allowed to coagulate. The coagulated blood was centrifuged, and the serum was separated, aliquoted (500 µl), and stored at −80°C, until use for MASP-1, MASP-2, MASP-3, Map-44, and Map-19 concentration determinations.

The concentrations of MASP-1, MASP-2, MASP-3, Map-44, and Map-19 were measured in according to published previously (8, 12, 13). The assays used for protein determinations were monoclonal antibody-based time-resolved immunofluorometric assays (TRIFMAs) and were carried out in partnership with the Institute of Medical Microbiology and Immunology, University of Aarhus, Aarhus. The human MASP-1 assay was based on competition from MASP-1 in serum with the interaction between anti-MASP-1 antibody and a fragment of MASP-1 coated onto microtitre wells. In the case of MASP-2 concentration ("sandwich ELISA"), rat anti-MASP-2 mAb (clone 8B5) was used for coating while biotinylated rat anti-MASP-2/MAp19 mAb (clone 6G12). MASP-3, Map-44, and Map-19 was determined by sandwich

TABLE 1 | MASP-1, MASP-2, MASP-3, MAp-44, and MAp-19 serum concentrations in patients with cervical lesions and cancer.

	CIN-1 (n = 52)	CIN-2 (n = 73)	CIN-3 (n = 141)	Ca (n = 78)	p
MASP-1 (ng/mL) median (IQR)	5,636 (3,758–8,129)	6,083 (3,823–8,422)	4,714 (3,319–6,839)	6,435 (3,971–9,074)	0.012
MASP-2 (ng/mL) median (IQR)	232.2 (163–386)	264.5 (190–418)	282.5 (204–410)	354.4 (234–570)	0.001
MASP-3 (ng/mL) median (IQR)	3,846 (2,750–5,212)	3,984 (3,181–5,180)	4,053 (2,947–5,071)	3,954 (2,705–5,142)	0.829
Map-44 (ng/mL) median (IQR)	1,695 (1,343–2,248)	1,787 (1,471–2,271)	1,710 (1,434–2,099)	1,866 (1,598–2,171)	0.246
Map-19 (ng/mL) median (IQR)	214.2 (152–289)	239.3 (162–318)	234.4 (167–298)	309.9 (219–487)	0.025

IQR, Interquartile range; CIN, Cervical intraepithelial neoplasia; Ca, Cancer.

ELISA using specific antibodies. All the assays used Eu^{3+}-labeled streptavidin (Perkin Elmer, USA)—for detection. All the antibodies were kindly provided by Prof. Jens C. Jensenius (Aarhus University, Denmark).

Data were analyzed as frequency and contingency tables. The Kolmogorov–Smirnov test was used to assess the data distribution. Central tendency was expressed as mean and standard deviation or median and interquartile range (IQR), and the Mann–Whitney test was used to compare numerical data. A receiver-operator characteristic curve (ROC) was also calculated for MASP-2. Results were considered statistically significant at $p < 0.05$. GraphPad Prism 7.0 software was used for statistical analysis.

TABLE 2 | Association between MASP-1, MASP-2, MASP-3, MAp-44, and MAp-19 serum concentrations and clinical evolution in patients with cervical lesions.

	Without death or relapse	With death or relapse	P*
MASP-1 (ng/mL) median	5,144	6,206	0.069
MASP-2 (ng/mL) median	273.7	382.4	0.002
MASP-3 (ng/mL) median	3,960	3,846	0.58
Map-44 (ng/mL) median	1,739	1,814	0.76
Map-19 (ng/mL) median	239.7	299.5	0.025

**Mann–Whitney test.*

RESULTS

The serum concentration of MASP-1, MASP-2, MASP-3, MAp-44, and MAp-19 proteins in the investigated groups is presented in **Table 1**. Significantly higher MASP-2, MASP-1, and MAp-19 serum were observed in patients with invasive cancer compared to other groups ($p < 0.025$). However, no significant differences were observed for MASP-3 and MAp-44 levels.

Regarding clinical evolution, 41 (11.9%; mean age 51.4 years) patients died within 24–48 months. Surviving patients had a mean age of 34.8 years. When serum concentrations were evaluated, median MASP-2 levels were higher among patients who died than among those who survived (439.4 ng/ml × 278.3 ng/mL; $p < 0.0001$). For MASP-1 (6988 ng/mL vs. 5110 ng/mL; $p = 0.0035$) and MAp-19 (366 ng/mL vs. 234 ng/mL; $p = 0.012$), the same trend was observed. Serum concentration of MASP-3 and MAp-44 were not significantly different between the two groups. When patients who died and those who experienced relapse of CIN or cancer during follow-up were considered, only MASP-2 and MAp-19 were significantly different (**Table 2**).

ROC curve was used to show the sensitivity and specificity for MASP-2 serum concentrations in relation to the prognosis of cervical cancer progression. High levels of MASP-2 (>291.9 ng/mL) showed a sensitivity of 71.3 and a specificity of 63.2 for worse prognosis of cervical lesions.

DISCUSSION

Our study demonstrates that MASP-2, MASP-1, and MAp-19 could have a role in the progression of cervical cancer. Patients diagnosed with invasive cancer showed a significant increase in the concentrations of these lectin pathway components. In another study conducted by our group, we failed to establish the relationship between serum concentration of MBL and the evolution of cervical intraepithelial neoplasias (10). These novel findings indicate possible involvement of the lectin pathway in the immunopathogenesis of cervical cancer, although it can result, in part, from activation of the complement system due to the presence of tumor cells. In fact, the participatory role of lectin pathway components in defense against pathogens such as viruses, bacteria, or fungi is much better known and studied: MASPs deficiencies are associated with increased infection susceptibility, and increased levels are associated with tissue injury (14). However, studies about its role in the development of cancer are scarce.

In a study of colorectal cancer, Ytting et al. (10) observed higher MASP-2 serum concentrations in patients with cancer, although no differences for *MASP2* genotypes were detected between patients with colorectal cancer and healthy controls. Furthermore, serum levels of MASP-2 have been associated with post-operative infections, recurrent cancer, and poor survival in colorectal cancer patients (9). These findings suggest that increased MASP-2 serum concentrations may occur due to factors other than genetics and that MASP-2 may play a role in cancer development and disease outcome. Corroborating these observations, in our study high MASP-2 serum concentrations were related to worse prognosis in cervical cancer and interestingly, they were mainly altered in patients who died and/or had disease recurrence. MASP-2 is produced in hepatocytes, and its promoter is regulated by cytokines such as interleukin (IL)-1b and IL-6 or transcription factor STAT3 (15).It is possible that tumor tissue releases mediators that may increase serum levels of MASP-2, however this is a hypothesis that needs to be clarified. Studying genetic polymorphism and MASP-2 serum levels in patients with ovarian cancer, Swierzko et al. (9) concluded that the expression of MBL and MASP-2 is altered in ovarian cancer, possibly indicating involvement of the lectin pathway of complement in the disease. Similar results of increased MASP-2 serum levels were described in children with tumors of the central nervous system (16) and in patients with acute lymphoblastic leukemia and non-Hodgkin's lymphoma (16).

In our study, MASP-1 serum concentrations were significantly higher in cancer patients than in other studied groups. The normal MASP-1 concentration in serum/plasma is approximately 20-fold higher than that of MASP-2 (13). It is known that MASP-1 activates MASP-2 in heterocomplexes of large oligomeric MBL and produces 60% of the C2b responsible for C3 convertase formation (17). Additionally, MASP-1 was reported to be essential for the development of autoimmune-associated inflammatory tissue injury by activating the alternative complement pathway in an experimental model of inflammatory arthritis (18). There are no studies on MASP-1 concentrations in cancer.

Complement system and macrophages collaborate synergistically to maintain progression of angiogenesis, and create conditions of carcinogenesis such as dysregulation of mitogenic signaling pathways, cellular proliferation, angiogenesis, resistance to apoptosis, and escape from immuno-surveillance. Macrophages release mediators that modulate inflammation and acquired immunity response. In addition, promote angiogenesis, tissue remodeling and tissue repair (19). The tumor growth is sustained by the infiltration of M2-tumor-associated macrophages, and high levels of C3a and C5a. Macrophages have receptors for both C3a and C5a on their cell surface, and this specific binding affects the functional modulation and angiogenic properties (19). High levels of MASP-2 and MASP-1 may increase activation of the complement system by the lectin pathway, thereby augmenting the release of C5a, a potent anaphylatoxin that activates cellular responses involved in tumor growth and progression (20). During cervical lesion progression, the number of M2 macrophages is significantly increased. The aggregation of M2 is a key event in the pathological process of carcinogenesis (21). M2 macrophages increase vascular endothelial growth factor (VEGF) and metalloprotease-9 secretion to aid in tissue repair. On the other hand, complement system activation by tumors may result in basement membrane disruption, tumor growth, and metastasis (22). *In vivo*, HPV does not bind directly to cells but requires contact with the basement membrane. This contact can be accomplished by microabrasions on the cervical surface, which reveal the basement membrane. The most plausible receptor of the major capsid protein (L1) of HPV appears to be the tissue-specific heparin sulfate proteoglycan, which belongs to the basement membrane (23, 24). It is possible that patients with higher serum levels of MASP-1 and/or MASP-2 present exacerbate activation of complement leading to the disturbance of the basement membrane, and ultimately to its damage or rupture and consequently, tumor invasion.

Interestingly, HPV protein (E2, E6, E7) action on *IL10* gene leads to increased IL-10 levels which in turn increases HPV E6 and E7 expression, leading to a vicious cycle (3, 22). IL-10 is an anti-inflammatory cytokine that modulates cytokine synthesis and exerts effects on resident and circulating immune cells, suppressing the immune system; however, their role in cancer remains controversial (3). On the other hand, activation of complement system is clearly an inflammatory process that acts to protect the host. However, to date, the majority of studies on cancer and the lectin pathway have shown a relation with worse prognosis when serum levels of components of this pathway were increased (9, 16). Future studies should investigate how complement interacts with the basement membrane and tumor tissue along with the influence of cytokine network on this system.

The limitations of this study are due to its cross-sectional study design, which prevented the use of serial dosages of the lectin pathway components over time to evaluate the stability of component concentrations throughout disease progression. Thus, future investigations evaluating the role of the different components of the lectin pathway, including collectins, ficolins and MASPs in the evolution of cervical lesions should be encouraged. In addition, our study did not include a healthy control group, for obvious reason, since it would be very difficult to obtain a group of women without HPV infection, either for ethical reasons or lack of lab tests to prove this condition. Thus, we believe that CIN-1 was the appropriate comparison group for our study, especially considering that such patients show good immune response against HPV and generally (>90%) do not progress to cancer (2).

In conclusion, our study shows that high MASP-2, MASP-1, and MAp-19 serum levels are associated with cervical cancer progression and worse disease prognosis. Future investigations should clarify the role of these complement components in cervical cancer immunopathogenesis.

AUTHOR CONTRIBUTIONS

CM and NdC: protocol and project development, data collection or management, and manuscript writing and editing; RN: protocol and project development, data analysis, and manuscript writing and editing; HM: protocol and project development, laboratorial assays, and manuscript writing and editing; JJ, ST, and IM-R: protocol and project development, and manuscript writing and editing.

REFERENCES

1. Bosch FX, Broker TR, Forman D, Moscicki AB, Gillison ML, Doorbar J, et al. Comprehensive control of human papillomavirus infections and related diseases. *Vaccine* (2013) 31 (Suppl. 7):H1–31. doi: 10.1016/j.vaccine.2013.10.003
2. Doorbar J, Quint W, Banks L, Bravo IG, Stoler M, Broker TR, et al. The biology and life-cycle of human papillomaviruses. *Vaccine* (2012) 30 (Suppl. 5):F55–70. doi: 10.1016/j.vaccine.2012.06.083
3. Berti FCB, Pereira APL, Cebinelli GCM, Trugilo KP, Brajão de Oliveira K. The role of interleukin 10 in human papilloma virus infection and progression to cervical carcinoma. *Cytokine Growth Factor Rev.* (2017) 34:1–13. doi: 10.1016/j.cytogfr.2017.03.002
4. Stanley MA. Epithelial cell responses to infection with human papillomavirus. *Clin Microbiol Rev.* (2012). 25:215–22. doi: 10.1128/CMR.05028-11
5. Bordignon V, Di Domenico EG, Trento E, D'Agosto G, Cavallo I, Pontone M, et al. How human papillomavirus replication and immune evasion strategies take advantage of the host DNA damage repair machinery. *Viruses* (2017) 9:390. doi: 10.3390/v9120390
6. Berraondo P, Minute L, Ajona D, Corrales L, Melero I, Pio R. Innate immune mediators in cancer: between defense and resistance. *Immunol Rev.* (2016) 274:290–306. doi:doi: 10.1111/imr.12464
7. Degn SE, Jensen L, Olszowski T, Jensenius JC, Thiel S. Co-complexes of MASP-1 and MASP-2 associated with the soluble pattern-recognition molecules drive lectin pathway activation in a manner inhibitable by MAp44. *J Immunol.* (2013) 191:1334–45. doi: 10.4049/jimmunol.1300780
8. Degn SE, Jensen L, Gál P, Dobó J, Holmvad SH, Jensenius JC, et al. Biological variations of MASP-3 and MAp44, two splice products of the MASP1 gene involved in regulation of the complement system. *J Immunol Methods* (2010) 361:37–50. doi: 10.1016/J.JIM.2010.07.006
9. Swierzko AS, Szala A, Sawicki S, Szemraj J, Sniadecki M, Sokolowska A, et al. Mannose-Binding Lectin (MBL) and MBL-associated serine protease-2 (MASP-2) in women with malignant and benign ovarian tumours. *Cancer Immunol Immunother.* (2014) 63:1129–40. doi: 10.1007/s00262-014-1579-y
10. Ytting H, Christensen IJ, Steffensen R, Alsner J, Thiel S, Jensenius JC, et al. Mannan-binding lectin (MBL) and MBL-associated serine protease 2 (MASP-2) genotypes in colorectal cancer. *Scand J Immunol.* (2011) 73:122–7. doi: 10.1111/j.1365-3083.2010.02480.x
11. Maestri C, Nisihara R, Ramos G, Mendes H, Messias-Reason IJ, Carvalho N. Mannose binding lectin is not acting as a biomarker for the progression of pre-invasive lesions of invasive cervical cancer. *Med Princ Pract.* (2017) 330:530–4. doi: 10.1159/000485037
12. Møller-Kristensen M, Jensenius JC, Jensen L, Thielens N, Rossi V, Arlaud G, et al. Levels of mannan-binding lectin-associated serine protease-2 in healthy individuals. *J Immunol Methods* (2003) 282:159–67. doi: 10.1016/j.jim.2003.08.012
13. Thiel S, Jensen L, Degn SE, Nielsen HJ, Gál P, Dobó J, et al. Mannan-binding lectin (MBL)-associated serine protease-1 (MASP-1), a serine protease associated with humoral pattern-recognition molecules: normal and acute-phase levels in serum and stoichiometry of lectin pathway components. *Clin Exp Immunol.* (2012) 169:38–48. doi: 10.1111/j.1365-2249.2012.04584.x
14. Beltrame MH, Boldt ABW, Catarino SJ, Mendes HC, Boschmann SE, Goeldner I, et al. MBL-associated serine proteases (MASPs) and infectious diseases. *Mol Immunol.* (2015) 67:85–100. doi: 10.1016/j.molimm.2015.03.245
15. Unterberger C, Hanson S, Klingenhoff A, Oesterle D, Frankenberger M, Endo Y, et al. Stat3 is involved in control of MASP2 gene expression. *Biochem Biophys Res Commun.* (2007) 364:1022–5. doi: 10.1016/J.BBRC.2007.10.114
16. Fisch UP, Zehnder A, Hirt A, Niggli F, Simon A, Ozsahin H, et al. Mannan-binding lectin (MBL) and MBL-associated serine protease-2 in children with cancer. *Swiss Med Wkly.* (2011) 141:w1319. doi: 10.4414/smw.2011.13191
17. Degn S, Jensen L, Hansen A, Duman D, Tekin M, Jensenius JC, et al. Mannan-binding lectin-associated serine protease (MASP)-1 is crucial for lectin pathway activation in human serum, whereas neither MASP-1 nor MASP-3 is required for alternative pathway function. *J Immunol.* (2012) 189:3957–69. doi: 10.4049/jimmunol.1201736
18. Banda NK, Takahashi M, Levitt B, Glogowska M, Nicholas J, Takahashi K, et al. Essential role of complement mannose-binding lectin-associated serine proteases-1/3 in the murine collagen antibody-induced model of inflammatory arthritis. *J Immunol.* (2010) 185:5598–606. doi: 10.4049/jimmunol.1001564
19. Khan MA, Assiri AM, Broering DC. Complement and macrophage crosstalk during process of angiogenesis in tumor progression. *J Biomed Sci.* (2015) 22:58. doi: 10.1186/s12929-015-0151-1
20. Markiewski MM, Deangelis RA, Benencia F, Ricklin-Lichtsteiner SK, Koutoulaki A, Gerard C, et al. Modulation of the anti-tumor immune response by complement. *Nat Immunol.* (2008) 9:1225–35. doi: 10.1038/ni.1655
21. Song D, Li H, Li H, Dai J. Effect of human papillomavirus infection on the immune system and its role in the course of cervical cancer (Review). *Oncol Lett.* (2015) 10:600–6. doi: 10.3892/ol.2015.3295
22. Deligeoroglou E, Giannouli A, Athanasopoulos N, Karountzos V, Vatopoulou A, Dimopoulos A, et al. HPV infection: immunological aspects and their utility in future therapy. *Infect Dis Obstet Gynecol.* (2013) 2013:540850. doi: 10.1155/2013/540850
23. Schiller JT, Day PM, Kines RC. Current understanding of the mechanism of HPV infection. *Gynecol Oncol.* (2010) 118 (Suppl. 1):S12–7. doi: 10.1016/j.ygyno.2010.04.004
24. Joyce JG, Tung J-S, Przysiecki CT, Cook JC, Lehman ED, Sands JA, et al. The L1 major capsid protein of human papillomavirus type 11 recombinant virus-like particles interacts with heparin and cell-surface glycosaminoglycans on human keratinocytes. *J Biol Chem.* (1999) 274:5810–22. doi: 10.1074/JBC.274.9.5810

7

Spontaneous Remission in Paroxysmal Nocturnal Hemoglobinuria—Return to Health or Transition into Malignancy?

*Eva-Stina Korkama[1], Anna-Elina Armstrong[2], Hanna Jarva[1,3] and Seppo Meri[1,3]**

[1] *Immunobiology Research Program, Department of Bacteriology and Immunology, University of Helsinki, Helsinki, Finland,* [2] *Coagulation Disorder Unit, Helsinki University Hospital Comprehensive Cancer Center, Helsinki, Finland,* [3] *Helsinki University Hospital Laboratory (HUSLAB), Helsinki, Finland*

Correspondence:
Seppo Meri
seppo.meri@helsinki.fi

Paroxysmal nocturnal hemoglobinuria (PNH) is an acquired syndrome characterized by intravascular hemolysis, thrombosis, and bone marrow failure. The disease is caused by a mutation in the *PIG-A* gene that leads to the lack of glycosylphosphatidylinositol-anchored complement regulatory molecules CD55 and CD59 on affected blood cell surfaces. In previous studies, spontaneous clinical remissions have been described. The disease manifestations are very heterogeneous, and we wanted to examine if true remissions and disappearance of the clone occur. In a follow-up of a nation-wide cohort of 106 Finnish patients with a PNH clone, we found six cases, where the clone disappeared or was clearly diminished. Two of the patients subsequently developed leukemia, while the other four are healthy and in clinical remission. According to our data, spontaneous remissions are not as frequent as described earlier. Since the disappearance of the PNH cell clone may indicate either a favorable or a poor outcome—remission or malignancy—careful clinical monitoring in PNH is mandatory. Nevertheless, true remissions occur, and further studies are needed to understand the immunological background of this phenomenon and to obtain a better understanding of the natural history of the disease.

Keywords: paroxysmal nocturnal hemoglobinuria, aplastic anemia, spontaneous remission, leukemia

INTRODUCTION

Paroxysmal nocturnal hemoglobinuria (PNH) is an acquired syndrome characterized by intravascular hemolysis, thrombosis, and bone marrow (BM) failure (1). The disease is caused by a mutation in the *PIG-A* gene that leads to the lack of glycosylphosphatidylinositol (GPI)-anchored molecules, including the complement regulatory proteins CD55 and CD59 from the surface of a clonal lineage of blood cells (2–4). In addition, rare forms of PNH with mutations in the CD59 gene have been described indicating the key role of the absence of CD59 in the disease (5, 6).

The diagnosis of PNH is made by analyzing GPI-anchored molecules or the anchor itself on blood cells by flow cytometry. The disease course is often unpredictable, and the therapeutic options are limited. While in previous studies spontaneous remissions have been reported to occur in up to 15–30% of cases (7, 8), there are only few detailed case reports published on these patients. Recently, four cases of spontaneous remission were described in two different studies (9, 10), but doubts exist whether remissions really occur in PNH patients. In particular, it would be important to distinguish true remissions from other developing disorders, especially from malignancy, because in both cases the PNH diagnostics may give a negative result.

Because of the variable clinical course of PNH, we wanted to explore whether true spontaneous remissions occur in PNH in the Finnish patient material that we have collected during a long period of time. A nation-wide study of all PNH patients diagnosed in Finland since 1995 and an extended follow-up time (up to 20 years) have provided a unique opportunity to perform a detailed analysis of the course of the disease in our patients.

PATIENTS AND METHODS

In a nation-wide project, we collected patients from all Health Care Districts in Finland (with a total population of 5.6 million). The sources of information included the Helsinki University Central Hospital Laboratory (HUSLAB) databases, flow cytometry analysis of red blood cells (RBCs) and leukocytes, patients' medical records, and a patient questionnaire. The patients were evaluated until September 2016, and the remission cases were followed until June 2017. In total, 106 patients with a CD59-deficient cell clone in flow cytometry were included in the study.

Besides the flow cytometry analysis the laboratory parameters included levels of hemoglobin (Hb), lactate dehydrogenase, haptoglobin, erythrocytes, leukocytes, platelets, inflammation markers (CRP, ESR), D-dimer, fibrinogen, coagulation factor VIII, creatinine, and ventricular natriuretic peptide. In addition, the glomerular filtration rates and BM analyses were performed. The clinical data included the symptoms and conditions attributable to PNH: hemoglobinuria, thrombotic events, infections, fatigue, renal failure, pulmonary hypertension, abdominal pain, dysphagia, dyspnea, erectile dysfunction, anemia, and the co-existence of PNH with aplastic anemia (AA), myelodysplastic syndrome (MDS), or leukemia.

An ethical permission for the study was provided by the coordinating ethical committee at the Helsinki University Hospital Health Care District. A research permission was also obtained from the National Institute of Health and Welfare (THL, Helsinki, Finland), and the patients gave written informed consents for the study.

RESULTS

In a cohort of 106 Finnish patients with a PNH clone, we found 6 cases, where the clone disappeared or clearly diminished (to a level equal or below 1.5%). Two of the six patients subsequently developed leukemia (acute myeloid leukemia and chronic myelomonocytic leukemia), while the other four are in clinical remission (**Table 1**).

Patient number 1 was diagnosed with AA in 1986 during a twin pregnancy. The patient had pre-eclampsia and a cesarean section was performed. The PNH diagnosis was made by Ham's test in 1990 at the age of 23 years. The first flow cytometry test was performed in 2001 (24% CD59-negative erythrocytes) (**Figure 1A**). The patient was first treated with steroids without any positive outcome and with androgens for 2 years. In 1994, the patient was diagnosed with multiple sclerosis. In the mid 90s, the

TABLE 1 | Patients and treatments.

	Age at PNH diagnosis (year)	Age at AA/BM failure diagnosis (year)	Treatment
Patient 1	23 years (1990)[a]	19 years (1986)	Androgens, corticosteroids
Patient 2	56 years (1998)	Hypoplastic BM 57 years (1999)	Androgens, corticosteroids
Patient 3	24 years (1998)	21 years (1995)	Antithymocyte globulin, prednisolone, cyclosporine, granulocyte growth factor
Patient 4	25 years (1998)	19 years (1992)	Cyclosporine, androgens
Patient 5	43 years (2000)	43 years (2000)	Antithymocyte globulin, prednisolone, cyclosporine
Patient 6	44 years (1998)	43 years (1997)	Prednisolone, cyclosporine

PNH, paroxysmal nocturnal hemoglobinuria; AA, aplastic anemia; BM, bone marrow.
[a]Diagnosis by Ham's test. First flow cytometry in 2001. For further clinical information, please see the text.

patient got several blood transfusions and twice more in 2005 and 2006. No thrombotic complications occurred. The patient was given anticoagulation treatment. Low molecular-weight heparin was used postoperatively after a gynecologic operation in 2006, and since 2008 the patient used aspirin. In 2012, erythrocytes, monocytes, and neutrophils were analyzed by the flow cytometry test, and no PNH clone was detected. The patient had no longer signs of hemolysis. In the same year, however, the patient was diagnosed with MDS and later with acute myeloid leukemia. The patient died of leukemia in 2013 at the age of 45 years.

Case 2 (female) was diagnosed with PNH in 1998 at the age of 56 years (30% CD59-negative erythrocytes by flow cytometry). At the time of diagnosis, the Hb level was 70 g/L, and the numbers of leukocytes 2.5×10^9/L and platelets 6×10^9/L. The patient had a tendency for bruising, petechiae, and bleeding on probing. In 1999, the patient's BM sample showed hypoplastic features. The patient was treated with corticosteroids from 1998 until 2005. Androgen treatment was stopped because of elevated liver values. The CD59-negative erythrocyte clone peaked in 1998 after which it gradually declined. In 1999, the patient received cyclosporine treatment, which had a good effect on the anemia. In 2007, the patient recurrently developed anemia and thrombocytopenia. At that time, the RBCs had a normal CD59 expression level on flow cytometry (**Figure 1B**). The BM sample showed myelodysplastic changes and a systemic mastocytosis with c-*KIT* mutation was observed. In 2010, the patient was diagnosed with chronic myelomonocytic leukemia and azacytidine treatment was started. In 2011, the patient died because of acute ischemic heart disease during the leukemia treatment.

Case 3 (female) was diagnosed with AA in 1995 at the age of 21 years. At the time of diagnosis, the Hb level was 50 g/L, leukocytes 1.9×10^9/L, and platelets 8×10^9/L. The patient was treated with antithymocyte globulin, prednisolone, cyclosporine, and granulocyte growth factor. In 1996, 8% of the erythrocytes were CD59 deficient. When the flow cytometry was performed next time in 1998, 50% of the erythrocytes was type I CD59-deficient cells and 30% type II (partially CD59 deficient) cells (**Figure 1C**). No thrombotic complications or bleeding have occurred at any time of the disease history. The lactate dehydrogenase level was

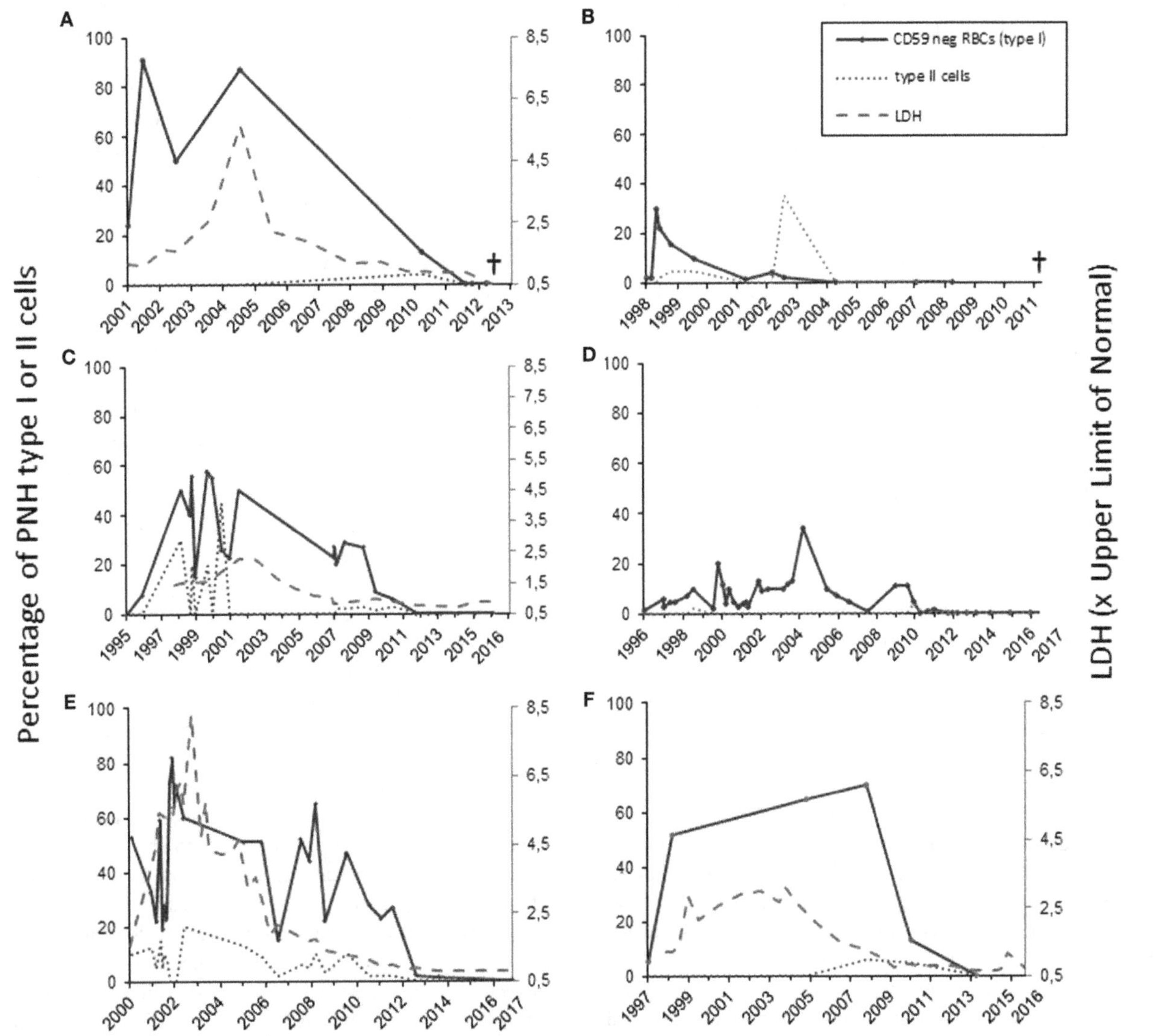

FIGURE 1 | The percentage of totally and partially CD59-deficient red blood cells in patients 1–6 [**(A–F)**, respectively]. For patients 1, 3, 5, and 6 who had intravascular hemolysis, the lactate dehydrogenase levels (LD) are shown at right on the *Y*-axis as values in relation to the upper limit of normal **(A,C,E,F)**. Patients 1 and 2 **(A,B)** suffered from leukemia and subsequently died. Patients 3–6 are in remission.

elevated earlier, but has been normal since 2006 (**Figure 1C**). The patient had two deliveries, in 2003 and 2007. During the first delivery, the patient was given blood transfusions and suffered from postpartum endometritis. The second delivery was without complications. In the 1990s, the patient had periods of hemoglobinuria. In 2012, the cyclosporine treatment was stopped, and only 0.2% of the erythrocytes were CD59 negative. Since 2013 the expression of CD59 has been normal on erythrocytes and the GPI-negative clone in neutrophils and monocytes has been 0.3–0.6% and the patient is symptom free.

Patient 4 (male) was diagnosed with AA in 1992, and the PNH diagnosis was made in 1998 when the patient was 25 years old (10% CD59-negative erythrocytes in flow cytometry). Before that the patient had had a small CD59-negative RBC clone (1.7–7%) since 1996. In 1992, the patient got several RBC and platelet transfusions. Cyclosporine and androgen treatment were started in 1992 with a good response leading to recovery from the cytopenias. The androgen treatment was discontinued in 2003 and cyclosporine treatment in 2012. Since then the patient has had no symptoms, and the laboratory parameters have been in the normal range. In 2010, CD59 expression on the erythrocytes was normal. In later controls, the expression has been either fully normal or the CD59-negative erythrocyte cell clone has been small (between 0.2 and 1.4%) (**Figure 1D**). The GPI-negative clone in neutrophils and monocytes has been in the range 0.2–1.5%.

Case 5 (male) was diagnosed with AA and PNH in 2000 at the age of 43 years. Fifty-three percent of the erythrocytes were totally CD59 deficient. In addition, 10% had a decreased expression (type II cells). In the BM sample, the cellularity was 25–30%

of normal. At the time of diagnosis, the Hb level was 54 g/L, neutrophils 0.3 × 10^9/L, and platelets 26 × 10^9/L. The patient was initially treated with prednisolone for a short time. Later, the patient was given antithymocyte globulin treatment and cyclosporine for 1 year. Initially, the response to the immunosuppressive treatment was not sufficient, and an allogeneic stem cell transplantation with register donor was already being planned. In 2002, the transplantation was canceled because of a late response to the treatment. At that point, the Hb level was 122 g/L, neutrophils 0.77 × 10^9/L, and platelets 96 × 10^9/L. The patient had hemolysis and hemoglobinuria, fatigue, and erectile dysfunction. No thrombotic complications occurred. The anemia was compensated, and there was no transfusion dependency. Since 2009 the patient has been symptom free and the lab values stable, Hb level 155 g/L. The PNH clone has been declining (**Figure 1E**). In 2017, it was below 1% in both RBCs and neutrophils.

Patient 6 (male) was diagnosed with AA at the age of 43 years in 1997. At that time, the patient had pancytopenia and 5.4% of RBCs were CD59 deficient. The patient was treated with cyclosporine with a good response. In 1998, the size of the PNH clone was 52%. The patient had tendency for bruising, hemoglobinuria, and erectile dysfunction, but no thrombosis. Since 2009 the LD values normalized, and the patient did not report hemoglobinuria any more. In 2010, the size of the PNH clone had already clearly diminished, and in 2013, it was 0.3% in RBCs and 0.8% in neutrophils (**Figure 1F**).

Among all the six patients, the median time from the diagnosis until the remission was 12.5 years (range 6–15 years). For the two patients who developed leukemia, the diagnosis was made 26 and 12 years after the initial PNH/AA diagnosis, respectively. In one patient, the CD59-deficient cell clone disappeared 3 years earlier, and for the other one in the same year leukemia was diagnosed. For all six patients, the median CD59-deficient RBC clone size was 64% at highest (range 30–91%) (**Figure 1**). Four of the patients had classical PNH with signs of hemolysis. None of the patients received eculizumab therapy since it was not available at the time of diagnosis. All patients had underlying AA or another type of BM failure. Four of the patients were treated with cyclosporine, three with androgens, and five with corticosteroids. Two of the remission cases also got antithymocyte globulin, and one was given granulocyte growth factor. None of the patients was heavily transfusion dependent.

DISCUSSION

Paroxysmal nocturnal hemoglobinuria is a potentially serious illness with variable manifestations and outcomes. Reliably defined complete remissions from the disease have only rarely been described, and doubt exists whether a permanent cure from the disease can occur. In Finland, it has been possible to conduct a nation-wide study because it has a relatively small population (5.6 million) with a comprehensive public healthcare system, where rare cases are centralized to specialized healthcare. Thus, for this study, we were able to collect all patients diagnosed with PNH from a period of over 20 years, altogether 106 PNH patients. Indeed, among these we found six cases, where the PNH cell clones disappeared. In four cases, this was accompanied with spontaneous clinical remission, as well. By contrast, in two other cases—showing apparently the disappearance of the PNH clone—the disease developed into malignancy.

Our data show that spontaneous remissions are not as frequent as previously described, and the disappearance of the PNH cell clone can be related to dramatically different outcomes. In a Spanish patient cohort, spontaneous remission was reported to occur in as many as 30% of the patients (17/56), but the cases were not characterized further, and the spontaneous remission was not defined (8). We considered that the patients were in remission when they had no clinical signs of disease (i.e., no cytopenias, signs of hemolysis, or thrombosis) and no flow cytometry evidence for PNH. For the latter, a threshold level of 1.5% for GPI-anchor negative RBCs was employed, because levels lower than this may be artifacts due to staining or transportation. Small PNH-like clones may also be seen in healthy individuals (11). In a British material from the year 1995, spontaneous clinical remissions were reported in 15% of the patients (12/80) (7). The patients had a negative Ham's test. In five cases, flow cytometry was later performed, and in all cases, the RBCs expressed normal levels of GPI-linked proteins. However, possible misdiagnoses with the earlier less specific Ham's test cannot be excluded.

Nevertheless, as our study shows, true remissions occur, but the patients need to be carefully followed up for a potential emergence of malignancy. Among the six patients, where the PNH clone disappeared, four are healthy and have no treatment. The actual mechanisms or the reasons for the remissions are unknown. They may be spontaneous, have an immunological background, or be related to therapy. A proposed explanation has been that the PNH clone has a finite lifespan and that normal stem cells are capable of repopulating the BM (7). Recently, a case was described, where a decrease in the PNH clone did not restore normal hematopoiesis but instead was associated with clonal replacement (9). Notably, however, in this case, the PNH clone did not disappear but remained at a 15% level. All of our six patients had an underlying BM failure. Patients received treatments (e.g., cyclosporine, androgens, steroids, CSF, or antithymocyte globulin) that may also have affected the PNH cell clone or the cell clone could have lost its growth advantage (12) after repopulating the BM.

Paroxysmal nocturnal hemoglobinuria has previously been considered to be a monoclonal disorder, and the expansion of the GPI-deficient clone has been explained by extrinsic factors (13). Recent studies have shown that multiple clones are present, and a number of additional somatic mutations in the PNH clones have been detected (14, 15). The latter may lead to clonal selection. Partially, CD59-deficient type II cells are thought to emerge because of only a partially defective or absent PIG-A enzyme. As PNH is currently regarded as a multiclonal disease with clonal hierarchy (14) and a large number of cells are involved, a repairing mutation can not be the explanation for remission. In our view, the most likely possibility is that the immune system is eliminating cells through complement attack and/or by the formation of antibodies or by a cell-mediated immune response. If antibodies against cells develop, as may occur after blood transfusions, the clearance of CD59-negative cells could be further boosted. Cells lacking CD59 and CD55 would, after all, be more susceptible to complement-mediated clearance. Some antibodies may even be targeted against unique epitopes on GPI-anchor deficient cells.

Paroxysmal nocturnal hemoglobinuria is known to be a very variable disease, and this is also typical among the remission cases. The fact that the clone disappears may be related to different outcomes, total recovery, or BM suppression and development of leukemia. This provides a challenge to the clinician. Careful follow-up is needed to determine the direction to which the disease is progressing. Further studies on the mechanisms of spontaneous remissions could also provide clues for finding a curative treatment for PNH in the future.

AUTHOR CONTRIBUTIONS

E-SK performed the research, analyzed data, and wrote the initial draft of the manuscript. HJ and SM designed and supervised the research, revised, and approved the manuscript. A-EA provided clinical information, reviewed, and approved the manuscript.

ACKNOWLEDGMENTS

This work was supported by grants from Sigrid Jusélius Foundation, Signe and Ane Gyllenberg Foundation, Helsinki University Hospital Funds (EVO), and Alexion Pharmaceuticals Inc. The sponsors support science in general and had no role in gathering, analyzing, or interpreting the data. E-SK is a PhD candidate at University of Helsinki, and this work is submitted in partial fulfillment of the requirement for the PhD degree.

REFERENCES

1. Parker C, Omine M, Richards S, Nishimura J, Bessler M, Ware R, et al. Diagnosis and management of paroxysmal nocturnal hemoglobinuria. *Blood* (2005) 106(12):3699–709. doi:10.1182/blood-2005-04-1717
2. Pangburn MK, Schreiber RD, Muller-Eberhard HJ. Deficiency of an erythrocyte membrane protein with complement regulatory activity in paroxysmal nocturnal hemoglobinuria. *Proc Natl Acad Sci U S A* (1983) 80(17):5430–4. doi:10.1073/pnas.80.17.5430
3. Holguin MH, Fredrick LR, Bernshaw NJ, Wilcox LA, Parker CJ. Isolation and characterization of a membrane protein from normal human erythrocytes that inhibits reactive lysis of the erythrocytes of paroxysmal nocturnal hemoglobinuria. *J Clin Invest* (1989) 84(1):7–17. doi:10.1172/JCI114172
4. Nicholson-Weller A, March JP, Rosenfeld SI, Austen KF. Affected erythrocytes of patients with paroxysmal nocturnal hemoglobinuria are deficient in the complement regulatory protein, decay accelerating factor. *Proc Natl Acad Sci U S A* (1983) 80(16):5066–70. doi:10.1073/pnas.80.16.5066
5. Yamashina M, Ueda E, Kinoshita T, Takami T, Ojima A, Ono H, et al. Inherited complete deficiency of 20-kilodalton homologous restriction factor (CD59) as a cause of paroxysmal nocturnal hemoglobinuria. *N Engl J Med* (1990) 323(17):1184–9. doi:10.1056/NEJM199010253231707
6. Nevo Y, Ben-Zeev B, Tabib A, Straussberg R, Anikster Y, Shorer Z, et al. CD59 deficiency is associated with chronic hemolysis and childhood relapsing immune-mediated polyneuropathy. *Blood* (2013) 121(1):129–35. doi:10.1182/blood-2012-07-441857
7. Hillmen P, Lewis SM, Bessler M, Luzzatto L, Dacie JV. Natural history of paroxysmal nocturnal hemoglobinuria. *N Engl J Med* (1995) 333(19):1253–8. doi:10.1056/NEJM199511093331904
8. Munoz-Linares C, Ojeda E, Fores R, Pastrana M, Cabero M, Morillo D, et al. Paroxysmal nocturnal hemoglobinuria: a single Spanish center's experience over the last 40 yr. *Eur J Haematol* (2014) 93(4):309–19. doi:10.1111/ejh.12346
9. Babushok DV, Stanley N, Xie HM, Huang H, Bagg A, Olson TS, et al. Clonal replacement underlies spontaneous remission in paroxysmal nocturnal haemoglobinuria. *Br J Haematol* (2017) 176(3):487–90. doi:10.1111/bjh.13963
10. Ferla V, Zaninoni A, Fattizzo B, Fermo E, Gianelli U, Barcellini W. Paroxysmal nocturnal hemoglobinuria with spontaneous clinical remission. *Eur J Intern Med* (2017) 43:e11–4. doi:10.1016/j.ejim.2017.04.011
11. Hu R, Mukhina GL, Piantadosi S, Barber JP, Jones RJ, Brodsky RA. PIG-A mutations in normal hematopoiesis. *Blood* (2005) 105(10):3848–54. doi:10.1182/blood-2004-04-1472
12. Bessler M. Paroxysmal nocturnal hemoglobinuria: the price for a chance. *Schweiz Med Wochenschr* (1996) 126(45):1912–21.
13. Young NS, Calado RT, Scheinberg P. Current concepts in the pathophysiology and treatment of aplastic anemia. *Blood* (2006) 108(8):2509–19. doi:10.1182/blood-2006-03-010777
14. Shen W, Clemente MJ, Hosono N, Yoshida K, Przychodzen B, Yoshizato T, et al. Deep sequencing reveals stepwise mutation acquisition in paroxysmal nocturnal hemoglobinuria. *J Clin Invest* (2014) 124(10):4529–38. doi:10.1172/JCI74747
15. Schubert J, Roth A. Update on paroxysmal nocturnal haemoglobinuria (PNH): on the long way to understand the principles of the disease. *Eur J Haematol* (2015) 94(6):464–73. doi:10.1111/ejh.12520

8

Reference Intervals of Factor H and Factor H-Related Proteins in Healthy Children

Anna E. van Beek[1,2], Angela Kamp[1], Simone Kruithof[1], Ed J. Nieuwenhuys[3], Diana Wouters[1†], Ilse Jongerius[1], Theo Rispens[1], Taco W. Kuijpers[2,4] and Kyra A. Gelderman[3]*

[1] Department of Immunopathology, Sanquin Research and Landsteiner Laboratory of the Academic Medical Centre, University of Amsterdam, Amsterdam, Netherlands, [2] Department of Pediatric Hematology, Immunology and Infectious Diseases, Emma Children's Hospital, Academic Medical Centre, Amsterdam, Netherlands, [3] Sanquin Diagnostic Services, Amsterdam, Netherlands, [4] Department of Blood Cell Research, Sanquin Research and Landsteiner Laboratory of the Academic Medical Centre, University of Amsterdam, Amsterdam, Netherlands

Correspondence:
Kyra A. Gelderman
k.gelderman@sanquin.nl

†Present address:
Diana Wouters, Centre for Infectious Disease Control, National Institute for Public Health and the Environment, Bilthoven, Netherlands

Complement is activated as part of the innate immune defense against invading pathogens. Also, it helps to remove apoptotic debris and immune complexes from the circulation. Impaired complement function due to aberrant plasma levels of complement proteins may be indicative for complement-mediated diseases or can be involved in susceptibility for infections. To determine whether plasma levels are abnormal, reference intervals (RIs) are used from adult healthy donors. Since many complement-mediated diseases have an onset during childhood, it is important to know whether these RIs can be extrapolated to children. RIs of Factor H (FH), the crucial fluid-phase regulator, and the FH-related proteins (FHRs), its homologous counterparts, are unknown in healthy children. While FH is measured to diagnose and monitor therapy of patients with atypical hemolytic uremic syndrome, recent studies also implicated increased plasma levels of FHRs in disease. Here, we investigated the levels of FH and FHRs in healthy children using recently developed specific ELISAs. We found that levels of FH, FHR-2, and FHR-3 were equal to those found in healthy adults. Levels of FHR-4A and FHR-5 were lower in children than in adults. However, only the FHR-5 levels associated with age. The RIs of these FH family proteins now serve to support the interpretation of plasma levels in prospective and retrospective studies that can be used for routine diagnostic and monitoring purposes including pediatric patient samples.

Keywords: normal ranges, complement, complement factor H, factor H-related proteins, pediatrics, diagnostics, reference intervals

INTRODUCTION

Complement is part of innate immunity, comprising a powerful cascade of proteins able to eradicate invading pathogens and is important for removal of apoptotic debris and immune complexes from the circulation. Complement activation is tightly controlled and regulator proteins make sure that bystander damage to healthy host cells is kept to a minimum. Within the population, there is variation in the expression levels of these proteins and other complement components, leading to different steady-state complement activities in healthy individuals (1). Assessment of abnormal circulating levels can help to diagnose complement-mediated diseases such as atypical hemolytic uremic syndrome (aHUS) and differences in expression levels can help in understanding the susceptibility for infectious diseases as described in retrospective studies (2).

To discriminate between normal and abnormal levels, and to interpret retrospective studies, clinical laboratory reference intervals (RIs) are needed. As many complement-mediated diseases can have their onset during childhood, it is important to know whether adult levels can be extrapolated toward pediatric patients. For proteins such as C3 and C4, it has been determined that the normal ranges can be different in childhood compared to adults and between different ethnicities, and as such, adjusted RIs may be used (3–6). No pediatric RIs are known of Factor H (FH) and the FH-related proteins (FHRs), of which their plasma levels associate with various diseases.

Factor H is a crucial regulator of the alternative complement pathway and protects human host cells from unwanted complement activation. Genetic variants in complement regulator FH are associated with multiple diseases. Such variants can either alter protein functionality or induce variation in levels of expression. Many have been described to associate with aHUS or age-related macular degeneration, affecting the regulating function of FH (7, 8). However, some genetic variants result in lower (insufficient) circulating levels of FH (9–11). Differences in steady-state FH protein levels are associated with susceptibility for meningococcal disease and have recently been implicated as a marker of cardiovascular risk in chronic Chagas disease (12, 13). In general, low expression of complement regulators, such as FH, would make an individual more prone for chronic inflammation but more protected against infectious diseases, while high expression rather associates with risk of infectious diseases but less chronic inflammation (14).

Apart from FH, the FH protein family also includes the short splice variant of FH, FH-like-1 (FHL-1), and the FH-related (FHR) proteins, named FHR-1, FHR-2, FHR-3, FHR-4, and FHR-5, all of which are encoded by their own gene. FHR-4A and FHR-4B are the two splice variants of *CFHR4*, but FHR-4A is the only circulating variant found in human serum (15). While FHRs share homology with FH in its surface binding domains, they lack domains similar to SCR1-4 in FH and FHL-1, and for that reason are believed to have no complement-regulatory activity (16). Although limited data are available on the *in vivo* function of FHRs, many have shown associations of complement-mediated diseases with these FHR genes due to their copy number variations (17, 18), internal duplications (19–21), fusion proteins (22–26), or polymorphisms (27–30).

In addition, recent developments in the determination of circulating FHR levels in adults have led to the discovery of new associations with disease. FHR-1 levels were shown to be increased during IgA nephropathy (31, 32), although the authors report much higher levels than we and others have published (33, 34). FHR-3 levels were shown to be elevated during sepsis (35) and in systemic lupus erythematosus, rheumatoid arthritis, and polymyalgia rheumatica (36). Although Schäfer et al. did not find increased FHR-3 levels in aHUS patients, a recent study demonstrated increased levels in a larger, well-characterized cohort (36, 37). FHR-2 and FHR-4A levels have, so far, not been studied except in healthy donors, although FHR-2 and FHR-4A are implicated in the acute phase of bacterial infections (van Beek et al., manuscript in preparation) (15, 33, 38). FHR-5 levels were shown to be decreased in patients with C3 glomerulonephropathy (C3G) (39) and was recently identified as an independent risk factor for IgA nephropathy (32, 40). In summary, assessment of FHR protein levels contributes to the understanding of various diseases.

To investigate whether different RIs should be used for FH and the FHRs in children, we assessed the circulating levels in a cohort of healthy Dutch children and adolescents (all referred to as children), covering various age categories. These RIs now serve to support the interpretation of plasma levels in retrospective studies that include children. Moreover, they can be used for routine diagnostic and monitoring purposes in pediatric patient samples.

MATERIALS AND METHODS

Samples

Serum samples were obtained from anonymous, healthy children from a previous study, in accordance with Dutch regulations and approved by the Sanquin Ethical Advisory Board in accordance with the Declaration of Helsinki (41). Samples from adult healthy donors (n = 124 for FH and FHR-3, n = 120 for FHR-1, 2, 4A, and 5) were collected and measured during previous studies (15, 33, 35).

ELISAs

All ELISAs were performed as previously described for an adult healthy donor cohort (15, 33, 35). Briefly, the FH ELISA uses anti-FH.16, a monospecific mAb directed against SCR16-17, as a coat and goat anti-human-FH antiserum as detection. FHR-1/1 homodimers were measured using anti-FH.02 (directed against SCR20 of FH and cross-reactive to SCR5 of FHR-1) both as catching and detecting mAb. FHR-1/2 homodimers were also caught by anti-FH.02, but detected with a commercially available anti-FHR-2 (R&D Systems). FHR-2/2 homodimer levels, as well as total levels of FHR-1 and FHR-2 were calculated based on the observed levels of FHR-1/1 and FHR-1/2 dimers. The FHR-3 ELISA uses anti-FHR-3.1 (cross-reactive to FHR-4A) as a coating mAb and anti-FHR-3.4 (cross-reactive to FH) as a detecting mAb. FHR-4A was measured by catching with the monospecific mAb anti-FHR-4A.04 and detecting with rabbit anti-FHR-3 antiserum. FHR-5 homodimers were measured using two monospecific mAbs, anti-FHR-5.1 and anti-FHR-5.4. Two control sera were included in each plate to ensure limited inter assay variation.

Statistics

GraphPad Prism software v7 was used to analyze data and perform statistics (GraphPad Software, La Jolla, CA, USA). Significant differences were assessed by unpaired t-test. Correlations were assessed with a parametric Pearson's correlation test.

RESULTS

With this study, we obtained more insight in the normal ranges of FH and the FHRs in children. For this, we used a cohort of 110 healthy children, of which 53% were females (**Table 1**). The subjects were evenly distributed across the age categories, aged 7 months up to 251 months (20.9 years) (41). We compared the levels in children to the levels that we previously found in adult healthy Dutch donors (15, 33, 35).

TABLE 1 | General cohort characteristics.

Cohort	*n*	Mean age (years)
Total children	110	10.3
Males	52 (47%)	9.2
Females	58 (53%)	11.2
Age group (years)	**Males (*n*)**	**Females (*n*)**
0–3	8	1
3–6	13	13
6–9	8	8
9–12	3	9
12–15	8	7
15–18	5	17
18–21	7	3

We investigated the plasma levels of FH and the FHRs in these healthy children (**Figure 1**). We observed that the levels of FH and FHR-3 were similar between the two genders and independent of age (**Figures 1A,G**). Indeed, the levels are equal to those previously found in adult healthy Dutch donors (**Table 2**) (35).

Next, FHR-1 and FHR-2 were assessed using dimer-specific ELISAs (**Figures 1B,C**). The levels of FHR-1/1 homodimers were independent of age and gender, although we did find a minor, but significant, difference when comparing the FHR-1/1 levels to adults (**Table 2**, difference between means = 1.2 μg/mL) (33). FHR-1/2 heterodimers and FHR-2/2 homodimers were also found to be independent of age and gender but were similar to the adult healthy donors (**Figure 1D**; **Table 2**). This implied that only the FHR-1 plasma levels differed from the adults. Indeed, when we calculated the concentrations of total FHR-1 and FHR-2 monomers, only FHR-1 levels were significantly lower [difference between means = 1.3 μg/mL (33 nM)] than the healthy adults (**Figures 1E,F**; **Table 2**).

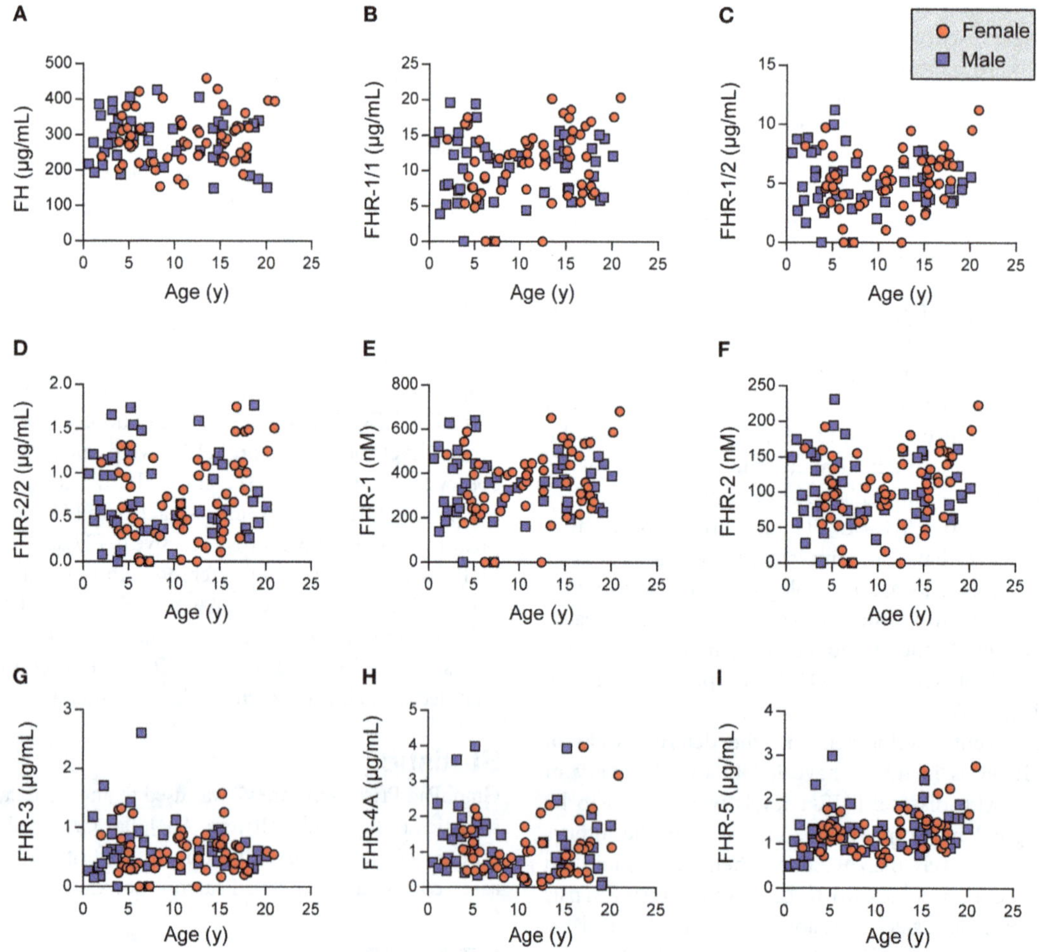

FIGURE 1 | Factor H (FH) family proteins in healthy children. **(A–C,G–I)** Show FH and FHRs as assessed by in-house ELISA. **(D–F)** Indicate calculated FHR-1 and FHR-2 levels. **(D,F)** Samples lacking FHR-1 (likely *CFHR1* deficient) were excluded. Females are indicated by red circles, males by blue squares. Data were analyzed using Pearson's correlation and unpaired *t*-tests (**Table 2**).

TABLE 2 | Factor H (FH) family normal ranges characteristics.

		FH (μg/mL)	FHR-1/1 (μg/mL)[b]	FHR-1/2 (μg/mL)[b]	FHR-2/2 (μg/mL)[a,b]	FHR-1 (nM)[a,b]	FHR-2 (nM)[a,b]	FHR-3 (μg/mL)[b]	FHR-4A (μg/mL)	FHR-5 (μg/mL)
Median	Male	286	11.2	5.1	0.6	351	96	0.58	0.92	1.2
	Female	279	11.5	5.4	0.6	362	105	0.54	0.91	1.2
IQR (25%)	Male	237.5	7.0	3.7	0.39	243	73	0.36	0.54	0.93
	Female	237.3	7.2	3.6	0.34	245	65	0.34	0.46	0.92
IQR (75%)	Male	426.5	13.5	6.7	1.1	439	150	0.81	1.6	1.48
	Female	459.5	14.4	7.0	1.1	469	223	0.74	1.3	1.47
95% range	Male	150–420	0–20	0–11	0–1.8	0–637	0–219	0–2.3	0.1–4.0	0.5–2.8
	Female	157–445	0–20	0–11	0–1.6	0–669	0–209	0–1.5	0.1–3.6	0.6–2.7
Gender difference	Unpaired *t*-test (*P* value)	0.84	0.28	0.75	0.87	0.51	1.00	0.42	0.26	0.99
Children vs age	Pearson *r*	0.00	0.13	0.07	0.03	0.12	0.06	−0.14	−0.03	0.29
	R squared	0.00	0.02	0.00	0.00	0.01	0.00	0.02	0.00	0.09
	P value	0.97	0.20	0.48	0.73	0.22	0.54	0.15	0.76	0.002
Children vs adults	Unpaired *t*-test (*P* value)	0.655	0.030	0.444	0.870	0.0498	0.873	0.100	<0.0001	<0.0001
	Difference between means (μg/mL)	4.114	1.219	0.2173	−0.0095	32.66 nM	0.9862 nM	0.0952	1.438	0.3863

[a]*Values of FHR-2/2 homodimers, and total levels of FHR-1 and FHR-2 monomers are calculated based on measured levels of FHR-1/1 homodimers and FHR-1/2 heterodimers.*
[b]*Donors lacking FHR-1, FHR-2 (in the adult donor cohort) or FHR-3 were excluded from correlations and unpaired t-tests*

We recently demonstrated that FHR-4A is the only circulating form of FHR-4 and that no FHR-4B could be observed in serum (15). Therefore, we measured only FHR-4A in the children and found that FHR-4A levels were lower than expected based on levels found in adult healthy donors (**Figure 1H; Table 2**). It would, therefore, be expected that the levels showed an association with age. Surprisingly, the FHR-4A levels did neither show an association with age, nor with gender, in the children.

Last, we assessed the levels of FHR-5/5 homodimers. Similar to the other FHR proteins, FHR-5 levels were independent of gender. However, the levels did increase with age (**Figure 1I, Table 2**), being approximately 0.5 μg/mL lower in the youngest children than in the oldest children. While the younger children indeed showed significantly lower levels, the older children presented with levels equal to the adult healthy donors.

As the *CFHR* genes originated as part of segmental duplications of the *CFH* gene, it would be possible that protein expression is similarly regulated (42). Therefore, we investigated whether FH plasma levels associated with plasma levels of the FHRs. We saw an association between FH and FHR-1/1 homodimer levels in adult donors, when they carry two copies of *CFHR1* (r = 0.62, P < 0.0001), in contrast to those who carry only 1 copy of *CFHR1* (r = 0.09, P = 0.67) (33, 35). Children who most likely carry two copies of *CFHR1* [expressing > 10.1 μg/mL FHR-1/1 homodimers, as determined by ROC analysis (area under the curve = 0.97)] showed a similar association (r = 0.49, P < 0.0001) (33). No association between FH and other FHR levels was noted. As a general conclusion, we observed no remarkable differences compared to adult circulating levels of FH family proteins.

DISCUSSION

We have determined RIs for FH and FHR-1 to 5 in Dutch healthy children. We were able to interpret the circulating levels of these FH family proteins in relation to adult healthy donors, which we have previously assessed (15, 33, 35). We found differences in some but not all of these proteins in the healthy children when compared with adults.

In contrast to FHR-1, FHR-4A, and FHR-5, no remarkable observations were made when analyzing the circulating levels of FH, FHR-2, and FHR-3. The three proteins were independent of age and gender, confirming a previous study on FH in Brazilian children (43). FH levels were previously found to be low in neonates, suggesting that plasma levels reach adult ranges within the first 6 months after birth (44, 45). Unfortunately, no sera were available from children below the age of 6 months. Future studies should test cord blood and plasma of neonates for the presence of FHRs at birth and early infancy to investigate these protein levels in more detail.

FHR-1 levels were independent of age and gender. We did observe lower FHR-1 levels than previously seen in adults, although the biological relevance may be disputed. FHR-3 levels were also trending toward significance, indicating that a minor difference in the copy number variation in *CFHR3/CFHR1* between the two cohorts might be affecting the results (33, 35).

We found lower FHR-4A levels in children than in adults, even though FHR-4A did not associate with age of the children. Our group demonstrated previously that FHR-4A is stable up to at least 10 freeze-thaw cycles (15). However, we cannot exclude the possibility that long-term storage of these samples may have suffered from breakdown of FHR-4A when kept at −30°C (15). New studies on more recent samples are needed to confirm or disprove this possible explanation.

For FHR-5, we observed an increase with age, indicating that normal ranges for FHR-5 are low in the youngest children and that RIs may need to be adjusted accordingly. As FHR-5 levels positively associated with severity of IgA nephropathy in adults (32), and as IgA nephropathy is the main nephropathy in children (46), measurements of FHR-5 in a pediatric cohort will be highly informative to further study the role of FHR-5 in this nephropathy.

This study represents the most complete assessment of FH family proteins to date in a cohort of healthy children providing RIs. These RIs can now be used to interpret serum levels in prospective and retrospective studies that include children and used for routine diagnostic and monitoring purposes in pediatric patient samples. Ideally, each laboratory should adapt these RIs for their own assays.

AUTHOR CONTRIBUTIONS

AB, DW, TK, and KG designed research. AB, AK, SK, and EN performed research. AB, IJ, TR, TK, and KG analyzed data and wrote the paper. All authors critically reviewed the manuscript, gave final approval of the version to be published, and agreed to be accountable for all aspects of the work in ensuring that questions related to the accuracy or integrity of any part of the work are appropriately investigated and resolved.

FUNDING

Research leading to these results has received funding from the European Union's seventh Framework program under EC-GA no. 279185 (EUCLIDS; www.euclids-project.eu). The funders had no role in study design, data collection and analysis, decision to publish, or preparation of the manuscript.

REFERENCES

1. Harris CL, Heurich M, Rodriguez de Cordoba S, Morgan BP. The complotype: dictating risk for inflammation and infection. *Trends Immunol* (2012) 33:513–21. doi:10.1016/j.it.2012.06.001
2. Davila S, Wright VJ, Khor CC, Sim KS, Binder A, Breunis WB, et al. Genome-wide association study identifies variants in the CFH region associated with host susceptibility to meningococcal disease. *Nat Genet* (2010) 42:772–6. doi:10.1038/ng.640
3. Jolliff CR, Cost KM, Stivrins PC, Grossman PP, Nolte CR, Franco SM, et al. Reference intervals for serum IgG, IgA, IgM, C3, and C4 as determined by rate nephelometry. *Clin Chem* (1982) 28:126–8.
4. Roach B, Kim Y, Jerome E, Michael AF. Influence of age and sex on serum complement components in children. *Am J Dis Child* (1981) 135:918–20.
5. Kardar GA, Oraei M, Shahsavani M, Namdar Z, Kazemisefat GE, Haghi Ashtiani MT, et al. Reference intervals for serum immunoglobulins IgG, IgA, IgM and complements C3 and C4 in Iranian healthy children. *Iran J Public Health* (2012) 41:59–63.
6. Norman ME, Gall EP, Taylor A, Laster L, Nilsson UR. Serum complement profiles in infants and children. *J Pediatr* (1975) 87:912–6. doi:10.1016/S0022-3476(75)80904-8
7. Kavanagh D, Goodship TH, Richards A. Atypical hemolytic uremic syndrome. *Semin Nephrol* (2013) 33:508–30. doi:10.1016/j.semnephrol.2013.08.003
8. Toomey CB, Johnson LV, Bowes Rickman C. Complement factor H in AMD: bridging genetic associations and pathobiology. *Prog Retin Eye Res* (2018) 62:38–57. doi:10.1016/j.preteyeres.2017.09.001
9. Triebwasser MP, Roberson EDO, Yu Y, Schramm EC, Wagner EK, Raychaudhuri S, et al. Rare variants in the functional domains of complement factor H are associated with age-related macular degeneration. *Investig Opthalmol Vis Sci* (2015) 56:6873. doi:10.1167/iovs.15-17432
10. Dragon-Durey MA, Frémeaux-Bacchi V, Loirat C, Blouin J, Niaudet P, Deschenes G, et al. Heterozygous and homozygous factor H deficiencies associated with hemolytic uremic syndrome or membranoproliferative glomerulonephritis: report and genetic analysis of 16 cases. *J Am Soc Nephrol* (2004) 15:787–95. doi:10.1097/01.ASN.0000115702.28859.A7
11. Ansari M, McKeigue PM, Skerka C, Hayward C, Rudan I, Vitart V, et al. Genetic influences on plasma CFH and CFHR1 concentrations and their role in susceptibility to age-related macular degeneration. *Hum Mol Genet* (2013) 22:4857–69. doi:10.1093/hmg/ddt336
12. Haralambous E, Dolly SO, Hibberd ML, Litt DJ, Udalova IA, O'dwyer C, et al. Factor H, a regulator of complement activity, is a major determinant of meningococcal disease susceptibility in UK Caucasian patients. *Scand J Infect Dis* (2006) 38:764–71. doi:10.1080/00365540600643203
13. Lidani KCF, Sandri TL, Andrade FA, Bavia L, Nisihara R, Messias-Reason IJ. Complement Factor H as a potential atherogenic marker in chronis Chagas disease. *Parasite Immunol* (2018) 40(7):e12537. doi:10.1111/pim.12537
14. Heurich M, Martinez-Barricarte R, Francis NJ, Roberts DL, Rodriguez de Cordoba S, Morgan BP, et al. Common polymorphisms in C3, factor B, and factor H collaborate to determine systemic complement activity and disease risk. *Proc Natl Acad Sci U S A* (2011) 108:8761–6. doi:10.1073/pnas.1019338108
15. Pouw RB, Brouwer MC, Van Beek AE, Józsi M, Barlow PN, Sim RB, et al. Complement factor H-related protein 4A is the dominant circulating splice variant of CFHR4. *Front Immunol* (2018) 9:729. doi:10.3389/fimmu.2018.00729
16. Medjeral-Thomas N, Pickering MC. The complement factor H-related proteins. *Immunol Rev* (2016) 274:191–201. doi:10.1111/imr.12477
17. Kubista KE, Tosakulwong N, Wu Y, Ryu E, Roeder JL, Hecker LA, et al. Copy number variation in the complement factor H-related genes and age-related macular degeneration. *Mol Vis* (2011) 17:2080–92.
18. Cantsilieris S, White SJ, Richardson AJ, Guymer RH, Baird PN. Comprehensive analysis of copy number variation of genes at chromosome 1 and 10 loci associated with late age related macular degeneration. *PLoS One* (2012) 7:e35255. doi:10.1371/journal.pone.0035255
19. Tortajada A, Yébenes H, Abarrategui-garrido C, Anter J, García-fernández JM, Martínez-barricarte R, et al. C3 glomerulopathy-associated CFHR1 mutation alters FHR oligomerization and complement regulation. *J Clin Invest* (2013) 123:2434–46. doi:10.1172/JCI68280
20. Gale DP, de Jorge EG, Cook HT, Martinez-Barricarte R, Hadjisavvas A, McLean AG, et al. Identification of a mutation in complement factor H-related protein 5 in patients of Cypriot origin with glomerulonephritis. *Lancet* (2010) 376:794–801. doi:10.1016/S0140-6736(10)60670-8
21. Medjeral-Thomas N, Malik TH, Patel MP, Toth T, Cook HT, Tomson C, et al. A novel CFHR5 fusion protein causes C3 glomerulopathy in a family without Cypriot ancestry. *Kidney Int* (2014) 85:933–7. doi:10.1038/ki.2013.348
22. Xiao X, Ghossein C, Tortajada A, Zhang Y, Meyer N, Jones M, et al. Familial C3 glomerulonephritis caused by a novel CFHR5-CFHR2 fusion gene. *Mol Immunol* (2016) 77:89–96. doi:10.1016/j.molimm.2016.07.007
23. Chen Q, Wiesener M, Eberhardt HU, Hartmann A, Uzonyi B, Kirschfink M, et al. Complement factor H-related hybrid protein deregulates complement in dense deposit disease. *J Clin Invest* (2014) 124:145–55. doi:10.1172/JCI71866
24. Malik TH, Lavin PJ, Goicoechea de Jorge E, Vernon KA, Rose KL, Patel MP, et al. A hybrid CFHR3-1 gene causes familial C3 glomerulopathy. *J Am Soc Nephrol* (2012) 23:1155–60. doi:10.1681/ASN.2012020166
25. Valoti E, Alberti M, Tortajada A, Garcia-Fernandez J, Gastoldi S, Besso L, et al. A novel atypical hemolytic uremic syndrome-associated hybrid CFHR1/CFH gene encoding a fusion protein that antagonizes factor H-dependent complement regulation. *J Am Soc Nephrol* (2015) 26:209–19. doi:10.1681/ASN.2013121339
26. Togarsimalemath SK, Sethi SK, Duggal R, Le Quintrec M, Jha P, Daniel R, et al. A novel CFHR1-CFHR5 hybrid leads to a familial dominant C3 glomerulopathy. *Kidney Int* (2017) 92(4):876–87. doi:10.1016/j.kint.2017.04.025
27. Westra D, Vernon Ka, Volokhina EB, Pickering MC, van de Kar NC, van den Heuvel LP. Atypical hemolytic uremic syndrome and genetic aberrations in

the complement factor H-related 5 gene. *J Hum Genet* (2012) 57:459–64. doi:10.1038/jhg.2012.57

28. Abrera-Abeleda Ma, Nishimura C, Smith JLH, Sethi S, McRae JL, Murphy BF, et al. Variations in the complement regulatory genes factor H (CFH) and factor H related 5 (CFHR5) are associated with membranoproliferative glomerulonephritis type II (dense deposit disease). *J Med Genet* (2006) 43:582–9. doi:10.1136/jmg.2005.038315
29. Bernabéu-Herrero ME, Jiménez-Alcázar M, Anter J, Pinto S, Sánchez Chinchilla D, Garrido S, et al. Complement factor H, FHR-3 and FHR-1 variants associate in an extended haplotype conferring increased risk of atypical hemolytic uremic syndrome. *Mol Immunol* (2015) 67:276–86. doi:10.1016/j.molimm.2015.06.021
30. Monteferrante G, Brioschi S, Caprioli J, Pianetti G, Bettinaglio P, Bresin E, et al. Genetic analysis of the complement factor H related 5 gene in haemolytic uraemic syndrome. *Mol Immunol* (2007) 44:1704–8. doi:10.1016/j.molimm.2006.08.004
31. Tortajada A, Gutiérrez E, Goicoechea de Jorge E, Anter J, Segarra A, Espinosa M, et al. Elevated factor H-related protein 1 and factor H pathogenic variants decrease complement regulation in IgA nephropathy. *Kidney Int* (2017) 92(4):953–63. doi:10.1016/j.kint.2017.03.041
32. Medjeral-thomas NR, Lomax-browne HJ, Beckwith H, Willicombe M, Mclean AG, Brookes P, et al. Circulating complement factor H-related proteins 1 and 5 correlate with disease activity in IgA nephropathy. *Kidney Int* (2017) 92:942–52. doi:10.1016/j.kint.2017.03.043
33. van Beek AE, Pouw RB, Brouwer MC, van Mierlo G, Geissler J, Ooijevaar-De Heer P, et al. Factor H-related (FHR)-1 and FHR-2 form homo- and heterodimers, while FHR-5 circulates only as homodimer in human plasma. *Front Immunol* (2017) 8:1328. doi:10.3389/fimmu.2017.01328
34. Kopczynska M, Zelek W, Touchard S, Gaughran F, Di Forti M, Mondelli V, et al. Complement system biomarkers in first episode psychosis. *Schizophr Res* (2017). doi:10.1016/j.schres.2017.12.012
35. Pouw RB, Brouwer MC, Geissler J, van Herpen LV, Zeerleder SS, Wuillemin WA, et al. Complement factor H-related protein 3 serum levels are low compared to factor H and mainly determined by gene copy number variation in CFHR3. *PLoS One* (2016) 11:e0152164. doi:10.1371/journal.pone.0152164
36. Schäfer N, Grosche A, Reinders J, Hauck S, Pouw RB, Kuijpers TW, et al. Complement regulator FHR-3 is elevated either locally or systemically in a selection of autoimmune diseases. *Front Immunol* (2016) 7:1–16. doi:10.3389/fimmu.2016.00542
37. Pouw RB, Delgado IG, Lera AL, Rodríguez de Córdoba S, Wouters D, Kuijpers TW, et al. High complement factor H-related (FHR)-3 levels are associated with the atypical hemolytic-uremic syndrome-risk allele CFHR3*B. *Front Immunol* (2018) 9:848. doi:10.3389/fimmu.2018.00848
38. Hebecker M, Józsi M. Factor H-related protein 4 activates complement by serving as a platform for the assembly of alternative pathway C3 convertase via its interaction with C3b protein. *J Biol Chem* (2012) 287:19528–36. doi:10.1074/jbc.M112.364471
39. Vernon Ka, Goicoechea de Jorge E, Hall AE, Fremeaux-Bacchi V, Aitman TJ, Cook HT, et al. Acute presentation and persistent glomerulonephritis following streptococcal infection in a patient with heterozygous complement factor H-related protein 5 deficiency. *Am J Kidney Dis* (2012) 60:121–5. doi:10.1053/j.ajkd.2012.02.329
40. Zhu L, Guo W, Shi S, Liu L, Lv J, Medjeral-thomas NR, et al. Circulating complement factor H-related protein 5 levels contribute to development and progression of IgA nephropathy. *Kidney Int* (2018) 94(1):150–8. doi:10.1016/j.kint.2018.02.023
41. Lepage N, Huang SHS, Nieuwenhuys E, Filler G. Pediatric reference intervals for immunoglobulin G and its subclasses with Siemens immunonephelometric assays. *Clin Biochem* (2010) 43:694–6. doi:10.1016/j.clinbiochem.2010.02.003
42. Cantsilieris S, Nelson BJ, Huddleston J, Baker C, Harshman L, Penewit K. Recurrent structural variation, clustered sites of selection, and disease risk for the complement factor H (CFH) gene family. *Proc Natl Acad Sci U S A* (2018) 115(19):E4433–42. doi:10.1073/pnas.1717600115
43. De Paula PF, Barbosa JE, Junior PR, Ferriani VPL, Latorre MRDO, Nudelman V, et al. Ontogeny of complement regulatory proteins – concentrations of factor H, factor I, C4b-binding protein, properdin and vitronectin in healthy children of different ages and in adults. *Scand J Immunol* (2003) 58:572–7. doi:10.1046/j.1365-3083.2003.01326.x
44. Sonntag J, Brandenburg U, Polzehl D, Strauss E, Vogel M, Dudenhausen JW, et al. Complement system in healthy term newborns: reference values in umbilical cord blood. *Pediatr Dev Pathol* (1998) 1:131–5. doi:10.1007/s100249900016
45. Davis CA, Vallota EH, Forristal J. Serum complement levels in infancy: age related changes. *Pediatr Res* (1979) 13:1043–6. doi:10.1203/00006450-197909000-00019
46. Wenderfer SE, Gaut JP. Glomerular diseases in children. *Adv Chronic Kidney Dis* (2017) 24:364–71. doi:10.1053/j.ackd.2017.09.005

9

The C3dg Fragment of Complement is Superior to Conventional C3 as a Diagnostic Biomarker in Systemic Lupus Erythematosus

Anne Troldborg[1,2], Lisbeth Jensen[3], Bent Deleuran[1,3], Kristian Stengaard-Pedersen[1,2], Steffen Thiel[3] and Jens Christian Jensenius[3]*

[1] Department of Rheumatology, Aarhus University Hospital, Aarhus, Denmark, [2] Institute of Clinical Medicine, Aarhus University, Aarhus, Denmark, [3] Department of Biomedicine, Aarhus University, Aarhus, Denmark

***Correspondence:**
Anne Troldborg
annetrol@rm.dk

Introduction/objectives: In 2012, hypocomplementemia was included in the classification criteria of systemic lupus erythematosus (SLE). The suggested measurement of C3 or C4 often reflect disease activity poorly. Our objective was to establish an assay measuring C3dg, which is generated following complement activation, and to evaluate the assay in a cross-sectional SLE cohort.

Method: We included SLE patients (n = 169) and controls (n = 170) and developed a modified C3dg assay where C3dg fragments were separated from the large plasma proteins by polyethylene glycol (PEG), and the supernatant containing the C3dg fragment was used for analysis in an antibody-based sandwich-type assay. Gel permeation chromatography and western blotting were used to establish the optimal conditions for PEG precipitation.

Results: 16% PEG was optimal for separating C3dg from C3 and the larger protein fragments. The assay showed a high degree of stability when using EDTA plasma, and measurements correlated well with commercially available complement activation assays. SLE patients had higher concentrations in plasma of C3dg than controls ($p < 0.05$). ROC analysis showed that the C3dg activation fragment of C3 with an AUC of 0.96 (CI 0.94–0.98) was superior to C3 (AUC 0.52) in differentiating between patients and controls.

Conclusion: Our results present a modified assay for the measurement of C3dg. We demonstrate that C3dg was superior to conventional C3 measurements in discriminating SLE patients from controls. We suggest that C3dg should be considered as a complement activation measurement in the SLE classification criteria.

Keywords: complement system, complement activation, systemic lupus erythematosus, biomarker, diagnostics

INTRODUCTION

Systemic lupus erythematosus (SLE) is an autoimmune disease involving loss of tolerance to self-antigens, which is manifested in the production of autoantibodies and deposition of complement-fixing immune complexes in injured tissue (1). Activation of the complement system has for decades been known as a significant contributor to SLE pathogenesis (2). However, not all mechanisms leading to complement activation are understood.

In 2012, new classification criteria of SLE were published by the SLICC group (Systemic Lupus International Collaborating Clinics) (3), and expert consensus included low complement protein 3 and 4 (C3 and C4) or low CH50 [complement hemolytic activity (4)] in the classification criteria. There is no explanation for this choice, but it reflects what has been done in the clinic for years. No suggestions of type of assays were given for the measurements of C3, C4, and CH50 in relation to the classification criteria.

The complement system, comprising more than 40 soluble and membrane bound proteins, is activated through three pathways: the classical, the alternative, and the lectin pathway (5). The classical and the lectin pathways are activated through pattern recognition. Serine proteases bound to a pattern-recognition molecule are activated upon recognition of a fitting pattern and through several enzymatic reactions this lead to the activation of the classical and lectin pathway C3-convertase (C4b2a) (6). The alternative pathway is in a state of constant activation, but is at the same time inhibited. There is a continuous hydrolyzes of C3 in the circulation, which potentially can lead to complement activation *via* the alternative pathway of complement activation. Under normal circumstances, this process is inhibited both in the circulation and at the cell surface (7, 8).

There are several ways to measure complement activation. One way is quantification of C3 and C4 protein (9) or fragments of the cleaved complement factors, e.g., C5a or C3a (10). Other assays estimate capacity of erythrocyte lysis (11) or estimate the level of soluble membrane attack complex (12, 13).

The central component in complement activation is C3 (14). When activated, C3 is cleaved into two fragments: C3a and C3b (14). C3b is further cleaved by factor I into iC3b and finally to C3dg and C3c (14). The smallest fragments C3a has a short half-live (15), while the larger fragment C3dg (37 kDa) has a longer plasma half-life of 4 h (16). C3c showed a shorter half-life than C3dg. Because of its size, C3dg can relatively easy be separated by size from the larger C3 molecules that also comprise the C3dg part [C3, C3(H_2O), C3b, and iC3b]. These molecules will collectively here be termed C3′. A method for measuring the C3 split product C3dg was previously introduced using precipitation with 11% polyethylene glycol (PEG) to separate C3dg from C3′ (17). It has, however, not gained routine use. The same is the case for the modified rocket immuno-electrophoresis (18). The so-called double-decker rocket immuno-electrophoresis is used in a few clinical laboratories despite its technical challenges (19).

Our objective was to optimize an assay for the measurement of C3dg using precipitation with PEG followed by C3dg determination in the supernatant by immune assays. Furthermore, to evaluate if C3dg was superior to conventional C3 in discriminating between SLE patients and healthy controls in a cross-sectional cohort of SLE patients.

MATERIALS AND METHODS

Patients

A cross-sectional cohort of 169 SLE patients were included consecutively at the out-patient clinic at the Department of Rheumatology, Aarhus University Hospital (November, 2015 to August, 2016). Inclusion criteria were fulfilment of the 1997 American College of Rheumatology (ACR) classification criteria for SLE (20), age 18 or above, understanding and speaking Danish. Exclusion criteria were infection, ongoing cancer treatment, and incapacitation. After written consent, clinical data including disease activity, SLE disease activity index (SLEDAI) (21), accumulated organ damage, SLICC/ACR (22), and treatment information were collected. Serum and plasma samples for research purposes were drawn at the same time as samples for routine biochemical assessments. Control samples ($n = 170$) were collected from blood donors at the blood bank of Aarhus University Hospital, Denmark (December, 2014 to January, 2015) as previously described (23).

Blood collected in EDTA plasma tubes (8 ml) and polystyrene serum tubes (10 ml) (Alere #367525 and #367896) were centrifuged at 2,000 *g* for 10 min. Plasma and serum were collected and frozen immediately at −80°C. Maximum time from blood drawing until freezing was 2 h.

Assays for C3dg

Time-Resolved Immuno Fluorometric Assay (TRIFMA)

A standard for the assay was generated by activation of serum according to the recommendations of the study group for the manufacture of the International Complement Standard #2 (24). Ten milliliters of serum were incubated for 4 h at 37°C after the admixture of 1 ml heat aggregated human IgG (#007815; CSL Behring GmbH, Germany, 10 mg/ml TBS, aggregated at 63°C for 1 h) and 0.1 g zymosan (Sigma #Z4250). The activation was stopped by adding 550 µl 0.4 M EDTA and 200 µl Futhan (Sigma, 10 mg/ml H_2O). Following precipitation with 11% PEG 6000 (w/v), the sample was centrifuged at 10,000 *g* 4°C for 30 min. The supernatant was collected and used as standard for the assay.

The standard curve was made by dilution of the activated serum standard 1/300 in Tris-buffered saline [0.14 M NaCl, 10 mM Tris, 14 mM sodium azide, with 0.05% (v/v) Tween 20 (TBS/Tween)], and further seven threefold dilutions.

Test samples (EDTA plasma) were pre-diluted 1/4 in TBS, and 40 µl was added to 60 µl TBS, 10 mM EDTA. Samples were kept on ice throughout mixing and dilution to inhibit complement activation. One hundred microliters of 32% PEG in H_2O (w/v) were admixed and samples incubated for 1 h followed by centrifugation at 4,000 *g* 4°C for 15 min. The supernatants were withdrawn and diluted 1/200 in TBS/Tween, reaching a 2,000-fold dilution of the starting plasma sample. Duplicates of 100 µl were added to Fluoro Nunc MaxiSorb microtiter plates (Nunc, #437958 or #43791) previously coated by incubation overnight at room temperature (RT) with 100 µl rabbit anti-human C3dg (DAKO cat. no. A0063), mistakenly termed "anti-human C3d" (confirmed by correspondence with DAKO), at 5 µg/ml PBS and blocked by incubation with HSA at 1 mg HSA/ml TBS followed by wash with TBS-Tween. After each step, the wells were washed three times with TBS/Tween. Development after incubation overnight at 4°C was with the same anti-C3dg antibody as used for coating only now the antibody was biotinylated as previously described (25). One hundred microliters of biotin-anti-C3dg,

1 μg/ml TBS/Tween, were added to the wells and incubated 2 h at RT. After washing, 25 ng of Eu^{3+}-streptavidin (Perkin Elmer #1244-360) in 100 μl TBS/Tween, 25 μM EDTA was added and incubated for 1 h at RT. After washing, 200 μl enhancement buffer (Ampliqon laboratory reagents #Q99800) was added to each well. Plates were read by time-resolved fluorometry using a DELFIA-reader Victor5 + (Perkin Elmer®) full TRIFMA protocol can be found Data Sheet 2 in Supplementary Material.

Enzyme-Linked Immune Sorbent Assay (ELISA)

The assay was also tested in an ELISA format identical to the above, except after incubation with biotinylated antibody and wash, 100 μl horseradish peroxidase (HRP)–streptavidin (DAKO #PO397) diluted 1/500 in TBS/Tween was added and incubated 1 h at RT. After washing, 100 μl substrate (Sigma #P4922-capsules and #A9941-tablets) was added and incubated for 30 min at 37°C. Plates were read at 405 nm on Victor5+ full ELISA protocol can be found Data Sheet 1 in Supplementary Material.

Assay for C3′

The assay was performed analogous to the C3dg TRIFMA (excluding PEG precipitation). Wells were coated with rabbit anti-human C3c (DAKO #Q0368, 1 μg/ml TBS), and the development was with the same antibody biotinylated in-house at 1 μg/ml. The standard curve was constructed with dilutions of the serum pool assigned a value of 1 AU C3/ml. The test plasma samples were diluted 750,000-fold in TBS/Tw, 5 mM EDTA.

Optimizing the PEG Precipitation

Plasma proteins were precipitated with increasing concentrations of PEG from 10 to 19% (w/v). Precipitations were done as in the assay described above with PEG being added at 20–38% (w/v). C3dg in the supernatants was estimated as described above.

Gel Permeation Chromatography (GPC)

Samples of serum, supernatant of PEG precipitated activated serum and EDTA-plasma supernatant after precipitation with either 11 or 16% PEG (w/v), were subjected to GPC on a Superose 6 10/300 GL column (GE Healthcare). The running buffer was TBS/Tween, 5 mM EDTA. Samples were diluted 1:1 in buffer and 200 μl was loaded on the column. Fractions of 0.25 ml were collected in pure polystyrene microtiter plates (Nunc #249570), which were pre-blocked by incubation with TBS-Tween. C3dg in the fractions was quantified as described above.

Western Blots

Samples of supernatants and precipitates after admixture of PEG were added to 1/4 volume sodium dodecyl sulfate-polyacrylamide gel electrophoresis (SDS-PAGE) sample buffer [30 mM Tris–HCl, 10% (v/v) glycerol, 8 M urea, 3% (w/v) SDS, 0.1% (w/v) bromophenol blue, pH 8.9]. TBS/Tween was added to reach the desired sample volume (30–45 μl). One-tenth volume of dithiothreitol (DDT), 0.6 M, was added to the samples to be reduced, and iodoacetic acid, 1.4 M, 1/10 vol, was added to all samples applied to gels containing both reduced and non-reduced samples. Samples were denatured at 100°C for 3 min. Proteins were separated on 4–15% gradient gels (Bio-Rad, Criterion TGX gels #567-1083). Following electrophoresis, the proteins were blotted onto nitrocellulose membranes (Bio-Rad #170-4159). The membranes were then blocked by incubation for 30 min at RT in TBS with 0.1% Tween (v/v), washed, and developed with polyclonal rabbit anti-human-C3dg (DAKO #0063) at 1 μg/ml or polyclonal rabbit anti-human-C3c (DAKO #0368) in primary buffer [Tris-buffered saline, 1 mM EDTA, pH 7.4, with 1 mg human serum albumin (CSL Behring #109697) and 100 μg human IgG (CSL Behring #007815) per ml]. Membranes were subsequently washed and incubated with HRP-conjugated goat anti-rabbit IgG antibody (DAKO #P0448) diluted 1/3,000 in secondary buffer (TBS/Tween, 100 μg human IgG/ml, 1 mM EDTA, pH 7.4). After washing, the blots were developed with SuperSignal West Dura extended-duration substrate (Pierce), and emission recorded by a charge-coupled device camera.

Storage, Freeze/Thaw, and Diurnal Variation

To test the stability of the assay, regarding handling of samples, we initially tested both serum and EDTA plasma. Samples were tested after 0, 1 h, and 5 h at RT, and at 1 and 5 h at 37°C. Blood collected in EDTA was left for 5 h at RT or 5 h at 37°C before centrifugation and collection of plasma.

To test the stability of the samples to freezing/thawing cycles, a pool of EDTA plasma was aliquoted in 500 μl samples, frozen at −80°C, and thawed 1–9 times. Each thaw cycle was 1 h at RT.

Influence of diurnal variation on complement activation was investigated on six healthy individuals with samples taken at 4 h intervals through 24 h.

Comparison With Commercial Assays

Immunoassays were bought from Hycult Biotech, estimating a C3c neo determinant (# HK368-02), Nordic Biosite, estimating a C3d neo determinant (#KSP-305) and Quidel, estimating C4d (#A008). Seventeen SLE samples and seventeen controls were randomly picked and run on all assays according to the manufacture's description.

Twelve SLE patients were randomly picked to have C3d measured at the hospital of Vejle, Denmark, using a double-decker rocket immuno-electrophoresis method (19).

Statistics

Checking the data for normality by Q–Q plots and histograms revealed that Gaussian distribution could not be assumed. Log-transformation did not improve normality significantly. Therefore, non-parametric tests were used for the statistical analysis. The Mann–Whitney *U*-test was used for comparison of plasma levels of the proteins in patients and controls and correlation analysis was performed calculating Spearman's rank correlation coefficient. For comparison of repeated measurements, the Kruskal–Wallis test was used. p-Values <0.05 were considered statistically significant. Stata version 12 and GraphPad Prism software package (version 6.0) were used for data management and statistical calculations.

Ethics

Clinical investigations were conducted according to the Declaration of Helsinki. The Danish Data Protection Agency and The Regional Committee on Health Research Ethics approved the study (case #1-10-72-214-13).

RESULTS

Patients and Controls

The cohort of SLE patients (**Table 1**) was comparable to other Caucasian cohorts. Controls had a mean age of 45 (SD 15) at inclusion and 90% were female making them comparable to our SLE cohort with respect to age and gender.

Assay

To test whether the activation of our standard was successful, we ran GPC of non-activated serum and supernatant of PEG-precipitated serum (**Figure 1A**). Before activation (red) most C3dg is found in the large fragments (C3′), whereas after activation and precipitation of the activated serum, the supernatant (blue) contained only the smaller C3dg fragment. We further PEG-precipitated EDTA plasma to find out which PEG% would be the best to separate C3dg from C3′ (**Figure 1B**) and found a plateau at 16% PEG, suggesting this would be the optimal concentration.

To compare the previously suggested PEG concentration of 11% (w/v) to our choice of 16% (w/v), we ran GPCs of samples after precipitation with both PEG concentrations (**Figure 1C**) (17). Using 16% PEG-precipitation reduced the C3′ peak (blue **Figure 1C**) and showed the supernatant predominantly contained C3dg.

We then investigated the efficiency of precipitation with 11 and 16% PEG by western blotting. The result shown in **Figure 1D** illustrate that 16% PEG is superior to 11% in precipitating all fragments larger than C3dg. We observed that both free C3dg and larger C3dg-containing components, C3′, were present in the supernatant after PEG-precipitation with 11% (lane 2), whereas precipitation with 16% PEG (lane 1) yielded a much cleaner separation of free C3dg from the other components, supporting the results illustrated in **Figures 1B,C**. A more detailed analysis by western blot is presented in Figure S1 in Supplementary Material in which fragments of C3 is visualized in different samples developed with either anti-C3c or anti-C3d antibodies.

We observed that the concentration of C3dg in serum increased with both the time and the temperature to which the samples were exposed (**Figure 2A**). By contrast, no significant increase in C3dg was seen in EDTA plasma (**Figure 2B**). Freeze–thaw cycles of EDTA-plasma showed an increase in C3dg concentration in samples after four freeze–thaw cycles ($p < 0.05$) (**Figure 2C**). The concentration of C3dg in plasma did not display significant diurnal variation ($p = 0.19$) (**Figure 2D**).

The performance of our assay was compared to three commercially available assays for complement activation products (**Figures 2E–G**). Significant correlations ($p < 0.05$) were observed with all assays. Furthermore, our C3dg results were compared with the results obtained by double-decker rocket immunoelectrophoresis on plasma from 12 randomly picked patients (**Figure 2H**) ($r = 0.74, p < 0.05$).

As ELISA is used more frequently than TRIFMA, it was considered expedient to subject the analysis of the PEG supernatants to assay by ELISA. The results were similar when comparing the two assays ($r = 0.91, p < 0.0001$) (**Figure 3**).

TABLE 1 | Systemic lupus erythematosus patient demographics.

Patient demographics	
Patient number	169
Age at inclusion, mean (SD)	45.4 (14.9)
Age at diagnosis, mean (SD)	33.5
Gender F (%)	90
Ethnicity: Caucasian (%)	97
American College of Rheumatology (ACR) criteria (cumulative)	
Number of ACR criteria, mean (SD)	6.3 (1.2)
Malar rash (ACR1) (%)	65.7
Discoid lupus (ACR2) (%)	5.3
Photosensitivity (ACR3) (%)	67.5
Oral/nasal ulcers (ACR4) (%)	44.4
Arthritis (ACR5) (%)	91.7
Serositis (ACR6) (%)	34.9
Nephritis (ACR7) (%)	31.4
CNS (ACR8) (%)	8.4
Hematological (ACR9) (%)	89.9
Immunological (ACR10) (%)	90.5
ANA (ACR11) (%)	98.2
Clinical and biochemical data at time of inclusion	
SLE disease activity index at inclusion, mean (SD)	3.9 (3.3)
SLICC, mean (SD)	0.9 (1.2)
Treatment at time of inclusion	
Hydroxychloroquine treatment (%)	79.6
Prednisolone treatment (%)	57.4
Other immuno-suppressives (%)	39.5

Complement Activation in SLE Patients and Controls

No significant difference was observed between SLE patients and controls for C3′, the value routinely determined as the C3 concentration ($p = 0.211$, **Figure 4A**). SLE patients showed higher C3dg concentrations in plasma compared with controls ($p < 0.0001$, **Figure 4B**). The C3dg/C3′ ratio was calculated for SLE patients and controls and showed a clear difference ($p < 0.0001$, **Figure 4C**).

C3dg and SLEDAI did not show any correlation ($r = 0.03$, $p = 0.71$). C3dg/C3′ correlated to SLEDAI ($r = 0.28, p < 0.001$) as did C3 ($r = -0.49, p < 0.001$), which was no surprise, since C3 is part of the SLEDAI score.

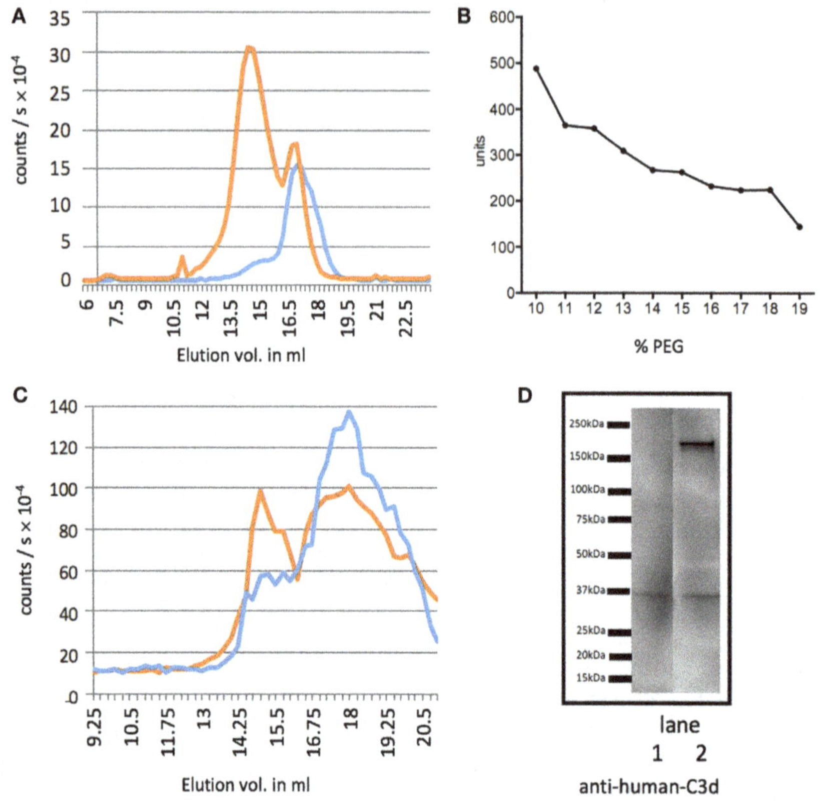

FIGURE 1 | Separation of C3dg from the larger C3 fragments. Measurements of C3 molecules encompassing the determinants of the segment C3dg, i.e., C3 and all degradation molecules containing this part of C3. **(A)** The figure illustrates C3dg measurement on gel permeation chromatography (GPC) fractions of serum before activation (red line) and supernatant of polyethylene glycol (PEG)-precipitated activated serum (blue line). **(B)** Test for the optimal concentration of PEG for precipitation. Increasing concentrations of PEG were added to EDTA plasma and C3dg was estimated in the supernatants. **(C)** GPC of supernatant after precipitation of EDTA plasma with 11% (red) and 16% (blue) PEG. C3dg in the fractions was measured. The 11% supernatant shows two major peaks, the first corresponding to C3 and larger C3 components, and the second corresponding to free C3dg. After precipitation with 16% PEG the first was significantly reduced. Panel **(D)** shows the results of western blotting of supernatants of EDTA-plasma precipitated with 16% (lane 1) or 11% (lane 2) PEG. The samples (corresponding to 0.1 µl plasma) were run non-reduced on the SDS-PAGE. The blot was developed with anti-C3d antibody. It can be seen that the 11% PEG supernatant still contains appreciable amounts of larger C3dg-encompassing molecules. This was repeated three times with similar results.

ROC-curves were made based on the measurements of C3, C3dg, and C3dg/C3 (**Figure 5**). C3dg was superior in separating patients from controls with an area under the curve of 0.96 (CI 0.94–0.98) (**Figures 5A,B**). When estimating sensitivity and specificity based on different cutoffs, C3dg yielded the best combination of both high sensitivity and high specificity (**Figure 5C**), revealing a much larger complement turnover in SLE patients than reflected by the C3 measurements.

DISCUSSION

Low complement C3, C4, and CH50 were introduced into the classification criteria of SLE in 2012 (3), reflecting an international acceptance of the importance of complement in the diagnosis. However, in many cases of SLE, low C3 or C4 poorly reflect disease activity, as patients often present with low levels irrespectively of disease activity (26, 27). Our newly developed C3dg assay was clearly superior to the conventional C3 measurement in discriminating SLE patients from controls both with regards to specificity and sensitivity. Thus, C3dg may be a valuable diagnostic biomarker in SLE.

Instead of simply estimating C3 or C4 and interpreting low levels as evidence for complement activation or consumption, it seems more relevant to directly evaluate ongoing complement activation. Several assays have been published for estimating complement activation products without being widely implemented. With a half-life of 4 h, C3dg is an ideal candidate for evaluating ongoing complement activation. As mentioned in the Section "Introduction," some procedures for estimating C3dg use precipitation of large proteins with PEG, followed by various assays for measurement of C3dg in the supernatant, have been published. The PEG concentration suggested in the first paper describing this idea (17), i.e., 11%, has been used in all the subsequent reports. We here re-addressed this issue and as illustrated with both GPC and western blot (**Figures 1B–D**), it appears expedient to increase the PEG concentrations to separate the large C3 components, here termed C3′, from C3dg (**Figure 1**). The PEG-C3dg assay has also been applied to samples from SLE patients. Significantly higher levels of C3dg have consistently

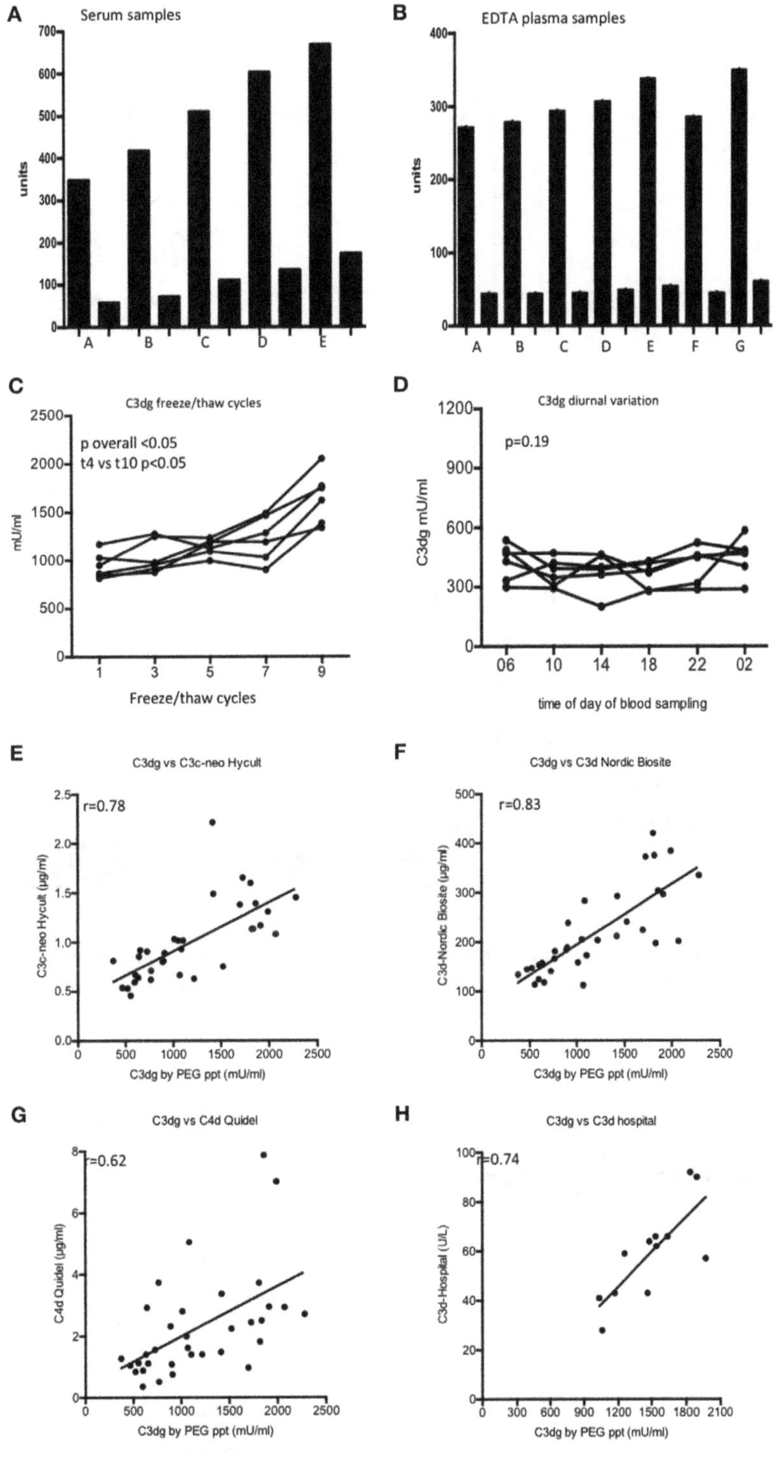

FIGURE 2 | C3dg measured on samples handled in different ways from the time of blood withdrawal until measurement. **(A)** shows the result using serum and **(B)** shows the results using EDTA plasma. Each sample was diluted 100 (tall columns) and 1,000-fold (short columns). **(A)** Samples frozen $t = 0$, **(B)** samples frozen after 60 min at room temperature (RT), **(C)** samples frozen after 60 min at 37°C, **(D)** samples frozen $t = 5$ h at RT, **(E)** samples frozen $t = 5$ h 37°C, **(F)** EDTA plasma left 1 h at RT before centrifugation, **(G)** EDTA plasma left 5 h at RT before centrifugation. **(C)** The samples were tested for sensitivity to freeze/thaw cycles using six EDTA plasma samples. Samples were frozen up to 10 times each followed by thawing at RT for 1 h. C3dg was measured after 2nd, 4th, 6th, 8th, and 10th thawing. **(D)** C3dg diurnal variation. Six controls had blood drawn at six time points during 24 h, and C3dg was estimated. For comparison of the repeated measurements, the Kruskal–Wallis test was used. **(E)** Comparison between our assay and enzyme-linked immune sorbent assay (ELISA) kit from Hycult Biotech (C3c-neo determinants). **(F)** Comparison with ELISA kit from Nordic Biocite (C3d). **(G)** Comparison to ELISA kit from Quidel (C4d). 34 samples [17 systemic lupus erythematosus (SLE) and 17 controls] were analyzed in all kits. **(H)** Twelve randomly chosen SLE samples had C3d measured using the double rocket immuno-electrophoresis (19). The same samples were measured in our C3dg assay. To assess the correlation between the assays, Spearman correlation was used.

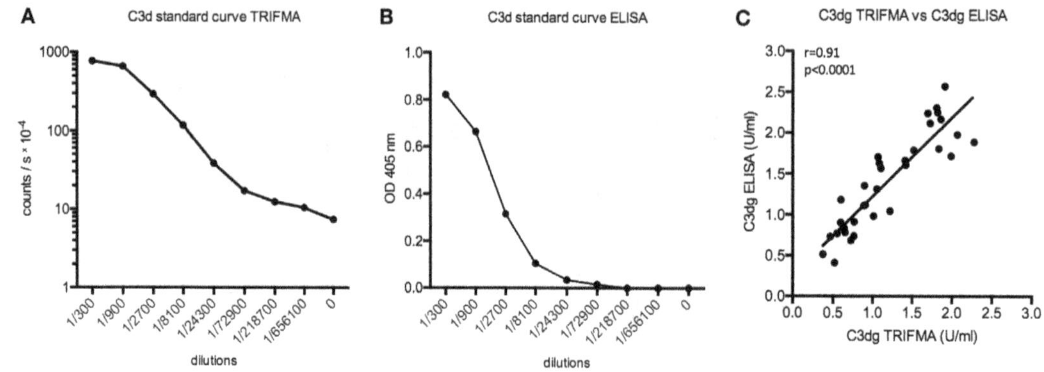

FIGURE 3 | Time-resolved immuno fluorometric assay (TRIFMA) and enzyme-linked immune sorbent assay (ELISA) C3dg assays compared. **(A)** shows the standard curve of the assay carried out using europium-label (TRIFMA) and **(B)** as ELISA. **(C)** Correlation (Spearman) between measurements of C3dg on EDTA plasma samples using our assay as TRIFMA and as ELISA.

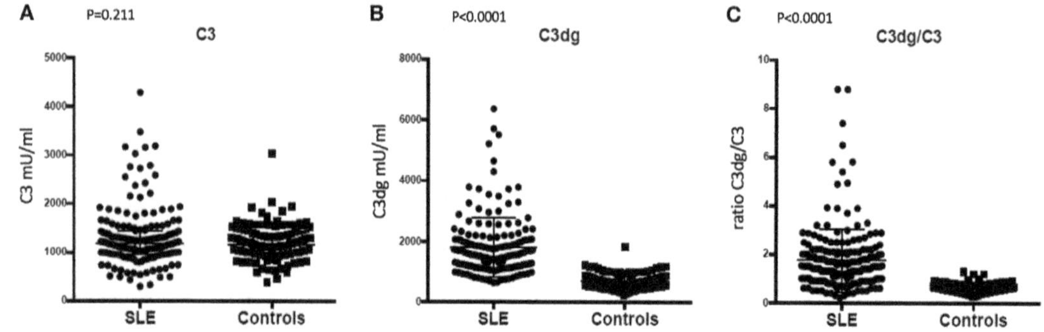

FIGURE 4 | Comparison of concentrations in plasma of **(A)** C3, **(B)** C3dg, and **(C)** C3dg/C3 ratio in systemic lupus erythematosus (SLE) patients and healthy controls (measured by time-resolved immuno fluorometric assay). The Mann–Whitney *U* test was used for the comparison.

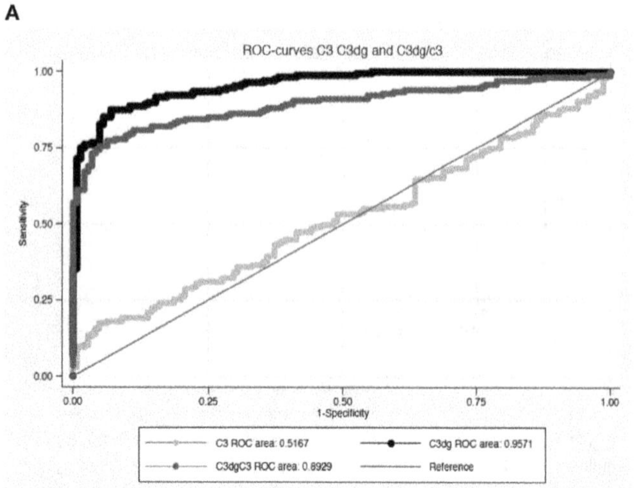

B

```
                          ROC                    -Asymptotic Normal--
               Obs       Area     Std. Err.      [95% Conf. Interval]
---------------------------------------------------------------------
C3             312     0.5167       0.0327       0.45250      0.58083
C3dg           312     0.9571       0.0100       0.93748      0.97671
C3dg/C3        312     0.8929       0.0190       0.85561      0.93022
---------------------------------------------------------------------
Ho: area(C3) = area(C3dg) = area (C3dg/C3)
    Chi2(2) = 3.75.08          prop>chi2 = 0.0000
```

C

	Cut-off	Sensitivity (%)	Specificity (%)	LR+	LR-
C3	900 (mU/ml)	80	14	0.98	1.04
	1400 (mU/ml)	28	79	1.47	0.88
C3dg	1000 (mU/ml)	87	90	8.45	0.14
	1100 (mU/ml)	84	94	15.2	0.17
C3dg/C3	0.85 (ratio)	80	89	5.38	0.26
	1.00 (ratio)	67	97	16.1	0.35

FIGURE 5 | Separation of systemic lupus erythematosus patients from controls using C3, C3dg, and C3dg/C3. **(A)** demonstrates ROC-curves for C3 (light gray), C3dg (black), and C3dg/C3 (dark gray). **(B)** represents calculations of area under the curve with 95% confidence intervals for each of the curves in **Figure 1B**. **(C)** shows calculations of sensitivity, specificity, and likelihood ratios for C3, C3dg, and C3dg/C3 using two different cutoffs for each measurement.

been reported in patients compared with controls (11, 17, 19, 26, 28, 29). Also, the improvement gained using the C3dg/C3 ratio have been reported (11). Considering the sizable literature on this subject, it seems surprising that C3dg assays have received little clinical attention.

The C3dg estimation proved stable using EDTA-plasma. It is clear, however, that even with the addition of EDTA, complement activation is not completely inhibited unless samples are kept cold and not thawed multiple times. This underlines the necessity of handling samples similarly when comparing cohorts (30). Control samples were stored for approximately a year longer than patient samples, and at least for EDTA plasma, storage at minus 80°C seemed to stop complement activation, as controls displayed considerable lower C3dg than patients. Another concern, when using blood for measurements is whether or not the component of interest displays diurnal variation. This is the case for several proteins and hormones (31, 32). We, however, observed no significant diurnal variation in complement activation reflected by C3dg.

The plasma concentration of C3 and C4 show inter-individual variation (33). Concentrations depend to a large extend on synthesis; however, SLE patients often show low levels of C4 due to a partial genetic defect (34, 35). Low C4, therefore, does not necessarily reflect consumption. Thus, it is dubious to use a single complement measurement for diagnostic/clinical purposes. Intuitively, therefore, it makes sense to use the C3dg/C3′ ratio, as previously suggested by Röther et al. (29). If initial concentration of intact complement components influences the concentration upon activation, it is reasonable to correct for this by calculating the C3dg/C3 ratio. Whether this measurement can be used for clinical purposes, e.g., to rule out a flare, remains to be tested on a prospective cohort. We demonstrated that the use of C3, as suggested in the SLE classification criteria, was not optimal for the SLE diagnosis. We found that C3dg was significantly higher in SLE patients than in healthy controls, whereas this was not the case for C3. C3dg showed superiority with regard to both sensitivity and specificity compared with C3. The performance of C3dg as a criterion for classification of SLE should be further evaluated by comparing SLE with other diseases.

The study raises the question of why most SLE patients have higher C3dg concentrations in plasma than controls (**Figure 4**). It likely indicates that in most patients there is complement turnover, even under conditions where patients are regarded as having inactive disease (36). The alternative pathway is an essential amplification loop in the activation of the complement system (37, 38). We know that lack of control of the alternative pathway potentially leads to devastating disease (39, 40). A possible explanation for higher C3dg in patients could be a relative lack of inhibition of the alternative pathway, making it easier to tip the balance to non-inhibition in cases of infection, cancer, sun exposure, and trauma, all known causes of SLE flares. Studies on lupus-prone mice have demonstrated exacerbation of disease with inadequate cell level complement inhibition (41). In line with this, low factor H has been associated with lupus nephritis (42). Another possible explanation could be anti-C3-antibodies. As reported by Vasilev et al., anti-C3-antibodies bind to the C3c part of C3 and thus bind C3, iC3b, C3b, and C3c (43). The antibodies likely compete for the same binding site as factor H, thereby hindering inhibition at the cell surface (43). Thus, one would expect patients with anti-C3-antibodies to have higher levels of C3dg because of more complement activation. Future studies are warranted to elucidate this in SLE patients.

We present a modified assay for measuring C3dg. The assay is simple, inexpensive, and stable. The estimation of C3dg directly reflects complement turnover independently of activation pathway. The assay differentiated excellently between SLE patients and healthy controls. We propose that C3dg measurements should be evaluated as a standard complement activation measurement in patients with SLE particularly with respect to classification.

AUTHOR CONTRIBUTIONS

AT and LJ performed the laboratory experiments. AT was in charge of collecting blood samples and handling the blood samples after they were drawn. AT, BD, and KS-P handled patient inclusion and clinical assessments. ST and JJ developed the assays used in the project and supervised laboratory procedures. AT, ST, JJ, and KS-P wrote the manuscript. All authors participated in the editing of the article.

ACKNOWLEDGMENTS

The authors would like to acknowledge all patients participating in the project. We thank Kristina Nilsson-Ekdahl for generous advice and help comparing C3dg assays.

FUNDING

The Danish Rheumatism Association (Grant nr: R122-A3031) and Aase and Ejnar Danielsens Fond supported the project.

REFERENCES

1. Bao L, Cunningham PN, Quigg RJ. Complement in lupus nephritis: new perspectives. *Kidney Dis (Basel)* (2015) 1:91–9. doi:10.1159/000431278
2. Sturfelt G, Truedsson L. Complement and its breakdown products in SLE. *Rheumatology (Oxford)* (2005) 44:1227–32. doi:10.1093/rheumatology/keh719
3. Petri M, Orbai A-M, Alarcón GS, Gordon C, Merrill JT, Fortin PR, et al. Derivation and validation of the systemic lupus international collaborating clinics classification criteria for systemic lupus erythematosus. *Arthritis Rheum* (2012) 64:2677–86. doi:10.1002/art.34473
4. Costabile M. Measuring the 50% haemolytic complement (CH50) activity of serum. *J Vis Exp* (2010) 37:1923. doi:10.3791/1923
5. Bajic G, Degn SE, Thiel S, Andersen GR. Complement activation, regulation, and molecular basis for complement-related diseases. *EMBO J* (2015) 34:2735–57. doi:10.15252/embj.201591881
6. Kjaer TR, Le LTM, Pedersen JS, Sander B, Golas MM, Jensenius JC, et al. Structural insights into the initiating complex of the lectin pathway of complement activation. *Structure* (2015) 23:342–51. doi:10.1016/j.str.2014.10.024
7. Meri S, Pangburn MK. Discrimination between activators and nonactivators of the alternative pathway of complement: regulation via a sialic acid/polyanion binding site on factor H. *Proc Natl Acad Sci U S A* (1990) 87:3982–6. doi:10.1073/pnas.87.10.3982
8. Zewde N, Gorham RD, Dorado A, Morikis D. Quantitative modeling of the alternative pathway of the complement system. *PLoS One* (2016) 11:e0152337. doi:10.1371/journal.pone.0152337
9. Nived O, Sturfelt G. ACR classification criteria for systemic lupus erythematosus: complement components. *Lupus* (2004) 13:877–9. doi:10.1191/0961203304lu2027oa
10. Mollnes TE, Kirschfink M. Complement analysis in clinic and research. *Adv Exp Med Biol* (2006) 586:361–80. doi:10.1007/0-387-34134-X_24
11. Ekdahl KN, Norberg D, Bengtsson AA, Sturfelt G, Nilsson UR, Nilsson B. Use of serum or buffer-changed EDTA-plasma in a rapid, inexpensive, and easy-to-perform hemolytic complement assay for differential diagnosis of systemic lupus erythematosus and monitoring of patients with the disease. *Clin Vaccine Immunol* (2007) 14:549–55. doi:10.1128/CVI.00486-06
12. Mollnes TE, Lea T, Frøland SS, Harboe M. Quantification of the terminal complement complex in human plasma by an enzyme-linked immunosorbent assay based on monoclonal antibodies against a neoantigen of the complex. *Scand J Immunol* (1985) 22:197–202. doi:10.1111/j.1365-3083.1985.tb01871.x
13. Morgan BP. The membrane attack complex as an inflammatory trigger. *Immunobiology* (2016) 221:747–51. doi:10.1016/j.imbio.2015.04.006
14. Merle NS, Church SE, Fremeaux-Bacchi V, Roumenina LT. Complement system part I – molecular mechanisms of activation and regulation. *Front Immunol* (2015) 6:262. doi:10.3389/fimmu.2015.00262
15. Norda R, Schött U, Berséus O, Akerblom O, Nilsson B, Ekdahl KN, et al. Complement activation products in liquid stored plasma and C3a kinetics after transfusion of autologous plasma. *Vox Sang* (2012) 102:125–33. doi:10.1111/j.1423-0410.2011.01522.x
16. Teisner B, Brandslund I, Grunnet N, Hansen LK, Thellesen J, Svehag SE. Acute complement activation during an anaphylactoid reaction to blood transfusion and the disappearance rate of C3c and C3d from the circulation. *J Clin Lab Immunol* (1983) 12:63–7.
17. Perrin LH, Lambert PH, Miescher PA. Complement breakdown products in plasma from patients with systemic lupus erythematosus and patients with membranoproliferative or other glomerulonephritis. *J Clin Invest* (1975) 56:165–76. doi:10.1172/JCI108065
18. Bourke BE, Moss IK, Maini RN. Measurement of the complement C3 breakdown product C3d by rocket immunoelectrophoresis. *J Immunol Methods* (1982) 48:97–108. doi:10.1016/0022-1759(82)90214-9
19. Brandslund I, Siersted HC, Svehag SE, Teisner B. Double-decker rocket immunoelectrophoresis for direct quantitation of complement C3 split products with C3d specificities in plasma. *J Immunol Methods* (1981) 44:63–71. doi:10.1016/0022-1759(81)90107-1
20. Hochberg MC. Updating the American College of Rheumatology revised criteria for the classification of systemic lupus erythematosus. *Arthritis Rheum* (1997) 40:1725. doi:10.1002/art.1780400928
21. Bombardier C, Gladman DD, Urowitz MB, Caron D, Chang CH. Derivation of the SLEDAI. A disease activity index for lupus patients. The committee on prognosis studies in SLE. *Arthritis Rheum* (1992) 35:630–40. doi:10.1002/art.1780350606
22. Gladman DD, Goldsmith CH, Urowitz MB, Bacon P, Fortin P, Ginzler E, et al. The Systemic Lupus International Collaborating Clinics/American College of Rheumatology (SLICC/ACR) damage index for systemic lupus erythematosus international comparison. *J Rheumatol* (2000) 27:373–6.
23. Troldborg A, Hansen A, Hansen SWK, Jensenius JC, Stengaard-Pedersen K, Thiel S. Lectin complement pathway proteins in healthy individuals. *Clin Exp Immunol* (2017) 188(1):138–47. doi:10.1111/cei.12909
24. Bergseth G, Ludviksen JK, Kirschfink M, Giclas PC, Nilsson B, Mollnes TE. An international serum standard for application in assays to detect human complement activation products. *Mol Immunol* (2013) 56:232–9. doi:10.1016/j.molimm.2013.05.221
25. Mao S-Y. Biotinylation of antibodies. *Methods Mol Biol* (2010) 588:49–52. doi:10.1007/978-1-59745-324-0_7
26. Charlesworth JA, Peake PW, Golding J, Mackie JD, Pussell BA, Timmermans V, et al. Hypercatabolism of C3 and C4 in active and inactive systemic lupus erythematosus. *Ann Rheum Dis* (1989) 48:153–9. doi:10.1136/ard.48.2.153
27. Birmingham DJ, Irshaid F, Nagaraja HN, Zou X, Tsao BP, Wu H, et al. The complex nature of serum C3 and C4 as biomarkers of lupus renal flare. *Lupus* (2010) 19:1272–80. doi:10.1177/0961203310371154
28. Manzi S, Rairie JE, Carpenter AB, Kelly RH, Jagarlapudi SP, Sereika SM, et al. Sensitivity and specificity of plasma and urine complement split products as indicators of lupus disease activity. *Arthritis Rheum* (1996) 39:1178–88. doi:10.1002/art.1780390716
29. Röther E, Lang B, Coldewey R, Hartung K, Peter HH. Complement split product C3d as an indicator of disease activity in systemic lupus erythematosus. *Clin Rheumatol* (1993) 12:31–5. doi:10.1007/BF02231555
30. Pfeifer PH, Kawahara MS, Hugli TE. Possible mechanism for in vitro complement activation in blood and plasma samples: futhan/EDTA controls in vitro complement activation. *Clin Chem* (1999) 45:1190–9.
31. Thompson DK, Sloane R, Bain JR, Stevens RD, Newgard CB, Pieper CF, et al. Daily variation of serum acylcarnitines and amino acids. *Metabolomics* (2012) 8:556–65. doi:10.1007/s11306-011-0345-9
32. Kage A, Fenner A, Weber B, Schöneshöfer M. Diurnal and ultradian variations of plasma concentrations of eleven adrenal steroid hormones in human males. *Klin Wochenschr* (1982) 60:659–66. doi:10.1007/BF01716798
33. Sebastián-Gámbaro MA, Lirón-Hernández FJ, Fuentes-Arderiu X. Intra- and inter-individual biological variability data bank. *Eur J Clin Chem Clin Biochem* (1997) 35:845–52.
34. Lintner KE, Wu YL, Yang Y, Spencer CH, Hauptmann G, Hebert LA, et al. Early components of the complement classical activation pathway in human systemic autoimmune diseases. *Front Immunol* (2016) 7:36. doi:10.3389/fimmu.2016.00036
35. Yih Chen J, Ling Wu Y, Yin Mok M, Jan Wu Y-J, Lintner KE, Wang C-M, et al. Effects of complement C4 gene copy number variations, size dichotomy, and C4A deficiency on genetic risk and clinical presentation of systemic lupus erythematosus in east Asian populations. *Arthritis Rheumatol* (2016) 68:1442–53. doi:10.1002/art.39589
36. Swaak AJ, Hannema A, Vogelaar C, Boom FA, van Es L, van Aalst R, et al. Determination of the half-life of C3 in patients and its relation to the presence of C3-breakdown products and/or circulating immune complexes. *Rheumatol Int* (1982) 2:161–6. doi:10.1007/BF00286138
37. Harboe M, Ulvund G, Vien L, Fung M, Mollnes TE. The quantitative role of alternative pathway amplification in classical pathway induced terminal complement activation. *Clin Exp Immunol* (2004) 138:439–46. doi:10.1111/j.1365-2249.2004.02627.x
38. Harboe M, Garred P, Karlstrøm E, Lindstad JK, Stahl GL, Mollnes TE. The down-stream effects of mannan-induced lectin complement pathway activation depend quantitatively on alternative pathway amplification. *Mol Immunol* (2009) 47:373–80. doi:10.1016/j.molimm.2009.09.005
39. Tan PL, Bowes Rickman C, Katsanis N. AMD and the alternative complement pathway: genetics and functional implications. *Hum Genomics* (2016) 10:23. doi:10.1186/s40246-016-0079-x
40. DeZern AE, Brodsky RA. Paroxysmal nocturnal hemoglobinuria: a complement-mediated hemolytic anemia. *Hematol Oncol Clin North Am* (2015) 29:479–94. doi:10.1016/j.hoc.2015.01.005

41. Miwa T, Zhou L, Maldonado MA, Madaio MP, Eisenberg RA, Song W-C. Absence of CD59 exacerbates systemic autoimmunity in MRL/lpr mice. *J Immunol* (2012) 189:5434–41. doi:10.4049/jimmunol.1201621
42. Wang F, Yu F, Tan Y, Song D, Zhao M. Serum complement factor H is associated with clinical and pathological activities of patients with lupus nephritis. *Rheumatology (Oxford)* (2012) 51:2269–77. doi:10.1093/rheumatology/kes218
43. Vasilev VV, Noe R, Dragon-Durey MA, Chauvet S, Lazarov VJ, Deliyska BP, et al. Functional characterization of autoantibodies against complement component C3 in patients with lupus nephritis. *J Biol Chem* (2015) 16: 25343–55. doi:10.1074/jbc.M115.647008

10

Complement Activation as a Helping Hand for Inflammophilic Pathogens and Cancer

Marcin Okrój[1] and Jan Potempa[2,3]**

[1] Department of Medical Biotechnology, Intercollegiate Faculty of Biotechnology, University of Gdańsk and Medical University of Gdańsk, Gdańsk, Poland, [2] Department of Oral Immunology and Infectious Diseases, University of Louisville School of Dentistry, Louisville, KY, United States, [3] Faculty of Biochemistry, Biophysics and Biotechnology, Jagiellonian University, Kraków, Poland

***Correspondence:**
Marcin Okrój
marcin.okroj@gumed.edu.pl
Jan Potempa
jspote01@louisville.edu

The complement system, an evolutionarily ancient component of innate immunity, is capable of protecting hosts from invading pathogens, either directly, by lysis of target cells, or indirectly, by mobilization of host immune mechanisms. However, this potentially cytotoxic cascade must be tightly regulated, since improperly controlled complement can damage healthy cells and tissues. The practical importance of this axis is highlighted when impairment of complement regulators or bacterial mechanisms of complement evasion result in pathogenic conditions. Recognition of complement as a "double-edged sword" is widely acknowledged, but another, currently underappreciated aspect of complement function has emerged as an important player in homeostatic balance—the dual outcome of complement-mediated inflammation. In most cases, the proinflammatory properties of complement are beneficial to the host. However, certain pathogens have developed the ability to utilize local inflammation as a source of nutrients and as a way to establish a niche for further colonization. Such a strategy can be illustrated in the example of periodontitis. Interestingly, certain tumors also seem to benefit from complement activation products, which promote a proangiogenic and immunosuppressive microenvironment.

Keywords: inflamation, periodontits, cancer, *Porphyromonas gingivalis*, complement activation

INTRODUCTION

The term "inflammo-*philic*" (=loving or attracting inflammation) was introduced in 2014 by George Hajishengallis to describe dysbiotic microbiome on the tooth surface below the gum line, which thrive in the inflammatory environment of periodontal pockets (1). Remarkably, as described in details later in this review, bacteria responsible for initiation and progression of periodontitis (periodontopathogens) have the unique ability to manipulate the complement system to disengage bacterial clearance from inflammation.

In general, the local inflammatory response to bacterial and fungal pathogens triggered by complement activation is absolutely essential to eliminate invaders (2, 3). Therefore, all successful pathogens developed a large variety of means to interfere with complement activation and/or hinder complement-dependent bacterial clearance mechanisms (2–6) (**Table 1**). Unfortunately, if inflammatory reaction triggered by pathogens escape the control it becomes highly detrimental to the host as illustrated by invasive candidiasis [*Candida albicans* (7)], meningitis [*Neisseria meningitidis* (8)], and sepsis [*N. meningitidis* (8), *Staphylococcus aureus* (9), and *Streptococcus pyogenes* (10)]. It needs to be kept in mind that an overwhelming inflammatory response and a dysregulated immune response to these infections is by no means the manifestation of an

TABLE 1 | Exemplary complement evasion strategies used by microbes.

Mechanism	Organism	Protein or molecule/*Host target*
Recruitment of host soluble complement inhibitors: -> support of proteolytic cleavage of C3b and C4b, acceleration of convertases' decay	*Streptococcus pyogenes*	M protein family (b) *Factor H* *C4BP* FH-binding proteins: fibronectin-binding protein (FbaA) (b) and streptococcal collagen-like protein 1 (Scl1)(b) *Factor H* *FH-related protein 1*
	Escherichia coli	OmpA: Outer membrane protein (b) *C4BP*
	Moraxella catarrhalisis	Usp1, 2: Ubiquitous surface protein 1 and 2 (b) *C4BP*
	Borrelia burgdorferi	BbCRASP-1 (b) *Factor H*
	Candida albicans	Gpm1p (b) *C4BP*
	Streptococcus pneumoniae	PspC (b) *Factor H*
Physical barrier preventing Fc receptors on phagocytes to contact complement-derived opsonins on bacteria	*Streptococcus pyogenes*	hyaluronic acid capsule (b)
Blocking of receptor of complement components on immune cells	*Staphylococcus aureus*	Chemotaxis inhibitory protein of *Staphylococcus aureus (CHIPS) (s)* *C5aR*
Proteolytic inactivation of complement components	*Streptococcus pyogenes*	ScpA (s) *C3a, C5a*
		SpeB (s) *C1 inhibitor, C2, C3, C4, C5a C6, C7, C8, C9*
	Pseudomonas aeruginosa	*Pseudomonas* elastase (PaE) (s) *C3*
	Staphylococcus aureus	Staphylokinase (s) *C3b*
	Serratia marcescens	56kDa protease (s) *C5a*
	Porphyromonas gingivalis	*gingipains (s)* *C3,C4,C5*
	Tannerella forsythia	Mirolysin (s) *Mannan binding lectin (MBL), ficolins, C4, C5*
Blocking of classical pathway initiation	*Streptococcus pyogenes*	endopeptidase O (PepO) (s) *IgG-C1q interaction* IdeS/Mac-1 (s) *IgG (degradation)*
	Staphylococcus aureus	Staphylococcal protein A (SpA) (b) *Ig (binding)*
	Streptococcus sp. gr. G	Protein G (b) *Ig (binding)*
Interference/function-blocking of complement components	*Streptococcus pyogenes*	streptococcal inhibitor of complement (SIC) (s) *C5b-7*
		Vitronectin binding proteins (VnBPs) (b) *Vitronectin – C9 polymerization*

(Continued)

TABLE 1 | Continued

Mechanism	Organism	Protein or molecule/*Host target*
	Staphylococcus aureus	extracellular fibrinogen-binding protein (Efb) (s) *C3*
		staphylococcal superantigen-like protein 7 (SSL-7) (s) *C5*
		Staphylococcal complement inhibitor (SCIN) (s) *blocking of AP and CP/LP C3 convertases*
	Borrelia burgdorferi	CD59-like protein (b) *C8, C9*
Moonlighting proteins	*Streptococcus pyogenes*	GAPDH (b),(s) *binds and sequesters C5a*
	Filifactor alocis	Acetylornithine transaminase (FACIN) (b) *binding to C3 and activated C3 in complex with factor B*

(s), soluble protein/molecule.
(b), surface—bound protein/molecule. For original references see the review articles with reference numbers 2–6.

inflammophilic character of these pathogens since the controlled, local inflammation is protective against these pathogens (9). Therefore, the pathogenic strategy to endure inflammation but in the same time to take advantage of it, seems to be limited to periodontopathogens. It is fascinating that the apparently similar strategy is employed by cancer and in both cases exploitation of the complement system underlines pathology.

COMPLEMENT SYSTEM

The complement system is one of the oldest mechanisms of immunity. Its essential components, such as the C3 molecule, have existed through more than 500 million years of evolution (11). A primitive complement system probably appeared in the common ancestor of eumetazoa, and its original role was limited to opsonization and the induction of inflammation. Genetic events like the duplication-based appearance of pathway specific components (e.g., factor B and C2) and the gain of terminal pathway constituents (C5–C9) allowed the primodal complement system to evolve into a an advanced and complex defense system capable not only of promoting osmotic lysis of target cells, anaphylaxis, and phagocytosis, but also of crosstalk with other systems (e.g., coagulation) and signaling pathways (e.g., Toll-like receptors) involved in the maintenance of bodily homeostasis (12, 13). There are three independent complement cascades, the evolutionarily older alternative and lectin pathway (with basic elements like C3, MASPs, and factor B existing in invertebrates) and the relatively younger classical pathway developed in jawed vertebrates (11). The alternative complement pathway is constitutively active at a low level due to the spontaneous breakdown of C3 into anaphylatoxin C3a and the active C3b fragment, which activate downstream steps in the cascade. Therefore, propagation of the alternative pathway does not depend on specific activation but relies on the lack of inhibition by numerous endogenous regulators that differentiate self and non-self surfaces. This mechanism ensures constant monitoring of the body. In contrast to the alternative pathway, the classical and lectin pathways require specific stimuli, such as antibodies, C-reactive protein, phosphatydylserine, or certain sugar moieties, to be present on the surface of target cells (14–16). The upstream components of both pathways, including C1q, mannan binding protein (MBL), and the ficolins, act as sensors and thus can be considered soluble pattern recognition molecules (PRMs) (17, 18). All pathways converge at the level of the central complement molecule C3. C3 is processed by enzymatic complexes called complement convertases into C3a anaphylatoxin and the C3b fragment, which in turn forms C5 convertases. C5 convertases cleave the C5 molecule into C5a anaphylatoxin and the C5b fragment, which initiates the common terminal pathway. Binding of C6, C7, C8, and C9 leads to formation of the membrane attack complex (MAC), which targets the cell membrane and causes osmotic lysis. A schematic representation of the complement system is shown in **Figure 1**.

The binding of antibodies as a stimulus for the initiation of the complement cascade bridges the innate and adaptive immune systems. Moreover, opsonins like C3b and their degradation products act as natural adjuvants, contributing to proper presentation of antigens to lymphocytes and providing a co-stimulatory and anti-apoptotic signal for B cells (19). Deficiencies of complement, while relatively rare, emphasize the importance of this multifunctional protein cascade (20). The exact symptoms that develop depend on precisely which complement components are lacking or impaired. Deficiencies in essential components of the alternative pathway and the terminal pathway result in higher susceptibility to recurrent bacterial infections, especially these caused by Neisseriae and incidence peak up in early childhood (20). The lack of early components of the classical pathway predisposes to systemic lupus erythematosus (SLE), a disease in which

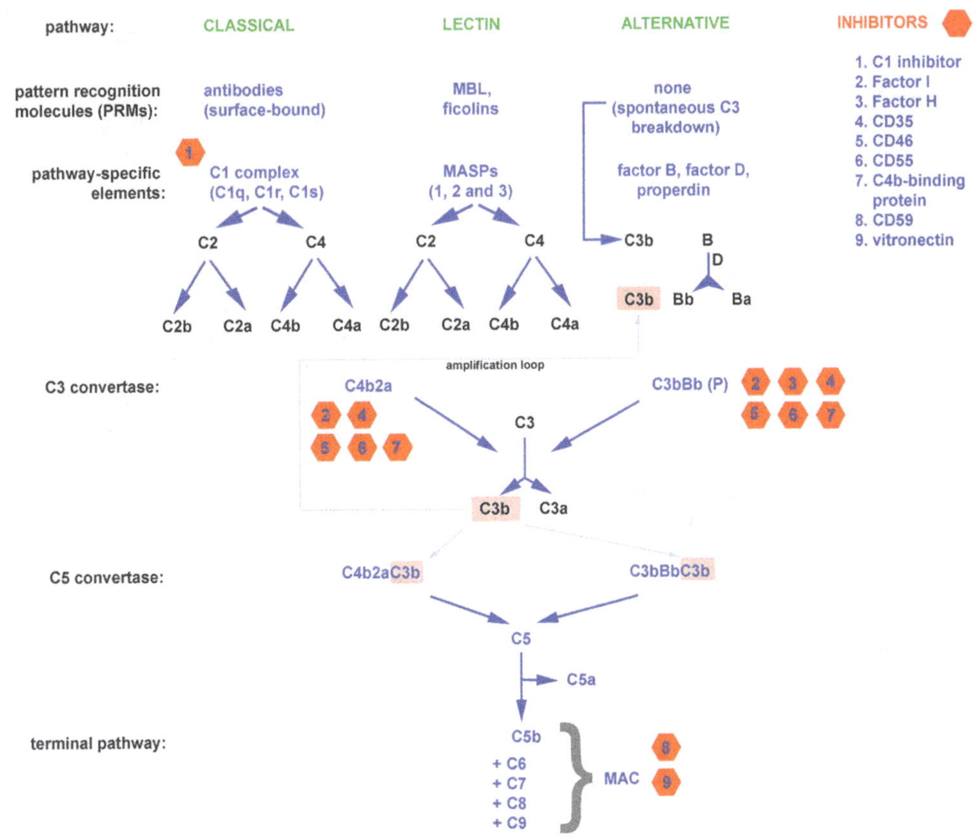

FIGURE 1 | A simplified representation of the complement system, divided into pattern recognition molecules (PRMs), pathway specific and common components as well as inhibitors.

the scavenging function of complement is impaired, and thus debris from dying cells persists and can act as a source of autoantigens (21). Autoimmune diseases that stem from direct damage of cells and tissues typically arise from deficiencies in complement inhibitors that normally protect the host from excessive or misguided complement attacks (22). These include C3 glomerulopathies, atypical hemolytic uremic syndrome (aHUS), age-related macular degeneration (AMD), paroxysmal nocturnal hemoglobinuria (PHN), and many more (20). Paradoxically, a deficiency of functional complement inhibitors such as factor H (the main soluble inhibitor of the alternative pathway) can also result in a deficiency of complement activation. Factor H is the main soluble inhibitor of alternative pathway, which prevents propagation of cascade beyond the spontaneous breakdown of C3 and formation of C3 convertase (**Figure 1**). The lack of such inhibitor fuels a positive feedback mechanism that unproductively depletes complement and leaves the host without an important line of defense (23). On the other hand, unwanted complement activation is an effector mechanism in many inflammatory diseases, including rheumatoid arthritis (24), diabetic nephropathy (25), and ischemia/reperfusion injury (26). All these examples support a perception of the complement system as a "double-edged sword," where a proper balance is pivotal for maintaining protection while avoiding autoimmunity. Both microbial infections and tumors influence this physiological equilibrium and employ two main strategies for survival in a complement-saturated microenvironment.

STRATEGY #1: TO COUNTERACT COMPLEMENT

Innate immunity relies on recognition of a spectrum of pathogen-associated molecular patterns (PAMPs), invariable molecular determinants typical for the most common invaders, including lipopolysaccharide (LPS), lipoteichoic acid, flagellin, double-stranded RNA, β1-3 glucan, N-formylmethionine peptides, and many more. The constant region of the antibody heavy chain (Fc) also falls into this category of molecules. Pathogen-associated molecular patterns (PAMPs) bind to specific receptors on innate immune cells and activate effector mechanisms such as complement or antibody-dependent cell cytotoxicity (ADCC). Molecules that sense PAMPs and trigger immune system activation are called pattern recognition receptors (PRRs) and include Toll-like receptors (TLRs), C-type lectins, and NOD-like receptors. Soluble molecules, which exert an analogical role are termed as PRMs and the most upstream components of the classical and lectin pathways (C1 complex, MBL, and ficolins) belong to this group (18). Complement is therefore a multispecific and powerful defense system against pathogens that is theoretically capable of eliminating every cell unless constrained by endogenous complement inhibitors. In practice, since complement co-evolved with pathogens over millions of years, pathogens have developed various mechanisms to evade complement attack. Pathogens employ a variety of tactics for this purpose, including proteolytic cleavage of complement components, mimicking and hijacking host complement inhibitors, inactivation of the C3 molecule, preventing of complement-mediated activation of immune cells, depletion of antibodies, and unproductive exhaustion of early complement components [reviewed in (2, 4, 27–29)]. Selected examples of abovementioned strategies are given in **Table 1**.

Similarly to bacterial, fungal, or viral pathogens expressing PAMPs, tumor cells are visible to the immune system due to changes in their mutational or metabolic status, which is reflected by changes in the expression of cell surface molecules. The presentation of epitopes derived from mutated proteins (so-called neoantigens) within MHC I molecules (30) as well as the peroxidation of membrane lipids or changed patterns of glycosylation distinguish tumor cells from normal cells.

Spontaneous fixation of complement onto the surface of tumor cells is of low physiological relevance due to the low titer of naturally occurring antitumor antibodies and the expression of complement inhibitors by tumor cells (31). The introduction of antitumor monoclonal antibodies, which is considered a breakthrough in tumor immunology, enabled researchers to use the cytotoxic potential of the complement system to combat cancer (32). Complement-activating therapeutics like the anti-CD20 antibodies rituximab and ofatumumab are first-line therapies in the treatment of B cell malignancies. However, certain patients fail to respond or only partially respond to antitumor antibodies, and one possible explanation is the unfavorable ratio of the molecular target (e.g., CD20) to membrane-bound complement inhibitors on the surface of tumor cells (33, 34). Successful experiments in which bispecific antibodies against CD20 and CD55 were used (35) or in which complement inhibitors were silenced (36) support the theory that inhibition of complement by tumor cells is an important mechanism of cancer resistance. Expression of membrane-bound

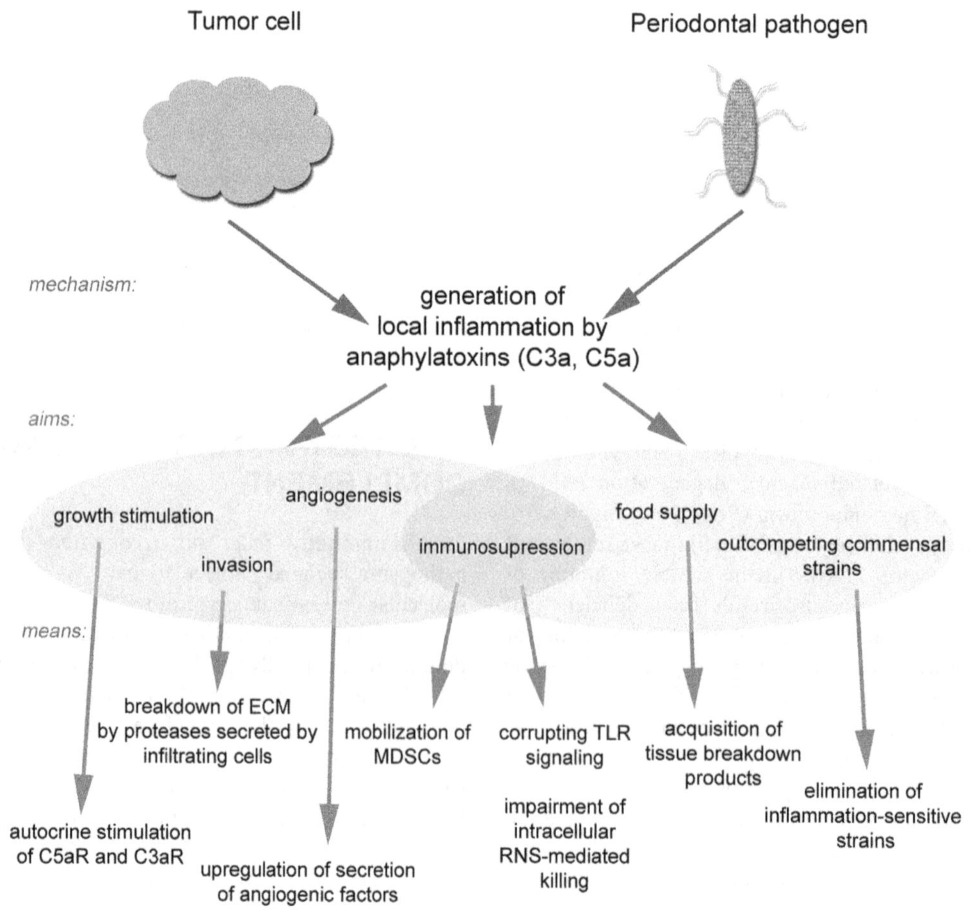

FIGURE 2 | A schematic drawing of strategies utilized by tumor cells and inflammophilic bacteria to subvert complement activation.

complement inhibitors like CD35 (Complement receptor 1, CR1), CD46, CD55, and CD59 is typical for nucleated cells, and the majority of cell types express at least one of these molecules. In contrast, the production of soluble complement inhibitors such as factor I, factor H, C4b-binding protein (C4BP) is usually the domain of liver hepatocytes, and there are only few extrahepatic sources of fluid-phase complement regulators (37). However, the expression of soluble complement inhibitors by tumor cells has been described, and it seems to provide an additional level of protection, as shown in an *in vitro* model of non-small lung cancer cell (NSCLC) lines expressing factor I, C4BP, and factor H (38). The tumor-supporting effect of endogenous factor H expressed by NSCLC cells was shown *in vivo* in a mouse xenograft model (39, 40). Further evidence for the pro-tumor effect of soluble complement inhibitors comes from analysis of tissue microarrays of breast cancer specimens. Expression of factor I was positively correlated with tumor size, de-differentiation score (Nottingham scale), and poor prognosis (cancer-specific survival and recurrence-free survival) (41). Other investigators reported a correlation between factor I expression and tumor aggressiveness in cutaneous squamous cell carcinoma (42). In addition to expressing soluble complement inhibitors, tumor cells can also hijack these proteins from the plasma. Horl et al. showed that blocking factor H binding to the surface of leukemia cells increased the cytotoxicity of rituximab (43) and ofatumumab (44). Although factor H is an inhibitor of the alternative complement pathway, it plays a role in enhancing the complement cascade when it is initiated via the classical pathway (such as by antitumor antibodies) at the level of C3b formation. C3b gives rise to an amplification loop (**Figure 1**) due to the formation of alternative convertases, which are targets for factor H. Points of action of particular complement inhibitors are indicated in **Figure 1**. Another possible way to increase tumor cell resistance to complement attack is removal of the MAC from the surface, a process dependent on endocytosis or active rearrangement of the cell membrane mediated by phosphorylation of essential signaling proteins (45).

The logical consequence of complement inhibition by microbes and tumor cells at various stages of the cascade is a more aggressive and more drug-resistant phenotype, as discussed above. However, the picture is not as simple as it may originally seem, and another strategy used by pathogens and tumor cells to evade complement has been described.

STRATEGY #2: TO EXPLOIT THE COMPLEMENT SYSTEM

Low oxygen concentration is a feature of rapidly growing solid tumors, which cannot develop the vasculature necessary for the efficient supply of nutrients to proliferating neoplastic cells. Therefore, the expanding tumor mass sooner or later develops hypoxic cores. Normal cells are equipped with a sensor of oxygen concentration that works at the transcriptional level. Hypoxia-inducible factor Iα (HIF-1α) can stabilize the p53 tumor suppressor, triggering either apoptotic signaling or metabolic reprogramming of the cell (46). Both of these processes lead to changes in the molecules expressed at the cell surface, which has the effect of making the tumor cell visible to the immune system. Previous studies with human umbilical vein endothelial cells (HUVECs) revealed that these cells activate the classical complement pathway in response to hypoxia and as well as during subsequent reoxygenation. At the same time, HUVECs increased their surface expression of two membrane-bound complement inhibitors, CD46 and CD55 (47), which induce the proteolytic cleavage of activated complement components C3b and C4b, respectively, and the dissociation of the corresponding complement convertases. Another study showed a 3.6-fold increase in HUVEC expression of complement receptor 1 (CR1 or CD35) after 48 h of hypoxia (48). These results suggest that endothelial cells actively counteract complement activation under hypoxic conditions, and therefore the expression of complement inhibitors in hypoxic NSCLC cells was studied (49). These cells not only expressed membrane-bound complement inhibitors but also produced soluble inhibitors of complement, including C4BP and factors I and H (38). In contrast to HUVECs, NSCLCs significantly downregulated the mRNA expression of all complement inhibitors tested except CD59 after 24 h of hypoxia, but a drop in the mRNA expression of soluble complement inhibitors was detected as early as 6 h after hypoxic challenge. Importantly, this rapid decrease did not correspond to the number of dying cells, which did not significantly increase in first 24 h (49). The conclusion is that unlike endothelial cells, NSCLCs do not utilize protection mechanisms that prevent the deposition of early complement components during hypoxia, but they do maintain expression of CD59, which protects from the terminal stages of complement attack (the insertion of the MAC into the membrane) (47–49).

From the research reviewed above, it has become apparent that lung cancer cells may benefit from the propagation of local inflammation mediated by C3a and C5a. Possible scenarios include the production of proangiogenic and growth factors by tumor-infiltrating lymphocytes and macrophages as well as the mobilization of immune suppressor cells that impair tumor antigen presentation (50–53). Indirect support for this hypothesis comes from studies done by Ajona et al. who reported elevated C4d deposition in lung tumors and its correlation with decreased survival (54). Moreover, high levels of soluble C4d in the plasma could discriminate between patients with benign pulmonary nodules and lung cancer (55), and were associated with reduced survival of individuals with early and advanced lung cancer. C4d levels in the plasma were also reduced after surgical removal of the tumor (54). C4d is an end degradation product of the activated C4b molecule, a hallmark of classical complement pathway activation. For that reason, one can assume that the survival and malignant potential of NSCLC cells is based on stimulation of complement. Indeed, anaphylatoxin C5a is one of the key players in complement-mediated support of lung cancer growth. Corrales et al. found that C5 deposition and subsequent C5a generation in NSCLC cells was much higher than in non-malignant bronchial epithelial cells in the presence of serum (56). Interestingly, tumor cells but not non-transformed cells produced endogenous C5, and C5a generation took place even in the absence of serum. C5a levels in the plasma of lung cancer patients were also found to be elevated, similarly to C4d levels. C5a also stimulated migration and tube formation by HUVECs *in vitro*. Finally, the impact of C5a was tested in a syngenic mouse model of 3LL lung cancer. Microvessel density was compared in 3LL tumors in mice treated with a C5a receptor (C5aR) antagonist. Tumors in the mice treated with the C5aR antagonist showed significantly fewer microvessels (56). Additionally, C5a signaling positively influenced the recruitment of myeloid-derived suppressor cells (MDSCs; CD11b^{+}, Ly6c^{+}), as blockade of C5aR reduced the number of MDSCs in tumor-bearing mice. The authors also found decreased expression of molecules associated with an immunosuppressive state and silencing of the immune response (ARG1, CTLA-4, IL-10, LAG3, and PD-L1) in C5aR antagonist-treated mice (57–59).

Importantly, the first evidence for the impact of C5a on the mobilization of MDSCs into the tumor mass was shown by Markiewski et al. in the TC-1 tumor model, a lung epithelial cell line expressing human papilloma virus (HPV) E6 and E7 antigens (60). The authors found that C5aR-deficient mice developed smaller tumors than wild-type littermates, and the same effect was observed when a C5aR antagonist was administered. However, in this model, the slower rate of tumor growth in C5aR antagonist-treated animals was not dependent on tumor cell proliferation/apoptosis or angiogenesis, as evidenced by analysis of end-point tumor specimens. Conversely, there were differences in the infiltration of tumor tissue by cytotoxic T cells, the main effectors of the antitumor immune response. Profiling of MDSCs isolated from tumors and spleens of C5aR-deficient, tumor-inoculated animals confirmed that C5a contributes to the accumulation of MDSCs in peripheral lymphoid organs and their migration into tumors. Of note, MDSCs isolated from mice with disabled C5aR signaling were less able to suppress T cell proliferation *in vitro*. This deficiency was linked to lower production of reactive oxygen species (ROS) and reactive nitrogen species (RNS) in mononuclear MDSC from C5aR-deficient animals.

Similarly to lung cancer cells, endogenous C5a generation by pancreatic and colon cancer cells was later reported. These cells processed C5 with a cell surface-expressed serine protease and expressed C5aR, suggesting autocrine activation of complement (61). In ovarian cancer, endogenous production of complement components and autocrine stimulation of the anaphylatoxin receptors C3aR and C5aR was suggested to be an important mechanism supporting tumor growth (62). The observed effect was independent of infiltration by cytotoxic T cells, since experiments with silenced expression of C3 yielded the same result (i.e., reduced tumor growth) in CD8 T cell-sufficient and -deficient mice. A direct effect of C3aR and C5aR agonists on proliferation, migration, and invasion of tumor cells has also been reported. Finally, quantification of C3 mRNA in tumors from patients with ovarian cancer showed that overall survival in patients with low tumor expression of C3 was more than double that of patients with high expression of C3 in the tumor (62).

In recent years, there has also been growing evidence for the pro-tumor activity of anaphylatoxins and anaphylatoxin receptors in either tumor cells or the tumor stroma in multiple tumors types, including melanoma, breast, ovarian, cervical, colon, and intestinal cancer, as well as sarcoma [reviewed in (63)]. Interestingly, in addition to the larger body of work focusing on the role of C3a and C5a in promoting tumor growth, recent studies have described a pro-tumor effect of factor B silencing (64) as well as a complement-independent enhancement of tumor growth, adhesion, and angiogenesis by C1q produced by the tumor stroma (65). The concept of complement activation supporting tumor growth provided the rationale for combined inhibition of C5a and PD-1 (66, 67), suggesting that targeting complement may be an effective anticancer treatment. These novel discoveries may be perceived as contradictory to the acknowledged theory that complement inhibits tumor growth. For example, NSCLC cells, which have been shown to benefit from C5a generation (56), were previously shown to form smaller tumors in a mouse xenograft model when their endogenous expression of the complement inhibitor factor H was silenced (40). In addition, potent complement activators such as the anti-CD20 immunotherapeutics rituximab and ofatumumab are first-line therapies for treatment of B cell malignancies (33). Notably, solid and circulating tumors have different requirements for growth. While sold tumors are typically depend on angiogenesis, migration, degradation of extracellular matrix, liquid tumors originate in the bone marrow, peripheral blood, or lymph nodes, which are rich in both nutrients and complement. Even solid tumors of the same origin can differ one from another in their mutational status, basal expression of growth factors and metalloproteinases, and metabolic rate. All of these parameters can influence the overall effect of complement activation on tumorigenesis and/or tumor progression. Finally, tumor cells often produce both complement activators and complement inhibitors. Thus, it seems as though tumor cells actively regulate the complement system depending on microenvironmental conditions, rather than simply avoiding constitutive inhibition or activation of complement (68).

Despite the extremely long phylogenetic distance between eukaryotic cells and bacteria, some prokaryotes have acquired strategies similar to tumor cells, which utilize the host inflammatory status to create favorable survival conditions. Bacterial growth in the human body is less dependent on neovascularization than tumor growth, and in contrast to tumor cells, bacteria do not have to overcome internal mechanisms controlling proliferation. Moreover, most bacteria can stand much harsher conditions than eukaryotic cells in terms of pH, oxygen tension, temperature, concentration of metabolites, *etc.* Nevertheless, the common feature between bacteria and tumor cells is the demand for nutrients and certain microelements. While solid tumors induce angiogenesis to acquire a source of nutrients, bacteria can successfully utilize products from the breakdown of local tissue. Therefore, tissue-destructive processes linked to local inflammation form permissive conditions for prokaryotic pathogens, which can survive immune attack. An additional benefit of this strategy is the elimination of inflammation-sensitive bacterial species (human commensals or normal microflora) that normally compete within the same niche (69, 70).

INFLAMMOPHILIC CHARACTER OF PORPHYROMONAS GINGIVALIS, WHICH PROPELS PERIODONTISIS

One of the most well-documented examples of bacteria hijacking host immunity to create an environmental niche occurs in periodontitis, a chronic inflammatory disease characterized by dysbiosis that results in degradation of the gingiva and tooth-supporting bone and ultimately leads to tooth loss (1). Periodontal disease begins from dental plaque, a microbial matrix colonizing the gum line usually as a result of inefficient oral hygiene (71). The next stage, gingivitis, is characterized by local inflammatory response to microbial plaque. The switch between non-destructive gingivitis and destructive periodontitis involve dysbiosis of the normal oral microbiome. The dysbiotic process results from an imbalance of homeostasis caused by so-called keystone pathogens (72). A keystone pathogen is usually a microorganism of low abundance that induces changes in the composition of the local microflora by introducing a new selective pressure, such as inflammation. In periodontitis, the keystone pathogen is *Porphyromonas gingivalis.* However, as shown by studies in mice, this Gram-negative bacteria cannot establish periodontitis by itself, but requires commensal microbes. These microbes are then converted from a symbiotic into a dysbiotic community. Pivotal experiments showed that bone loss was reduced when C3aR- or C5aR-deficient mice were inoculated with *P. gingivalis* and that no changes in the oral microbiota were observed in these knockout mice after *P. gingivalis* inoculation, in contrast to wild-type mice (69). As some tumor cells generate C5a through their surface enzymes, so does *P. gingivalis.* It is equipped with gingipains, outer membrane-anchored bacterial surface arginine-specific proteases with C5 convertase-like activity (73, 74). Importantly, gingipains release C5a from C5, but at higher concentrations, they degrade the larger fragment (C5b), thus preventing MAC formation (75). C3 and C4 complement proteins are also degraded by high concentrations of gingipains. Thus, human serum pre-incubated with clinical strains of *P. gingivalis* but not mutants lacking gingipains is devoid of bactericidal activity (74, 76). Additionally, gingipains interact with the C1 complex and increase its deposition onto bacteria surfaces (74). Based on these findings, one can postulate a biphasic effect of *P. gingivalis* proteolytic enzymes. A low abundance of bacteria initiates the classical complement pathway, but increasing numbers of bacteria results in the degradation of crucial complement components, leading to osmotic lysis. C5 is present in gingival crevicular fluid at concentration corresponding to 70% of that in serum and the active C5a anaphylatoxin can be locally released by convertases and bacterial proteases (77). C5a is a strong inflammatory mediator that increases vascular permeability and attracts and modulates the function of neutrophils, monocytes, and mast cells. All these events are considered antimicrobial events. Paradoxically, *P. gingivalis*' strategy for immune subversion by proinflammatory C5a involves targeted immunosuppression of macrophages. C5a affects intracellular killing of engulfed *P. gingivalis* by RNS and corrupts the crosstalk between C5aR and TLR2, one of the most important PRMs in antibacterial innate immunity (73). At the same time, C5aR-TLR2 crosstalk results in release of proinflammatory cytokines such as IL-1β, IL-6, and TNF-α, which accelerate bone resorption and thus contributes to the pathological mechanism of periodontitis. Similarly, *P. gingivalis* spoils intracellular killing mechanism but not proinflammatory activity of neutrophils by degradation of TLR2 adaptor molecule MyD88 provoked by concomitant activation of TLR2 and C5aR (78).

Another functional similarity between *P. gingivalis* and tumor cells, which produce either complement inhibitors or complement components, is the fact that *P. gingivalis* not only possesses the proteolytic machinery to generate C5a but also expresses a unique enzyme, peptidyl arginine deiminase (PPAD), which can citrullinate the C-terminal arginine in C5a, a modification that results in substantial loss of anaphylatoxin chemotactic activity (79). This suggests that the evolutionary goal of pathogens like *P. gingivalis* is not constitutive activation or inhibition of the complement system, but rather the ability to actively control complement status depending on its current needs. As a keystone pathogen, *P. gingivalis* is a low-abundance species that plays a major role in remodeling the local microbiota community (69). Following establishment of *P. gingivalis* infection, a succession of other dysbiotic species proliferates in the periodontal plaque. Some express their own complement inhibitors, such as *Tannerella forsythia,* which produces karilysin and mirolysin (80, 81), *Filifactor alocis,* which produces FACIN (82), and *Prevotella intermedia,* which produces interpain A (83). Of note, interpain A works in concert with gingipains in the initial stages of infection, as both proteins activate the C1 complex and increase its deposition onto the cell surface. A dysbiotic bacterial community may promote a transcriptomic response that further improves bacterial fitness by regulation of nutrient acquisition and expression of virulence factors (84). This process resembles the crosstalk between tumor cells and the stroma, at least to a certain extent. Tumor cells can drive the polarization of infiltrating immune cells (e.g., into M2 macrophages), which in turn benefit the tumor cells by, for example, expressing angiogenic cytokines (85, 86). In addition, carcinoma-associated fibroblasts (CAF), which differentiate from normal fibroblasts upon stimulation by cancer-derived cytokines such as TGF-β, have emerged as important players in cancer progression and metastasis (87, 88).

CONCLUDING REMARKS

The role of the complement system in combating bacteria and cancer is more complicated than was initially believed. Certain pathogens have evolved the ability not only to evade complement attack but also to use it as a tool for establishing their own niche, while remaining protected from complement-mediated lysis. Such a strategy seems to be widespread in nature and has been adopted by both bacteria and tumor cells (**Figure 2**). It seems likely that additional pathogenic strategies remain to be discovered, and thus one must be careful when designing complement-based therapeutics. On the other hand, anti-complement approaches may be effective in the treatment of infections caused by inflammophilic microbes.

AUTHOR CONTRIBUTIONS

All authors listed have made a substantial, direct and intellectual contribution to the work, and approved it for publication.

FUNDING

MO is supported by National Science Centre Poland, grant number 2014/14/E/NZ6/00182. JP is supported by National Science Centre Poland, grant number 2016/21/B/NZ1/00292 and NIH/NICDR grant number DE 022597.

REFERENCES

1. Hajishengallis G. The inflammophilic character of the periodontitis-associated microbiota. *Mol Oral Microbiol.* (2014) 29:248–57. doi: 10.1111/omi.12065
2. Ermert DML. Catch me if you can: *Streptococcus* pyogenes Complement Evasion Strategies. *J Innate Immun.* (2018) 11:3–12. doi: 10.1159/000492944
3. Heesterbeek DAC, Angelier ML, Harrison RA, Rooijakkers SHM. Complement and bacterial infections: from molecular mechanisms to therapeutic applications. *J Innate Immun.* (2018) 10:455–64. doi: 10.1159/000491439
4. Blom AM, Hallstrom T, Riesbeck K. Complement evasion strategies of pathogens-acquisition of inhibitors and beyond. *Mol Immunol.* (2009) 46:2808–17. doi: 10.1016/j.molimm.2009.04.025
5. Thammavongsa V, Kim HK, Missiakas D, Schneewind O. Staphylococcal manipulation of host immune responses. *Nat Rev Microbiol.* (2015) 13:529–43. doi: 10.1038/nrmicro3521
6. Pietrocola G, Nobile G, Rindi S, Speziale P. *Staphylococcus aureus* manipulates innate immunity through own and host-expressed proteases. *Front Cell Infect Microbiol.* (2017) 7:166. doi: 10.3389/fcimb.2017.00166
7. Duggan S, Leonhardt I, Hunniger K, Kurzai O. Host response to *Candida albicans* bloodstream infection and sepsis. *Virulence* (2015) 6:316–26. doi: 10.4161/21505594.2014.988096
8. Johswich K. Innate immune recognition and inflammation in *Neisseria meningitidis* infection. *Pathog Dis.* (2017) 75. doi: 10.1093/femspd/ftx022
9. Lupu F, Keshari RS, Lambris JD, Coggeshall KM. Crosstalk between the coagulation and complement systems in sepsis. *Thromb Res.* (2014) 133 (Suppl. 1):S28–31. doi: 10.1016/j.thromres.2014.03.014
10. Reglinski M, Sriskandan S. The contribution of group A streptococcal virulence determinants to the pathogenesis of sepsis. *Virulence* (2014) 5:127–36. doi: 10.4161/viru.26400
11. Nonaka M. Evolution of the complement system. *Subcell Biochem.* (2014) 80:31–43. doi: 10.1007/978-94-017-8881-6_3
12. Hajishengallis G, Lambris JD. Crosstalk pathways between Toll-like receptors and the complement system. *Trends Immunol.* (2010) 31:154–63. doi: 10.1016/j.it.2010.01.002
13. Amara U, Flierl MA, Rittirsch D, Klos A, Chen H, Acker B, et al. Molecular intercommunication between the complement and coagulation systems. *J Immunol.* (2010) 185:5628–36. doi: 10.4049/jimmunol.0903678
14. Biro A, Rovo Z, Papp D, Cervenak L, Varga L, Fust G, et al. Studies on the interactions between C-reactive protein and complement proteins. *Immunology* (2007) 121:40–50. doi: 10.1111/j.1365-2567.2007.02535.x
15. Nauta AJ, Trouw LA, Daha MR, Tijsma O, Nieuwland R, Schwaeble WJ, et al. Direct binding of C1q to apoptotic cells and cell blebs induces complement activation. *Eur J Immunol.* (2002) 32:1726–36. doi: 10.1002/1521-4141(200206)32:6<1726::AID-IMMU1726>3.0.CO;2-R
16. Kouser L, Madhukaran SP, Shastri A, Saraon A, Ferluga J, Al-Mozaini M, et al. Emerging and novel functions of complement protein C1q. *Front Immunol.* (2015) 6:317. doi: 10.3389/fimmu.2015.00317
17. Bohlson SS, Fraser DA, Tenner AJ. Complement proteins C1q and MBL are pattern recognition molecules that signal immediate and long-term protective immune functions. *Mol Immunol.* (2007) 44:33–43. doi: 10.1016/j.molimm.2006.06.021
18. Ricklin D, Hajishengallis G, Yang K, Lambris JD. Complement: a key system for immune surveillance and homeostasis. *Nat Immunol.* (2010) 11:785–97. doi: 10.1038/ni.1923
19. Mongini PK, Jackson AE, Tolani S, Fattah RJ, Inman JK. Role of complement-binding CD21/CD19/CD81 in enhancing human B cell protection from Fas-mediated apoptosis. *J Immunol.* (2003) 171:5244–54. doi: 10.4049/jimmunol.171.10.5244
20. Grumach AS, Kirschfink M. Are complement deficiencies really rare? Overview on prevalence, clinical importance and modern diagnostic approach. *Mol Immunol.* (2014) 61:110–7. doi: 10.1016/j.molimm.2014.06.030
21. Leffler J, Bengtsson AA, Blom AM. The complement system in systemic lupus erythematosus: an update. *Ann Rheum Dis.* (2014) 73:1601–6. doi: 10.1136/annrheumdis-2014-205287
22. Ballanti E, Perricone C, Greco E, Ballanti M, Di Muzio G, Chimenti MS, et al. Complement and autoimmunity. *Immunol Res.* (2013) 56:477–91. doi: 10.1007/s12026-013-8422-y
23. Pickering MC, Cook HT. Translational mini-review series on complement factor H: renal diseases associated with complement factor H: novel insights from humans and animals. *Clin Exp Immunol.* (2008) 151:210–30. doi: 10.1111/j.1365-2249.2007.03574.x
24. Okroj M, Heinegard D, Holmdahl R, Blom AM. Rheumatoid arthritis and the complement system. *Ann Med.* (2007) 39:517–30. doi: 10.1080/07853890701477546
25. Bus P, Chua JS, Klessens CQF, Zandbergen M, Wolterbeek R, van Kooten C, et al. Complement activation in patients with diabetic nephropathy. *Kidney Int Rep.* (2018) 3:302–13. doi: 10.1016/j.ekir.2017.10.005
26. Markiewski MM, Lambris JD. The role of complement in inflammatory diseases from behind the scenes into the spotlight. *Am J Pathol.* (2007) 171:715–27. doi: 10.2353/ajpath.2007.070166
27. Lambris JD, Ricklin D, Geisbrecht BV. Complement evasion by human pathogens. *Nat Rev Microbiol.* (2008) 6:132–42. doi: 10.1038/nrmicro1824
28. Potempa M, Potempa J. Protease-dependent mechanisms of complement evasion by bacterial pathogens. *Biol Chem.* (2012) 393:873–88. doi: 10.1515/hsz-2012-0174
29. Zipfel PF, Wurzner R, Skerka C. Complement evasion of pathogens: common strategies are shared by diverse organisms. *Mol Immunol.* (2007) 44:3850–7. doi: 10.1016/j.molimm.2007.06.149
30. DuPage M, Mazumdar C, Schmidt LM, Cheung AF, Jacks T. Expression of tumour-specific antigens underlies cancer immunoediting. *Nature* (2012) 482:405–9. doi: 10.1038/nature10803
31. Jurianz K, Ziegler S, Garcia-Schuler H, Kraus S, Bohana-Kashtan O, Fishelson Z, et al. Complement resistance of tumor cells: basal and induced mechanisms. *Mol Immunol.* (1999) 36:929–39. doi: 10.1016/S0161-5890(99)00115-7
32. Murawski N, Pfreundschuh M. New drugs for aggressive B-cell and T-cell lymphomas. *Lancet Oncol.* (2010) 11:1074–85. doi: 10.1016/S1470-2045(10)70210-2
33. Okroj M, Osterborg A, Blom AM. Effector mechanisms of anti-CD20 monoclonal antibodies in B cell malignancies. *Cancer Treat Rev.* (2013) 39:632–9. doi: 10.1016/j.ctrv.2012.10.008
34. Takei K, Yamazaki T, Sawada U, Ishizuka H, Aizawa S. Analysis of changes in CD20, CD55, and CD59 expression on established rituximab-resistant B-lymphoma cell lines. *Leuk Res.* (2006) 30:625–31. doi: 10.1016/j.leukres.2005.09.008
35. Macor P, Secco E, Mezzaroba N, Zorzet S, Durigutto P, Gaiotto T, et al. Bispecific antibodies targeting tumor-associated antigens and neutralizing complement regulators increase the efficacy of antibody-based immunotherapy in mice. *Leukemia* (2015) 29:406–14. doi: 10.1038/leu.2014.185
36. Mamidi S, Hone S, Teufel C, Sellner L, Zenz T, Kirschfink M. Neutralization of membrane complement regulators improves complement-dependent effector functions of therapeutic anticancer antibodies targeting leukemic cells. *Oncoimmunology* (2015) 4:e979688. doi: 10.4161/2162402X.2014.979688

37. Schlaf G, Demberg T, Beisel N, Schieferdecker HL, Gotze O. Expression and regulation of complement factors H and I in rat and human cells: some critical notes. *Mol Immunol.* (2001) 38:231–9. doi: 10.1016/S0161-5890(01)00045-1
38. Okroj M, Hsu YF, Ajona D, Pio R, Blom AM. Non-small cell lung cancer cells produce a functional set of complement factor I and its soluble cofactors. *Mol Immunol.* (2008) 45:169–79. doi: 10.1016/j.molimm.2007.04.025
39. Ajona D, Castano Z, Garayoa M, Zudaire E, Pajares MJ, Martinez A, et al. Expression of complement factor H by lung cancer cells: effects on the activation of the alternative pathway of complement. *Cancer Res.* (2004) 64:6310–8. doi: 10.1158/0008-5472.CAN-03-2328
40. Ajona D, Hsu YF, Corrales L, Montuenga LM, Pio R. Down-regulation of human complement factor H sensitizes non-small cell lung cancer cells to complement attack and reduces *in vivo* tumor growth. *J Immunol.* (2007) 178:5991–8. doi: 10.4049/jimmunol.178.9.5991
41. Okroj M, Holmquist E, Nilsson E, Anagnostaki L, Jirstrom K, Blom AM. Local expression of complement factor I in breast cancer cells correlates with poor survival and recurrence. *Cancer Immunol Immunother.* (2015) 64:468–78. doi: 10.1007/s00262-015-1658-8
42. Riihila P, Nissinen L, Farshchian M, Kivisaari A, Ala-Aho R, Kallajoki M, et al. Complement factor I promotes progression of cutaneous squamous cell carcinoma. *J Invest Dermatol.* (2014) 135:579–88. doi: 10.1038/jid.2014.376
43. Horl S, Banki Z, Huber G, Ejaz A, Windisch D, Muellauer B, et al. Reduction of complement factor H binding to CLL cells improves the induction of rituximab-mediated complement-dependent cytotoxicity. *Leukemia* (2013) 27:2200–8. doi: 10.1038/leu.2013.169
44. Horl S, Banki Z, Huber G, Ejaz A, Mullauer B, Willenbacher E, et al. Complement factor H-derived short consensus repeat 18-20 enhanced complement-dependent cytotoxicity of ofatumumab on chronic lymphocytic leukemia cells. *Haematologica* (2013) 98:1939–47. doi: 10.3324/haematol.2013.089615
45. Donin N, Jurianz K, Ziporen L, Schultz S, Kirschfink M, Fishelson Z. Complement resistance of human carcinoma cells depends on membrane regulatory proteins, protein kinases and sialic acid. *Clin Exp Immunol.* (2003) 131:254–63. doi: 10.1046/j.1365-2249.2003.02066.x
46. Courtnay R, Ngo DC, Malik N, Ververis K, Tortorella SM, Karagiannis TC. Cancer metabolism and the Warburg effect: the role of HIF-1 and PI3K. *Mol Biol Rep.* (2015) 42:841–51. doi: 10.1007/s11033-015-3858-x
47. Collard CD, Vakeva A, Bukusoglu C, Zund G, Sperati CJ, Colgan SP, et al. Reoxygenation of hypoxic human umbilical vein endothelial cells activates the classic complement pathway. *Circulation* (1997) 96:326–33. doi: 10.1161/01.CIR.96.1.326
48. Collard CD, Bukusoglu C, Agah A, Colgan SP, Reenstra WR, Morgan BP, et al. Hypoxia-induced expression of complement receptor type 1 (CR1, CD35) in human vascular endothelial cells. *Am J Physiol.* (1999) 276:C450–8. doi: 10.1152/ajpcell.1999.276.2.C450
49. Okroj M, Corrales L, Stokowska A, Pio R, Blom AM. Hypoxia increases susceptibility of non-small cell lung cancer cells to complement attack. *Cancer Immunol Immunother.* (2009) 58:1771–880. doi: 10.1007/s00262-009-0685-8
50. Murdoch C, Giannoudis A, Lewis CE. Mechanisms regulating the recruitment of macrophages into hypoxic areas of tumors and other ischemic tissues. *Blood* (2004) 104:2224–34. doi: 10.1182/blood-2004-03-1109
51. Angelo LS, Kurzrock R. Vascular endothelial growth factor and its relationship to inflammatory mediators. *Clin Cancer Res.* (2007) 13:2825–30. doi: 10.1158/1078-0432.CCR-06-2416
52. Gately S, Li WW. Multiple roles of COX-2 in tumor angiogenesis: a target for antiangiogenic therapy. *Semin Oncol.* (2004) 31:2–11. doi: 10.1053/j.seminoncol.2004.03.040
53. Leek RD, Harris AL. Tumor-associated macrophages in breast cancer. *J Mammary Gland Biol Neoplasia* (2002) 7:177–89. doi: 10.1023/A:1020304003704
54. Ajona D, Pajares MJ, Corrales L, Perez-Gracia JL, Agorreta J, Lozano MD, et al. Investigation of complement activation product c4d as a diagnostic and prognostic biomarker for lung cancer. *J Natl Cancer Inst.* (2013) 105:1385–93. doi: 10.1093/jnci/djt205
55. Ajona D, Okroj M, Pajares MJ, Agorreta J, Lozano MD, Zulueta JJ, et al. Complement C4d-specific antibodies for the diagnosis of lung cancer. *Oncotarget* (2018) 9:6346–55. doi: 10.18632/oncotarget.23690
56. Corrales L, Ajona D, Rafail S, Lasarte JJ, Riezu-Boj JI, Lambris JD, et al. Anaphylatoxin c5a creates a favorable microenvironment for lung cancer progression. *J Immunol.* (2012) 189:4674–83. doi: 10.4049/jimmunol.1201654
57. Pakkala S, Owonikoko TK. Immune checkpoint inhibitors in small cell lung cancer. *J Thorac Dis.* (2018) 10:S460–7. doi: 10.21037/jtd.2017.12.51
58. Draghiciu O, Lubbers J, Nijman HW, Daemen T. Myeloid derived suppressor cells-an overview of combat strategies to increase immunotherapy efficacy. *Oncoimmunology* (2015) 4:e954829. doi: 10.4161/21624011.2014.954829
59. Okamura T, Fujio K, Sumitomo S, Yamamoto K. Roles of LAG3 and EGR2 in regulatory T cells. *Ann Rheum Dis.* (2012) 71 (Suppl. 2):i96–100. doi: 10.1136/annrheumdis-2011-200588
60. Markiewski MM, DeAngelis RA, Benencia F, Ricklin-Lichtsteiner SK, Koutoulaki A, Gerard C, et al. Modulation of the antitumor immune response by complement. *Nat Immunol.* (2008) 9:1225–35. doi: 10.1038/ni.1655
61. Nitta H, Murakami Y, Wada Y, Eto M, Baba H, Imamura T. Cancer cells release anaphylatoxin C5a from C5 by serine protease to enhance invasiveness. *Oncol Rep.* (2014) 32:1715–9. doi: 10.3892/or.2014.3341
62. Cho MS, Vasquez HG, Rupaimoole R, Pradeep S, Wu S, Zand B, et al. Autocrine effects of tumor-derived complement. *Cell Rep.* (2014) 6:1085–95. doi: 10.1016/j.celrep.2014.02.014
63. Reis ES, Mastellos DC, Ricklin D, Mantovani A, Lambris JD. Complement in cancer: untangling an intricate relationship. *Nat Rev Immunol.* (2018) 18:5–18. doi: 10.1038/nri.2017.97
64. Riihila P, Nissinen L, Farshchian M, Kallajoki M, Kivisaari A, Meri S, et al. Complement component C3 and complement factor B promote growth of cutaneous squamous cell carcinoma. *Am J Pathol.* (2017) 187:1186–97. doi: 10.1016/j.ajpath.2017.01.006
65. Bulla R, Tripodo C, Rami D, Ling GS, Agostinis C, Guarnotta C, et al. C1q acts in the tumour microenvironment as a cancer-promoting factor independently of complement activation. *Nat Commun.* (2016) 7:10346. doi: 10.1038/ncomms10346
66. Ajona D, Ortiz-Espinosa S, Moreno H, Lozano T, Pajares MJ, Agorreta J, et al. A combined PD-1/C5a blockade synergistically protects against lung cancer growth and metastasis. *Cancer Discov.* (2017) 7:694–703. doi: 10.1158/2159-8290.CD-16-1184
67. Wang Y, Sun SN, Liu Q, Yu YY, Guo J, Wang K, et al. Autocrine complement inhibits IL10-dependent T-cell-mediated antitumor immunity to promote tumor progression. *Cancer Discov.* (2016) 6:1022–35. doi: 10.1158/2159-8290.CD-15-1412
68. Stasilojc G, Osterborg A, Blom AM, Okroj M. New perspectives on complement mediated immunotherapy. *Cancer Treat Rev.* (2016) 45:68–75. doi: 10.1016/j.ctrv.2016.02.009
69. Hajishengallis G, Liang S, Payne MA, Hashim A, Jotwani R, Eskan MA, et al. Low-abundance biofilm species orchestrates inflammatory periodontal disease through the commensal microbiota and complement. *Cell Host Microbe* (2011) 10:497–506. doi: 10.1016/j.chom.2011.10.006
70. Walker AW, Sanderson JD, Churcher C, Parkes GC, Hudspith BN, Rayment N, et al. High-throughput clone library analysis of the mucosa-associated microbiota reveals dysbiosis and differences between inflamed and non-inflamed regions of the intestine in inflammatory bowel disease. *BMC Microbiol.* (2011) 11:7. doi: 10.1186/1471-2180-11-7
71. Kinane DF, Peterson M, Stathopoulou PG. Environmental and other modifying factors of the periodontal diseases. *Periodontol* (2006) 40:107–19. doi: 10.1111/j.1600-0757.2005.00136.x
72. Hajishengallis G, Darveau RP, Curtis MA. The keystone-pathogen hypothesis. *Nat Rev Microbiol.* (2012) 10:717–25. doi: 10.1038/nrmicro2873
73. Wang M, Krauss JL, Domon H, Hosur KB, Liang S, Magotti P, et al. Microbial hijacking of complement-toll-like receptor crosstalk. *Sci Signal.* (2010) 3:ra11. doi: 10.1126/scisignal.2000697
74. Popadiak K, Potempa J, Riesbeck K, Blom AM. Biphasic effect of gingipains from *Porphyromonas gingivalis* on the human complement system. *J Immunol.* (2007) 178:7242–50. doi: 10.4049/jimmunol.178.11.7242
75. Wingrove JA, DiScipio RG, Chen Z, Potempa J, Travis J, Hugli TE. Activation of complement components C3 and C5 by a cysteine proteinase (gingipain-1) from *Porphyromonas (Bacteroides) gingivalis*. *J Biol Chem.* (1992) 267:18902–7.

76. Okuda K, Kato T, Naito Y, Ono M, Kikuchi Y, Takazoe I. Susceptibility of *Bacteroides gingivalis* to bactericidal activity of human serum. *J Dent Res.* (1986) 65:1024–7. doi: 10.1177/00220345860650070601
77. Schenkein HA, Genco RJ. Gingival fluid and serum in periodontal diseases. I. Quantitative study of immunoglobulins, complement components, and other plasma proteins. *J Periodontol.* (1977) 48:772–7. doi: 10.1902/jop.1977.48.12.772
78. Maekawa T, Krauss JL, Abe T, Jotwani R, Triantafilou M, Triantafilou K, et al. *Porphyromonas gingivalis* manipulates complement and TLR signaling to uncouple bacterial clearance from inflammation and promote dysbiosis. *Cell Host Microbe* (2014) 15:768–78. doi: 10.1016/j.chom.2014.05.012
79. Bielecka E, Scavenius C, Kantyka T, Jusko M, Mizgalska D, Szmigielski B, et al. Peptidyl arginine deiminase from *Porphyromonas gingivalis* abolishes anaphylatoxin C5a activity. *J Biol Chem.* (2014) 289:32481–7. doi: 10.1074/jbc.C114.617142
80. Jusko M, Potempa J, Mizgalska D, Bielecka E, Ksiazek M, Riesbeck K, et al. A metalloproteinase mirolysin of *Tannerella forsythia* inhibits all pathways of the complement system. *J Immunol.* (2015) 195:2231–40. doi: 10.4049/jimmunol.1402892
81. Jusko M, Potempa J, Karim AY, Ksiazek M, Riesbeck K, Garred P, et al. A metalloproteinase karilysin present in the majority of *Tannerella forsythia* isolates inhibits all pathways of the complement system. *J Immunol.* (2012) 188:2338–49. doi: 10.4049/jimmunol.1101240
82. Jusko M, Miedziak B, Ermert D, Magda M, King BC, Bielecka E, et al. FACIN, a double-edged sword of the emerging periodontal pathogen filifactor alocis: a metabolic enzyme moonlighting as a complement inhibitor. *J Immunol.* (2016) 197:3245–59. doi: 10.4049/jimmunol.1600739
83. Potempa M, Potempa J, Kantyka T, Nguyen KA, Wawrzonek K, Manandhar SP, et al. Interpain A, a cysteine proteinase from *Prevotella intermedia*, inhibits complement by degrading complement factor C3. *PLoS Pathog.* (2009) 5:e1000316. doi: 10.1371/journal.ppat.1000316
84. Hajishengallis G. Periodontitis: from microbial immune subversion to systemic inflammation. *Nat Rev Immunol.* (2015) 15:30–44. doi: 10.1038/nri3785
85. Santoni M, Massari F, Amantini C, Nabissi M, Maines F, Burattini L, et al. Emerging role of tumor-associated macrophages as therapeutic targets in patients with metastatic renal cell carcinoma. *Cancer Immunol Immunother.* (2013) 62:1757–68. doi: 10.1007/s00262-013-1487-6
86. Yang Y, Ye YC, Chen Y, Zhao JL, Gao CC, Han H, et al. Crosstalk between hepatic tumor cells and macrophages via Wnt/beta-catenin signaling promotes M2-like macrophage polarization and reinforces tumor malignant behaviors. *Cell Death Dis.* (2018) 9:793. doi: 10.1038/s41419-018-0818-0
87. Bremnes RM, Donnem T, Al-Saad S, Al-Shibli K, Andersen S, Sirera R, et al. The role of tumor stroma in cancer progression and prognosis: emphasis on carcinoma-associated fibroblasts and non-small cell lung cancer. *J Thorac Oncol.* (2011) 6:209–17. doi: 10.1097/JTO.0b013e3181f8a1bd
88. Paulsson J, Micke P. Prognostic relevance of cancer-associated fibroblasts in human cancer. *Semin Cancer Biol.* (2014) 25:61–8. doi: 10.1016/j.semcancer.2014.02.006

11

A New Tool for Complement Research: *In vitro* Reconstituted Human Classical Complement Pathway

Michele Mutti, Katharina Ramoni, Gábor Nagy†, Eszter Nagy† and Valéria Szijártó†*

Arsanis Biosciences, Vienna, Austria

***Correspondence:**
Michele Mutti
michele.mutti@arsanis.com

***†Present Address:**
Gábor Nagy,
Eszter Nagy, and Valéria Szijártó,
Independent Researchers, Vienna, Austria

The complement, as part of the innate immune system, represents the first line of defense against Gram-negative bacteria invading the bloodstream. The complement system is a zymogen cascade that ultimately assemble into the so-called membrane attack complex (MAC), which lyses Gram-negative bacteria upon insertion into the outer membrane. Traditionally, serum has been used as complement source, for example to study the bactericidal activity of monoclonal antibodies or antibodies raised upon vaccination. Due to the significant donor to donor variability, as well as susceptibility of complement factors to handling and storage conditions, assay reproducibility using human serum is low. Moreover, the presence of pre-existing antibodies and antimicrobial compounds are confounding factors. To remove antibodies from human serum, we applied κ/λ-light chain specific affinity chromatography, however the method severely reduced the complement activity due to the depletion of complement components. Therefore, we attempted to reconstitute human complement—namely the alternative (rAP) and the classical (rCP) pathways—from purified complement factors. We found that adding C1-inhibitor to the mixture was essential to maintain a stable and functional C1 and thus to generate an active rCP. We further confirmed the functionality of the rCP by testing the complement-dependent bactericidal activity of a human monoclonal antibody, A1124 against an *E. coli* clinical isolate belonging to the ST131 clonal complex, and that of a polyclonal IVIg against a laboratory *E. coli* strain (MG1655) not expressing LPS O-antigen and capsule. Although the alternative pathway did not have any bactericidal activity by itself, it enhanced MAC deposition induced by rCP and increased the overall bactericidal activity against the ST131 *E. coli* strain. In conclusion, we report for the first time the successful *in vitro* reconstitution of the classical pathway of the human complement to establish a serum-free, complement dependent bactericidal assay. This system offers high level of standardization and could support the study of the complement in different research fields.

Keywords: C1-INH, bactericidal activity, monoclonal Ab, classical pathway, alternative pathway, *E. coli* ST131, MG1655, complement system

INTRODUCTION

As part of the innate immunity, the complement system is one of the first lines of defense against Gram-negative pathogens. Besides its direct bactericidal activity, the activation of the complement system stimulates phagocytosis and triggers pro-inflammatory signaling. The three different pathways—alternative, classical and lectin—converge into the terminal pathway (TP) that leads to the assembly of the C5b-9 complex, also called Membrane Attack Complex (MAC). The alternative pathway (AP) is spontaneously activated on the pathogen surface. The classical (CP) and lectin pathways (LP), are induced by an initial receptor-ligand recognition on the target surface. In case of the CP, the antigen-antibody complex (or immune complex, IC) activates the complement cascade by binding to C1, a complex formed by C1q, C1r, and C1s. In the LP, various lectins recognize specific sugar structures on the microbial surface and activate the Mannose Binding Protein-Associated Serine Proteases (MASPs) (1). Both CP and LP are negatively regulated by the C1 inhibitor (C1-INH), which sequesters and inhibits C1r, C1s, and MASPs (2). In the absence of C1-INH, C1 undergoes spontaneous activation (3, 4). Cleavage and activation of the various complement factors leads to the formation of the C5 convertase cleaving C5 to C5a and C5b, initiating the terminal pathway. C5b, attached to the target surface, associates with C6, C7, and C8 and induces the polymerization of C9 monomers, forming the MAC. MAC is a pore forming complex able to insert into lipid membranes, including the outer membrane of Gram-negative pathogens to induce membrane damage and cell lysis.

The different complement pathways interact with each other establishing a complex network in the serum (1, 5, 6). This complexity is further increased by the presence of additional serum bactericidal factors that may act in concert with the complement, or work independently against the invading pathogens (7–9). Therefore, it is difficult to dissect the contribution of the different complement pathways to the bactericidal action of the serum. It is especially relevant for studies using human serum as complement source due to the heterogeneity of the pre-existing antibody repertoires against human pathogens (10) and complement activity (11). While previous studies reported the successful reconstitution *in vitro* of the alternative pathway from individual components (12, 13), up to our knowledge, there have been no reports of a functionally active reconstituted classical pathway, particularly not to study its bactericidal activity.

We aimed to establish an *in vitro* model system with purified human complement components that allows studying complement without confounding factors.

METHODS AND MATERIALS

Bacterial Strains and Media

E. coli strains 81009 (14, 15) and MG1655 (16) were grown in LB or on Trypticase soy agar (TSA) plates (bioMérieux). To prepare overnight cultures, a single colony was inoculated in LB and incubated at 37 °C with agitation at 200 RPM overnight. Mid-log-phase bacterial cultures were obtained by diluting the overnight cultures 1:100 in LB and incubating at 37°C at 200 RPM until the cultures reached an OD_{600} of ~0.5.

Complement Factors, Sera, and Reagents

Rabbit erythrocytes, Gelatin Veronal Buffer with or without EDTA, as well as the complement factors C3 (A113c), H (A137), I (A138), B (A135), P (A139), C5 (A120), C6 (A123), C7 (A124), C8 (A125), C9 (A126), C1 (A098), C2 (A112), C4 (A105c), and C1-INH (A140) were purchased from CompTech. Dullbecco's phosphate-buffer saline (DPBS) without (14190144) or with calcium and magnesium (14040133) was obtained from ThermoFisher Scientific. Human serum albumin (HSA) (Albiomin, 200 g/L) was from Biotest. The monoclonal antibody A1124, a humanized IgG1 targeting the LPS O25b-antigen of *E. coli* ST131-H30 strains, as well as an isotype-matched control mAb were expressed in CHO cells as described by Guachalla et al. (17). Blood was taken from healthy volunteers into Vacutainer® clot activator tube (367896, Becton Dickinson and Company), and the off-the-clot normal human serum (NHS) was separated by centrifugation and aliquots were stored at −80°C until use. ClairYG® (50 mg/mL) was obtained from LFB-Biomedicaments.

Determination of Complement Activity

The complement activity was measured by commercial ELISA-based kits from Eurodiagnostica detecting C5b-9 deposition specific to classical (Wieslab COMPL CP310 RUO), alternative (Wieslab COMPL AP330 RUO) and MBP (Wieslab COMPL MP320 RUO) pathways according to manufacturer's instructions. Hemolytic activity of the complement was determined using rabbit erythrocytes according to the manufacturer's instructions using NHS as positive control.

Removal of Antibodies From Human Serum

To remove antibodies from NHS, κ/λ-light chain specific affinity chromatography was employed. The matrix was prepared by mixing three parts of κ-light chain specific beads with one part of λ-light chain specific beads (083310 and 084910, respectively, Life Technology). To avoid clogging of the resin, NHS was spin-filtered before incubating with double volume of resin at 4°C for 10 min. The supernatant was separated from the matrix by centrifugation (Ig depleted serum, Ig-dep). As control, equivalent volume of serum was treated identically but without the chromatography matrix (mock). Both Ig-depleted and mock sera were concentrated with Vivaspin 500 (10,000 MWCO PES, Sartorius). The dilution factor was determined based on absorbance measurement at 405, 490, and 650 nm, compared to that of untreated serum. To remove beads, fibers and precipitates, the samples were spin-filtered. Bound antibodies were recovered by washing the resin with DPBS with Ca/Mg, eluting with 0.1 M glycine pH 2.0 buffer and neutralizing with 1 M Tris pH 8.0. This immunoglobulin fraction was concentrated with Vivaspin 20 (10,000 MWCO PES, Sartorius) followed by Vivaspin 500 and finally spin-filtered. In all cases Ultrafree™-MC Centrifugal Filter Devices 0.22 μm (EMD Millipore) was employed for spin-filtration. Samples were stored at −80°C.

Preparation of Fab Fragment of Human IVIg

Fab fragments of human IVIg (ClairYg®) were prepared by digestion with agarose-immobilized papain (20341, ThermoFisher) according to the manufacturer's instructions. DPBS with 10 mM EDTA pH 7.0 was used as buffer. The uncleaved Igs and Fc fragments were removed by using MabSelect Sure® (17543801, GE Healthcare) according to the manufacturer's instructions. The flow-through, containing the Fabs, was buffer exchanged in DPBS, concentrated (Vivaspin 500, Sartorius) and spin filtered (Ultrafree™-MC Centrifugal Filter Devices 0.22 μm; EMD Millipore) to ensure sterility. An untreated aliquot of ClairYg® was buffer exchanged and treated the same way to be used as control. The concertation of both Fab and full IgG in DPBS was determined by bicinchoninic acid (BCA) assay (23225, ThermoFisher).

Surface Staining of *E. Coli*

To detect surface binding antibodies, 10^8 CFU/ml bacteria were incubated with various concentration of ClairYg® or its Fab fragments, followed by incubation with secondary detection reagent Alexa Fluor 488 goat anti-human IgG Fcγ or Alexa Fluor 488 goat anti-human Fab_2 (109-546-170 and 109-546-097 respectively, Jackson Immuno) and stained with 5 μM SYTO 62 nucleic acid stain (S11344, ThermoFisher). Samples were measured in a CytoFLEX flow cytometer (Beckman Coulter) and data were analyzed using the FCS Express Flow 5 (*De Novo* Software).

Immunoblotting

Samples diluted 1:400 in Laemmli buffer were separated on Mini-PROTEAN TGX 4-20% gels (4561096 or 4561094, Bio Rad) and blotted onto 0.22 μm nitrocellulose membrane using the high MW program of the TransBlot Turbo system (Bio Rad). The membrane was blocked in 5 % skim milk in Tris Buffered Saline (TBS, Fischer scientific), incubated with 1:50,000 diluted horseradish peroxidase (HRP) conjugated goat anti-human IgG (H+L) (109-035-088, Jackson ImmunoResearch) and 1:50,000 HRP conjugated goat anti-human albumin (PA1-28334, Pierce). To detect C4 cleavage, the membrane was incubated with goat anti-human C4 serum (1:2,000, A205, CompTech) as primary antibody and with donkey IgG-HRP anti-goat-IgG (1:40,000, 6420-05, Southern Biotech) as secondary antibody. Blots were developed with Amersham ECL Prime solution reagent (GE Healthcare).

Determination of C1q and MBL2 Levels in Human Sera

Concentrations of C1q and MBL2 were determined by ELISA using a commercial kit according to the manufacturer's instructions (HK356 and HK323, respectively, HycultBiotech). The serum samples were diluted 1:200 for C1q and 1:50 for MBL2 determination. The Ig depleted sera and the eluates were diluted according to the estimated protein concentrations.

Preparation of C1/C1-INH Mixture

C1-INH was concentrated to about 2 mg/mL (Vivaspin 500, Sartorius), mixed with about 0.2–0.4 mg/mL C1 and 25 mg/mL HSA, and incubated for 10 min on ice. This mixture or C1 alone was dialyzed twice against DPBS with Ca/Mg at 4°C for 3 h followed by concentration to ∼1.3 mg/mL of C1 (Vivaspin 500, Sartorius). In the C1/C1-INH mixture, the C1-INH to C1 ratio was 1.8 times the physiological ratio. The samples were spin filtered to ensure sterility (Ultrafree™-MC Centrifugal Filter Devices 0.22 μm; EMD Millipore) and then aliquoted and stored at −80°C until use. At least of three different batches of C1/C1-INH were prepared and used.

Complementation Assay With C1q-Depleted Serum

C1 alone or premixed with C1-INH was incubated on ice or at 37°C for 60 min, and added to C1q-depleted serum (A300, CompTech). The activity of the classical pathway was measured with the ELISA-based kit described above.

C4 Cleavage Assay

Heat-aggregated IgG (HAGG) was generated by incubating ClairYg® in DPBS with Ca/Mg at 63°C for 30 min as described previously (18). C4 (200 μg/mL), HSA (20 mg/mL) and HAGG (750 μg/mL) were mixed on ice (final concentration indicated). C1 (67.5 μg/mL) combined with C1-INH at various final concentrations ranging between 68.5 and 685 μg/mL was added to the mixture. The concentration of Ca and Mg were kept constant at 0.45 mM and 0.25 mM, respectively. After 5 min on ice, the reaction was started by incubation at 37°C for 5 min. The reaction was stopped by boiling in reducing Laemmli buffer (1610737, BIORAD for 5 min. C4 cleavage was detected by immunoblotting as described above.

Reconstitution of the Human Complement

The alternative pathway (rAP) was reconstituted as reported by Schreiber et al. (12, 13). Briefly, C3, factor H and factor I were incubated for 30 min at 37°C. After cooling the mixture on ice, factor B, factor P, and the terminal pathway components C5, C6, C7, C8, and C9 were added. For the reconstitution of the rCP, C3 was incubated for 30 min at 37°C (analogous to treatment in rAP), cooled on ice, then TP components, C2, C4, and C1/C1-INH mixture were added, and then the solution was supplemented with DPBS and HSA. For the combination of the alternative and classical pathways (rAP+rCP), the alternative pathway was reconstituted as above, then TP components, C2, C4, and C1/C1-INH mixture were added, and finally the mixture was supplemented with DPBS and HSA. In all experiments the final concentration of Ca, Mg and HSA was 0.17 mM, 0.09 mM, and 25 mg/mL respectively. The proteins were added in the order described above. The final concentration of each factor matched the physiological concentration of 50% diluted human serum (3, 12): C3 at 600 μg/mL, C5 at 36 μg/mL, C6 at 32 μg/mL, C7 at 27 μg/mL, C8 at 27 μg/mL, C9 at 29.5 μg/mL, factor B at 100 μg/mL, factor D at 1 μg/mL, factor H at 235 μg/mL, factor I at 17 μg/mL, factor P at 10 μg/mL, C2 at 12.5 μg/mL, C4 at 200 μg/mL, C1 at 67.5 μg/mL and C1-INH at 120 μg/mL.

Activity of rCP With or Without C1-INH

When the rCP with or without C1-INH was tested, the preparations were treated as follows. Two mixtures of rCP with or without C1-INH were prepared simultaneously as described above, on ice and aliquoted into 5 tubes. One aliquot was snap frozen in liquid nitrogen and stored at −80°C. The remaining four aliquots were incubated at 37°C or on ice for 10 min or 60 min and then snap frozen. For measuring complement activity, the aliquots were thawed on ice at once and the assay was started immediately.

Bactericidal Assay

Survival of bacteria was assayed as described previously (19). Briefly, bacteria at about $\sim 5 \times 10^4$ CFU/mL (collected from mid-log phase culture) were added to the reconstituted complement and incubated at 37°C with agitation. After 3 h, surviving bacterial count was enumerated by plating. In case of *E. coli* strain MG1655, the final concentration of each factor matched the physiological concentration in 25% diluted human serum, while in assays with the *E. coli* strain 81009, the factors were set to 50% of the physiological concentration.

Stability of rCP

rCP mixture was divided into four aliquots; one was immediately frozen at −80°C (untreated control), one underwent 3 cycles of freeze and thaw, one was stored at 4°C for 48 h, and one was incubated at 37°C for 24 h before freezing at −80°C. On the day of the testing, the samples were thawed at once and their complement activity was compared with the ELISA based kit as described above.

Statistical Analysis

Data were analyzed with paired two-tailed *t*-test using GraphPad Prism version 6. Difference was considered statistically significant if $P < 0.05$.

RESULTS

Removal of Antibodies From Human Serum Impairs the Complement

First, we tested the possibility of removing antibodies from normal human serum (NHS) to generate a complement source devoid of pre-existing antibodies for studying complement-mediated bactericidal activity. We employed affinity chromatography with Ig light chain (κ and λ) specific resin to remove all isotypes of antibodies. Based on immunoblot analysis, no IgGs could be detected in the depleted sera (**Figure 1A**). Next, we determined whether Ig depletion affected the complement activity of the human serum samples. The four NHS tested had comparable classical and alternative pathway activities prior to depletion, however, all had reduced or no activity after incubation with the resin (**Figure 1B**). We detected both MBL2 and C1q in the elution fractions together with the antibodies (**Supplementary Figure 1**).

Given that depletion of antibodies from NHS was not possible without compromising the complement activity, we next attempted to reconstitute the classical and the alternative complement pathways *in vitro*.

In vitro Reconstitution of the Alternative Complement Pathway

First, we wanted to recapitulate the results of Schreiber et al. (12) reported four decades ago demonstrating the functional activity of reconstituted alternative pathway (rAP). We combined purified complement components in the following order: C3, factor H and factor I incubated at 37°C, then adding factor B, factor P, and the terminal pathway components C5, C6, C7, C8, and C9. As a measure of complement activity, we detected C5b-9 assembly by ELISA (**Figure 2**) or by the rabbit erythrocyte lysis assay (**Supplementary Figure 2**). The activity of the rAP measured by ELISA was in the range of the AP activity of untreated NHS samples and the rabbit RBC lytic activity of rAP was also comparable to that of NHS (**Supplementary Figure 2**). The activity in both assays was specific, as it was completely lost upon the exclusion of the C5 component from to the rAP mixture.

C1-INH Is Required to Preserve the Functionality of the Classical Pathway

Analogous to the generation of rAP, we attempted to reconstitute the classical pathway (rCP) by combining all factors from C1 to C9. First, C3 was incubated at 37°C, and cooled on ice before the terminal pathway components C5, 6, 7, 8 9, then C2, C4, and finally C1 were added at concentrations equivalent to those in 50% human serum. To test the stability of the reconstituted classical pathway, the mixture was preincubated for up to 60 min at 37°C, before being assayed for the C5b-9 deposition. To resemble the physiologic activation, we measured the activity of the classical pathway with an ELISA kit, with wells coated with IgM, mimicking the immunocomplexes. Surprisingly, we detected only a very low complement activity (approximately 20% that of human serum) that was even further decreased when the mixture was incubated on ice or was completely lost after incubation at 37°C (**Figure 3A**).

Since the rAP, that shares many components with the CP, was functionally active and stable, we focused our investigation on the components specific for the classical pathway, particularly C1. To assess the activity of C1, we employed a C1q depleted (C1q-dep) serum preparation that lacked any CP activity and supplemented this with C1. We found that C1 was able to rescue the classical pathway activity of the C1q depleted serum, but with decreased efficiency after pre-incubation of C1 at 37°C (**Figure 3B**). These data suggested that the purified C1 was functional, but it lost its ability to induce the C5b-9 deposition upon incubation at 37°C.

We speculated that the loss of C1 activity was due to the spontaneous activation of C1 itself. Therefore, we assessed whether the C1 inhibitor (C1-INH), a serine protease inhibitor naturally present in human serum, would be able to stabilize C1. Indeed, we observed that the supplementation of C1q-depleted serum with C1 pre-incubated at 37°C in the presence of C1-INH, fully restored the CP activity (**Figure 3B**). Hence, we added C1-INH to the rCP, and the experiment was repeated as

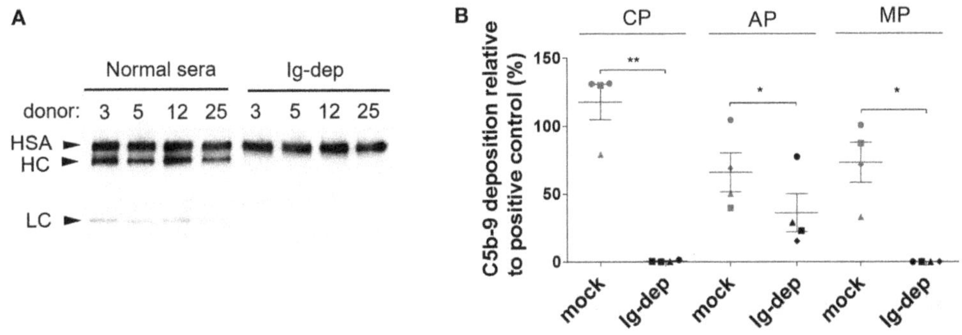

FIGURE 1 | Depletion of Ig from normal human serum. **(A)** IgG (Fcγ-heavy chain, HC and light chain, LC) was detected by immunoblotting in normal human serum (NHS) and in the corresponding sera depleted with light-chain specific resin (Ig-dep). Albumin (HSA) was used as loading control and detected with a specific antibody. **(B)** Classical (CP), alternative (AP), mannose-binding lectin (MP) pathway activity was measured by ELISA in sera depleted with light chain specific resin (Ig-dep), or in mock treated (mock) samples and compared to a positive control provided in the kit. Graph shows mean values obtained with sera from 4 donors ±SEM. C5b-9 deposition in Ig-dep was compared to the mock treated sample by two-tailed paired *t*-test (*$P < 0.05$; **$P < 0.01$). The circle, square, triangle and diamond represent donor #3, #5, #12, and #25, respectively.

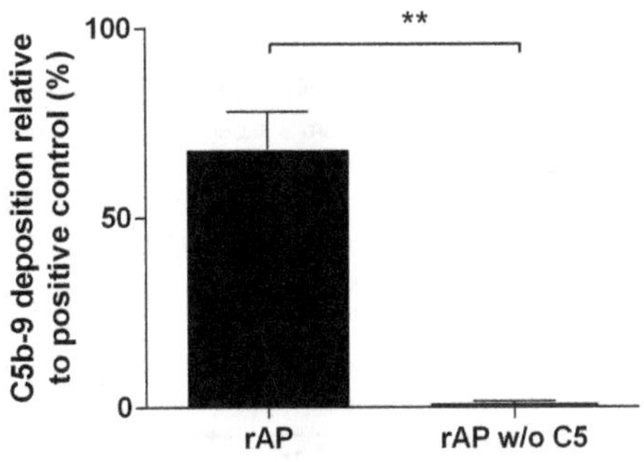

FIGURE 2 | Activity of reconstituted alternative pathway. The activity of the reconstituted alternative pathway with all factors (rAP) or without C5 (rAP w/o C5) was measured by ELISA. The bars show mean ± SEM of 3 independent experiments performed with duplicates. Results were compared with paired *t*-test (**$P < 0.01$).

described above. When adding C1-INH to the rCP, we observed a full classical pathway activity, in all the conditions tested (**Figure 3A**).

To monitor the C1 activity at the molecular level during the incubation of rCP, we detected C4 and C3 cleavage products by immunoblotting. We observed the proteolytic conversion of both C4 and C3 α chains to α'-chain in the absence, but not in the presence of C1-INH (**Figure 3A**). These data corroborated that spontaneous activation of C1 led to activation of the CP, which ultimately consumed the native complement factors in the mixture. On the other hand, in presence of C1-INH we did not observe any cleavage of C4 and C3, even after incubation for 1 h at 37°C (**Figure 3A**).

To examine whether the C1-INH concentration used in the assay still allows the specific activation of C1 initiated by immune complexes (IC), we monitored C4 cleavage triggered by heat-aggregated Ig. We found that even large excess of C1-INH (up to 10-fold the physiological C1-INH/C1 ratio) did not impair the specific activation of C1 (**Supplementary Figure 3**).

We also tested the stability of rCP upon freeze-thaw cycles or incubation at 37°C or at 4°C. As shown in **Supplementary Figure 4**, the rCP is resistant to three cycles of freeze and thaw, and stable at 4°C for 48 h, but incubation at 37°C for 24 h significantly impairs the complement activity.

rCP, Alone or in Combination With rAP, Is Functional and Induces a Strong Bactericidal Action

Next, we reconstituted the classical complement pathway in combination with rAP. Both rAP and rCP were functionally active when combined (rAP+rCP) (**Figure 4A**). However, when measuring the classical pathway activity in the combined system, it was lower than in the rCP alone (**Figure 4A**). These results suggested that components present in the rAP (partially) inhibit the classical pathway activity of rCP.

As proof of practical application, we tested the bactericidal activity of the rAP, rCP or their combination (rAP+rCP) against two different *Escherichia coli* strains in the presence of specific antibodies.

ST131 strain 81009 expressing the O25b LPS O-antigen and mAb A1124 specific for O25b (17) were co-incubated with the reconstituted complement. In presence of the rCP, we observed significant antibody-dependent bactericidal activity, while rAP alone did not support bacterial killing (**Figure 4B**). Interestingly, the mixture of rCP and rAP displayed enhanced bactericidal effect (**Figure 4B**).

Another *E. coli*, the K-12 strain MG1655, not expressing LPS O-antigen (rough), was incubated with a human IVIg preparation (ClairYg®) that was shown to contain antibodies binding to the surface of this strain (**Supplementary Figure 5**). In the presence of IVIg (500 μg/ml), the MG1655 strain was completely killed in rCP or rAP+rCP, while it survived in the rAP (**Figure 4C**). MG1655 also survived and even grew in rCP and rAP+rCP when incubated with ClairYg®-derived Fab,

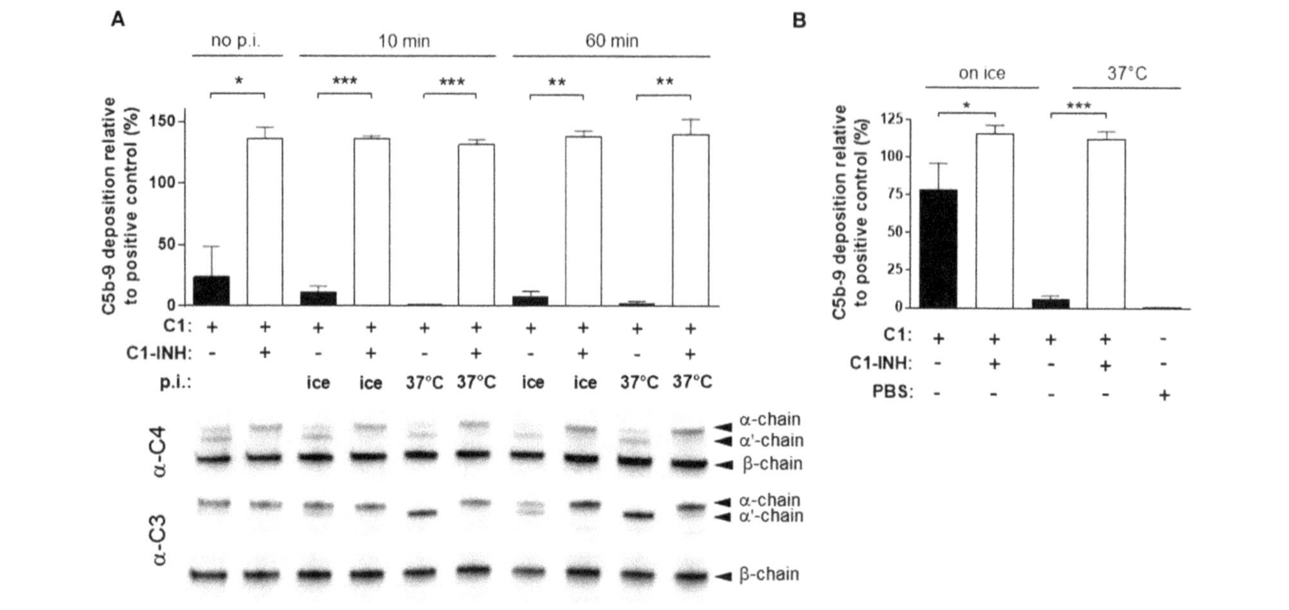

FIGURE 3 | Preserving C1 activity by C1-INH. **(A)** The activity of the reconstituted classical pathway (rCP) was measured by ELISA. rCP with or without C1-INH was pre-incubated (p.i.) for 10 min or 60 min, at 37°C or on ice, before testing for C5b-9 deposition. Graphs show mean ± SEM from 3 experiments, compared with two-tailed paired *t*-test ($^*P < 0.05$; $^{**}P < 0.01$; $^{***}P < 0.001$). The same samples were assayed for C4 and C3 cleavage by immunoblotting that is indicated by the appearance of the α'-chain. **(B)** C1 incubated for 1 h at 37°C or on ice was added to C1q-depleted serum. The classical pathway activity was measured by ELISA detecting C5b-9 deposition. The results are expressed as % of signal compared to the positive control. Graph shows mean ± SEM from 4 independent experiments compared with two-tailed paired *t*-test ($^*P < 0.05$; $^{***}P < 0.001$).

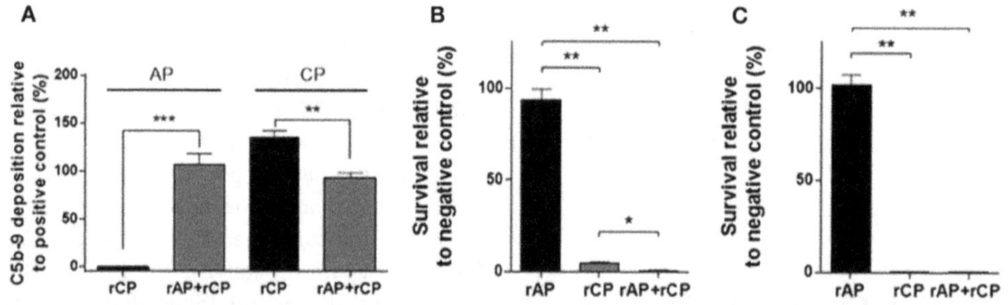

FIGURE 4 | Complement and bactericidal activity of *in vitro* reconstituted complement pathways. **(A)** ELISA detecting the alternative (AP) or classical (CP) pathway-dependent C5b-9 deposition by the *in vitro* reconstituted alternative (rAP) and classical pathway (rCP), alone or in combination (rAP+rCP). The results are expressed relative to positive control. Graphs show mean values ±SEM of 6 independent experiments analyzed with two-tailed paired *t*-test ($^{**}P < 0.01$; $^{***}P < 0.001$). **(B)** Survival of the *E. coli* strain 81009 in the presence of the reconstituted complement pathways with mAb A1124 after 180 min incubation. The survival is expressed relative to the survival with an unrelated control mAb. **(C)** Survival of the *E. coli* strain MG1655 in the presence of the reconstituted complement pathways with ClairYg® after 180 min incubation. The survival is expressed relative to the survival in presence of ClairYg®-derived Fab. Graphs **(B,C)** show mean ± SEM of 3 and 2 independent experiments, respectively, analyzed with two-tailed paired *t*-test ($^*P < 0.05$; $^{**}P < 0.01$).

corroborating that the bactericidal activity was not intrinsic to the rCP.

Low amounts of human IgG contamination was detected in all three mixtures of reconstituted complement (**Supplementary Figure 6**). Contaminants were—at least partially—introduced with the human albumin. Despite the presence of contaminating antibodies, we did not detect any specific, surface binding antibodies against the two *E. coli* strains (data not shown).

DISCUSSION

Serum bactericidal assay (SBA) is the gold standard *in vitro* assay to assess complement-dependent bactericidal activity of antibodies raised upon active immunization (10, 20) or applied as passive immunization (17). In SBA, human or rabbit serum is used as complement source and target bacteria are incubated in presence of specific antibodies or immune serum. In such assays, bacterial survival is

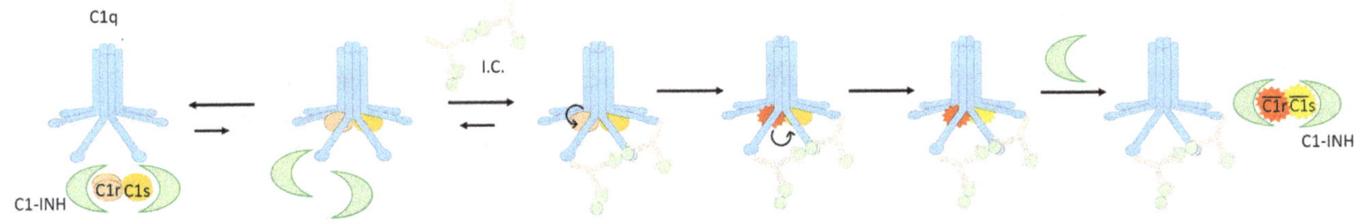

FIGURE 5 | Activation of C1 in presence of C1-INH and immunocomplexes. C1-INH reversibly inhibits in fluid phase the pro-C1r and pro-C1s, when they dissociates from C1-INH they can bind C1q, but this is disfavored. In presence of immunocomplexes (I.C.), the association of $C1r_2s_2$ to C1q is favored and stable, so C1q activates C1r which in turn cleaves C1s. Afterwards, the activated $C1r_2s_2$ (indicated as $\overline{C1r}$ and $\overline{C1s}$) is then displaced from C1q and irreversibily inhibited by C1-INH.

compared to those with a negative control antibody or non-immune serum as well as an inactivated complement source. Most often rabbit serum is preferred over human serum, because baby rabbit sera lack pre-existing antibodies (10, 20). Previous reports showed the possibility of depleting human serum from pre-existing antibodies by using Protein G affinity purification, with the drawback that C1q and C5 were significantly depleted during the process (21). Moreover, the method did not deplete IgM or IgA, two isotypes also able to activate the complement system (1, 22).

In this study, we aimed to establish a reproducible method with a complement source free of antibodies. First, we depleted human serum from all isotypes of immunoglobulins with a light chain specific resin. While we were able to remove the majority of IgGs, this treatment abolished activity of the classical and lectin pathways due to the non-specific depletion of C1q and MBL2, significantly impaired activity of the alternative pathway, and potentially depleted other complement factors by the resin.

In addition to antibodies, non-complement serum factors can also significantly contribute to the killing of bacteria in human serum (7, 8, 23). Therefore, we decided to test a bottom-up approach and reconstituted the complement system from its individual components. While reconstituted cytolytic alternative pathway was reported by two papers of Schreiber et al. ((12), (13)), up to our knowledge there are no reports of successful reconstitution of the complete classical pathway from C1 to C9, despite the significant amount of work put into reconstituting parts of it (24–31). We aimed to establish a method to reconstitute the classical pathway also in combination with the alternative pathway, to be used in studying complement mediated bactericidal activity. To make it available for the broader scientific community, we used commercially available factors purified from human serum.

First, we reproduced previous work of reconstitution of the alternative pathway (12). This was primarily done to confirm that the purified proteins were functionally active. The protocol was slightly modified with the addition of human serum albumin as carrier protein. The mixture of the AP components was active based on the detection of the C5b-9 complex measured by ELISA and the lysis of rabbit erythrocytes, and the activity was found comparable to that of human serum (32).

When we mixed the factors of the classical pathway, we detected very low CP activity. Furthermore, short incubation at 37°C (10 min) completely abolished this activity.

Apart from C1, C2 and C4, all components were already used and proved to be active in rAP, therefore we tested the activity of CP-specific factors. Importantly, the commercially available C1 is supplied with EDTA and protease inhibitors, which inhibit the activity of the complement factors, therefore, we had to remove these inhibitors by buffer exchange. This treatment could have affected activity or stability of the C1 or its components, like C1q. In line with this, C1 pre-incubated on ice was able to rescue the classical pathway in C1q-depleted serum, but not when pre-incubated at 37°C. This suggested that the buffer exchange *per se* was not responsible for the impairment of C1 activity, but rather affected its stability. Furthermore, we speculated that the lack of C5b-9 deposition in both rCP and C1q depleted serum was due to the spontaneous activation of C1r and C1s at 37°C. Indeed, in normal serum, the spontaneous activation of C1 is prevented by C1-INH that has a dual role; it inhibits irreversibly the zymogen form of C1s and C1r and in a reversible way the pro-zymogen form of C1r and C1s. In the presence of ICs, C1-INH disengages the pro-zymogens C1r and C1s, allowing their activation (4) (**Figure 5**). Thus, we tested whether C1-INH was able to maintain a functional C1 in an *in vitro* system as well without affecting the specific activity of C1. A previous study by Nielsen (33) showed that even large excess of C1-INH had no effect on the activation of C1 by immune complexes. However, the C1-INH preparation used in that work differed from the C1-INH available for us (34, 35). Therefore, we set up a method to detect the specific activation of C1 induced by heat-aggregated gamma globulins. We observed that even a 10-fold excess of the C1-INH did not impair the specific activation by IC.

Next, we showed that the classical pathway was fully rescued when C1q-depleted serum was supplemented with C1 co-incubated with C1-INH at 37°C. Likewise, the presence of C1-INH in rCP allowed full reconstitution of the classical pathway that was unchanged even after 1 h of incubation at 37°C. We confirmed that in the absence of C1-INH, C4 was promptly cleaved, even without specific activation. The cleavage of C4 led to the cleavage of C3 as well, but with a slower kinetics. The very low activity of the classical pathway in the rCP correlated well with the amount of native C3 in the mixture. On the other hand, when C1-INH was present, both C4 and C3 remained uncleaved (in native state). In conclusion, the very low level of C5b-9 deposition by rCP in the absence of C1-INH is due to the consumption of the downstream factors, rather than to C1 instability. An interesting indirect proof for the requirement of C1-INH in CP is the phenotype of hereditary angioedema (HAE) type I and II. In HAE low activity of C1-INH leads to the activation of the contact system (which induces edema) and the collateral spontaneous activation of C1 and consumption of C4 and C2 (36).

While rCP appeared to remain active after three freeze-thaw cycles and at 4°C for 48 h, incubation at 37°C impaired the complement activity, in agreement with the observation by Mollnes et al. (37).

When we combined alternative and classical pathways, we found both to be active alone and in combination in the ELISA-based complement activity assay. The lower CP activity of rAP+rCP compared to rCP alone could be explained by the presence of Factor H and I. Factor H acts as cofactor for factor I to cleave C3b and C4b, and it can block the induction of the downstream cascade (5). In addition, factor H alone could also displace C1 from the ligand, as shown by Kishore and Sim (38).

After confirming the activity of the reconstituted *in vitro* complement, we proved that this experimental system is suitable for studying the complement mediated bactericidal activity of monoclonal or polyclonal antibodies. Using an extra-intestinal pathogenic *E. coli* strain 81009, we found that the rCP was able to induce a strong and specific bactericidal activity in combination with the specific mAb, A1124. The bactericidal activity was further increased when alternative and classical pathways were combined. This confirms that although the alternative pathway alone does not induce bactericidal effect, it enhances the activity of the classical pathway through the amplification loop. Of note, in the ELISA based activity assay we did not observe an increase in the classical pathway activity when rCP was combined with rAP, however this was due to the use of different complement dilutions in the two assays: in the ELISA the complement mixture was diluted 1:101 (vs. the 1:2 dilution used in the bactericidal assay) and at such a high dilution the contribution of the alternative pathway could not be detected.

We found that IVIg ClairYg® contained a significant amount of antibodies against MG1655, as also reported by others (39); therefore it was used as a source of Abs to target this strain. MG1655 is a rough and non-encapsulated K-12 archetype strain, extremely sensitive to the bactericidal activity of the serum. In agreement with its sensitivity, the strain was completely killed in both rCP and rAP+rCP in the presence of ClairYg®. Despite of the low content of contaminating antibodies in the reconstituted complement pathways, we did not observe any killing when no ClairYg® was added to the mixture. In contrast with our data, the K-12 derivative strain, W1485, was previously shown to be killed by a reconstituted alternative pathway alone (12). However, the growth conditions used in the two studies were different, and previously also no carrier protein was added to the reconstituted mixture. Moreover, it cannot be excluded that the complement factors used previously differed in purity and potentially contained bactericidal proteins.

To our knowledge, this is the first report of the successful reconstitution of the classical pathway from individual components. In this model system, it is possible to strictly control the concentration of each component or to substitute a factor with a mutated version, as well as to supplement the assay with additional purified components, as demonstrated by adding a specific antibody. By adding lectins and MASPs to the C1/C1-INH mixture, we speculate that the system can be further complemented with the lectin pathway.

We propose that the method could have a broad applicability beyond the testing of complement mediated bactericidal activity of antibodies. It was proposed that new methods are needed to study the role of the complement in the activity of the anti-CD20 mAB, rituximab in non-Hodgkin lymphomas (40). As serum was reported to display great donor to donor heterogeneity in the killing of cancerous cells (41), the *in vitro* reconstituted complement may offer a simple method to be used in cancer studies. Similarly, this tool could be applied to study the role of the complement in viral pathogenesis (42), transplant rejection (43) and autoimmune diseases (44, 45).

AUTHOR CONTRIBUTIONS

MM performed the experiments. KR provided technical assistance. MM and VS designed the experiments. MM, VS, GN, and EN wrote the manuscript.

REFERENCES

1. Murphy K, Kenneth M, Travers P, Walport M, Janeway C. *Janeway's Immunobiology*. London: Garland Science (2008).
2. Beinrohr L, Dobó J, Závodszky P, Gál P. C1, MBL-MASPs and C1-inhibitor: novel approaches for targeting complement-mediated inflammation. *Trends Mol Med.* (2008) 14:511–21. doi: 10.1016/j.molmed.2008.09.009
3. Ziccardi RJ. A new role for C-1-inhibitor in homeostasis: control of activation of the first component of human complement. *J Immunol.* (1982) 128:2505–8. doi: 10.1371/journal.pcbi.1000778
4. Ziccardi RJ. Spontaneous activation of the first component of human complement (C1) by an intramolecular autocatalytic mechanism. *J Immunol.* (1982) 128:2500–4.
5. Merle NS, Church SE, Fremeaux-Bacchi V, Roumenina LT. Complement system part I - molecular mechanisms of activation and regulation. *Front Immunol.* (2015) 6:1–30. doi: 10.3389/fimmu.2015.00262
6. Merle NS, Noe R, Halbwachs-Mecarelli L, Fremeaux-Bacchi V, Roumenina LT. Complement System Part II: role in immunity. *Front Immunol.* (2015) 6:257. doi: 10.3389/fimmu.2015.00257
7. Berends ETM, Mohan S, Miellet WR, Ruyken M, Rooijakkers SHM. Contribution of the complement Membrane Attack Complex to the bactericidal activity of human serum. *Mol Immunol.* (2015) 65:328–35. doi: 10.1016/j.molimm.2015.01.020
8. Miajlovic H, Smith SG. Bacterial self-defence: how *Escherichia coli* evades serum killing. *FEMS Microbiol Lett.* (2014) 354:1–9. doi: 10.1111/1574-6968.12419

9. Zimmer J, Hobkirk J, Mohamed F, Browning MJ, Stover CM. On the functional overlap between complement and anti-microbial peptides. *Front Immunol.* (2015) 5:689. doi: 10.3389/fimmu.2014.00689
10. McIntosh EDG, Bröker M, Wassil J, Welsch JA, Borrow R. Serum bactericidal antibody assays - The role of complement in infection and immunity. *Vaccine* (2015) 33:4414–21. doi: 10.1016/j.vaccine.2015.07.019
11. Szijártó V, Guachalla LM, Hartl K, Varga C, Badarau A, Mirkina I, et al. Endotoxin neutralization by an O-antigen specific monoclonal antibody: a potential novel therapeutic approach against Klebsiella pneumoniae ST258. *Virulence* (2017) 8:1203–15. doi: 10.1080/21505594.2017.1279778
12. Schreiber RD, Morrison DC, Podack ER, Müller-Eberhard HJ, Schreiber BRD, Morrison DC, et al. Bactericidal activity of the alternative complement pathway generated from 11 isolated plasma proteins. *J Exp Med.* (1979) 149:870–82.
13. Schreiber RD, Müller-Eberhard HJ. Assembly of the cytolytic alternative pathway of complement from 11 isolated plasma proteins. *J Exp Med.* (1978) 148:1722–7.
14. Mutti M, Sonnevend Á, Pál T, Junttila S, Ekker H, Galik B, et al. Complete genome sequence of *Escherichia coli* 81009, a representative of the sequence Type 131 C1-M27 clade with a multidrug-resistant phenotype. *Genome Announc.* (2018) 6:e00056-18. doi: 10.1128/genomeA.00056-18
15. Szijártó V, Pal T, Nagy G, Nagy E, Ghazawi A, Al-Haj M, et al. The rapidly emerging ESBL-producing *Escherichia coli* O25-ST131 clone carries LPS core synthesis genes of the K-12 type. *FEMS Microbiol Lett.* (2012) 332:131–6. doi: 10.1111/j.1574-6968.2012.02585.x
16. Blattner FR, Plunkett G, Bloch CA, Perna NT, Burland V, Riley M, et al. The complete genome sequence of Escherichia coli K-12. *Science* (1997) 277:1453–62. doi: 10.1126/science.277.5331.1453
17. Guachalla LM, Hartl K, Varga C, Stulik L, Mirkina I, Malafa S, et al. Multiple modes of action of a monoclonal antibody against multidrug-resistant *Escherichia coli* Sequence Type 131- H 30. *Antimicrob Agents Chemother.* (2017) 61:e01428–e01417. doi: 10.1128/AAC.01428-17
18. Augener W, Grey HM. Studies on the mechanism of heat aggregation of human gamma-G. *J Immunol.* (1970) 105:1024–30.
19. Szijártó V, Guachalla LM, Visram ZC, Hartl K, Varga C, Mirkina I, et al. Bactericidal monoclonal antibodies specific to the lipopolysaccharide O antigen from multidrug-resistant *Escherichia coli* clone ST131-O25b:H4 elicit protection in mice. *Antimicrob Agents Chemother.* (2015) 59:3109–16. doi: 10.1128/AAC.04494-14
20. Santos GF, Deck RR, Donnelly J, Blackwelder W, Granoff DM. Importance of complement source in measuring meningococcal bactericidal titers. *Clin Diagn Lab Immunol.* (2001) 8:616–23. doi: 10.1128/CDLI.8.3.616-623.2001
21. Brookes C, Kuisma E, Alexander F, Allen L, Tipton T, Ram S, et al. Development of a large scale human complement source for use in bacterial immunoassays. *J Immunol Methods* (2013) 391:39–49. doi: 10.1016/j.jim.2013.02.007
22. Roos A, Bouwman LH, van Gijlswijk-Janssen DJ, Faber-Krol MC, Stahl GL, Daha MR. Human IgA activates the complement system via the mannan-binding lectin pathway. *J Immunol.* (2001) 167:2861–8. doi: 10.4049/jimmunol.167.5.2861
23. Stowell SR, Arthur CM, Dias-Baruffi M, Rodrigues LC, Gourdine J-P, Heimburg-Molinaro J, et al. Innate immune lectins kill bacteria expressing blood group antigen. *Nat Med.* (2010) 16:295–301. doi: 10.1038/nm.2103
24. Peitsch MC, Tschopp J, Kress A, Isliker H. Antibody-independent activation of the complement system by mitochondria is mediated by cardiolipin. *Biochem. J.* (1988) 249:495–500. doi: 10.1042/bj2490495
25. Prandini MH, Reboul, A, Colomb MG. Biosynthesis of complement C1 inhibitor by Hep G2 cells. Reactivity of different glycosylated forms of the inhibitor with C1s. *Biochem. J.* (1986) 237:93–8. doi: 10.1042/bj2370093
26. Reboul A, Bensa JC, Colomb MG. Characteristics of complement subcomponents C1r and C1s synthesized by Hep G2 cells. *Biochem. J.* (1986) 233:559–64.
27. Reboul A, Prandini MH, Colomb MG. Proteolysis and deglycosylation of human C1 inhibitor. Effect on functional properties. *Biochem J.* (1987) 244:117–21. doi: 10.1042/bj2440117
28. Schweinle JE, Hitchcock PJ, Tenner AJ, Hammer CH, Frank MM, Joiner KA. Interaction of Neisseria gonorrhoeae with classical complement components, C1-inhibitor, and a monoclonal antibody directed against the Neisserial H.8 antigen. *J. Clin Invest.* (1989) 83:397–403. doi: 10.1172/JCI113897
29. Strang CJ, Cholin S, Spragg J, Davis AE, Schneeberger EE, Donaldson VH, et al. Angioedema induced by a peptide derived from complement component C2. *J Exp Med.* (1988) 168:1685–98.
30. Suankratay C, Zhang Y, Jones D, Lint TF, Gewurz H. Enhancement of lectin pathway haemolysis by immunoglobulins. *Clin Exp Immunol.* (1999) 117:435–41. doi: 10.1046/J.1365-2249.1999.00996.X
31. Tacnet-Delorme P, Chevallier S, Arlaud GJ. Beta-amyloid fibrils activate the C1 complex of complement under physiological conditions: evidence for a binding site for A beta on the C1q globular regions. *J Immunol.* (2001) 167:6374–81. doi: 10.4049/jimmunol.167.11.6374
32. Seelen MA, Roos A, Wieslander J, Mollnes TE, Sjöholm AG, Wurzner R, et al. Functional analysis of the classical, alternative, and MBL pathways of the complement system: standardization and validation of a simple ELISA. *J Immunol Methods* (2005) 296:187–98. doi: 10.1016/j.jim.2004.11.016
33. Nielsen EW, Waage C, Fure H, Brekke OL, Sfyroera G, Lambris JD, et al. Effect of supraphysiologic levels of C1-inhibitor on the classical, lectin and alternative pathways of complement. *Mol Immunol.* (2007) 44:1819–26. doi: 10.1016/j.molimm.2006.10.003
34. Gauthier M, Patston PA. Reactivation of C1-inhibitor polymers by denaturation and gel-filtration chromatography. *Anal Biochem.* (1997) 248:228–33. doi: 10.1006/abio.1997.2133
35. Patston PA, Hauert J, Michaud M, Schapira M. Formation and properties of C1-inhibitor polymers. *FEBS Lett.* (1995) 368:401–4.
36. Csuka D, Veszeli N, Varga L, Prohászka Z, Farkas H. The role of the complement system in hereditary angioedema. *Mol Immunol.* (2017) 89:59–68. doi: 10.1016/j.molimm.2017.05.020
37. Mollnes TE, Garred P, Bergseth G. Effect of time, temperature and anticoagulants on *in vitro* complement activation: consequences for collection and preservation of samples to be examined for complement activation. *Clin Exp Immunol.* (1988) 73:484–8.
38. Kishore U, Sim RB. Factor H as a regulator of the classical pathway activation. *Immunobiology* (2012) 217:162–8. doi: 10.1016/J.IMBIO.2011.07.024
39. Schneider C, Smith DF, Cummings RD, Boligan KF, Hamilton RG, Bochner BS, et al. The human IgG anti-carbohydrate repertoire exhibits a universal architecture and contains specificity for microbial attachment sites. *Sci Transl Med.* (2015) 7:269ra1. doi: 10.1126/scitranslmed.3010524
40. Pierpont TM, Limper CB, Richards KL. Past, Present, and Future of Rituximab—The World's First Oncology Monoclonal Antibody Therapy. *Front Oncol.* (2018) 8:163. doi: 10.3389/fonc.2018.00163
41. Lei X, Liu C, Azadzoi K, Li C, Lu F, Xiang A, et al. A novel IgM–H-Ficolin complement pathway to attack allogenic cancer cells *in vitro*. *Sci Rep.* (2015) 5:7824. doi: 10.1038/srep07824
42. Stoermer KA, Morrison TE. Complement and viral pathogenesis. *Virology* (2011) 411:362–73. doi: 10.1016/J.VIROL.2010.12.045
43. Stites E, Le Quintrec M, Thurman JM. The complement system and antibody-mediated transplant rejection. *J Immunol.* (2015) 195:5525–31. doi: 10.4049/jimmunol.1501686
44. Chen M, Daha MR, Kallenberg CGM. The complement system in systemic autoimmune disease. *J Autoimmun.* (2010) 34:J276–J286. doi: 10.1016/j.jaut.2009.11.014
45. Vignesh P, Rawat A, Sharma M, Singh S. Complement in autoimmune diseases. *Clin Chim Acta* (2017) 465:123–30. doi: 10.1016/j.cca.2016.12.017

12

Intradialytic Complement Activation Precedes the Development of Cardiovascular Events in Hemodialysis Patients

Felix Poppelaars [1†], Mariana Gaya da Costa [1†], Bernardo Faria [1,2,3], Stefan P. Berger [1], Solmaz Assa [4], Mohamed R. Daha [1,5], José Osmar Medina Pestana [6], Willem J. van Son [1], Casper F. M. Franssen [1] and Marc A. Seelen [1]*

[1] Division of Nephrology, Department of Internal Medicine, University of Groningen, University Medical Center Groningen, Groningen, Netherlands, [2] Nephrology and Infecciology Group, INEB/I3S, University of Porto, Porto, Portugal, [3] Department of Nephrology, Hospital Braga, Braga, Portugal, [4] Department of Cardiology, University of Groningen, University Medical Center Groningen, Groningen, Netherlands, [5] Department of Nephrology, University of Leiden, Leiden University Medical Center, Leiden, Netherlands, [6] Nephrology Division, Federal University of São Paulo, São Paulo, Brazil

***Correspondence:**
Felix Poppelaars
felix.poppelaars@gmail.com

† These authors have contributed equally to this work

Background: Hemodialysis (HD) is a life-saving treatment for patients with end stage renal disease. However, HD patients have markedly increased rates of cardiovascular morbidity and mortality. Previously, a link between the complement system and cardiovascular events (CV-events) has been reported. In HD, systemic complement activation occurs due to blood-to-membrane interaction. We hypothesize that HD-induced complement activation together with inflammation and thrombosis are involved in the development of CV-events in these patients.

Methods: HD patients were followed for the occurrence of CV-events during a maximum follow-up of 45 months. Plasma samples were collected from 55 patients at different time points during one HD session prior to follow-up. Plasma levels of mannose-binding lectin, properdin and C3d/C3 ratios were assessed by ELISA. In addition, levels of von Willebrand factor, TNF-α and IL-6/IL-10 ratios were determined. An *ex-vivo* model of HD was used to assess the effect of complement inhibition.

Results: During median follow-up of 32 months, 17 participants developed CV-events. In the CV-event group, the C3d/C3-ratio sharply increased 30 min after the start of the HD session, while in the event-free group the ratio did not increase. In accordance, HD patients that developed a CV-event also had a sustained higher IL-6/IL-10-ratio during the first 60 min of the HD session, followed by a greater rise in TNF-α levels and von Willebrand factor at the end of the session. In the *ex-vivo* HD model, we found that complement activation contributed to the induction of TNF-α levels, IL-6/IL-10-ratio and levels of von Willebrand factor.

Conclusions: In conclusion, these findings suggest that early intradialytic complement activation predominantly occurred in HD patients who develop a CV-event during follow-up. In addition, in these patients complement activation was accompanied by a pro-inflammatory and pro-thrombotic response. Experimental complement inhibition revealed that this reaction is secondary to complement activation. Therefore, our data suggests that HD-induced complement, inflammation and coagulation are involved in the increased CV risk of HD patients.

Keywords: complement, kidney, cardiovascular risk, hemodialysis, biocompatibility, innate immunity, C1-inhibitor

INTRODUCTION

Renal replacement therapy (RRT) represents a cornerstone in the treatment of patients with end stage renal disease (ESRD). Hemodialysis (HD) remains the most common form of RRT (1). Despite being lifesaving, HD comes with a risk (2). The life expectancy and quality of life of patients on dialysis is inferior to the general population. Overall, HD has been associated with increased cardiovascular morbidity and mortality (3). Previous studies have suggested that the innate immune system plays a key role in the development of cardiovascular disease in HD patients (4).

The complement system is a major component of innate immunity and activation of this system induces an inflammatory response (5). Complement activation can occur via three pathways: the classical pathway (CP), lectin pathway (LP), and alternative pathway (AP). Regardless of the trigger, all pathways lead to the cleavage of C3 resulting in the formation of C3b, the large fragment and C3a, an anaphylatoxin. Ultimately, C3b is broken down progressively to iC3b and then to the more stable fragment C3d. The functions of the complement system were thought to be limited to opsonization and lysis of pathogens. However, nowadays this system is known to have numerous functions and complement has been shown to be involved in the pathogenesis of various diseases (6).

For decades, HD has been known to activate the complement system (7). In dialysis, complement activation is mainly caused by the interaction of blood with the HD membrane (4). Regardless of the efforts to improve biocompatibility, complement activation still occurs in HD, even with modern membranes (8–10). It has been hypothesized that complement activation leads to HD-induced inflammation and thereby increases the subsequent cardiovascular risk (4). In accordance, several studies have shown an association between complement and cardiovascular events (CV-event) (8, 11–14). However, the link between complement activation products and CV-events remains poorly characterized (15). Only Lines et al. reported an association in HD patients between soluble C5b-9 and cardiovascular risk (15). Furthermore, previous experimental studies proposed a link between HD-induced complement activation, pro-inflammatory cytokines, and the coagulation system (10, 16).

Abbreviations: AP, Alternative pathway; BSA, Body surface area; C5b-9, Membrane attack complex; CV-event, Cardiovascular event; ESRD, End stage renal disease; ELISA, Enzyme-linked immunosorbent assay; HD, Hemodialysis; IL-6, Interleukin 6; IL-10, Interleukin 10; LP, Lectin pathway; MBL, Mannose-binding lectin; RRT, Renal replacement therapy; PCI, Percutaneous coronary intervention; TNF-α, Tumor necrosis factor-α; vWF, Von Willebrand factor

We hypothesize that an unfavorable complement profile is seen in HD patients who will develop a CV-event. To investigate the mechanism of increased cardiovascular risk in HD, we measured complement activation, pro-inflammatory cytokines and pro-thrombotic factors during one HD session in patients that developed a CV-event during follow-up and compared this to patients without a CV-event during follow-up. Furthermore, we used an *ex-vivo* model of HD to further elucidate the role of complement activation as a trigger for inflammation and coagulation in HD.

MATERIALS AND METHODS

Study Population and Design

A cohort of 55 hemodialysis patients from Dialysis Center Groningen and the University Medical Center Groningen were followed for a maximum of 45 months. The original cohort was composed out of 109 patients; however, due to a lack of samples only 55 patients could be included for this study. The protocol has been previously described (2). In short, patients were included if the duration of HD therapy was longer than 3 months. Patients with severe heart failure (NYHA class IV) were excluded. Patient characteristics were extracted from patient records.

Dialysis Settings

Patients were on maintenance HD treatment for three times a week with a low-flux polysulfone hollow-fiber dialyzer (F8; Fresenius Care, Bad Homburg, Germany). The hemodialysis sessions lasted for 4 h. The blood and dialysate flow rates were 250–350 and 500 mL/min, respectively. A constant ultrafiltration rate was used. Dialysate composition was as follows: acetate, 3.0 mmol/L; bicarbonate, 34 mmol/L; calcium, 1.5 mmol/L; chloride, 108 mmol/L; glucose, 1.0 g/L; magnesium, 0.5 mmol/L; potassium, 1.0 or 2.0 mmol/L; sodium, 139 mmol/L The dialysate temperature was kept on 36.0 or 36.5°C. Blood samples were taken just before the start of the dialysis session, and after 30, 60, 180, and 240 min.

Definition of Endpoint

The end-point of the study was defined as the time to the first CV-event. CV-events included cardiac, cerebrovascular, or peripheral vascular events. Occurrence of a cardiac event was defined as a ischemic heart disease (unstable angina pectoris, myocardial infarction, Coronary Artery Bypass Grafting (CABG) and/or Percutaneous Coronary Intervention (PCI), sudden cardiac death and congestive heart failure. In order to classify as acute myocardial infarction, two out of the following three criteria had to be present: clinical status, elevated heart enzymes, and EKG changes. Cerebrovascular events were defined as stroke, ischemic insult, or newly diagnosed >70% stenosis of the extracranial carotid artery. Strokes and ischemic insults had to be verified by CT or MRI. Peripheral vascular disease was defined as having intermittent claudication with angiographically or sonographically proven stenosis >50% of the major arteries of the lower limbs or ulcers caused by atherosclerotic stenosis or surgery for this disorder. Transplantation was a censoring event and the transplantation date was considered as the final follow-up date (17).

Ex-vivo Model of Hemodialysis

An *ex-vivo* model of HD was used as previously described (18). In brief, a closed circuit was assembled using a pediatric polysulfone hollow-fiber dialyzer (FX paed; Fresenius Care, Germany) and blood lines (SN-Set ONLINEplus BVM 5008-R, Fresenius Care, Germany). The total volume of the circuit was approximately 50 mL. Perfusion was achieved using a Masterflex® peristaltic pump (Cole-Parmer, USA) and was flow-controlled (TS410 tubing flow module, Transonic systems Inc, USA) to reach a perfusion flow of approximately 140 to 160 mL/min. The temperature was kept constant at 37°C and controlled by an external heater. Whole blood was taken from healthy volunteers ($n = 3$) and anticoagulated with low-molecular weight heparin (1 U/mL). Initially, the circuit was primed with NaCl 0.9% and perfused for approximately 20 min to remove air bubbles. Prior to perfusion, the dialysate compartment was filled with NaCl 0.9% and closed. Next, freshly drawn heparinized blood was added to the circuit, while the same volume of the saline solution was discarded. The system was perfused with recirculating blood for 4 h. Samples were collected at the start of the perfusion and after 30, 60, 120, 180, and 240 min. To investigate the effect of complement inhibition, two consecutive sessions were performed for each healthy volunteer. During one session, 200 units of C1-inhibitor (Cinryze©, Viropharma, USA) were added to the blood prior to perfusion, whereas the other session without C1-inhibitor (C1-INH) served as a control.

Inflammatory Markers and Pro-thrombotic Factors

In the HD cohort, TNF-α was measured by Quantikine HS Human Immunoassay (R&D System Inc., USA). Furthemore, IL-6 and IL-10 were determined using a quantitative sandwich enzyme immunoassay technique (R&D System Inc., USA). Lastly, Von Willebrand Factor (vWF) was measured by enzyme-linked immunosorbent assay (Dakopatts, UK). In the *ex-vivo* HD model, TNF-α, IL-6, IL-10, and vWF were measured using a human magnetic luminex assay (R&D Systems Inc, USA) according to the manufacturer's instructions.

Quantification of Complement Proteins

C3d was measured by sandwich enzyme immunoassay as previously described (19). Quantitative antigenic assay for C3 was performed by the radial immunodiffusion technique with monospecific anti-sera (19). The C3d/C3 ratio was determined by dividing the C3d values in μg/mL by the C3 concentration in mg/mL. Additionally, Properdin and MBL concentrations were measured as described earlier (19, 20).

Statistics

Statistical analysis was performed using IBM SPSS 22.0 (IBM Corporation, Chicago, IL, USA). Normally distributed data are presented as mean ± standard deviation, whereas non-normally distributed data are shown as median with interquartile range. Nominal data are displayed as total number of patients with percentage [n (%)]. Differences between two groups were assessed with the student t-test, whereas the paired t-test was used to compare values of a single variable during different time points within the HD session. A one-way ANOVA was used when assessing for differences in multiple groups, followed by Bonferroni's *post-hoc* comparisons tests. The association between different variables and the incidence of CV-event were assessed by Cox proportional hazard regression. The Harrell's C statistic is the equivalent of the area under the ROC curve, if the outcome is binary (21).

Ethics

This study was performed in accordance to the Declaration of Helsinki and was approved by the Medical Ethical Committee from the University Medical Center Groningen. All participants signed informed written consent.

RESULTS

Patients Characteristics

Blood samples from 55 patients on maintenance HD were available, of which 35 were male and 20 female (**Table 1**). The mean age was 62 ± 15 years and baseline dialysis vintage was 1.2 years [IQR: 0.6–3.9 years]. The median follow-up of the study was 32 months and during this time 17 patients (31%) developed a CV-event, whereas 16 patients died (29%). In our study, the causes of death were cardiovascular (44%), infection (12.5%), discontinuation of the HD treatment (12.5%), or unknown (31%). Among the patients that developed CV-events, 35% had acute coronary syndrome, 17% needed coronary artery bypass surgery, 11% developed congestive heart failure, 17% had a cerebro-vascular accident and 17% developed peripheral vascular disease. Next, we created two different groups; the 17 patients that developed a CV-event during follow-up (CV-event group) and the 38 patients that remained event-free (event-free group).

Complement Activation in the HD Patients

To assess complement activation, we determined the C3d/C3-ratio in 55 patients during one HD session at the start of the follow-up. The C3d/C3-ratio at baseline was not statistically different between the patients that would develop a CV-event (7.0 ± 6.2) compared to the patients that would not (9.0 ± 7.4). Surprisingly, at the end of the HD session the C3d/C3-ratio was also not statistically different between the two groups (CV-event group: 11.8 ± 8.5, event-free group: 12.9 ± 10.0). However, when the intradialytic C3d/C3-ratios were compared between the two groups, clear differences were seen (**Figure 1** and **Table 1**). At 30 min intradialysis, there was a significant increase in the C3d/C3-ratio in the CV-event group compared to the patients who remained event-free. During these initial 30 min, the C3d/C3-ratio increased by 3.29 fold in the CV-event group and

TABLE 1 | Baseline characteristics of our study population of hemodialysis patients with and without a cardiovascular event.

		Patients			Univariable	
	All (n = 55)	**CV-event (n = 17)**	**No CV-event (n = 38)**	**P***	**St. beta**	**P#**
C3d/C3 RATIO						
0 min	5.9 [4.8–9.3]	5.6 [4.7–8.1]	6.1 [4.8–11.5]	0.2	−0.02	0.6
30 min	9.8 [7.3–17.0]	12.0 [10–33.5]	8.4 [6.8–13.4]	**0.01**	0.05	**0.002**
60 min	8.4 [5.4–12.4]	7.8 [4.4–11.9]	8.9 [5.6–16.2]	0.2	−0.04	0.2
120 min	8.6 [5.5–14.5]	7.4 [5.2–12.7]	9.1 [5.6–16.4]	0.3	−0.03	0.3
240 min	8.4 [5.8–17.9]	8.6 [5.9–20.0]	8.3 [5.8–17.9]	0.8	−0.04	0.8
DEMOGRAPHICS						
Age, years	62.7 ± 15.8	66.5 ± 11.4	61.0 ± 17.2	0.2	0.01	0.3
Male gender, n (%)	35 (63)	11 (64)	24 (63)	0.9	−0.22	0.6
Current diabetes, n (%)	10 (18)	5 (29)	5 (13)	0.2	0.51	0.3
Hypertension, n (%)	48 (87)	14 (82)	34 (89)	0.2	−0.99	0.1
Cardiovascular history, n (%)	11 (20)	5 (29)	6 (15)	0.2	0.64	0.2
BSA, m^2	1.8 ± 0.3	1.7 ± 0.5	1.9 ± 0.2	0.08	−2.04	**0.02**
HEMODIALYSIS						
Dialysis vintage, months	14.1 [7.3–47.3]	12.2 [8.6–50.4]	16.4 [4.7–47.5]	0.5	0.002	0.8
Ultrafiltration volume, L	2.5 ± 0.7	2.4 ± 0.6	2.5 ± 0.7	0.9	0.00	0.7
Ultrafiltration rate, ml/kg/h	8.1 ± 2.3	7.9 ± 1.8	8.2 ± 2.5	0.7	−0.01	0.8
PRIMARY RENAL DISEASE, *n* (%)						
Hypertension	12 (22)	4 (23)	8 (21)	0.8	0.02	0.9
Diabetes	5 (9)	3 (17)	2 (5)	0.1	0.65	0.3
ADPKD	7 (13)	1 (6)	6 (16)	0.3	−0.96	0.3
FSGS	6 (11)	2 (12)	4 (10)	0.8	0.89	0.2
IgA nephropathy	3 (6)	0 (0)	3 (7)	0.2	−3.15	0.4
Chronic pyelonephritis	1 (2)	1 (6)	0 (0)	0.1	2.02	0.06
Glomerulonephrytis	6 (11)	1 (6)	5 (13)	0.4	−0.75	0.4
Other Diagnosis	9 (16)	3 (18)	6 (16)	0.8	0.35	0.6
Unknown	5 (9)	2 (12)	3 (7)	0.8	−0.34	0.9
LABORATORY MEASUREMENTS						
Hematocrit, %	34.4 ± 3.7	34.0 ± 4.2	34.6 ± 3.5	0.6	−5.98	0.3
HbA1C, mmol/mol	5.56 ± 0.9	5.7 ± 1.1	5.5 ± 0.8	0.4	0.17	0.4
Albumin, g/L	38 [37-41]	38 [37-41]	38 [36-42]	0.9	0.004	0.9
Calcium, mmol/L	2.32 ± 0.2	2.31 ± 0.1	2.32 ± 0.2	0.8	−0.55	0.6
Phosphate, mmol/L	1.74 ± 0.5	1.70 ± 0.4	1.75 ± 0.6	0.7	0.009	0.9
hsCRP, mg/L	5.5 [1.5–8.8]	5.0 [2.3–11.8]	5.8 [1.4–8.8]	0.5	0.01	0.3
MEDICATION						
Aspirin, n (%)	34 (62)	8 (47)	26 (68)	0.2	−0.80	0.09
Calcium channel blockers, n (%)	12 (22)	4 (23)	8 (21)	0.8	−0.14	0.7
β-Blocker, n (%)	31 (56)	10 (59)	21 (55)	0.8	0.24	0.6
ACE inhibitor, n (%)	5 (9)	1 (5)	4 (10)	0.6	−0.44	0.6
AT2–receptor antagonists, n (%)	8 (14)	2 (12)	6 (16)	0.7	−0.41	0.6
Statin, n (%)	13 (24)	2 (12)	11 (29)	0.2	−0.88	0.2
Diuretics, n (%)	5 (9)	2 (12)	3 (7)	0.7	1.11	0.2

P indicates P-value for the difference in baseline characteristics between the patient with and without a cardiovascular-event. Differences were tested by Student's t-Test or Mann–Whitney U test for continuous variables and with χ^2 test for categorical variables. Data are presented as mean ± SD or median [IQR]. P# indicates P-value for univariate Cox-regression for the occurrence of CV-event. Data are presented as beta coefficient with corresponding P-value.*

CV, cardiovascular; BSA, body surface area; ADPKPD, autosomal dominant polycystic disease; FSGS, focal segmental glomerulosclerosis; HbA1c, Hemoglobin A1c; hsCRP, high sensitive C-reactive protein; ACE inhibitor, angiotensin-converting-enzyme inhibitor; AT2-receptor antagonists, Angiotensin II receptor antagonists.

by only 1.26 fold in the event-free group ($P < 0.01$). In addition, Cox regression analysis was performed to assess the association between C3d/C3 ratio at 30 min and occurrence of a CV-event (**Table 2**). In the crude model, C3d/C3 ratios were associated with a hazard ratio of 1.06 (95% CI 1.02-1.09; $P < 0.001$). After adjustment for age and gender, variables with $P < 0.1$

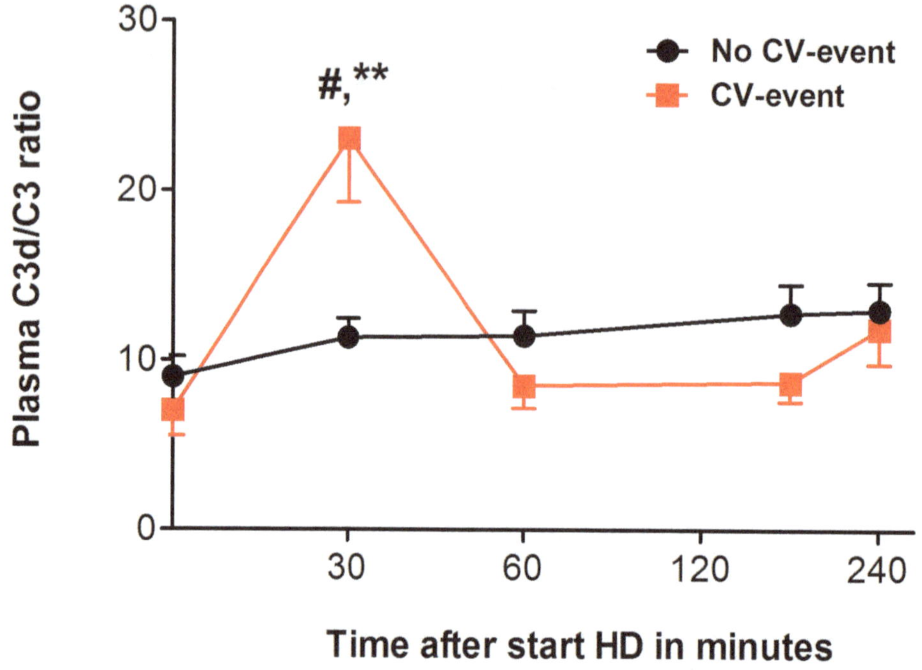

FIGURE 1 | The C3d/C3-ratio during hemodialysis. Course of plasma C3d/C3 ratio in patients that developed a cardiovascular event (CV-event) during follow-up and in those that remained CV-event free (no CV-event). The data is presented as mean ± SEM and C3d/C3-ratio was calculated by dividing the C3d values (μg/mL) by the C3 levels (in mg/mL). The C3d/C3-ratio was determined at the start of hemodialysis session and 30, 60, 180 and 240 min after. Differences between the two groups were assessed by the student *t*-test and a one-way ANOVA followed by Bonferroni's *post-hoc* comparisons tests was used to compare C3d/C3 ratios at different time points within one group (**$P < 0.01$). The hashtag above the bars denotes a significant difference between the two groups (#$P < 0.05$), whereas the asterisk above the bars denotes a significant difference compared to baseline within the group. The number of subject is 17 in the "CV-event group" and 38 in the "No CV-event group".

TABLE 2 | Associations of intradialytic complement activation with outcome.

	Cardiovascular events		
	C3d/C3 ratio at 30 min		
	HR	**95% CI**	***P***
Model 1	1.06	1.02–1.09	<0.001
Model 2	1.06	1.03–1.09	0.001
Model 3	1.04	1.01–1.08	0.03
Model 4	1.06	1.02–1.09	0.001
Model 5	1.07	1.02–1.09	0.002

Model 1: crude. Model 2: adjusted for age and gender. Model 3: adjusted for BSA, aspirin and primary chronic pyelonephritis. Model 4: adjusted for DM, cardiovascular history and hypertension. Model 5: adjusted for HD vintage , UF rate and UF volume.
Data are presented as hazard ratio (HR) plus 95% confidence interval (CI). BSA, body surface area; DM, diabetes mellitus; HD, Hemodialysis; UF, ultrafiltration rate.

in univariate analysis (BSA, chronic pyelonephritis as primary renal disease and use of aspirin), cardiovascular risk factors (CV history, DM and hypertension) or characteristics of HD (Ultrafiltration rate, ultrafiltration volume and dialysis vintage), the association between C3d/C3 ratio at 30 min and CV-event remained significant. Subsequently, the Harrell's-C statistics was determined to further confirm the potential relationship between complement activation and CV-events. Plasma C3d/C3 ratio at 30 min had a Harrell's-C statistics of 0.71 (95% CI 0.55–0.88; $P = 0.01$).

We next set out to assess the contribution of the AP and LP to HD-induced complement activation. Due to a lack of samples, properdin and MBL levels were measured in a subgroup of 30 patients (**Figure 2**). In this subgroup, there were 11 patients in the CV-event group and 19 patients in the event free group. MBL and properdin levels were comparable between the two groups at the start and at the end of the HD session. Conversely, at 30 min intradialysis, MBL levels decreased significantly in the event-free group but not in the CV-event group ($P < 0.05$). Furthermore, properdin levels were significantly lower at 30 min in the CV-event group, compared to the event-free group. To summarize, MBL consumption was seen in the event-free group implying LP activation, while lower properdin levels were observed in the CV-event group suggesting AP activation.

Inflammatory and Pro-thrombotic Factors in the HD Patients

We determined cytokines and Von Willebrand factor (vWF) to investigate if complement activation during HD was accompanied by a pro-inflammatory response and a pro-thrombotic state. During HD, distinct time-courses for levels of vWF were observed between the two groups (**Figure 3**). In the CV-event group, vWF levels increased steadily during the session

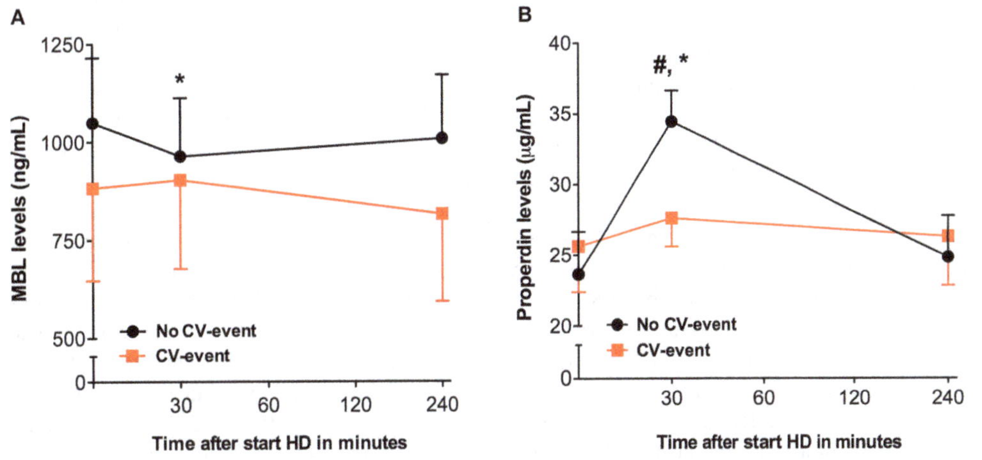

FIGURE 2 | Intradialytic levels of properdin and Mannose-binding lectin. Course of plasma mannose-binding lectin (MBL) and properdin in patients that developed a cardiovascular event (CV-event) during follow-up and in those that remained CV-event free (no CV-event). The data is presented as mean ± SEM. **(A)** The levels of MBL were determined at the start of hemodialysis session and 30 and 240 min after. **(B)** The levels of properdin were determined at the start of hemodialysis session and 30 and 240 min after. Differences between the two groups were assessed by the student *t*-test and a one-way ANOVA followed by Bonferroni's *post-hoc* comparisons tests was used to compare levels at different time points within one group (*$P < 0.05$). The hashtag above the bars denotes a significant difference between the two groups (#$P < 0.05$), whereas the asterisk above the bars denotes a significant difference compared to baseline within the group. The number of subject is 11 in the "CV-event group" and 19 in the "No CV-event group".

($P < 0.05$). Furthermore, compared to the event-free group, the CV-event group had significantly higher levels of vWF at 180 and 240 min intradialysis ($P < 0.05$). Cytokines such as tumor necrosis factor-α (TNF-α) may initiate inflammation and are therefore believed to play a role in dialysis-related cardiovascular risk. Levels of TNF-α rose significantly during the HD session in both groups (**Figure 4A**). In the CV-event group, levels peaked at 180 min after the start of the HD session ($P < 0.01$) and were significantly higher than in the event-free group ($P < 0.05$). Furthermore, in the event-free group, the maximum TNF-α levels were reached at the end of the session ($P < 0.001$).

To evaluate the relation between anti-inflammatory cytokines and pro-inflammatory cytokines, we determined the IL-6/IL-10 ratio (**Figure 4B**). Interestingly, IL-6/IL-10 ratios were the highest in both groups at the start of the HD session and showed a decreasing trend during the dialysis session, although not significant compared to baseline. Moreover, at 60 min intradialysis an important decrease in the IL-6/IL-10 ratio occurred in the event-free group, indicating a shift toward a less inflammatory profile. However, IL-6/IL-10 ratios remained elevated in the HD patients that developed a CV-event during follow-up, revealing a significant difference between the groups at this time point ($P < 0.05$). Overall, enhanced levels of pro-inflammatory and pro-thrombotic mediators seem to prelude the development of CV-events in HD patients.

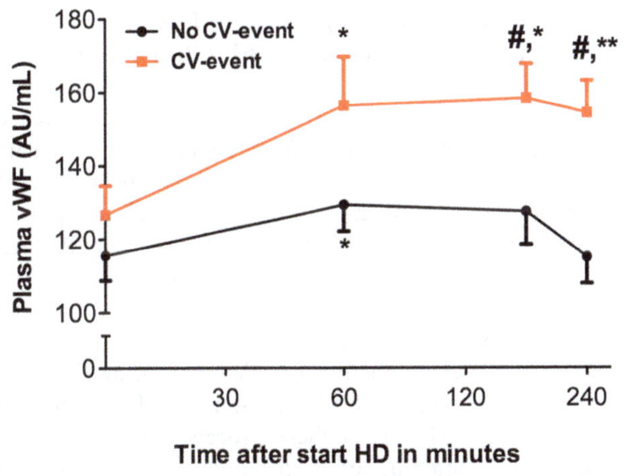

FIGURE 3 | Levels of von Willebrand factor during hemodialysis. Course of von Willebrand factor (vWF) in patients that developed a cardiovascular event (CV-event) during follow-up and in those that remained CV-event free (no CV-event). The data is presented as mean ± SEM. vWF was determined at the start of hemodialysis session and 60, 180 and 240 min after the start of the session. Differences between the two groups were assessed by the student *t*-test and a one-way ANOVA followed by Bonferroni's *post-hoc* comparisons tests was used to compare levels at different time points within one group (*$P < 0.05$, **$P < 0.01$). The hashtag above the bars denotes a significant difference between the two groups (#$P < 0.05$), whereas the asterisk above the bars denotes a significant difference compared to baseline within the group. The number of subject is 17 in the "CV-event group" and 38 in the "No CV-event group".

Ex-vivo Model of Hemodialysis

To further evaluate the effect of HD-induced complement activation on inflammation and coagulation, we used an *ex-vivo* model of HD. During the 4 h of perfusion, the C3d/C3 ratio increased progressively from 4.7 ± 0.6 at baseline to 55.8 ± 12.5 after 240 min (**Figure 5A**). MBL and properdin levels were determined to discriminate between complement activation via the AP and/or the LP. Both MBL and properdin levels decreased significantly over time. After 4 h, MBL levels were reduced by 55.2% ($P < 0.05$) and properdin levels by 34.4%, respectively (**Figure 5**). We next assessed inflammatory and pro-thrombotic factors. Similarly to complement activation, the HD model resulted in a significant increase in TNF-α, IL-6/IL-10 ratio, and vWF levels after 240 min of dialysis (**Figure 6**).

Finally, we evaluated the effect of complement inhibition in our model to test if complement activation acts as a trigger for inflammation and coagulation in HD. C1-INH was added and significantly reduced C3d/C3 ratios compared to controls, namely from 55.8 ± 13 to 33.1 ± 24 (**Figure 5A**; $P < 0.05$). HD-induced consumption of properdin and MBL was not prevented by the use of C1-INH.Furthermore, TNF-α levels were 1654 ± 631 ng/mL after 240 min in the control session, while in the session with C1-INH levels were reduced to 48.7 ± 74.7 ng/mL(**Figure 6A**). Correspondingly, a similar trend was seen after 240 min in the IL-6/IL-10 ratio (control session 1086 ± 630 pg/mL, C1-INH session 51 ± 78 pg/mL; **Figure 6C**) and for vWF levels (control session: 98.2 ± 22.7 pg/mL, C1-INH session: 1.7 ± 3.3 pg/mL) when the control session was compared to C1-INH session (**Figure 6B**). To summarize, C1-INH addition was able to inhibit HD-induced complement activation and thereby reduce vWF, TNF-α and IL-6/IL-10 by 98, 97, and 95% respectively.

DISCUSSION

Hemodialysis treatment comes with the balance between the dangers of advanced uremia and the inherent risks related to this form of RTT (22, 23). The higher cardiovascular risk seen in this population is not only related to ESRD but it is also associated with the HD procedure itself (2). Innate immunity has been proposed to be the missing link in the mechanism of CV-events in HD patients (4). We observed distinct differences in molecular profiles during HD of patients that will later develop CV-events compared to those who remained event-free during follow-up. At the start of dialysis, a unique peak in complement activation was only seen in patients in the CV-event group. Furthermore, enhanced inflammation and coagulation accompanied the complement activation seen in HD patient that will develop CV-events. Moreover, these processes arose long before the actual development of the CV-event. Altogether these three elements showed different dynamics, with complement activation possibly initiating these processes. In accordance, complement inhibition in our *ex-vivo* model not only decreased complement activation but also diminished pro-inflammatory and pro-thrombotic mediators.

Despite significant advances in the biocompatibility of HD membranes, complement activation remains an undesired but relevant issue (8, 15). Higher levels of complement components as well as loss of complement inhibitors have been associated with a higher risk for cardiovascular disease in HD patients (8, 11–14). Recently, complement activation prior to a HD session was associated with the occurrence of CV-events in HD patients (15). Here, we showed that activation of C3 during dialysis is linked to the development of CV-events. Our study is the first, to our knowledge, to assess the relationship between intradialytic complement activation and subsequent outcome. In accordance, previous studies have shown that activation of the complement system peaks during the first 15 to 30 min of the HD session (24). However, the mechanism by which complement activation increases the risk for cardiovascular disease remains largely unknown.

The LP and AP initiate complement activation during HD (25, 26). In our study, we only found MBL consumption in the event-free group, implying that this decrease is actually beneficial. In accordance, MBL has been proposed to be involved in the removal of atherogenic particles, thereby decreasing atherosclerosis. Our previous data showed that higher MBL levels in HD patients were associated with protection against cardiovascular disease (9). We also found a rise in properdin levels in the event-free group. Properdin, unlike other complement factors, is produced by leukocytes, predominately neutrophils (27). Therefore, the increase in properdin is presumably the result of leukocyte activation by the HD membrane leading to degranulation (28). Since, this rise was not seen in the CV-event group, we speculate this was due to properdin consumption by AP activation in these patients.

We found higher TNF-α levels and IL-6/IL-10 ratios in patients that would develop a CV-event. TNF-α and IL-6 are potent cytokines that can initiate a powerful pro-inflammatory reaction (29, 30). If this response is not contained, it can lead to hypotension, organ dysfunction, and eventually result in death. Elevated levels of these cytokines have also been related to an increased risk for CV-events in the general population and in HD patient (31–34). In contrast, IL-10 is a major anti-inflammatory cytokine with the ability to suppress the production and secretion of pro-inflammatory mediators in leukocytes, thereby effectively controlling the inflammation (35). The IL-6/IL-10 ratio has previously been linked to outcome after inflammatory disorders and to the development of HD-induced left ventricular dysfunction (36–38). In *ex-vivo* models, the induction of IL-6 during the bio-incompatibility reaction was shown to be completely complement-dependent, while the induction of TNF-α was only partially complement-dependent (16). In addition, in a primate model of HD, complement inhibition lead to enhanced levels of IL-10, demonstrating the relationship between the two systems (39).

Thrombosis is a key element in the development of cardiovascular disease. Previously, Péquériaux et al. reported that vWF is a good predictor of CV-events in patients undergoing RRT (40). Von Willebrand factor is a glycoprotein involved in hemostasis but vWF is also a marker of endothelial cell activation (41). We found significantly higher levels of vWF in the group of patients who developed CV-events, which could be evidence of a prothrombotic state. vWF is produced in endothelial cells and megakaryocytes, but also stored in the granules of platelets (42). Considering our *ex-vivo* lacks endothelial cells, the vWF is most likely derived from platelets. The release of vWF could either be the direct effect of complement activation or via C5a-activated leukocytes (43, 44). The link between the complement system and thrombosis is not new in HD (45). Complement receptors on leukocytes are important for the formation of platelet-leukocytes complexes, which contributes to thrombotic processes (46). In addition, complement activation during HD induces the production of pro-coagulation factors (47). Moreover, plasma levels of C3 correlated with a denser clot structure in HD patients (48).

The complement system is a strong mediator of the bioincompatibility reaction. Therefore, we proposed that

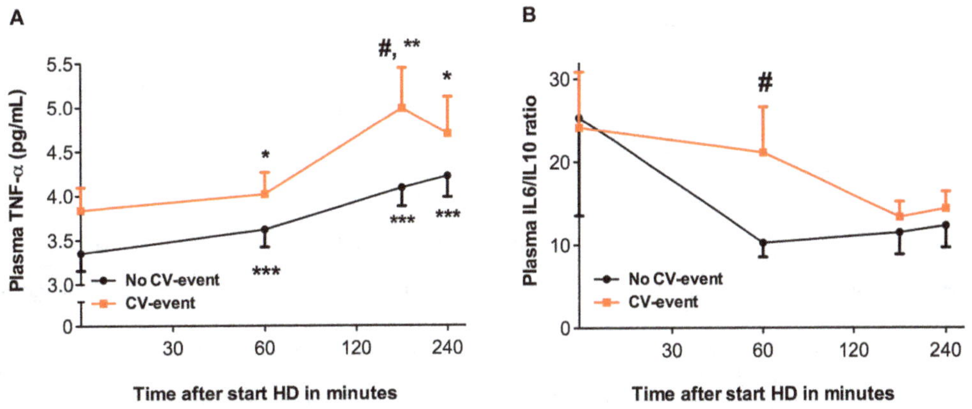

FIGURE 4 | Levels of tumor necrose factor alpha and the ratio of interleukin-6 to interleukin-10 during hemodialysis. Course of tumor necrose factor alpha (TNF-α) and ratio of interleukin-6 (IL-6) to interleukin-10 (IL-10) in patients that developed a cardiovascular event (CV-event) during follow-up and in those that remained CV-event free (no CV-event). The data is presented as mean ± SEM. **(A)** The levels of TNF-α were determined at the start of hemodialysis session and 60, 180 and 240 min after the start of the session. **(B)** Levels IL-6 and IL-10 were determined at the start of hemodialysis session and 60, 180, and 240 min after. The IL-6/IL- 10 ratio was calculated by dividing the IL-6 (in pg/mL) values by the IL-10 levels (in pg/mL). Differences between the two groups were assessed by the student *t*-test and a one-way ANOVA followed by Bonferroni's *post-hoc* comparisons tests was used to compare levels at different time points within one group. (*$P < 0.05$, **$P < 0.01$, ***$P < 0.001$). The hashtag above the bars denotes a significant difference between the two groups (#$P < 0.05$), whereas the asterisk above the bars denotes a significant difference compared to baseline within the group. The number of subject is 17 in the "CV-event group" and 38 in the "No CV-event group".

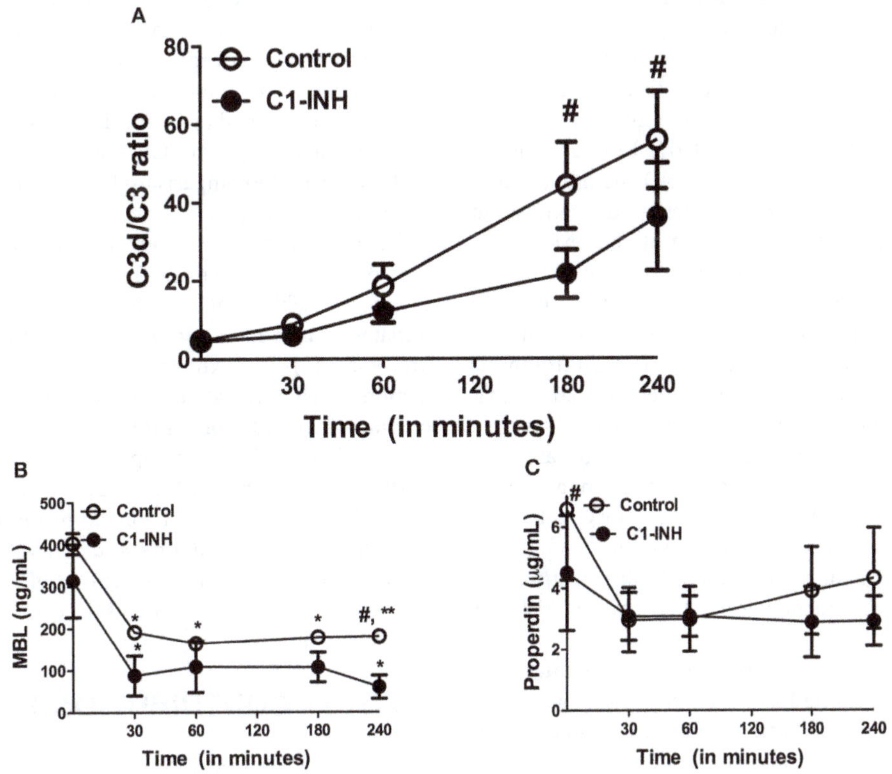

FIGURE 5 | Complement levels during *ex vivo* hemodialysis. Two different sessions were performed with whole blood of three healthy donors; one session with C1-inhibitor (C1-INH) and one session without, the control session. The data is presented as mean ± SEM. **(A)** C3d/C3 ratios were measured to determine complement activation. **(B)** MBL levels significantly decrease over time during the session. **(C)** Properdin levels were reduced during the session, although not significantly. Differences between the two groups were assessed by the student *t*-test and a one-way ANOVA followed by Bonferroni's *post-hoc* comparisons tests was used to compare levels at different time points within one group (*$P < 0.05$, **$P < 0.01$). The hashtag above the bars denotes a significant difference between the two groups (#$P < 0.05$), whereas the asterisk above the bars denotes a significant difference compared to baseline within the group.

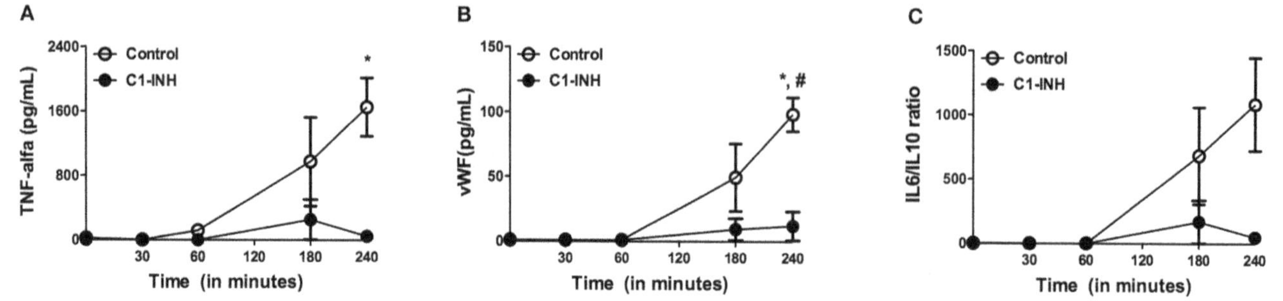

FIGURE 6 | Levels of tumor necrose factor alpha, ratio of interleukin-6 to interleukin-10 and vWF during *ex vivo* hemodialysis. Two different sessions were performed with whole blood of three healthy donors; one session with C1-inhibitor (C1-INH) and one session without, the control session. The data is presented as mean ± SEM. **(A)** TNF-α levels significantly increased in the control session, but not in the session with C1-INH. **(B)** Correspondingly, vWF showed a significant rise in the control session, while C1 INH additionlead to significantly lower levels. **(C)** The IL-6/IL-10 ratio progressively increased over time, although not statistically significant. Differences between the two groups were assessed by the student *t*-test and a one-way ANOVA followed by Bonferroni's *post-hoc* comparisons tests was used to compare levels at different time points within one group ($^*P < 0.05$). The hashtag above the bars denotes a significant difference between the two groups ($\#P < 0.05$), whereas the asterisk above the bars denotes a significant difference compared to baseline within the group.

complement activation has an essential role in orchestrating the inflammatory response in HD. In accordance with the result observed in the HD patients; our *ex-vivo* model demonstrated that the dialyzer induces complement activation, inflammation and enhances coagulation. We then wondered if HD-induced inflammation could be attenuated by complement inhibition. Addition of C1-INH to the *ex-vivo* HD model significantly diminished HD-induced complement activation and also almost completely abolished the induction of TNF-α levels, L-6/IL-10 ratios and vWF levels. Similarly, Kourtzelis et al, also demonstrated in an *ex vivo* model of HD the induction of coagulation during 2 h of perfusion. In their study, compstatin was used to block complement activation at the level of C3 (10). We postulate that HD-induced complement activation results in the formation of anaphylatoxins, thereby resulting in the activation of peripheral blood mononuclear cell and platelets initiating a pro-inflammatory and pro-thrombotic response. Previously, several reports demonstrated that bioincompatibility-induced inflammation relies mainly on complement, whereas granulocyte enzyme release was predominantly C3-dependent, leukocyte activation and pro-thrombotic mediators were largely dependent on C5 (16, 46). Altogether, our results support the hypothesis of the complement system as a key component in HD-induced inflammation and coagulation, which subsequently leads to a higher risk for CV-events.

We are aware that our study has strengths and limitations. Although the study has a long follow up, the samples were only collected during a single hemodialysis session. Our study could have benefited from a second assessment of these parameters during another dialysis session in the same patients, to assess reproducibility and increase reliability. Furthermore, while complement activation was seen in the patients during HD as well as in our *ex-vivo* model, clear differences were present. Moreover, in patients a significant peak of complement activation was seen during the first 30 min of HD. In contrast, in our *ex-vivo* model a continuous rise of complement activation was seen until the end of the session. Obviously these discrepancies arise due to the differences of *in-vivo* to *ex-vivo*. For instance, in the *ex-vivo* model blood recirculates without re-entering the human body, therefore it lacks the interaction with endothelial cells, liver and other organs. Lastly, the size of our cohort could be considered small and therefore might impact the statistical analysis. However, due to the long follow up, we achieved a relatively high number of CV-events which increases the power of the study in the comparisons between the CV-event group and the event free group.

There is a growing body of data supporting a role for the complement system in the development of cardiovascular disease. Ekdahl et al. proposed that complement activation initiates an inflammatory cascade and amplifies pro-thrombotic processes (4). For the first time, to our knowledge, we demonstrated intradialytic differences in complement activation, inflammation and a pro-thrombotic factor in HD patients that will develop a CV-event compared to HD patients that will not. Furthermore, we showed that complement inhibition during HD resulted in decreased levels of the pro-inflammatory and pro-thrombotic mediators. Future studies have to determine what the ideal target is to inhibit complement in HD to attenuate these processes and to determine if this decreases the risk of CV-events in HD patients.

AUTHOR CONTRIBUTIONS

FP, MG, MD, CF, and MS research idea and study design. FP, MG and SA data acquisition. FP, MG, BF, SB, MD, JM, WvS, CF, and MS data analysis/interpretation. FP and MG statistical analysis and wrote the manuscript. All authors were involved in editing the final manuscript. All authors read and approved the final manuscript.

REFERENCES

1. Robinson BM, Akizawa T, Jager KJ, Kerr PG, Saran R, Pisoni RL. Factors affecting outcomes in patients reaching end-stage kidney disease worldwide: differences in access to renal replacement therapy, modality use, and haemodialysis practices. *Lancet* (2016) 388:294–306. doi: 10.1016/S0140-6736(16)30448-2
2. Assa S, Hummel YM, Voors AA, Kuipers J, Westerhuis R, de Jong PE, et al. Hemodialysis-induced regional left ventricular systolic dysfunction: prevalence, patient and dialysis treatment-related factors, and prognostic significance. *Clin J Am Soc Nephrol.* (2012) 7:1615–23. doi: 10.2215/CJN.00850112
3. Weiner DE, Tighiouart H, Amin MG, Stark PC, MacLeod B, Griffith JL, et al. Chronic kidney disease as a risk factor for cardiovascular disease and all-cause mortality: a pooled analysis of community-based studies. *J Am Soc Nephrol.* (2004) 15:1307–15. doi: 10.1097/01.ASN.0000123691.46138.E2
4. Ekdahl KN, Soveri I, Hilborn J, Fellström B, Nilsson B. Cardiovascular disease in haemodialysis: role of the intravascular innate immune system. *Nat Rev Nephrol.* (2017) 13:285–96. doi: 10.1038/nrneph.2017.17
5. Nilsson B, Ekdahl KN, Mollnes TE, Lambris JD. The role of complement in biomaterial-induced inflammation. *Mol Immunol.* (2007) 44:82–94. doi: 10.1016/j.molimm.2006.06.020
6. Ricklin D, Hajishengallis G, Yang K, Lambris JD. Complement: a key system for immune surveillance and homeostasis. *Nat Immunol.* (2010) 11:785–97. doi: 10.1038/ni.1923
7. Craddock PR, Fehr J, Brigham KL, Kronenberg RS, Jacob HS. Complement and leukocyte-mediated pulmonary dysfunction in hemodialysis. *N Engl J Med.* (1977) 296:769–774. doi: 10.1056/NEJM197704072961401
8. Poppelaars F, Gaya da Costa M, Berger SP, Assa S, Meter-Arkema AH, Daha MR, et al. Strong predictive value of mannose-binding lectin levels for cardiovascular risk of hemodialysis patients. *J Transl Med.* (2016) 14:236. doi: 10.1186/s12967-016-0995-5
9. Poppelaars F, Gaya da Costa M, Berger SP, Assa S, Meter-Arkema AH, Daha MR, et al. Erratum to: strong predictive value of mannose-binding lectin levels for cardiovascular risk of hemodialysis patients. *J Transl Med.* (2016) 14:236. doi: 10.1186/s12967-016-1004-8
10. Kourtzelis I, Markiewski MM, Doumas M, Rafail S, Kambas K, Mitroulis I, et al. Complement anaphylatoxin C5a contributes to hemodialysis-associated thrombosis. *Blood* (2010) 116:631–9. doi: 10.1182/blood-2010-01-264051
11. Buraczynska M, Ksiazek P, Wacinski P, Zukowski P, Dragan M, Bednarek-Skublewska A. Complement receptor 1 gene polymorphism and cardiovascular disease in dialyzed end-stage renal disease patients. *Hum Immunol.* (2010) 71:878–82. doi: 10.1016/j.humimm.2010.06.001
12. Buraczynska M, Ksiazek P, Zukowski P, Benedyk-Lorens E, Orlowska-Kowalik G. Complement factor H gene polymorphism and risk of cardiovascular disease in end-stage renal disease patients. *Clin Immunol.* (2009) 132:285–90. doi: 10.1016/j.clim.2009.04.005
13. Kishida K, Kishida N, Arima M, Nakatsuji H, Kobayashi H, Funahashi T, et al. Serum C1q- binding adiponectin in maintenance hemodialysis patients. *BMC Nephrol.* (2013) 14:50. doi: 10.1186/1471-2369-14-50
14. Satomura A, Endo M, Fujita T, Ohi H, Ohsawa I, Fuke Y, et al. Serum mannose-binding lectin levels in maintenance hemodialysis patients: impact on all-cause mortality. *Nephron Clin Pract.* (2006) 102:c93–9. doi: 10.1159/000089666
15. Lines SW, Richardson VR, Thomas B, Dunn EJ, Wright MJ, Carter AM. Complement and cardiovascular disease - the missing link in haemodialysis patients. *Nephron* (2015) 132:5–14. doi: 10.1159/000442426
16. Lappegard KT, Christiansen D, Pharo A, Thorgersen EB, Hellerud BC, Lindstad J, et al. Human genetic deficiencies reveal the roles of complement in the inflammatory network: lessons from nature. *Proc Natl Acad Sci USA.* (2009) 106:15861–6. doi: 10.1073/pnas.0903613106
17. Assa S, Gansevoort RT, Westerhuis R, Kobold ACM, Voors AA, de Jong PE, et al. Determinants and prognostic significance of an intra-dialysis rise of cardiac troponin I measured by sensitive assay in hemodialysis patients. *Clin Res Cardiol.* (2013) 102:439–45. doi: 10.1007/s00392-013-0551-8
18. Rodríguez-Sanz A, Sánchez-Villanueva R, Domínguez-Ortega J, Fiandor AM, Ruiz MP, Trocoli F, et al. Mechanisms involved in hypersensitivity reactions to polysulfone hemodialysis membranes. *Artif Organs.* (2017) 41:E285–95. doi: 10.1111/aor.12954
19. Hempel JCJC, Poppelaars F, Gaya Da Costa M, Franssen CFMCFM, De Vlaam TPGTPG, Daha MRMR, et al. Distinct *in vitro* complement activation by various intravenous iron preparations. *Am J Nephrol.* (2017) 45:49–59. doi: 10.1159/000451060
20. Damman J, Seelen MA, Moers C, Daha MR, Rahmel A, Leuvenink HG, et al. Systemic complement activation in deceased donors is associated with acute rejection after renal transplantation in the recipient. *Transplantation* (2011) 92:163–9. doi: 10.1097/TP.0b013e318222c9a0
21. Austin PC, Steyerberg EW. Interpreting the concordance statistic of a logistic regression model: relation to the variance and odds ratio of a continuous explanatory variable. *BMC Med Res Methodol.* (2012) 12:82. doi: 10.1186/1471-2288-12-82
22. Slinin Y, Greer N, Ishani A, MacDonald R, Olson C, Rutks I, et al. Timing of dialysis initiation, duration and frequency of hemodialysis sessions, and membrane flux: a systematic review for a KDOQI clinical practice guideline. *Am J Kidney Dis.* (2015) 66:823–36. doi: 10.1053/j.ajkd.2014.11.031
23. Mcintyre CW, Rosansky SJ. Starting dialysis is dangerous: how do we balance the risk? *Kidney Int.* (2012) 82133:382–7. doi: 10.1038/ki.2012.133
24. Chenoweth DE. Complement activation during hemodialysis: clinical observations, proposed mechanisms, and theoretical implications. *Artif Organs.* (1984) 8:281–90. doi: 10.1111/j.1525-1594.1984.tb04291.x
25. DeAngelis RA, Reis ES, Ricklin D, Lambris JD. Targeted complement inhibition as a promising strategy for preventing inflammatory complications in hemodialysis. *Immunobiology* (2012) 217:1097–105. doi: 10.1016/j.imbio.2012.07.012
26. Mares J, Richtrova P, Hricinova A, Tuma Z, Moravec J, Lysak D, et al. Proteomic profiling of blood-dialyzer interactome reveals involvement of lectin complement pathway in hemodialysis-induced inflammatory response. *Proteomics Clin Appl.* (2010) 4:829–38. doi: 10.1002/prca.201000031
27. Lubbers R, van Essen MF, van Kooten C, Trouw LA. Production of complement components by cells of the immune system. *Clin Exp Immunol.* (2017) 188:183–94. doi: 10.1111/cei.12952
28. Schmaldienst S, Hö WH. Degranulation of polymorphonuclear leukocytes by dialysis membranes—the mystery clears up? mediators involved in neutrophil degranulation include. *Nephrol Dial Transpl.* (2000) 15:1909–10. doi: 10.1093/ndt/15.12.1909
29. Kalliolias GD, Ivashkiv LB. TNF biology, pathogenic mechanisms and emerging therapeutic strategies. *Nat Rev Rheumatol.* (2015) 12:49–62. doi: 10.1038/nrrheum.2015.169
30. Hunter CA, Jones SA. IL-6 as a keystone cytokine in health and disease. *Nat Immunol.* (2015) 16:448–57. doi: 10.1038/ni.3153
31. Pai JK, Pischon T, Ma J, Manson JE, Hankinson SE, Joshipura K, et al. Inflammatory markers and the risk of coronary heart disease in men and women. *N Engl J Med.* (2004) 351:2599–610. doi: 10.1056/NEJMoa040967
32. Zimmermann J, Herrlinger S, Pruy A, Metzger T, Wanner C. Inflammation enhances cardiovascular risk and mortality in hemodialysis patients. *Kidney Int.* (1999) 55:648–58. doi: 10.1046/j.1523-1755.1999.00273.x
33. Barreto DV, Barreto FC, Liabeuf S, Temmar M, Lemke HD, Tribouilloy C, et al. Plasma interleukin-6 is independently associated with mortality in both hemodialysis and pre-dialysis patients with chronic kidney disease. *Kidney Int.* (2010) 77:550–6. doi: 10.1038/ki.2009.503
34. Stenvinkel P, Ketteler M, Johnson RJ, Lindholm B, Pecoits-Filho R, Riella M, et al. IL-10, IL-6, and TNF-α: central factors in the altered cytokine network of uremia—The good, the bad, and the ugly. *Kidney Int.* (2005) 67:1216–33. doi: 10.1111/j.1523-1755.2005.00200.x
35. Ouyang W, Rutz S, Crellin NK, Valdez PA, Hymowitz SG. Regulation and functions of the IL-10 family of cytokines in inflammation and disease. *Annu Rev Immunol.* (2011) 29:71–109. doi: 10.1146/annurev-immunol-031210-101312
36. Assa S, Hummel YM, Voors AA, Kuipers J, Westerhuis R, Groen H, et al. Hemodialysis-induced regional left ventricular systolic dysfunction and inflammation: a cross-sectional study. *Am J Kidney Dis.* (2014) 64:265–73. doi: 10.1053/j.ajkd.2013.11.010

37. Sapan HB, Paturusi I, Jusuf I, Patellongi I, Massi MN, Pusponegoro AD, et al. Pattern of cytokine (IL-6 and IL-10) level as inflammation and anti-inflammation mediator of multiple organ dysfunction syndrome (MODS) in polytrauma. *Int J Burns Trauma.* (2016) 6:37–43.
38. Ng PC, Li K, Wong RPO, Chui K, Wong E, Li G, et al. Proinflammatory and anti-inflammatory cytokine responses in preterm infants with systemic infections. *Arch Dis Child Fetal Neonatal Ed.* (2003) 88:209–13. doi: 10.1136/fn.88.3.F209
39. Reis ES, DeAngelis RA, Chen H, Resuello RRG, Ricklin D, Lambris JD. Therapeutic C3 inhibitor Cp40 abrogates complement activation induced by modern hemodialysis filters. *Immunobiology* (2015) 220:476–82. doi: 10.1016/j.imbio.2014.10.026
40. Pequeriaux NC, Fijnheer R, Gemen EF, Barendrecht AD, Dekker FW, Krediet RT, et al. Plasma concentration of von Willebrand factor predicts mortality in patients on chronic renal replacement therapy. *Nephrol Dial Transplant.* (2012) 27:2452–7. doi: 10.1093/ndt/gfr735
41. Sioulis A, Malindretos P, Makedou A, Makris P, Grekas D. Coagulation factors as biological risk markers of endothelial dysfunction. Association with the thrombotic episodes of chronic hemodialysis patients. *Hippokratia* (2009) 13:237–41.
42. Lenting PJ, Christophe OD, Denis CV. von Willebrand factor biosynthesis, secretion, and clearance: connecting the far ends. *Blood* (2015) 125:2019–28. doi: 10.1182/blood-2014-06-528406
43. Gralnick HR, Williams SB, McKeown LP, Magruder L, Hansmann K, Vail M, et al. Platelet von Willebrand factor. *Mayo Clin Proc.* (1991) 66:634–40. doi: 10.1016/S0025-6196(12)60524-2
44. Stokes KY, Granger DN. Platelets: a critical link between inflammation and microvascular dysfunction. *J Physiol.* (2012) 590:1023–34. doi: 10.1113/jphysiol.2011.225417
45. Amara U, Rittirsch D, Flierl M, Bruckner U, Klos A, Gebhard F, Lambris JD, Huber-Lang M. Interaction between the coagulation and complement system. *Adv Exp Med Biol.* (2008) 632:71–9. doi: 10.1007/978-0-387-78952-1_6
46. Bergseth G, Lambris JD, Mollnes TE, Lappegård KT. Artificial surface-induced inflammation relies on complement factor 5: proof from a deficient person. *Ann Thorac Surg.* (2011) 91:527–33. doi: 10.1016/j.athoracsur.2010.10.084
47. Innes A, Farrell AM, Burden RP, Morgan AG, Powell RJ. Complement activation by cellulosic dialysis membranes. *J Clin Pathol.* (1994) 47:155–8. doi: 10.1136/jcp.47.2.155
48. Schuett K, Savvaidis A, Maxeiner S, Lysaja K, Jankowski V, Schirmer SH, et al. A potent mortality risk factor in patients on hemodialysis. *J Am Soc Nephrol.* (2017) 28:1622–30. doi: 10.1681/ASN.2016030336

13

The Role of Complement Activating Collectins and Associated Serine Proteases in Patients with Hematological Malignancies, Receiving High-Dose Chemotherapy and Autologous Hematopoietic Stem Cell Transplantations (Auto-HSCT)

*Anna S. Świerzko[1], Mateusz Michalski[1], Anna Sokołowska[1], Mateusz Nowicki[2], Łukasz Eppa[1], Agnieszka Szala-Poździej[1], Iwona Mitrus[3], Anna Szmigielska-Kapłon[4], Małgorzata Sobczyk-Kruszelnicka[3], Katarzyna Michalak[3], Aleksandra Gołos[5], Agnieszka Wierzbowska[4], Sebastian Giebel[3], Krzysztof Jamroziak[5], Marek L. Kowalski[6], Olga Brzezińska[6,7], Steffen Thiel[8], Jens C. Jensenius[8], Katarzyna Kasperkiewicz[9] and Maciej Cedzyński[1]**

***Correspondence:**
Maciej Cedzyński
mcedzynski@cbm.pan.pl

[1] Laboratory of Immunobiology of Infections, Institute of Medical Biology, Polish Academy of Sciences, Łódź, Poland, [2] Department of Hematology, Copernicus Memorial Hospital in Łódź Comprehensive Cancer Center and Traumatology, Łódź, Poland, [3] Department of Bone Marrow Transplantation and Oncohematology, Cancer Center and Institute of Oncology, Gliwice, Poland, [4] Department of Hematology, Medical University of Łódz, Łódź, Poland, [5] Department of Hematology, Institute of Hematology and Transfusion Medicine, Warsaw, Poland, [6] Department of Immunology and Allergy, Medical University of Łódz, Łódź, Poland, [7] Department of Rheumatology, Medical University of Łódz, Łódź, Poland, [8] Department of Biomedicine, Aarhus University, Aarhus, Denmark, [9] Department of Microbiology, University of Silesia, Katowice, Poland

We conducted a prospective study of 312 patients (194 with multiple myeloma, 118 with lymphomas) receiving high-dose conditioning chemotherapy and autologous hematopoietic stem cell transplantation (auto-HSCT). Polymorphisms of *MBL2* and *MASP2* genes were investigated and serial measurements of serum concentrations of mannose-binding lectin (MBL), CL-LK collectin and MASP-2 as well as activities of MBL-MASP-1 and MBL-MASP-2 complex were made. Serum samples were taken before conditioning chemotherapy, before HSCT and once weekly after (totally 4-5 samples); in minority of subjects also 1 and/or 3 months post transplantation. The results were compared with data from 267 healthy controls and analyzed in relation to clinical data to explore possible associations with cancer and with chemotherapy-induced medical complications. We found a higher frequency of MBL deficiency-associated genotypes (LXA/O or O/O) among multiple myeloma patients compared with controls. It was however not associated with hospital infections or post-HSCT recovery of leukocytes, but seemed to be associated with the most severe infections during follow-up. Paradoxically, high MBL serum levels were a risk factor for prolonged fever and some infections. The first possible association of *MBL2* gene 3′-untranslated region polymorphism with cancer (lymphoma) in Caucasians was noted. Heterozygosity for *MASP2* gene +359 A>G mutation was relatively frequent in lymphoma patients who experienced bacteremia during hospital stay. The median concentration of CL-LK was higher in myeloma patients compared with healthy subjects. Chemotherapy induced marked increases in serum MBL and MASP-2 concentrations, prolonged for several weeks and relatively slighter decline in CL-LK level within 1 week. Conflicting findings on the influence of MBL on infections following chemotherapy of myeloma and lymphoma have been reported. Here we found no evidence for an association between MBL deficiency and infection during the short period of neutropenia following conditioning treatment before HSCT. However, we noted a possible protective effect of MBL during follow-up, and suspected that to be fully effective when able to act in combination with phagocytic cells after their recovery.

Keywords: CL-LK, collectin, complement, hematopoietic stem cell transplantation (HSCT), mannose-binding lectin (MBL), MASP, mutliple myeloma, lymphoma

INTRODUCTION

Hematological cancers derive from various cells of the immune system. Multiple myeloma (MM), a plasma cell malignancy, is relatively common. It more often affects males than females and is usually diagnosed at age >55 years. Although incurable, treatment strategies including chemotherapy followed by autologous hematopoietic stem cell transplantation (auto-HSCT) allow marked prolongation of patients' life expectancy (1–5). The term "lymphoma" includes a variety of highly heterogeneous lymphoid malignancies. Hodgkin's lymphoma (HL) accounts for approximately 1/10 of all lymphomas at diagnosis. It is characterized by giant, multinucleated Reed-Sternberg and large mononuclear Hodgkin's cells (of B cell lineage). Incidence of HL peaks during early adulthood (20–34 years) and again at age >60 years; it is slightly commoner in males, and most newly diagnosed patients are successfully cured (6–9). Non-Hodgkin's lymphomas (NHL) are also more often diagnosed in men than in women (10–15). NHL usually arise from the B cells lineage (>40 subtypes; >80% of cases) although some T cell and NK cell lymphomas occur. Some NHL are histologically aggressive with a high mortality rate, but NHL are often curable when diagnosed and treated early.

Hematological malignancies obviously compromise the host immune response. Intensive chemotherapy and/or radiotherapy, adds further immunosuppression (mostly due to profound and prolonged neutropenia). High-dose chemotherapy and auto-HSCT is the standard first-line treatment for younger patients with multiple myeloma as well as standard second-line treatment in patients with Hodgkin's lymphoma and aggressive non-Hodgkin's lymphomas (1, 6, 10, 16).

Due to severe immunocompromise caused by both the disease and therapy, patients are at a high risk of morbidity and mortality due to infections. It is estimated that up to 80% of patients have fever, and more than one third suffer from well-defined infections (17–19). Septicemia is the commonest type of infection, and some patients are affected by pneumonia or alimentary tract infections (19). Post-HSCT reconstitution of bone marrow after conditioning therapy is usually attained in ~3 weeks, but full recovery of functional leukocytes takes longer (20, 21). During the period of aplasia, patients have to be isolated, carefully monitored and receive prophylactic/supportive medication (4, 18, 22).

Complement is a complex system of numerous components that constitutes a crucial branch of the immune response. It protects from a variety of infections and takes part in clearance of host cells undergoing apoptosis, necrosis or neoplastic transformation. However, dysregulation of its activation may result in chronic or systemic inflammation and possibly promotion of tumor growth. Therefore, involvement of complement may have opposing effects in cancer. Furthermore, some of its components may be considered as candidate diagnostic or prognostic biomarkers of the disease (23, 24).

Pattern recognition molecules known to activate complement *via* the lectin pathway are two collectins [mannose-binding lectin (MBL) and CL-LK, composed of two peptides: collectin-10 (CL-10, CL-L1) and collectin-11 (CL-11, CL-K1)] and ficolins (ficolin-1,-2,-3). They form complexes with MASP (MBL-associated serine proteases: MASP-1,-2,-3) and non-enzymatic related proteins (MAp19, MAp44) (25–27).

The aim of our investigation was to estimate possible association of complement-activating collectins (MBL, CL-LK) and associated serine proteases with cancer (MM, LYMPH) itself and with hospital infections after chemotherapy followed by auto-HSCT.

Single-nucleotide polymorphisms, localized to codons 52 (A/D), 54 (A/B), and 57 (A/C) of the first exon of the *MBL2* gene, influence both MBL serum level and its activity. The variant, dominant alleles (collectively designated O), are associated with lower MBL levels compared with the A (wild-type) one. Furthermore, promoter region polymorphisms (H/L and Y/X at positions−550 and−221, respectively) also determine MBL concentration to some extent, due to influence on gene expression. The O/O and LXA/O genotypes are considered to be associated with primary MBL deficiency [reviewed in (24)].

The role of MBL and clinical associations of its deficiency apparently depend on clinical context, patient's age, co-existence

Abbreviations: DLBCL, diffuse large B-cell lymphoma; HL, Hodgkin's lymphoma; HSCT, hematopoietic stem cell transplantation; LYMPH, lymphoma; MM, multiple myeloma; NHL, non-Hodgkin's lymphoma.

of other defects of the immune system, *etc.* Several reports and review papers suggested that *MBL2* A/O heterozygosity may be advantageous for the host. Relative high frequency of such genotypes in a variety of populations has been suspected to result from an evolutionary, selective trend (28–31). It was observed that *MBL2* O alleles (and especially O/O genotypes) are less common among centenarians than in general population. On the other hand, in this age group, a relatively low frequency of high MBL-producing haplotypes/genotypes was found. Similar trends were noted in octo- and nonagenarians (32, 33). Therefore, it was postulated that moderate MBL serum concentration may be favorable to healthy aging while both MBL deficiency and its hyper-reactivity may be deleterious for the host. The first was related to variety of infectious which, especially when severe or recurrent, may lead to the worsening of quality of life and therefore to shortening of life expectancy. On the other hand, high MBL may favor autoimmunity and/or promote tumorigenesis. The latter is often associated with cachexia and fatal outcome. That issue becomes even more complicated when some opposing effects are considered: MBL deficiency may be a risk factor for development of cancer (like childhood acute lymphoblastic leukemia) while high MBL may facilitate some intracellular pathogens to enter their target cells [reviewed in (24, 33)].

Originally, Peterslund et al. (34) found a strong relationship between MBL deficiency and serious infections in a relatively small group of patients suffering from hematological malignancies (n = 54, including 18 with MM and 13 with NHL). Many subsequent studies failed to reproduce the strength of this relationship although positive results were reported in some studies but not others. It is clear that MBL does not have a universal role in preventing infections following chemotherapy, but any influence or lack of it is still controversial. Further studies are therefore needed and should be carried out prospectively with substantial numbers of patients. We have investigated a large (n = 194) series of multiple myeloma patients and compared them with a more heterogeneous group of lymphoma patients (n = 118), as well as healthy controls (n = 267). In addition to MBL, we have also extended our investigations to include CL-LK and MASP-2 since those factors are also relevant to collectin-mediated complement activation.

MATERIALS AND METHODS

Patients and Controls

Three hundred and twelve patients suffering from hematological malignancies, undergoing auto-HSCT were recruited. This group included 194 persons diagnosed with multiple myeloma (MM; 95 females and 99 males; mean age: 58.9 ± 8.9 years), 27 with Hodgkin's lymphoma (HL; 6 females and 21 males; mean age: 40.8 ± 13.7) and 91 with non-Hodgkin's lymphomas (NHL; 40 females, 51 males; mean age: 51.6 ± 11.9). For analyses, HL and NHL groups were combined to form LYMPH (n = 118; mean age: 49.3 ± 13.1). The NHL group included patients with diffuse large B-cell lymphoma (DLBCL, n = 31), mantle cell lymphoma (MCL, n = 18), follicular lymphoma (FL, n = 13), Waldenström's macroglobulinemia (WM, n = 1), non-follicular (diffuse) lymphoma, unspecified (NFL, n = 21), marginal-zone lymphoma (mucosa-associated lymphoid tissue lymphoma, MALTL, n = 1), anaplastic large cell lymphoma, kinase negative (ALCL ALK-, n = 1), anaplastic large cell lymphoma, kinase positive (ALCL ALK+, n = 1), angioimmunoblastic T-cell lymphoma (AITL, n = 2), peripheral T-cell lymphoma (PTCL, n = 1), hepatosplenic T-cell lymphoma (HSTL, n = 1). In total, the group of patients included 141 females and 171 males; mean age was 55.2 ± 11.7 years; age range: 21–73). Basic demographic data are summarized in **Table 1**.

TABLE 1 | Basic characterisation of patients and controls.

	Group		
	Multiple myeloma (MM)	Lymphoma (LYMPH)	Control (C)
N	194	118	267
Sex (F/M)	95/99	46/72	174/93
Age (years)			
mean ± SD	58.9 ± 8.9	49.3 ± 13.1	48 ± 13
range	25-71	21–73	18–84
Conditioning therapy (n)	MEL-200 (156) MEL-140 (19) MEL-100 (7) Radiotherapy alone (12)	BEAM (88) BeAM (12) Bendamustine (4) CTX (13) TBC (1)	Not applicable
Complications (n)			Not applicable
Infections	74	72	
with bacteremia	45	35	
with no bacteremia	30	38	
Febrile neutropenia	39	10	
None of above	81	36	

With the exception of 12 persons suffering from MM undergoing radiotherapy alone, patients were treated with conditioning high-dose chemotherapy before transplantation (**Table 1**). In 28 patients (24 LYMPH and 4 MM), both chemotherapy and radiotherapy were used. Standard treatment for multiple myeloma was MEL-200 (melphalan at dosage 200 mg/m^2) although in some instances lower doses (MEL-140, MEL-100) were administered. The majority of LYMPH patients were treated with BEAM: carmustine (300 mg/m^2), etoposide (800 mg/m^2), cytarabine (1600 mg/m^2), melphalan (140 mg/m^2), accompanied, or not by radiotherapy. For the remaining, BeAM (carmustine replaced with bendamustine), bendamustine (alone or accompanied by radiation), cyclophosphamide (CTX) and radiotherapy or TBC combination (thiotepa, busulfan, cyclophosphamide) were used (**Table 1**).

During hospital stay, crucial clinical parameters like white blood cell (WBC) count, absolute neutrophil count (ANC), platelet (PLT) count, inflammatory markers [C-reactive protein (CRP), fibrinogen (FBG), and procalcitonin (PCT)] levels and incidence of complications [infections (associated with bacteremia or not), febrile neutropenia (FN); duration of fever >38°C] were recorded and used for analyses. Etiological agents of infections are listed in **Supplementary Table 1**.

One hundred age-matched controls (unrelated volunteers with no history of cancer, autoimmune diseases, or recurrence of infections) were recruited. Furthermore, DNA/serum samples from 167 healthy adult subjects collected for our previous projects were used, therefore control group included 267 individuals (174 females and 93 males; mean age: 48 ± 13; age range: 18–84). Basic data are presented in **Table 1**. The study was approved by the Ethics Committee of the Medical University of Lodz. The written informed consent from patients/controls was obtained. This work conforms to the provisions of the Declaration of Helsinki.

TABLE 2 | Frequency of *MBL2* genotypes (SNP located within promoter and exon 1) within major groups.

Genotype	Group		
	C	MM	LYMPH
A/A	180 (69.5)	132 (68)	80 (67.8)
YA/O	53 (20.5)	29 (14.9)	24 (20.3)
XA/O or O/O	26 (10)	33 (17)*	14 (11.9)

*Percentages are shown in parentheses. *p = 0.034; OR 1.84; 95%CI (1.06-3.19) (vs. C).*

Blood and Serum Samples

Blood samples for DNA extraction were taken into citrated tubes before chemotherapy and stored at −80°C. DNA was extracted with the use of GeneMATRIX Quick Blood Purification Kit (EURx Ltd, Gdansk, Poland), according to the manufacturer's protocol. Samples for serum isolation were taken into tubes with clot activator before chemotherapy (sample 1), before HSCT (sample 2; usually 3–7 days later) and once weekly till hospital discharge (sample 3: usually 7 days after HSCT; mean 7.0 ± 0.8; sample 4: usually 14 days after HSCT; mean 13.6 ± 1.2; in some patients sample 5: 21 days after HSCT; mean 20.3 ± 2). Sixty-three patients were additionally sampled~45 days (mean 45.3 ± 7.6; sample 45) while 59 were additionally sampled at ~100 days (mean 104.1 ± 19.3; sample 100) after HSCT, during control examination. Among them, 40 persons were sampled at "45" and "100" points. Sera were stored at −80°C until testing.

MBL2 Genotyping

Promoter (H/L, at position−550, rs11003125 and Y/X, at position−221, rs7096206) and exon 1 (A/D, codon 52, rs5030737; A/B, codon 54, rs1800450, and A/C, codon 57, rs1800451) single nucleotide polymorphisms of the *MBL2* gene were investigated as previously described (35). SNPs of the same gene, located within the 3′-untranslated region of the exon 4: Ex4-1483 T>C (rs10082466), Ex4-1260 C>T (rs56009657), Ex4-1067 G>A (rs10824792), Ex4-1064 G>T (rs35327474), Ex4-1063 G>T (rs35768126), Ex4-1047 T>G (rs12254577), Ex4-939 T>C (rs774307463), Ex4-901 A>G (rs2120132), Ex4-879 A>C (rs2120131), Ex4-845 C>T (rs2165813), Ex4-718 G>T (rs2099903) and Ex4-710 A>G (rs2099902) were investigated by direct sequencing. Briefly, PCRs were run on a C1000 Thermal Cycler (Bio-Rad, Hercules, CA, USA), using appropriate spanning primers (designed with the use of PRIMER3 software, http://bioinfo.ut.ee/primer3/):

forward: 5′-TTTCCCCATGGTTTTAATCTG-3′,

reverse: 5′-TCACTAAAACCACCAAAACAAGA-3′,

under the following conditions: 96°C for 5 min, then 35 cycles (96°C for 40 s, 60°C for 30 s, 72°C for 45 s) and finally 72°C for 5 min. The PCR products were purified with the help of EPPiC - Enzymatic Post-PCR Immediate Cleanup (A&A Biotechnology, Gdynia, Poland). Samples thus prepared were directly used as templates for sequencing, performed using the GeneAnalizer-3000 sequencer (Applied Biosystems, Foster City, CA, USA), reverse primer, BrightDyeTerminator Cycle Sequencing kit (NimaGen BV, Nijmegen, The Netherlands) and BDX64 Sequencing Enhancement Buffer (MCLab, San Francisco, CA, USA) according to the manufacturer's instructions. Sequence electropherograms were visually inspected to confirm base calling at the SNP sites using novoSNP (36).

MASP2 Genotyping

The presence of missense mutation +359 A>G (Asp120Gly) located within exon 3 of the *MASP2* gene, rs72550870) was investigated with the use of PCR-RFLP method, as described previously (37).

For an investigation of +1111 A>C (exon 10, Asp371Tyr, rs12711521) polymorphism, the PCR-RFLP procedure was employed. PCR reactions were run on a C1000 Thermal Cycler (Bio-Rad), using primers designed with the use of PRIMER3 software:

forward: 5′-TTATTTTCAGACCATGGGGG-3′,

reverse: 5′-TCTGGGTGGTTTCAAATTCC-3′.

The following conditions were applied: 95°C for 3 min, then 35 cycles (95°C for 30 s, 61°C for 20 s and 72°C for 30 s), followed by a final elongation (72°C for 5 min). After that, the PCR products were treated with MboI enzyme (Fermentas), (37°C, 2 h). The digestion products were further analyzed on a 6% polyacrylamide gel. The PCR product (522 bp) corresponding to C variant has two digestion sites while that corresponding to A allele has only one. Consequently, the first underwent cleavage into three (286, 176, and 60 bp) while the second was cleaved into two (286 and 237 bp) fragments.

MBL Quantification and Determination of MBL-MASP Activity

MBL concentration/activity was measured by ELISA based on binding to solid-phase mannan and detection using monoclonal anti-human MBL antibody (HYB131-1, BioPorto Diagnostics, Copenhagen, Denmark) as previously described (38). MBL-MASP-1 complex activity (39, 40) and MBL-MASP-2 activity (40, 41), were measured using a fluorescence method and an ELISA, respectively. VPR-AMC peptide (Bachem, Bubendorf, Switzerland) was used as the substrate for MASP-1 (39). Rabbit polyclonal anti-human C4c Abs (Dako, Glostrup, Denmark) and corresponding goat HRP-conjugated secondary antibodies (Dako) were used for detection of deposited C4 products after incubation of the serum sample on mannan-coated wells, for an estimation of MBL-MASP-2 complex activity (40). MBL deficiency was taken as 150 ng/ml (42, 43). "High" MBL concentration (>3000 ng/ml) was chosen based on the value

TABLE 3 | Frequency of *MBL2* genotypes (SNP located within exon 4 3′-UTR) within major groups.

Genotype	Polymorphism												Group		
	Ex4-710	Ex4-718	Ex4-845	Ex4-879	Ex4-901	Ex4-939	Ex4-1047	Ex4-1063	Ex4-1064	Ex4-1067	Ex4-1260	Ex4-1483	C ($n = 255$)	MM ($n = 194$)	LYMPH ($n = 118$)
gt1	A/A	G/G	C/C	A/A	A/A	T/T	T/T	G/G	G/G	A/A	C/C	T/T	95 (37.2)	59 (30.4)	28 (23.7)*
gt2	A/G	G/T	C/T	A/C	A/G	T/T	T/T	G/G	G/G	A/G	C/C	T/C	66 (25.9)	44 (22.7)	40 (33.9)
gt3	A/A	G/G	C/C	A/A	A/A	T/T	T/T	G/G	G/G	A/G	C/C	T/T	47 (18.4)	40 (20.6)	29 (24.6)
gt4	A/G	G/T	C/T	A/C	A/G	T/T	T/T	G/G	G/G	G/G	C/C	T/C	15 (5.9)	17 (8.8)	6 (5.1)
gt5	A/A	G/G	C/C	A/A	A/A	T/T	T/T	G/G	G/G	G/G	C/C	T/T	9 (3.5)	8 (4.1)	4 (3.4)
gt6	G/G	T/T	T/T	C/C	G/G	T/T	T/T	G/G	G/G	G/G	C/C	C/C	8 (3.1)	9 (4.6)	3 (2.5)
gt7	A/A	G/G	C/C	A/A	A/A	T/C	T/T	G/G	G/G	A/A	C/C	T/T	4 (1.6)	2 (1)	3 (2.5)
gt8	A/A	G/G	C/C	A/A	A/A	T/T	T/T	G/G	G/G	G/G	C/T	T/T	2 (0.8)	0	0
gt9	A/G	G/T	C/T	A/C	A/G	T/T	T/T	G/G	G/G	G/G	C/C	T/T	1 (0.4)	2 (1)	0
gt10	A/A	G/G	C/C	A/A	A/A	T/T	T/T	G/T	G/T	G/G	C/C	T/T	1 (0.4)	1 (0.5)	0
gt11	A/A	G/G	C/C	A/A	A/A	T/T	T/T	G/T	G/T	A/G	C/C	T/T	1 (0.4)	0	1 (0.8)
gt12	A/A	G/G	C/T	A/C	A/G	T/T	T/T	G/G	G/G	A/G	C/C	T/T	1 (0.4)	0	0
gt13	A/G	G/T	C/T	A/C	A/G	T/T	T/T	G/G	G/G	A/G	C/C	T/T	1 (0.4)	1 (0.5)	2 (1.7)
gt14	A/A	G/G	C/C	A/A	A/A	T/T	T/T	G/G	G/G	G/G	C/C	T/C	1 (0.4)	0	0
gt15	A/G	G/G	C/C	A/A	A/G	T/T	T/T	G/G	G/G	A/G	C/C	T/C	1 (0.4)	0	0
gt16	G/G	T/T	T/T	C/C	G/G	T/T	T/T	G/G	G/G	G/G	C/C	T/C	1 (0.4)	1 (0.5)	0
gt17	A/G	G/T	C/T	A/C	A/G	T/C	T/T	G/G	G/G	A/G	C/C	T/C	1 (0.4)	1 (0.5)	1 (0.8)
gt18	A/G	G/T	C/T	A/C	A/G	T/T	T/T	G/G	G/G	A/A	C/C	T/T	0	1 (0.5)	0
gt19	A/A	G/G	C/C	A/A	A/A	T/C	T/T	G/G	G/G	A/G	C/C	T/T	0	1 (0.5)	0
gt20	A/G	G/T	C/T	A/C	A/G	T/T	T/T	G/T	G/T	G/G	C/C	T/C	0	1 (0.5)	0
gt21	A/G	G/G	C/T	A/C	A/G	T/T	T/T	G/G	G/G	A/G	C/C	T/C	0	1 (0.5)	0
gt22	G/G	G/G	T/T	C/C	G/G	T/T	T/T	G/G	G/G	G/G	C/C	C/C	0	1 (0.5)	0
gt23	A/A	G/G	C/C	A/A	G/G	T/T	T/T	G/T	G/T	A/G	C/C	T/T	0	1 (0.5)	0
gt24	A/A	G/G	C/C	A/A	A/A	T/T	T/G	A/A	A/A	C/C	C/C	T/T	0	1 (0.5)	0
gt25	A/G	G/T	C/T	A/C	A/G	T/T	T/T	A/G	A/C	C/T	C/T	T/C	0	1 (0.5)	0
gt26	A/G	G/T	C/T	A/C	A/G	T/T	T/T	A/G	A/C	C/T	C/C	C/C	0	1 (0.5)	0
gt27	A/A	G/G	C/C	A/A	A/A	T/T	T/T	A/A	A/A	C/C	C/T	T/T	0	0	1 (0.8)

Percentages are shown in parentheses. Differences in comparison with gt1 are marked in red. *$^{*}p = 0.01$; OR 0.52; 95%CI (0.32-0.86) (vs. C).*

TABLE 4 | Frequency of *MASP2* genotypes (corresponding to polymorphisms +359 A>G and +1111 A>C SNP) within major groups.

Group	Polymorphism	
	+359 A/G	**+1111 A>C**
C	A/A: 233 (90)	A/A: 179 (69.6)
	A/G: 26 (10)	A/C: 69 (26.8)
	G/G: –	C/C: 9 (3.5)
MM	A/A: 175 (90.2)	A/A: 125 (64.4)
	A/G: 19 (9.8)	A/C: 65 (33.5)
	G/G: –	C/C: 4 (2.1)
LYMPH	A/A: 101 (85.6)	A/A: 91 (77.1)
	A/G: 17 (14.4)	A/C: 26 (22)*
	G/G: –	C/C: 1 (0.8)*

*Percentages are shown in parentheses. *Number of C allele carriers (A/C or C/C genotype) significantly lower in comparison with MM patients: p = 0.023; OR 1.86; 95% CI (1.11-3.13).*

corresponding to the 95th percentile determined for the control group (2978 ng/ml). For MBL-MASP-1 or-2 complex activities, the value of 1 U/ml was arbitrarily assigned for the standard serum (38, 40).

Assay for CL-LK

CL-LK concentration was determined by sandwich TRIFMA, as described (44). Mouse anti-human CL-10 monoclonal antibody (clone 4F97D) was used for coating while biotinylated rabbit anti-human CL-10 mAb (clone P1), followed by Eu^{3+}-labeled streptavidin (Perkin Elmer, Waltham, MA, USA) was used for detection. "Low" and "high" CL-LK levels were arbitrarily defined as <242 ng/ml (corresponding to the 10th percentile within control group) and >583 ng/ml (95th percentile determined for controls), respectively.

Assay for MASP-2

MASP-2 levels were determined by TRIFMA, as described by Moller-Kristensen et al. (45), with slight modification (37). Rat antibodies of clone 8B were used for coating, while those of clone 6G12 (biotinylated) were used for detection. "Low" and "high" MASP-2 levels (based on 10 and 95th percentiles within C group) were arbitrarily defined as <172 ng/ml and >627 ng/ml, respectively.

Statistical Analysis

The Statistica (version 13.1, Dell Poland) software package was used for data management and statistical calculations. The medians of protein concentrations were compared using the Mann-Whitney *U*-test. It was chosen because MBL, MASP-2, MBL-MASP-1, and MBL-MASP-2 values were not normally distributed (not shown). The same test was employed for CL-LK (normally distributed), to make the analyses comparable. Changes during hospital stay and after discharge were analyzed by Friedman's ANOVA test. The frequencies of low or high levels, as well as genotypes/alleles were compared by two-sided Fischer's exact test (or χ^2 when appropriate). Correlations were determined by Spearman's test. P <0.05 were considered statistically significant.

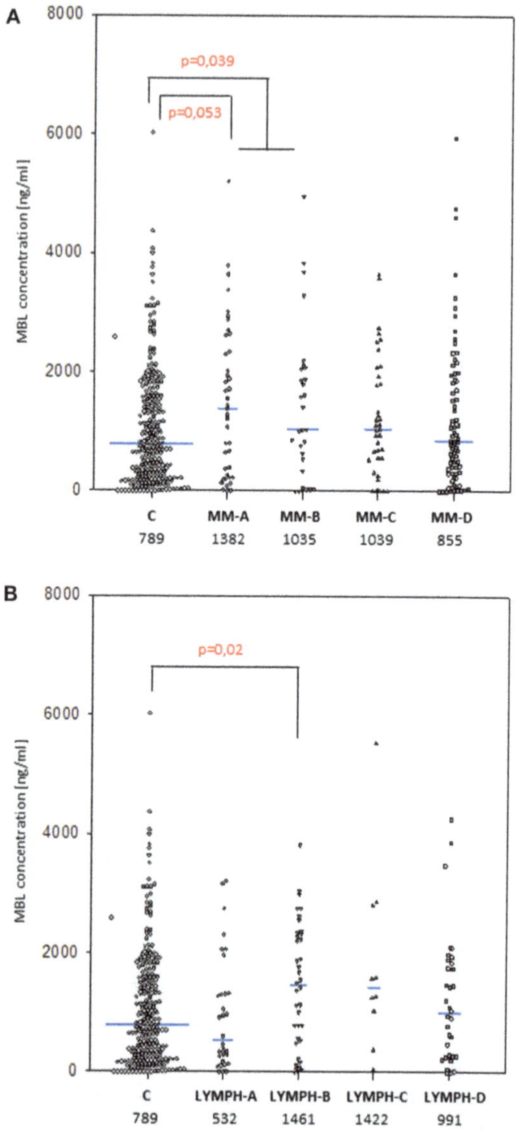

FIGURE 1 | Mannose-binding lectin serum concentrations in patients (before conditioning chemotherapy) and controls. Blue bars present median values (given below group descriptions). **(A)** controls (C) vs. multiple myeloma (MM) patients; **(B)** controls vs. lymphoma (LYMPH) patients. MM-A, LYMPH-A: patients who experienced infections with proven bacteremia; MM-B, LYMPH-B: patients who experienced infections with no bacteremia; MM-C, LYMPH-C: patients who experienced febrile neutropenia; MM-D, LYMPH-D: patients who experienced none of afore-mentioned complications during hospital stay.

RESULTS

MBL2 Gene Polymorphisms Located Within Promoter Region and Exon 1

The frequency of A/A homozygotes was similar in MM, LYMPH and C groups. However, MBL deficiency-associated genotypes

(LXA/O, O/O) were significantly more common in patients with multiple myeloma (**Table 2**). Those genotypes did not appear in the short term (2–3 weeks after HSCT) to be associated with higher susceptibility to infection as their frequency did not differ significantly between patients experiencing hospital infections/febrile neutropenia compared with patients free of those complications [MM: 15/114 (13.2%) vs. 18/80 (22.5%, $p = 0.12$); LYMPH: 10/82 (12.2%) vs. 4/36 (11.1%, $p = 1$)]. The high MBL-conferring genotypes (YA/YA) were associated with a trend toward more prolonged fever during the neutropenic period, with 47.1% of patients having fever of more than 4 days duration being YA/YA, compared with 24.1% having fever for less than 4 days and 30.1% who had no infection or FN. The LYMPH group differed from the MM patients in having a high frequency of the uncommon C allele (codon 57 SNP) (0.025 vs. 0.007 for C; $p = 0.049$), but this was not associated with hospital infections.

One hundred and two MM patients were followed-up for at least 6 months, of which six were hospitalized due to severe infections. One was O/O and 2 were LXA/O; two of them died. Other 3 persons (1 non-survivor) had A/A genotypes. Similarly, from 59 LYMPH patients that were followed-up, three had severe infections: two were MBL-deficient (O/O; one non-survivor) and one A/A (survivor).

MBL2 Gene Polymorphisms Located Within 3′-UTR Region (Exon 4)

Twelve polymorphic sites located within 3′-UTR region of the *MBL2* gene were analyzed. That allowed identification of 27 various genotypes, of which the 7 most common accounted for nearly 95% of controls and cases (**Table 3**). The genotype 1 (gt1) was commonest in the C and MM groups, but for the LYMPH group, genotype 2 was the most frequent. The difference between LYMPH and C groups with regard to genotype 1 (23.7 vs. 37.2%; $p = 0.01$) was statistically significant, possibly the first association of a *MBL2* gene 3′-untranslated region polymorphism with cancer to be observed in Caucasians.

MASP2 Gene Polymorphisms

When the +359 A>G mutation was investigated, no variant homozygote (and therefore MASP-2/MAp19 deficient) was found among individuals recruited to the study. The number of heterozygotes (**Table 4**) did not differ among the major (C, MM, LYMPH) groups, although a trend toward higher incidence of heterozygosity was noted within LYMPH group (**Table 4**). That primarily reflected relatively high frequency of A/G genotype among LYMPH patients who had bacteremia during hospital stay [8/34 (23.5%); $p < 0.04$ vs. C group].

For another *MASP2* SNP, +1111 A>C, no differences between patients and controls were found. However, this variant allele was commoner within the LYMPH patients than within the MM group ($p = 0.023$) (**Table 4**).

Serum MBL Concentration and Activity of Its Complexes With Serine Proteases

The median values determined for samples taken before chemotherapy did not differ significantly in either MM (1027 ng/ml; $n = 187$) or LYMPH (1072 ng/ml; $n = 116$) groups when compared with that found for healthy controls (789 ng/ml; $n = 265$) (**Figure 1**). However, the median was higher in MM patients who later experienced hospital infections (associated or not with bacteremia) and LYMPH patients who suffered from infections without bacteremia (**Figure 1A**).

As was expected from numerous other studies, the median serum MBL for males and females in the healthy controls were virtually identical (789 vs. 787 ng/ml), and the higher values

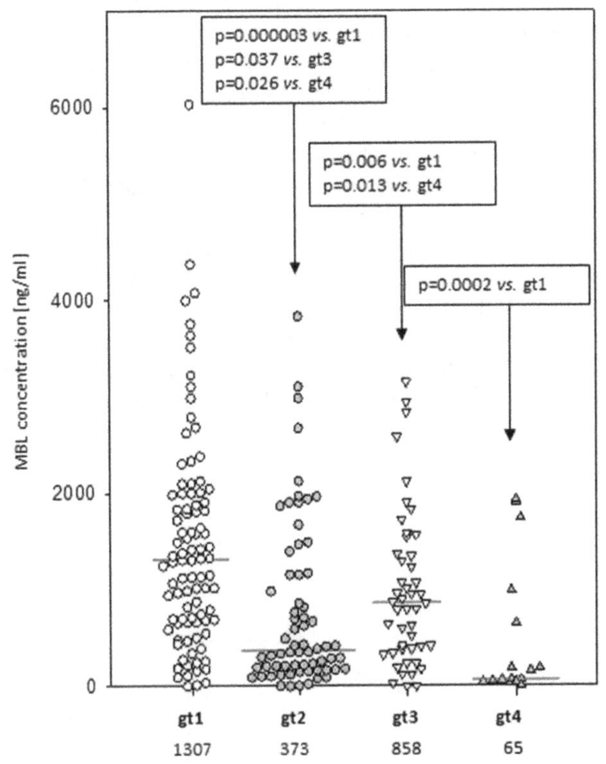

FIGURE 2 | Mannose-binding lectin serum concentrations in healthy controls carrying most common 3′-UTR *MBL2* genotypes (gt1-gt4; details are given in **Table 3**). Blue bars present median values (given below group descriptions).

TABLE 5 | Serum MBL concentrations in controls and patients (sample 1), corresponding to most common *MBL2* genotypes (basing on 3′-UTR polymorphisms).

Genotype	Group (n)	MBL concentration (ng/ml)		Statistical significance (vs. C)
		Median	IQR	
gt1	C (93)	1307	683–1969	–
	MM (59)	1681	804–2673	$p = 0.066$
	LYMPH (27)	1745	1039–2280	$p = 0.12$
gt2	C (66)	373	181–1154	-
	MM (41)	426	233–1213	$p = 0.53$
	LYMPH (40)	466	188–1479	$p = 0.67$
gt3	C (47)	858	384–1360	-
	MM (39)	1199	976–1858	$p = 0.016$
	LYMPH (28)	1285	880–1875	$p = 0.016$

found in the LYMPH group also showed no sex difference (1090 vs. 1054 ng/ml). However, male subjects in the MM group had significantly higher (1213 vs. 729 ng/ml; $p = 0.002$) values, and consequently male MM patients had higher average serum MBL than male controls ($p = 0.032$).

Despite well-known association between *MBL2* SNP located within promoter and exon 1 with MBL concentration (not shown), an influence of exon 4 polymorphisms has been observed. When the four most common genotypes were compared within the control group, significant differences in corresponding median MBL levels were found (**Figure 2**). Comparison of patients and controls showed MBL concentrations significantly higher in patients with genotype 3 for both MM and LYMPH groups (**Table 5**).

In both MM and LYMPH groups, MBL concentrations underwent significant changes ($p < 0.000001$; Friedman's ANOVA test) in relation to treatment (**Figure 3A**). The changes were generally more evident in persons experiencing complications during hospital stay (with the exception of LYMPH patients with bacteremias). (**Figure 3A**). Data from samples taken during control examinations (although from limited number of patients) demonstrated that the concentration of this lectin ~100 days post-HSCT practically returns to the initial (sample 1) value (**Figure 4A**). In the case of patients suffering from lymphomas, MBL increased more rapidly than in those with diagnosed MM, probably depending on chemotherapy used (BEAM vs. MEL) (**Figure 3A**). Again, a decrease was observed after discharge and data from sample 100 were comparable to those from sample 1 (**Figure 4A**).

Unexpectedly, very high MBL concentration (>3000 ng/ml) before treatment seemed to be associated with higher risk of hospital-acquired infection in MM patients. Such a high level of the protein was found in 9 of 71 (12.7%) MM patients who experienced infections, compared with 13 of 265 controls (4.9%; OR 2.81; $p = 0.029$). No such relationship was found for the LYMPH group (8/116 cases, 6.9%). No difference was found in the frequency of serum MBL deficiency (<150 ng/ml) between controls (17.7%) and patients (MM: 17.6%; LYMPH: 16.4%). independently of complications (not shown).

As expected, since correlation coefficients between serum MBL and activity of its complexes with MASP-1 or MASP-2 were ≥0.9, the latter activities gave similar results (**Supplementary Figure 1**). Moreover, observed MBL variations in MM patients, slightly but significantly, inversely correlated with variations in WBC, ANC, PLT counts (changes in leukocyte counts are demonstrated in **Figures 4D–F**). In contrast, relatively strong, positive correlations with concentrations of such markers of inflammation as CRP or PCT (but not FBG) were found

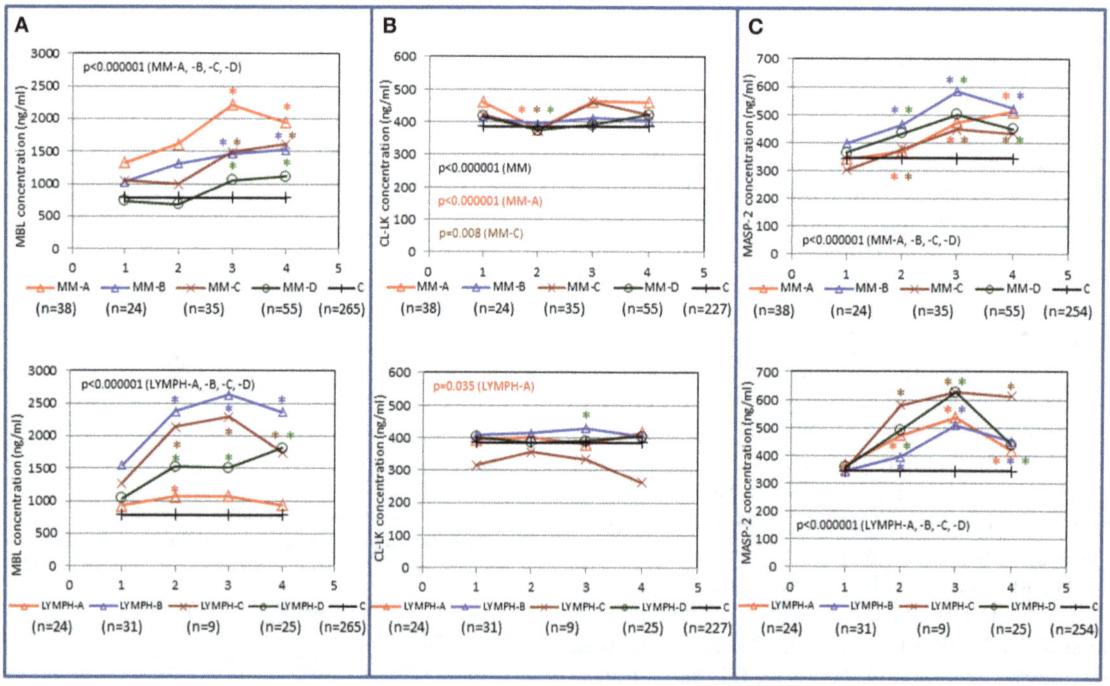

FIGURE 3 | Changes in concentrations of MBL **(A)**, CL-LK **(B)**, and MASP-2 **(C)** in patients, during treatment. 1–blood taken directly before conditioning chemotherapy; 2 – blood taken directly before autologous hematopoietic stem cell transplantation; 3–blood taken 1 week after HSCT; 4—blood taken 2 weeks after HSCT. Data from sample 5 (3 weeks after HSCT) are not shown due to relatively low number of cases within each subgroup. Median values for each time-point are presented. MM-A, LYMPH-A: patients who experienced infections with proven bacteremia; MM-B, LYMPH-B: patients who experienced infections with no bacteremia; MM-C, LYMPH-C: patients who experienced febrile neutropenia; MM-D, LYMPH-D: patients who experienced none of afore-mentioned complications during hospital stay. C—controls (sampled once). Statistics: given *p*-values regard to Friedman's ANOVA while asterisks (in colors corresponding to curves) mark significant differences in comparison with sample 1 (Wilcoxon's paired sample test). Graphs show data from complete sets (MBL levels measured in all 1-4 samples) only. Numbers of patients are given in parentheses.

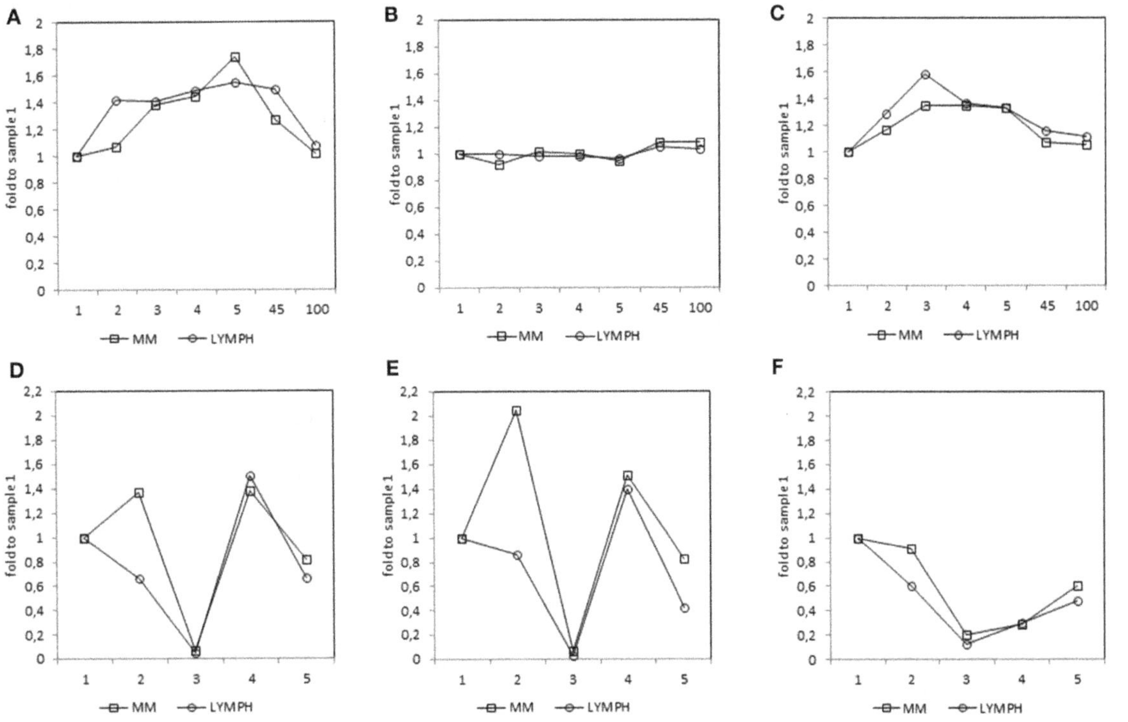

FIGURE 4 | Relative (median fold to sample 1) changes in concentrations of MBL **(A)**, CL-LK **(B)**, and MASP-2 **(C)** and blood morphology: white blood cells (WBC) count **(D)**, absolute neutrophil count (ANC) **(E)** and platelet (PLT) count **(F)** in patients, during treatment. 1—blood taken directly before conditioning chemotherapy; 2—blood taken directly before autologous hematopoietic stem cell transplantation; 3—blood taken 1 week (mean 7.0 ± 0.8 days) after HSCT; 4—blood taken 2 weeks after HSCT (mean 13.6 ± 1.2 days); 5—blood taken 3 weeks after HSCT (mean 20.3 ± 2 days); 45—blood taken 45 days after HSCT (mean 45.3 ± 7.6 days); 100—blood taken 100 days after HSCT (mean 104.1 ± 19.3 days).

(**Table 6**). It should be mentioned that WBC/ANC/PLT were checked routinely and regularly (taking samples 1-5 was coordinated with that) while concentrations of inflammatory proteins (especially FBG) were tested occasionally, in the case of morbid indications. Therefore, even relatively high correlation coefficient not always was associated with statistical significance (**Table 6**).

Concentration of CL-LK

The median level of CL-LK in pre-treatment samples from MM patients (423 ng/ml) was significantly higher than that from the control group (385 ng/ml; $p = 0.0002$) (**Figure 5A**) or the corresponding samples from LYMPH patients (388 ng/ml; $p = 0.009$). This difference did not seem to be associated with post-HSCT complications. No difference ($p = 0.56$) was found between healthy subjects and patients suffering from lymphoma (**Figure 5B**).

No significant differences in median CL-LK concentration between males and females were apparent in MM patients (420 vs. 429 ng/ml) or healthy controls (368 vs. 400 ng/ml). However, this value was significantly higher in LYMPH group females (430 vs. 371 ng/ml) compared with males ($p = 0.004$).

The highest CL-LK serum levels (>583 ng/ml) occurred as frequently among MM patients (7%) and LYMPH patients (6%) as controls (5.6%). However, low (<242 ng/ml) values were under-represented within the MM group (2.1%) compared with the C (5.6%, $p = 0.002$) or LYMPH (6%, $p = 0.037$) groups. It should be stressed that low CL-LK was found in none of the MM patients experiencing infections or febrile neutropenia (**Table 7**).

CL-LK concentration during treatment varied, but the changes noted were not so striking as for MBL. They were however significant when data from MM patients who suffered from bacteremia or FN were analyzed (Friedman's ANOVA: $p < 0.000001$ and $p = 0.008$, respectively) (**Figure 3B**). Within LYMPH group, variations were significant for persons affected by bacteremia only ($p = 0.035$). The level of CL-LK was generally lower at point 2 (before HSCT) compared with preceding and following samples. Interestingly, data from minority of patients who were sampled during control examinations suggested slight but significant increase of CL-LK at 45 and 100th days after HSCT (443 ng/ml; $n = 26$, $p = 0.016$ and 457 ng/ml; $n = 23$, $p = 0.048$ compared with data from sample 1). In the case of LYMPH, the median corresponding to samples 100 (384 ng/ml) was similar to that from samples taken before chemotherapy (**Figure 4B**).

Described variations were not associated with changes of blood cell counts or inflammatory markers (**Table 6**).

An incidental finding was a lack of detectable CL-LK in a healthy 45-year old woman. A repeat sample 2 months later yielded only a trace (<40 ng/ml). Sequencing of the *COLEC10* gene did not reveal homozygosity for any known variant allele

TABLE 6 | Correlations (Spearman's) between variations (samples 1–5) of concentrations/activities of tested proteins/complexes and selected clinical parameters (significant positive and inverse correlations marked with blue and red, respectively).

Tested factor	Blood cell counts			Markers of inflammation		
	WBC	ANC	PLT	CRP	FBG	PCT
A						
MBL	$r = -0.09$	$r = -0.11$	$r = -0.08$	$r = 0.09$	$r = 0.07$	$r = 0.12$
	$p = 0.013$	$p = 0.002$	$p = 0.029$	$p = 0.043$	$p = 0.63$	$p = 0.63$
	$n = 792$	$n = 784$	$n = 790$	$n = 518$	$n = 49$	$n = 20$
MBL-MASP-1	$r = -0.09$	$r = -0.11$	$r = -0.07$	$r = 0.08$	$r = 0.06$	$r = 0.14$
	$p = 0.015$	$p = 0.002$	$p = 0.052$	$p = 0.09$	$p = 0.69$	$p = 0.56$
	$n = 791$	$n = 783$	$n = 789$	$n = 517$	$n = 49$	$n = 20$
MBL-MASP-2	$r = -0.06$	$r = -0.09$	$r = -0.07$	$r = 0.1$	$r = 0.11$	$r = 0.12$
	$p = 0.11$	$p = 0.019$	$p = 0.072$	$p = 0.036$	$p = 0.46$	$p = 0.61$
	$n = 744$	$n = 736$	$n = 743$	$n = 487$	$n = 48$	$n = 20$
CL-LK	$r = -0.08$	$r = -0.09$	$r = -0.04$	$r = 0.1$	$r = 0.05$	$r = -0.13$
	$p = 0.022$	$p = 0.01$	$p = 0.21$	$p = 0.025$	$p = 0.76$	$p = 0.57$
	$n = 792$	$n = 784$	$n = 790$	$n = 518$	$n = 49$	$n = 20$
MASP-2	$r = -0.1$	$r = -0.09$	$r = -0.2$	$r = 0.2$	$r = -0.003$	$r = -0.08$
	$p = 0.004$	$p = 0.015$	$p < 0.000001$	$p = 0.000005$	$p = 0.98$	$p = 0.75$
	$n = 790$	$n = 782$	$n = 788$	$n = 516$	$n = 49$	$n = 20$
B						
MBL	$r = -0.03$	$r = -0.03$	$r = -0.09$	$r = 0.12$	$r = 0.03$	$r = 0.35$
	$p = 0.51$	$p = 0.53$	$p = 0.06$	$p = 0.044$	$p = 0.82$	$p = 0.015$
	$n = 463$	$n = 443$	$n = 462$	$n = 302$	$n = 72$	$n = 48$
MBL-MASP-1	$r = -0.02$	$r = 0.002$	$r = -0.07$	$r = 0.05$	$r = 0.06$	$r = 0.35$
	$p = 0.62$	$p = 0.97$	$p = 0.12$	$p = 0.41$	$p = 0.65$	$p = 0.014$
	$n = 462$	$n = 442$	$n = 461$	$n = 301$	$n = 72$	$n = 48$
MBL-MASP-2	$r = -0.005$	$r = 0.01$	$r = -0.08$	$r = 0.1$	$r = 0.15$	$r = 0.42$
	$p = 0.92$	$p = 0.84$	$p = 0.01$	$p = 0.071$	$P = 0.21$	$p = 0.003$
	$n = 441$	$n = 421$	$n = 440$	$n = 291$	$n = 71$	$n = 48$
CL-LK	$r = -0.02$	$r = 0.01$	$r = 0.06$	$r = 0.03$	$r = 0.05$	$r = 0.33$
	$p = 0.63$	$p = 0.77$	$p = 0.19$	$p = 0.56$	$p = 0.65$	$p = 0.02$
	$n = 463$	$n = 443$	$n = 462$	$n = 302$	$n = 72$	$n = 48$
MASP-2	$r = -0.27$	$r = -0.27$	$r = -0.31$	$r = 0.32$	$r = 0.13$	$r = 0.27$
	$p < 0.000001$	$p < 0.000001$	$p < 0.000001$	$p < 0.000001$	$p = 0.28$	$p = 0.066$
	$n = 463$	$n = 443$	$n = 462$	$n = 302$	$n = 72$	$n = 48$

A – patients suffering from multiple myeloma; B – patients suffering from lymphomas.

or "new" mutation when compared to the reference gene sequence (NCBI Reference Sequence: NC_000008.11, accessed from: https://www.ncbi.nlm.nih.gov/gene/10584) (not shown).

Concentration of MASP-2

No significant differences were found when pre-treatment median MASP-2 serum concentrations from MM (357 ng/ml) or LYMPH (359 ng/ml) were compared with that from healthy controls (344 ng/ml) (**Figure 6**). However, a higher value was observed in the subgroup of MM patients who had infections with no bacteremia (478 ng/ml, $p = 0.017$ vs. C group). Furthermore, median pre-treatment MASP-2 was higher in MM patients suffering from infections with Gram-positive bacteria (403 ng/ml) relative to those infected by Gram-negative bacteria (343 ng/ml; $p = 0.008$).

Within the control group, a significant sex difference in median MASP-2 level was found (372 vs. 330 ng/ml for males and females, respectively, $p = 0{,}019$). No such relationship was found in MM (360 vs. 352 ng/ml) or LYMPH (347 vs. 371 ng/ml) groups.

When the frequencies of high (>628 ng/ml) MASP-2 concentrations were compared, no significant difference between the groups was found (C: 5.1%, MM: 6.4%, LYMPH: 2.6%). Similarly, the incidence of low (<172 ng/ml) MASP-2 was similar among healthy subjects (10.2%), MM patients (13.4%), and LYMPH patients (13.8%).

MASP-2 concentrations underwent highly significant treatment-associated changes in both groups of patients, independently of complications (**Figure 3C**). There was again an increase after treatment, but the kinetics differed from those of MBL. One and three months after discharge, median MASP-2

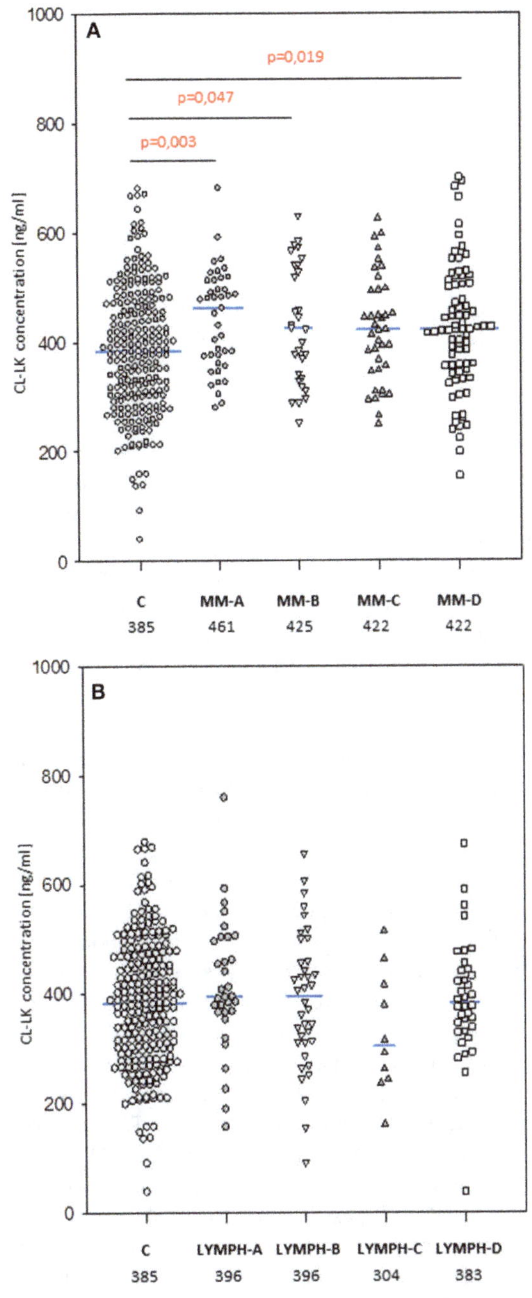

FIGURE 5 | Collectin CL-LK serum concentrations in patients (before conditioning chemotherapy) and controls. Blue bars present median values (given below group descriptions). **(A)** controls (C) vs. multiple myeloma (MM) patients; **(B)** controls vs. lymphoma (LYMPH) patients. MM-A, LYMPH-A: patients who experienced infections with proven bacteremia; MM-B, LYMPH-B: patients who experienced infections with no bacteremia; MM-C, LYMPH-C: patients who experienced febrile neutropenia; MM-A, LYMPH-A: patients who experienced none of afore-mentioned complications during hospital stay.

concentration in LYMPH patients was still higher than at point 1 (386 ng/ml, $n = 40$, $p = 0.0003$ and 419 ng/ml, $n = 36$, $p = 0.006$) while for MM group, the difference was insignificant (**Figure 4C**).

TABLE 7 | Frequency of low serum concentrations of collectin CL-LK in investigated groups (for MM and LYMPH groups: data from sample 1, taken before chemotherapy).

Group (*n*)	% of concentrations <242 ng/ml	Statistical significance (vs. C)
C (227)	9.7	-
MM (187)*	2.1	$p = 0.002$; OR 0.2; 95% CI (0.07-0.6)
MM-A (41)	0	$p = 0.031$; OR 0.11; 95% CI (0.007-1.85)
MM-B (30)	0	$p = 0.087$
MM-A+B (71)	0	$p = 0.003$; OR 0.06; 95% CI (0.004-1.07)
MM-C (38)	0	$p = 0.052$
MM-D (78)	5.1	$p = 0.25$
LYMPH (116)*	7.8	$p = 0.69$
LYMPH-A (32)	9.4	$p = 1$
LYMPH-B (38)	7.9	$p = 1$
LYMPH-A+B (70)	8.6	$p = 1$
LYMPH-C (10)	20	$p = 0.27$
LYMPH-D (36)	2.8	$p = 0.22$

**MM-A, LYMPH-A: patients who experienced infections with proven bacteremia; MM-B, LYMPH-B: patients who experienced infections with no bacteremia; MM-C, LYMPH-C: patients who experienced febrile neutropenia; MM-D, LYMPH-D: patients who experienced none of afore-mentioned complications during hospital stay.*

In both MM and LYMPH groups, MASP-2 correlated positively with CRP and inversely with WBC, ANC and PLT counts (**Table 6**). In contrast to MBL, serum MASP-2 concentrations did not differ between either group of patients and controls in relation to MASP-2 genotypes (**Table 8**).

DISCUSSION

Both cancer and its treatment impair immunity, but the role of MBL and the significance of its deficiency in this context are controversial since contrasting and apparently contradictory findings have been reported. Particular attention has focused on the effect of chemotherapy, both during the immediate neutropenic period and during longer periods of follow-up. Here we have demonstrated with a large series of multiple myeloma patients given similar therapy (and more heterogeneous lymphoma group), that MBL deficiency has no influence on the incidence of infections/febrile neutropenia. However, over a 6-month period of follow-up, MBL deficiency was over-represented in the small number of patients experiencing very severe infections. Our findings with a substantially larger series are not inconsistent with the studies of Molle et al. (46, 47) with a broadly similar group of myeloma patients.

These results could be interpreted as meaning MBL has little influence during the period of chemotherapy-induced cytopenia (and does not affect post-HSCT recovery of leukocytes, **Supplementary Figure 2**), but could have a protective effect when able to act in combination with phagocytic cells. That interpretation could explain why for patients receiving chemotherapy in general, MBL is found

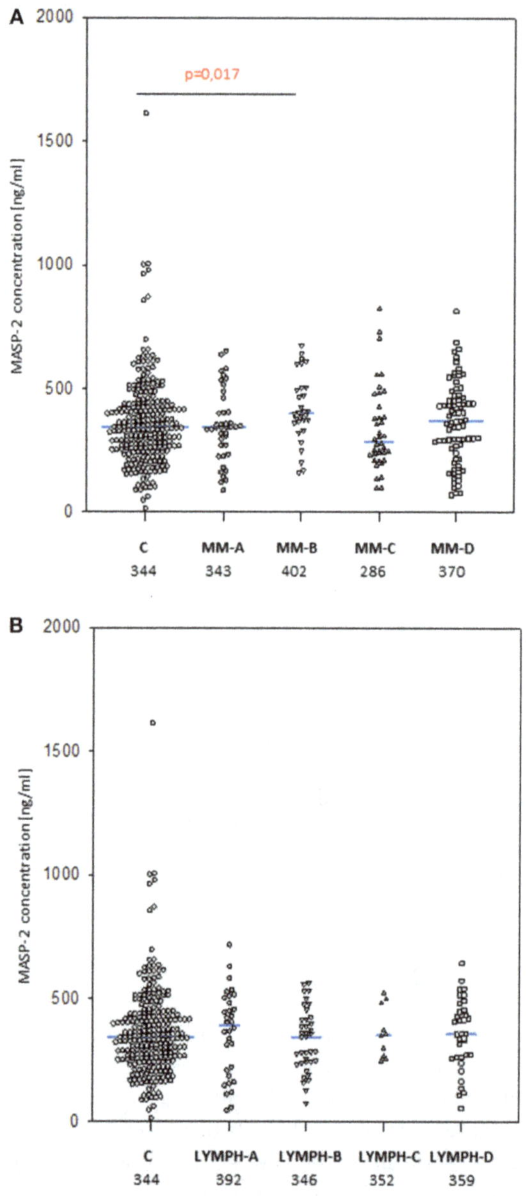

FIGURE 6 | MASP-2 serum concentrations in patients (before conditioning chemotherapy) and controls. Blue bars present median values (given below group descriptions). **(A)** controls (C) vs. multiple myeloma (MM) patients; **(B)**—controls vs. lymphoma (LYMPH) patients. MM-A, LYMPH-A: patients who experienced infections with proven bacteremia; MM-B, LYMPH-B: patients who experienced infections with no bacteremia; MM-C, LYMPH-C: patients who experienced febrile neutropenia; MM-A, LYMPH-A: patients who experienced none of afore-mentioned complications during hospital stay.

to be effective in studies with a medium to long follow-up period (48, 49) but ineffective in short-term follow-up studies (50, 51).

In this study we confirmed the observation of others that chemotherapy is generally followed by an increase in MBL concentration (46, 48, 52). We found that after several weeks it returns to the initial level. A new observation was an association between MBL deficiency and myeloma itself at the genetic level. Furthermore, our data suggest a protective effect of "gt1" from lymphoma. If and when confirmed, this would be the first association of a *MBL2* gene 3′-untranslated region polymorphism with cancer in Europeans [those SNPs were previously reported to have associations with breast or colon cancer in African-Americans but not in Caucasians (53, 54)]. The influence of 3′-end variant on serum MBL concentration was originally reported by Bernig et al. (53, 55). They suggested that Ex4-1067 A haplotype corresponds to high MBL. Indeed, in our study A/A homozygotes ("gt1" genotype) had higher median than A/G heterozygotes ("gt3") while, consequently, heterozygotes ("gt2") had higher values than G/G homozygotes ("gt4") (**Figure 2**). The Ex4-710/901/1067/1483 SNP were found to be components of a haplotype block (28, 54, 55). Our data (**Table 3**) are in agreement with that finding. Therefore, in general (although with very few exceptions), analyzing of one polymorphic site may provide information about the others (including also Ex4-718/845/879) (**Table 3**). Interestingly, the C allele corresponding to Ex4-1483 (associated with Ex4-1067 G) is responsible for interaction with miR-27a, a microRNA molecule which was suspected to predict lower MBL plasma concentration (54, 56). Again, it has been to some extent confirmed here: "gt1" and "gt3" carriers (T/T homozygotes) have generally higher MBL than "gt2" and "gt4" (T/C genotype) (**Figure 2**). Obviously, an interplay between 3′ block and 5′ one (promoter/5′-UTR/exon 1) has to be taken into account in considering genotype-phenotype relationships (28, 54, 56). For example, strong linkage disequilibria of Ex4-1067 with promoter H/L and Y/X SNP were proven [LDmatrix (https://analysistools.nci.nih.gov) (57)]. It is therefore noteworthy that the majority of "gt1" genotype carriers (74/95 controls and 61 of 87 patients) had YA/YA ("high MBL-producing") genotypes. Interestingly, the most prevalent 5′ end variant associated with "gt3" was YA/XA (34/47 controls and 52/69 patients; majority of remaining individuals carried at least one LXA allele) (not shown). That altogether confirms apparent links between Ex4-1067 A and promoter (position−221) Y alleles as well as G and X variants, respectively.

MBL, naturally complexed with MASP has been evidenced (employing animal model) to contribute to mobilization of hematopoietic cells from bone marrow to peripheral blood). That complex is able to trigger both complement and coagulation

TABLE 8 | Serum MASP-2 concentrations in controls and patients (sample 1), corresponding to *MASP2* genotypes (+1111 A>C SNP).

Genotype	Group (*n*)	MASP-2 concentrations (ng/ml)		Statistical significance (vs. C)
		Median	IQR	
A/A	C (171)	312	238–415	–
	MM (120)	320	231–404	$p = 0.83$
	LYMPH (89)	332	233–417	$p = 0.86$
A/C or C/C	C (73)	410	340–513	–
	MM (67)	437	335–544	$p = 0.46$
	LYMPH (27)	455	376–506	$p = 0.23$

systems activation, cross-talking in mobilization process (58–60). It has been suggested that MBL-deficient patients may be poor HSPC (hematopoietic stem progenitor cells) mobilizers even upon stimulation for transplantation (58, 59). It however has not been confirmed in our study: most of MBL deficient individuals (confirmed by both genotyping and MBL serum level) responded normally (not shown). It may be speculated that MBL deficiency is, at least partially, compensated by other lectin pathway-associated pattern-recognition molecules when MASP function is normal. Furthermore, it seems not to affect markedly recovery of leukocytes (at least when their counts recorded at ~14th day after HSCT, see **Supplementary Figure 2**).

Another collectin, CL-LK (as mentioned being a complex of CL-10 and CL-11), was found at higher concentrations in myeloma patients compared with controls. One and three months after discharge (samples 45 and 100) its level exceeded an initial one. However, no clinical significance of extremely high or low CL-LK was apparent. This is the first possible association of CL-LK with a hematological malignancy to have been noted. During hospital stay, CL-LK underwent marked changes in myeloma patients affected by bacteremia or febrile neutropenia suggesting involvement of this collectin in the immune response against some potentially life-threatening events.

The results of a retrospective study indicated that higher MASP-2 serum concentrations are associated with a longer event-free survival (EFS) in children with lymphoma (especially HL) (61). We have conducted a prospective study, and collected data from follow up longer than 3–6 months from a relatively low number of patients. Furthermore most of them survived that period and had no relapse so our results cannot easily be compared with the previous report. As with MBL, higher serum level of its associated serine protease-2 before chemotherapy seemed to be associated with hospital infections, at least in MM patients and Gram-positive bacterial agents. Earlier, *MASP2* variant allele (SNP at position +1111) was suggested to be protective against DLBCL (62). Among 31 DLBCL patients studied here, 7 (22.6%) were heterozygotes (no difference in comparison to C group). It should however be stressed that relatively high incidence of *MASP2* +359 A/G heterozygosity was noted among LYMPH patients who experienced bacteremia while relatively low - of +1111 A/C heterozygosity in LYMPH group in general. Both mentioned genotypes influence MASP-2 serum concentration (but not MBL-MASP-2 complex activity when measured as C4 cleaving potency; not shown). The *MASP2* +359 G variant abolishes the formation of the MBL-MASP-2 complex and heterozygotes present approx. half MASP-2 concentration in serum. However, this level suffices for full activity of the MBL pathway (37).

Cancers studied here seem in general to affect concentrations of complement activating collectins and MASP-2 disparately in males and females. As previously demonstrated by Troldborg et al. (63), MBL, CL-10, and CL-11 average levels do not differ between men and women while MASP-2 is higher in men. That was fully confirmed here for controls only. Neither in MM nor LYMPH group the latter differed depending on sex while MBL was found significantly higher in MM males compared with females and opposite effect was noted for CL-LK.

To summarize, we have studied the complex cross-talk between numerous endogenous and exogenous factors in the process of treating patients suffering from MM and LYMPH. Monitoring was started immediately before conditioning chemotherapy and continued for several weeks. The investigated factors, involved in activation of the complement and coagulation cascades, are undoubtedly important players in the events investigated, influencing disease/treatment course and outcome and also being influenced by disease itself and therapeutic procedures. Our data indicate multiple MBL involvements. We found its primary deficiency to be associated with MM risk but not hospital infections during cytopenia. Moreover, high MBL-conferring genotypes and high serum MBL were to some extent associated with adverse effects. Later, during follow-up, MBL deficiency seemed to predict higher morbidity and mortality due to infections. Additionally, we reported the first possible clinical association of a *MBL2* 3′-UTR polymorphism (protective effect of "gt1" from lymphoma) in Caucasians.

AUTHOR CONTRIBUTIONS

MC, KJ, AW, ASŚ co-authored the project and designed the study. ASŚ and MC planned and supervised experimental work which was done by ASŚ, AS, MM, AS-P, ŁE, and KK. AW, SG, and KJ supervised qualification and recruitment of patients and/or controls. MN, IM, AS-K, MS-K, KM, OB, and AG were responsible for patients' qualification, taking and collecting samples as well as collecting clinical data/follow-up. MLK and AG qualified controls, provided DNA/serum samples and corresponding clinical data. ST and JCJ produced anti-CL-10 and anti-MASP-2 monoclonal antibodies and discussed the data. MC and MM performed the statistical analysis. AS revised the data. MC wrote the original draft of the paper. All authors contributed to the manuscript revision/correction and approved the version to be submitted.

FUNDING

This work was supported by National Science Centre, Poland, grant UMO-2013/11/B/NZ6/01739.

ACKNOWLEDGMENTS

We are very grateful to Dr David C. Kilpatrick for critical reading of the manuscript and helpful discussion.

REFERENCES

1. Hari P. Recent advances in understanding multiple myeloma. *Hematol Oncol Stem Cell Ther*. (2017) 10:267–71. doi: 10.1016/j.hemonc.2017.05.005
2. Stevenson JD, Wall C, Patel A, Lim J. Multiple myeloma: a review. *Orthop Trauma* (2014) 28:187–93. doi: 10.1016/j.mporth.2014.05.007
3. Rölling C, Knap S, Bornhäuser M. Multiple myeloma. *Lancet* (2015) 385:2197–208. doi: 10.1016/S0140-6736(14)60493-1
4. Kumar SK, Rajkumar V, Kyle RA, van Duin M, Sonneveld P, Mateos MV, et al. Multiple myeloma. *Nat Rev Dis Primers* (2017) 3:17046:doi: 10.1038/nrdp.2017.46.
5. Brigle K, Rogers B. Pathobiology and diagnosis of multiple myeloma. *Semin Oncol Nurs*. (2017) 33:225–36. doi: 10.1016/j.soncn.2017.05.012
6. Shanbhag S, Ambinder AF. Hodgkin lymphoma: a review and update on recent progress. *CA Cancer J Clin*. (2018) 68:116–32. doi: 10.3322/caac.21438
7. Pileri SA, Ascani S, Leoncini L, Sabattini E, Zinzani PL, Piccaluga PP, et al. Hodgkin's lymphoma: the pathologist's viewpoint. *J Clin Pathol*. (2002) 55:162–76.
8. Townsend W, Linch D. Hodgkin's lymphoma in adults. *Lancet* (2012) 380:836–47. doi: 10.1016/S0140-6736(12)60035-X
9. Watkins MP, Fanale MA, Bartlett NL. SOHO state of the art updates and next questions: Hodgkin lymphoma. *Clin Lymphoma Myeloma Leuk*. (2018) 18:81–90. doi: 10.1016/j.clml.2018.01.001
10. Ninkovic S, Lambert J. Non-Hodgkin lymphoma. *Medicine* (2017) 45:297–304. doi: 10.1016/j.mpmed.2017.02.008
11. Warzocha K, Lech-Marańda E. Diagnosis and treatment of non-Hodgkin lymphomas. *Post N Med*. (2011) XXIV:567–76. Available online at: http://www.pnmedycznych.pl/wp-content/uploads/2014/09/pnm_2011_567_576.pdf
12. Shankland KR, Armitage JO, Hancock BW. Non-Hodgkin lymphoma. *Lancet* (2012) 380:848–57. doi: 10.1016/S0140-6736(12)60605-9
13. Lowry L, Linch D. Non-Hodgkin's lymphoma. *Medicine* (2013) 41:282–9. doi: 10.1016/j.mpmed.2013.03.008
14. Skarbek P, Turner D, Seftel M. Epidemiology of non-Hodgkin lymphoma. *Transfus Apher Sci*. (2013) 49:133–8. doi: 10.1016/j.transci.2013.07.014
15. Armitage JO, Gascoine RD, Lunning MA, Cavalli F. Non-Hodgkin lymphoma. *Lancet* (2017) 390:298–310. doi: 10.1016/S0140-6736(16)32407-2
16. Terpos E, on behalf of the International Myeloma Society. Multiple myeloma: clinical updates from the American Society of Hematology Annual Meeting 2016. *Clin Lymphoma Myeloma Leuk*. (2017) 17:329–39. doi: 10.1016/j.clml.2017.02.010
17. Safdar A, Armstrong D. Infections in patients with hematologic neoplasms and hematopoietic stem cell transplantation: neutropenia, humoral, and splenic defects. *Clin Infect Dis*. (2011) 53:798–06. doi: 10.1093/cid/cir492
18. Khayr W, Haddad RY, Noor SA. Infections in hematological malignancies. *Dis Mon*. (2012) 58:239–49. doi: 10.1016/j.disamonth.2012.01.001
19. Balletto E, Mikulska M. Bacterial infections in hematopoietic stem cell transplant recipients. *Mediterr J Hematol Infect Dis*. (2015) 7:e2015045. doi: 10.4084/MJHID.2015.045
20. Ogonek J, Kraij Juric M, Ghimire S, Varanasi PR, Holler E, Greinix H, et al. Immune reconstitution after allogeneic stem cell transplantation. *Front Immunol*. (2016) 7:507. doi: 10.3389/fimmu.2016.00507.
21. Pankratova OS, Chukhlovin AB. Time course of immune recovery and viral reactivation following hematopoietic stem cell transplantation. *Cell Therap Transplant*. (2016) 5:32–42. doi: 10.18620/ctt-1866-8836-2016-5-4-32-43
22. Ruhnke M, Arnold R, Gastmeier P. Infection control issues in patients with haematological malignancies in the era of multidrug-resistant bacteria. *Lancet Oncol*. (2014) 15:e606-9. doi: 10.1016/S1470-2045(14)70344-4
23. Markiewski M, Lambris JD. Is complement good or bad for cancer patients? a new perspective on an old dilemma. *Trends Immunol*. (2009) 30:286–92. doi: 10.1016/j.it.2009.04.002
24. Swierzko AS, Kilpatrick DC, Cedzynski M. Mannan-binding lectin in malignancy. *Mol Immunol*. (2012) 55:16–21. doi: 10.1016/j.molimm.2012.09.005
25. Kjaer TR, Le LTM, Pedersen JS, Sander B, Golas MM, Jensenius JC, et al. Structural insights into the initiating complex of the lectin pathway of complement activation. *Structure* (2015) 23:342–51. doi: 10.1016/j.str.2014.10.024
26. Henriksen ML, Madsen KL, Skjoedt K, Hansen S. Calcium-sensitive immunoaffinity chromatography: gentle and highly specific retrieval of a scarce plasma antigen, collectin-LK (CL-LK). *J Immunol Methods* (2014) 413:25–31. doi: 10.1016/j.jim.2014.07.006
27. Hansen SW, Ohtani K, Roy N, Wakamiya N. The collectins CL-L1, CL-K1 and CL-P1 and their roles in complement and innate immunity. *Immunobiology* (2016) 221:1058–67. doi: 10.1016/j.imbio.2016.05.012
28. Bernig T, Taylor JG, Foster CB, Staats B, Yeager M, Chanock SJ. Sequence analysis of the mannose-binding lectin (*MBL2*) gene reveals a high degree of heterozygosity with evidence of selection. *Genes Immun*. (2004) 5:461–76. doi: 10.1038/sj.gene.6364116
29. Seyfarth J, Garred P, Madsen HO. The "involution" of mannose-binding lectin. *Hum Mol Genet*. (2005) 14:2859–69. doi: 10.1093/hmg/ddi318
30. Verdu P, Barreiro LB, Patin E, Gessain A, Cassar O, Kidd JR, et al. Evolutionary insights into the high worldwide prevalence of *MBL2* deficiency alleles. *Hum Mol Genet*. (2006) 15:2650–8. doi: 10.1093/hmg/ddl193
31. Van de Geijn FE, Dolhain RJEM, van Rijs W, Willemsen SP, Hazes JMW, de Groot CJM. Mannose-binding lectin genotypes are associated with shorter gestational age. an evolutionary advantage of low MBL production genotypes? *Mol Immunol*. (2008) 45:1514–8. doi: 10.1016/j.molimm.2007.08.021
32. Tomaiuolo R, Ruocco A, Salapete C, Carru C, Baggio G, Franceschi C, et al Activity of mannose-binding lectin in centenarians. *Aging Cell* (2012) 11:394–400. doi: 10.1111/j.1474-9726.2012.00793.x
33. Scorza M, Liguori R, Elce A, Salvatore F, Castaldo G. Biological role of mannose-binding lectin: from newborns to centenarians. *Clin Chim Acta* (2015) 451(Pt A):78–81. doi: 10.1016/j.cca.2015.03.007
34. Peterslund NA, Koch C, Jensenius JC, Thiel S. Association between deficiency of mannose-binding lectin and severe infections after chemotherapy. *Lancet* (2001) 358:637–8. doi: 10.1016/S0140-6736(01)05785-3
35. Bak-Romaniszyn L, Szala A, Sokolowska A, Mierzwa G, Czerwionka-Szaflarska M, Swierzko AS, et al. Mannan-binding lectin deficiency in pediatric patients with inflammatory bowel disease. *Scand J Gastroenterol*. (2011) 46:1275–8. doi: 10.3109/00365521.2011.594087
36. Weckx S, Del-Favero J, Rademakers R, Claes L, Cruts M, De Jonghe P, et al. NovoSNP, a novel computational tool for sequence variation discovery. *Genome Res*. (2005) 15:436–42. doi: 10.1101/gr.2754005
37. Swierzko ASt, Cedzynski M, Domzalska-Popadiuk I, MacDonald SL, Borkowska-Klos M, et al. Mannan-binding lectin-associated serine protease-2 (MASP-2) in a large cohort of neonates and its clinical associations. *Mol Immunol*. (2009) 46:1696–701. doi: 10.1016/j.molimm.2009.02.022
38. Cedzynski M, Szemraj J, Swierzko AS, Bak-Romaniszyn L, Banasik M, Zeman K, et al. Mannan-binding lectin insufficiency in children with recurrent infections of the respiratory system. *Clin Exp Immunol*. (2004) 136:304–11. doi: 10.1111/j.1365-2249.2004.02453.x
39. Presanis JS, Hajela K, Ambrus G, Gal P, Sim RB. Differential substrate and inhibitor profiles for human MASP-1 and MASP-2. *Mol Immunol*. (2004) 40:921–9. doi: 10.1016/j.molimm.2003.10.013
40. Swierzko ASt, Szala A, Sawicki S, Szemraj J, Sniadecki M, Sokolowska A, et al. Mannose-Binding Lectin (MBL) and MBL-associated serine protease-2 (MASP-2) in women with malignant and benign ovarian tumours. *Cancer Immunol Immunother*. (2014) 11:1129–40. doi: 10.1007/s00262-014-1579-y
41. Petersen SV, Thiel S, Jensen L, Steffensen R, Jensenius JC. An assay for the mannan-binding lectin pathway of complement activation. *J Immunol Methods* (2001) 257:107–16. doi: 10.1016/S0022-1759(01)00453-7
42. Swierzko ASt, Szala A, Cedzynski M, Domzalska-Popadiuk I, Borkowska-Klos M, Jopek A, et al. Mannan-binding lectin genotypes and genotype-phenotype relationships in a large cohort of Polish neonates. *Hum Immunol*. (2009) 70:68–72. doi: 10.1016/j.humimm.2008.10.004
43. Swierzko ASt, Atkinson APM, Cedzynski M, MacDonald SL, Szala A, Domzalska-Popadiuk I, et al. Two factors of the lectin pathway of complement, L-ficolin and mannan-binding lectin, and their associations with prematurity, low birthweight and infections in a large cohort of Polish neonates. *Mol Immunol*. (2009) 46:551–8. doi: 10.1016/j.molimm.2008.07.025
44. Axelgaard E, Jensen L, Dyrlund TF, Nielsen HJ, Enghild JJ, Thiel S, et al. Investigations on collectin liver 1. *J Biol Chem*. (2013) 288:23407-20. doi: 10.1074/jbc.M113.492603

45. Moller-Kristensen M, Jensenius JC, Jensen L, Thielens N, Rossi V, Arlaud G, et al. Levels of mannan-binding lectin-associated serine protease-2 in healthy individuals. *J Immunol Methods* (2003) 282:159–67. doi: 10.1016/j.jim.2003.08.012
46. Molle I, Peterslund NA, Thiel S, Steffensen R. *MBL2* polymorphism and risk of severe infections in multiple myeloma patients receiving high-dose melphalan and autologous stem cell transplantation. *Bone Marrow Transpl.* (2006) 38:555–60. doi: 10.1038/sj.bmt.1705466
47. Molle I, Steffensen R, Thiel S, Peterslund NA. Chemotherapy-related infections in patients with multiple myeloma: associations with mannan-binding lectin genotypes. *Eur J Hematol.* (2006) 77:19–26. doi: 10.1111/j.1600-0609.2006.00669.x
48. Mullighan CG, Heatley SL, Danner S, Dean MM, Doherty K, Hahn U, et al. Mannose-binding lectin status is associated with risk of major infection following myeloablative sibiling allogeneic hemopoietic stem cell transplantation. *Blood* (2008) 112:2120–8. doi: 10.1182/blood-2007-07-100222
49. Horiuchi T, Gondo H, Miyagawa H, Otsuka J, Inaba S, Nagafuji K, et al. Association of MBL gene polymorphisms with major bacterial infection in patients treated with high-dose chemotherapy and autologous PBSCT. *Genes Immun.* (2005) 6:162–6. doi: 10.1038/sj.gene.6364165
50. Wong M, Ohrmalm L, Brollden K, Aust C, Hibberd M, Tolfvenstam T. Mannose-binding lectin 2 polymorphisms do not influence frequency and type of infection in adults with chemotherapy induced neutropaenia. *PLoS ONE* (2012) 7:e30819. doi: 10.1371/journal.pone.0030819
51. Bergmann OJ, Christiansen M, Laursen I, Bang P, Hansen NE, Ellegaard J, et al. Low levels of mannose-binding lectin do not affect occurrence of severe infections or duration of fever in acute myeloid leukaemia during remission induction therapy. *Eur J Haematol.* (2003) 70:91–7. doi: 10.1034/j.1600-0609.2003.00012.x
52. Kilpatrick DC, McLintock LA, Allan EK, Kopland M, Fujita T, Jordanides NE, et al. No strong relationship between mannan binding lectin or plasma ficolins and chemotherapy-related infections. *Clin Exp Immunol.* (2003) 134:279–84. doi: 10.1046/j.1365-2249.2003.02284.x
53. Bernig T, Boersma BJ, Howe TM, Welch R, Yadavalli S, Staats B, et al. The mannose-binding lectin (*MBL2*) haplotype and breast cancer: an association study in African-American and Caucasian women. *Carcinogenesis* (2007) 28:828–36. doi: 10.1093/carcin/bgl198
54. Zanetti KA, Haznadar M, Welsh JA, Robles AI, Ryan BM, McClary AC, et al. 3'UTR and functional secretor haplotypes in mannose-binding lectin 2 are associated with increased colon cancer risk in African Americans. *Cancer Res.* (2012) 72:1467–77. doi: 10.1158/0008-5472.CAN-11-3073
55. Bernig T, Breunis W, Brouwer N, Hutchinson A, Welch R, Roos D, et al. An analysis of genetic variation across the *MBL2* locus in Dutch Caucasians indicates that 3' haplotypes could modify circulating levels of mannose-binding lectin. *Hum Genet.* (2005) 118:404–15. doi: 10.1007/s00439-005-0053-5
56. Kalia N, Sharma A, Kaur M, Singh Kamboj S, Singh J. A comprehensive in silico analysis of non-synonymous and regulatory SNPs of human *MBL2* gene. *SpringerPlus* (2016) 5:811. doi: 10.1186/s40064-016-2 543-4
57. Machiela MJ, Chanock SJ. LDlink a web-based application for exploring population-specific haplotype structure and linking correlated alleles of possible functional variants. *Bioinformatics* (2015) 31:3555–7. doi: 10.1093/bioinformatics/btv402
58. Adamiak M, Abdelbaset-Ismail A, Suszynska M, Abdel-Latif A, Ratajczak J, Ratajczak MZ. Novel evidence that the mannan-binding lectin pathway of complement activation plays a pivotal role in triggering mobilization of hematopoietic stem/progenitor cells by activation of both the complement and coagulation cascades. *Leukemia* (2017) 31:262–65. doi: 10.1038/leu.2016.278
59. Adamiak M, Abdel-Latif A, Ratajczak MZ. Mannan binding lectin triggers mobilization of hematopoietic cells. *Oncotarget* (2017) 43:73368–9. doi: 10.18632/oncotarget.20705
60. Borkowska S, Suszynska M, Mierzejewska K, Ismail A, Budkowska M, Salata D, et al. Novel evidence that crosstalk between the complement, coagulation and fibrinolysis proteolytic cascades is involved in mobilization of hematopoietic stem/progenitor cells (HSPCs). *Leukemia* (2014) 28:2148–54. doi: 10.1038/leu.2014.115
61. Zehnder A, Fisch U, Hirt A, Niggli FK, Simon A, Ozsahin H, et al. Prognosis in pediatric hematologic malignancies is associated with serum concentration of mannose-binding lectin-associated serine protease-2 (MASP-2). *Pediatr Blood Cancer* (2009) 53:53–7. doi: 10.1002/pbc.22028
62. Hu W, Bassig BA, Xu J, Zheng T, Zhang Y, Berndt SI, et al. Polymorphisms in pattern-recognition genes in the innate immunity system and risk of non-Hodgkin lymphoma. *Environ Mol Mutagen* (2013) 54:72–7. doi: 10.1002/em.21739
63. Troldborg A, Hansen A, Hansen SWK, Jensenius JC, Stengaard-Pedersen K, Thiel S. Lectin complement pathway proteins in healthy individuals. *Clin Exp Immunol.* (2016) 188:138–47. doi: 10.1111/cei.12909

14

Sickening or Healing the Heart? The Association of Ficolin-1 and Rheumatic Fever

Sandra Jeremias Catarino [1], ***Fabiana Antunes Andrade*** [1], ***Angelica Beate Winter Boldt*** [1,2], ***Luiza Guilherme*** [3] ***and Iara Jose Messias-Reason*** [1*]

[1] Molecular Immunopathology Laboratory, Department of Medical Pathology, Clinical Hospital, Federal University of Paraná, Curitiba, Brazil, [2] Human Molecular Genetics Laboratory, Department of Genetics, Federal University of Paraná, Curitiba, Brazil, [3] Heart Institute (InCor), School of Medicine, University of São Paulo, São Paulo, Brazil

***Correspondence:**
Iara Jose Messias-Reason
iarareason@hc.ufpr.br

Rheumatic fever (RF) and its subsequent progression to rheumatic heart disease (RHD) are chronic inflammatory disorders prevalent in children and adolescents in underdeveloped countries, and a contributing factor for high morbidity and mortality rates worldwide. Their primary cause is oropharynx infection by *Streptococcus pyogenes*, whose acetylated residues are recognized by ficolin-1. This is the only membrane-bound, as well as soluble activator molecule of the complement lectin pathway (LP). Although LP genetic polymorphisms are associated with RF, *FCN1* gene's role remains unknown. To understand this role, we haplotyped five *FCN1* promoter polymorphisms by sequence-specific amplification in 193 patients (138 with RHD and 55, RF only) and 193 controls, measuring ficolin-1 serum concentrations in 78 patients and 86 controls, using enzyme-linked immunosorbent assay (ELISA). Patients presented lower ficolin-1 serum levels ($p < 0.0001$), but did not differ according to cardiac commitment. Control's genotype distribution was in the Hardy-Weinberg equilibrium. Four alleles (rs2989727: *c.−1981A*, rs10120023: *c.−542A*, rs10117466: *c.−144A*, and rs10858293: *c.33T*), all associated with increased *FCN1* gene expression in whole blood or adipose subcutaneous tissue ($p = 0.000001$), were also associated with increased protection against the disease. They occur within the **3C2* haplotype, associated with an increased protection against RF ($OR = 0.41$, $p < 0.0001$) and with higher ficolin-1 levels in patient serum ($p = 0.03$). In addition, major alleles of these same polymorphisms comprehend the most primitive **1* haplotype, associated with increased susceptibility to RF ($OR = 1.76$, $p < 0.0001$). Nevertheless, instead of having a clear-cut protective role, the minor *c.−1981A* and *c.−144A* alleles were also associated with additive susceptibility to valvar stenosis and mitral insufficiency ($OR = 3.75$, $p = 0.009$ and $OR = 3.37$, $p = 0.027$, respectively). All associations were independent of age, sex or ethnicity. Thus, minor *FCN1* promoter variants may play a protective role against RF, by encouraging bacteria elimination as well as increasing gene expression and protein levels. On the other hand, they may also predispose the patients to RHD symptoms, by probably contributing to chronic inflammation and tissue injury, thus emphasizing the dual importance of ficolin-1 in both conditions.

Keywords: *FCN1*, ficolin-1, polymorphism, haplotype, rheumatic fever, rheumatic heart disease

INTRODUCTION

Rheumatic fever (RF) is an immune-mediated disease occurring in genetically susceptible individuals, as a sequelae of group A (GAS) *Streptococcus pyogenes* pharyngitis. It affects predominantly children and adolescents in low-income and developing countries, where it remains a considerable public health problem (1, 2).

Five major manifestations reflect target tissue involvement in RF, including synovium (inflammatory arthritis), heart valves (endocarditis), brain (Sydenham's chorea), skin (erythema marginatum), and subcutaneous tissue (nodules). Repeated or severe RF episodes can result in permanent damage to the heart valves, leading to rheumatic heart disease (RHD), the most common acquired cardiovascular disease in young adults (3, 4). Rheumatic heart disease (RHD) is associated with high morbidity and mortality, causing 9 million disability-adjusted life years lost, 33 million cases (5) and 275,000 deaths each year (6). This multifactorial disorder involves multiple genetic and environmental factors, not yet fully elucidated. Well-designed case-control studies strive to unravel the genetic susceptibility to this disease, given that the only genome-wide association study done with RHD has rendered no relevant results (7).

Autoimmunity is known to play a role in the pathogenesis of RF and RHD, with tissue damage being mediated by autoantibodies resulting from molecular mimicry between GAS and heart tissue proteins. It has been shown that GAS molecules such as N-acetyl-β-D-glucosamine (GlcNAc) and M protein display cross reactivity with valve and myocellular contractile proteins of the host. GlcNAc is the immunodominant cell wall antigen of GAS, recognized by ficolins, molecules that comprise important pattern-recognition receptors (PRRs) of the complement (2, 5, 8, 9).

The complement system plays an important role, both in the defense against GAS infection, as well as in the development of autoimmunity in RHD. This system promptly responds to any pathogen, bridging innate and adaptive immune responses (10–14). Ficolins initiate one of the three complement activation pathways, known as the lectin pathway, along with collectins, as mannose-binding lectin (MBL). They occur in oligomeric structures of a basic homotrimer, where each chain is formed by a collagenous strand and a C-terminal fibrinogen-like recognition domain. The oligomers are complexed with homodimers of serine proteases (MASP-1 or MASP-2). Ficolin oligomers bind specific patterns of acetylated residues on the surface of pathogens or altered cells (8, 15). MASP-1 then autoactivates, transactivating MASP-2 leading to subsequent cleavage of downstream complement components [reviewed by Boldt et al. (16)]. The lectin pathway, along with the classical and alternative pathways, converge at the cleavage of C3 and C5, with subsequent C3b opsonization and pathogen phagocytosis or its destruction by membrane attack complex (MAC) pores on the cell membrane (17).

Three human ficolins have been described: ficolin-1 (M-ficolin), ficolin-2 (L-ficolin), and ficolin-3 (H-ficolin, Hakata antigen) (15). Unlike any other PRRs, ficolin-1 is expressed by myeloid cells, being found in monocytes, neutrophils and macrophages of the lung and spleen (8). It is also the only one that occurs in both soluble form (0.05–1.0 μg/mL in serum) and on the cell membrane (18–20). Apart from other acetylated residues, ficolin-1 has the unique ability to bind sialic acid to capsular polysaccharides of pathogens including *Streptococcus agalactiae,* as well as to the surface of immune cells (21, 22).

Ficolin-1 is encoded by the *FCN1* gene on chromosome 9q34 and contains nine exons. Among the several SNPs described for the *FCN1* gene, at least eight are associated with Ficolin-1 levels, four of them are located in the promoter and one in the first exon (23). Polymorphisms of collectin and ficolin genes have been repeatedly associated with infectious and autoimmune diseases (23–28). *FCN1* polymorphisms were associated with increased fatal outcome in patients with systemic inflammation (29), susceptibility to rheumatoid arthritis (28) and leprosy (26). Gene polymorphisms of the lectin pathway have already been associated with RF in case-control association studies with MBL (30–32), Ficolin-2 (33), and MASP-2 (34). Within this context, we are the first to investigate a membrane-bound molecule of the lectin pathway, able to activate the complement. More specifically, we evaluated the association of *FCN1* polymorphisms and haplotypes, as well as Ficolin-1 serum levels, with the susceptibility to RF and RHD.

MATERIALS AND METHODS

Subjects and Samples

This study was approved by the local medical ethics committee (CEP/HC 2658.265/2011-11). All patients and control subjects provided written informed consent in accordance with the *Declaration of Helsinki.* We investigated a total of 193 patients with a history of RF, all of them with ASO (anti streptolysin O) titers higher than 250 units, characterizing a precedent streptococcal infection and diagnosed according to Jones' modified criteria; 55 (28.5%) males and 138 (71.5%) females; with a mean age of 37 years (range = 7–76 years). Among them, 138 had RHD, confirmed by the transthoracic echocardiogram showing rheumatic involvement of the mitral or aortic valves (**Table 1**), and 55 did not present RHD, but had RF history and were designated as "rheumatic fever only" (RFo) patients. None of the patients presented other inflammatory disease, neoplasia, infective endocarditis, or other infections at the time their blood was collected. Values of high-sensitivity C-reactive protein (hs-CRP) levels, C3 levels and C4 levels, previously published by our group, are shown in **Table 1** (30). The control group included 193 blood donors from The Clinical Hospital of the University Federal of Paraná, with a mean age of 37 years (range = 18–64 years), 68 (35%) males, and 125 (65%) females.

Abbreviations: RF, Rheumatic Fever; RHD, Rheumatic Heart Disease; RFo, Rheumatic Fever only; *FCN1*, ficolin-1 gene; LP, Lectin Pathway; CRP, C-Reactive Protein; MAC, Membrane Attack Complex; GAS, Group A *Streptococcus*; LD, Linkage Disequilibrium; GlcNAc, N-acetyl-β-D-glucosamine; MBL, Mannose-binding lectin.

FCN1 Genotyping

DNA extraction from peripheral blood was performed using The QIAamp DNA Blood Mini Kit, QIAGEN (Hilden, Germany), following the manufacturer's instructions. The genotype method was adapted from a previously described multiplex PCR-SSP (sequence-specific amplification) method (30). Five *FCN1* single nucleotide polymorphisms (SNPs) were genotyped: rs2989727 SNP (*c.-1981G > A*) in the distal *FCN1* promoter, rs10120023 (*c.-542G > A*), rs17039495 (*c.-399G > A*), rs10117466 (c.*-144C > A*), and rs10858293 (*c.+33T > G*) SNPs in the proximal *FCN1* promoter, with primers listed in **Table S1**.

TABLE 1 | Clinical characteristics of patients.

Total patients	193
Males	55 (25.5%)
Females	138 (71.5%)
Mean age	37 years
Rheumatic fever only (RFo)	55 (28.5%)
Rheumatic heart disease (RHD)	138 (71.5%)
Mitral stenosis	83 (60.1%)
Aortic stenosis	25 (18.1%)
Tricuspid stenosis	4 (2.9%)
Mitral insufficiency	67 (48.5%)
Aortic insufficiency	41 (29.7%)
Tricuspid insufficiency	31 (22.5%)
hs-CRP level (mg/dL)	0.83* (0.03–26.10)
C3 level# (mg/dL)	109.2* (50.3–198)
C4 level# (mg/dL)	22.7* (6.82–45.4)

*hs-CRP, high-sensitivity C-reactive protein. Normal reference values for hs-CRP: <0.1 mg/dL, for C3: 82-160 mg/dL, for C4: 12-36 mg/dL. *mean; #Data already published by Schafranski et al. (30).*

*FCN1*_Prom-1981Af or *FCN1*_Prom-1981Gf were conjugated with the *FCN1*_*Prom_r* reverse primer to generate a fragment of 729 bp. PCR conditions were as follows: 0.2 µM of SSP primers, 1X Coral Load PCR buffer (Qiagen, Hilden, Germany), 1.6 mM $MgCl_2$ (Qiagen, Hilden, Germany), 0.5% glycerol, 0.2 mM deoxyribonucleoside triphosphate (dNTP) (Invitrogen, São Paulo, Brazil), 0.03 U/uL of Taq polymerase (Invitrogen, São Paulo, Brazil), 0.1 µg/mL DNA, ultrapure water for 15 µL. The amplification protocol starts with a 5 min denaturation step at 94°C, followed by 10 cycles of 20 s at 94°C, 30 s at 60°C, and 30 s at 72°C; 10 cycles of 20 s at 94°C, 30 s at 56°C, and 30 s at 72°C; 10 cycles of 20 s at 94°C, 30 s at 52°C, and 30 s at 72°C, concluding with 5 min at 72°C in the final DNA extension step.

*FCN1*_Prom-542Af or *FCN1*_Prom-542Gf were conjugated with the *FCN1*_Prom-144Ar or *FCN1*_Prom-144Cr to generate a fragment of 434 bp. PCR conditions differed from those previously mentioned as follows: 0.6 µM of SSP primers, 1.7 mM $MgCl_2$, and 1.5% glycerol. The amplification protocol differed from the previous one only by the annealing primer temperatures, which were 57°C in the first 10, 55°C in the next 10, and 53°C in the last 10 cycles.

*FCN1*_Prom-399Af or *FCN1*_Prom-399Gf were conjugated with the *FCN1*_Prom+33Gr or *FCN1*_Prom+33Tr to generate a fragment of 470 bp. PCR conditions differed from those previously noticed, as follows: 0.4 µM of SSP primers, 1.75 mM $MgCl_2$, 0.5% glycerol. The amplification protocol differed from the first one only by the annealing primer temperatures, which were 58°C in the first 10, 56°C in the next 10 and 54°C in the final 15 cycles.

Interpretation was based on the electrophoretic pattern of the amplified fragments, on agarose gels 1.5% stained with Sybrsafe (Invitrogen, São Paulo, Brazil). This bispecific PCR-SSP approach allows the identification of 8 haplotypes: **1 (GGGCG)*, **3A (AGGCG)*, **3A.3C2.A (AGGCT)*, **3A.3C2.B (AGACT)*,

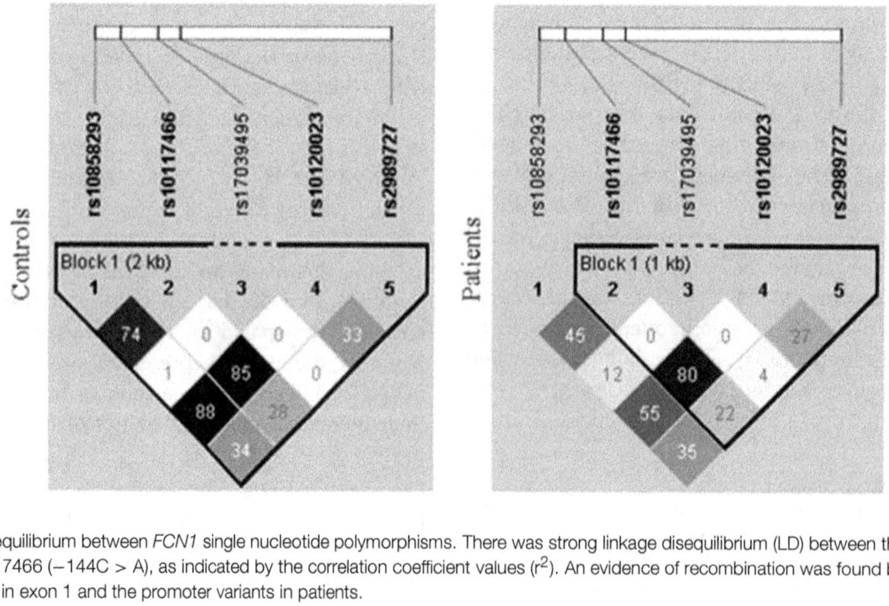

FIGURE 1 | Linkage disequilibrium between *FCN1* single nucleotide polymorphisms. There was strong linkage disequilibrium (LD) between the SNPs rs10120023 (−542G > A) and rs10117466 (−144C > A), as indicated by the correlation coefficient values (r^2). An evidence of recombination was found between the SNP rs10858293 (+33T > G) in exon 1 and the promoter variants in patients.

TABLE 2 | *FCN1* allele, genotype and haplotype frequencies and associations with RF.

SNP	**Controls *N* = 193 (%)**	**Patients *N* = 193 (%)**	**RFo patients *N* = 55 (%)**	**RHD patients *N* = 138 (%)**	Model	**Patients vs. controls OR [95% CI]**	***P* value (*Q* = 0.00185)**	**mRNA expression NES (GTex)**
rs2989727 (*c.−1981G > A*)	230 (59.6)	177 (45.9)	53 (48.2)	124 (44.9)	*A* x *G* *	**0.57 [0.43–0.76]**	**0.0002**	–
G/G	33 (17.1)	53 (27.5)	15 (27.3)	38 (27.5)	*A/A* x _	**0.42 [0.26–0.66]**	**<0.0001**	–
G/A	90 (46.6)	103 (53.4)	27 (49.1)	76 (55.1)	*A/_* x *G/G*	0.54 [0.33-0.89]	0.014 (ns)	–
A/A	70 (36.3)	37 (19.1)	13 (23.6)	24 (17.4)	*A/A* > *A/G* > *G/G*	**0.57 [0.42–0.76]**	**<0.0001**	0.32 (*P* = 5.5e−10) in AS
rs10120023 (*c.−542G > A*)	127 (32.9)	73 (18.9)	27 (24.5)	46 (16.7)	*A* x *G* *	**0.48 [0.34–0.66]**	**<0.0001**	–
G/G	84 (43.5)	132 (68.4)	33 (60.0)	99 (71.7)	*A/A* x __	–	ns	–
G/A	91 (47.2)	49 (25.4)	17 (30.1)	32 (23.2)	*A/_* x *G/G*	**0.36 [0.24–0.55]**	**<0.0001**	–
A/A	18 (9.3)	12 (6.2)	5 (9.9)	7 (5.1)	*A/A* > *A/G* > *G/G*	**0.49 [0.35–0.68]**	**<0.0001**	0.21 (*P* = 7.4e−8) in WB 0.24 (*P* = 0.000001) in AS
rs17039495 (*c.−399G > A*)	3 (0.8)	14 (3.6)	3 (2.7)	11 (4.0)	*A* x *G* *	4.8 [1.37–16.86]	0.012 (ns)	–
G/G	190 (98.4)	179 (92.7)	52 (94.5)	127 (92.0)	*A/_* x *G/G*	4.7 [1.3–16.7]	0.017 (ns)	–
G/A	3 (1.6)	14 (7.3)	3 (5.5)	11 (8.0)	–	–	–	–
rs10117466 (*c.−144C > A*)	114 (29.5)	61 (15.8)	23 (20.9)	38 (13.8)	*A* x *C* *	**0.45 [0.32–0.64]**	**0.000007**	–
C/C	92 (47.7)	141 (73.0)	36 (65.4)	105 (76.1)	*A/A* x __	–	ns	–
C/A	88 (45.6)	43 (22.3)	15 (27.3)	28 (20.3)	*A/_* x *C/C*	**0.36 [0.21–0.60]**	**<0.0001**	–
A/A	13 (6.7)	9 (4.7)	4 (7.3)	5 (3.6)	*A/A* > *A/C* > *C/C*	**0.53 [0.36–0.78]**	**0.001**	0.21 (*P* = 1.1e−7) in WB 0.24 (*P* = 0.000012) in AS
rs10858293 (*c.33G > T*)	131 (33.9)	90 (23.3)	29 (26.4)	61 (22.1)	*T* x *G* *	0.59 [0.43–0.81]	**0.0014**	–
G/G	83 (43.0)	114 (59.1)	30 (54.5)	84 (60.8)	*T/T* x __	0.49 [0.23–1.04]	0.064 (ns)	–
G/T	89 (46.1)	68 (35.2)	21 (38.2)	47 (34.1)	*T/_* x *G/G*	0.52 [0.35–0.78]	0.002 (ns)	–
T/T	21 (10.9)	11 (6.7)	4 (7.3)	7 (5.1)	*T/T* > *T/G* > *G/G*	**0.59 [0.43–0.81]**	**0.001**	0.2 (*P* = 6.2e−7) in WB 0.26 (*P* = 0.0000011) in AS
HAPLOTYPES								
**1 (GGGCG)*	156 (40.4)	209 (54.1)	57 (51.9)	152 (55.1)	Haplotype	**1.74 (1.31–2.32)**	**0.0002**	–
					Recessive	1.8 [1.13–3.02]	0.014 (ns)	–
					Dominant	**2.39 [1.5–3.8]**	**<0.0001**	–
					Additive	**1.76 [1.31–2.37]**	**<0.0001**	–
**3A (AGGCG)*	96 (24.9)	79 (20.5)	20 (18.2)	59 (21.4)	Any	–	ns	–

(Continued)

TABLE 2 | Continued

SNP	Controls $N = 193$ (%)	Patients $N = 193$ (%)	RFo patients $N = 55$ (%)	RHD patients $N = 138$ (%)	Model	Patients vs. controls OR [95% CI]	*P* value ($Q = 0.00185$)	mRNA expression NES (GTex)
*3C2 (AAGAT)	111 (28.8)	55 (14.2)	20 (18.2)	35 (12.7)	Haplotype	**0.41 [0.29–0.59]**	**<0.0001**	–
					Recessive	0.37 [0.13–1.06]	0.063 (ns)	–
					Dominant	**0.34 [0.22–0.53]**	**<0.0001**	–
					Additive	**0.41 [0.28–0.59]**	**<0.0001**	–
*3A.3C2.B (AGACT)	3 (0.8)	14 (3.6)	3 (2.7)	11 (4.0)	Haplotype	4.81 (1.37–16.86)	0.0118 (ns)	–
					Dominant	4.701 [1.32–16.69]	0.017 (ns)	–
*3C1 (AAGCT)	13 (3.4)	10 (2.6)	3 (2.7)	7 (2.5)	Any	–	Ns	–
*3A.3C2.A (AGGCT)	4 (1.0)	11 (2.8)	3 (2.7)	8 (2.9)	Dominant	2.76 [0.86–8.86]	0.087	–
*3C2.3A (AAGAG)	3 (0.8)	6 (1.6)	3 (2.7)	3 (1.1)	Any	–	Ns	–
*3B2 (AAGCG)	0	2 (0.5)	1 (0.9)	1 (0.3)	Any	–	ns	–

NES, Normalized effect size; AS, adipose subcutaneous tissue; WB, whole blood; ns, not significant Bonferroni corrected significance level $q^* = 0.001851852$.
The values shown in bold correspond to significant values.

**3B2 (AAGCG), *3C1 (AAGCT), *3C2 (AAGAT), and *3C2.3A (AGGCG),* as previously described (26).

Ficolin-1 Measurement

Ficolin-1 serum concentrations were measured in 78 patients and 86 controls using enzyme-linked immunosorbent assay (ELISA) SEA786Hu Cloud-Clone Corp. (Texas, USA).

Statistics

Allele, haplotype and genotype frequencies were obtained by direct counting (the phase between distantly situated SNPs could be deduced due to the strong LD between the variants, and were verified with the Expectation-Maximization algorithm implemented in the PLINK software. Exact tests of Guo and Thompson for testing the hypothesis of Hardy-Weinberg equilibrium were accomplished using ARLEQUIN v.3.5.2.2 (http://cmpg.unibe.ch/software/arlequin35/). The investigated polymorphisms were evaluated for regulatory effects on gene expression, using information from The Genotype-Tissue Expression (GTEx) Project. Associations with alleles were tested by the Exact Fisher test using the SISA quantitative skill tables and including genotypes and haplotypes, by multivariate binary logistic regression with the software package STATA v. 9.2. Correction for associated demographic factors (sex, age) and clinical factors were applied in the reduced logistic regression model where sample size was adequate, and p-values $\leq 5\%$ were considered significant. Distributions of ficolin-1 levels were tested for normality with the Shapiro-Wilk test. Since ficolin-1 levels presented a non-normal distribution, the two-tailed Mann-Whitney test was used to compare ficolin-1 levels between groups (GraphPad Prism v.7.03).

RESULTS

FCN1 Alleles and Haplotypes Association With RF

Genotype distribution was in equilibrium with the Hardy-Weinberg model in both controls and patients, except for SNPs rs10120023 ($c.{-542G} > A$) and rs10117466 ($c.{-144C} > A$) in patients ($p = 0.017$ and $p = 0.024$, respectively). A total of eight haplotypes were found in patients and seven, in controls. The phase between the variants in the proximal promoter was determined with bispecific PCR-SSP and the phase of these variants with the SNP $c.{-1981G} > A$ could be deduced due to a strong linkage disequilibrium (LD). Evidence for recombination was found between the SNP rs10858293 ($c.33G > T$) in exon 1 and promoter variants in patients (**Figure 1**).

The *c.−1981A, c.−542A, c.−144A,* and *c.33T* alleles were associated with an increased level of protection against RF, presenting an additive effect with homozygotes protecting more than heterozygotes. All four are also known to be associated with higher *FCN1* expression in adipose subcutaneous tissue. Three of them present the same effect in peripheral blood cells (GTex portal) (35). All the protective alleles occur within the **3C2* haplotype (*AAGAT*). As expected, this haplotype was also associated with increased protection against RF under the additive model ($OR = 0.41$, $p < 0.0001$). On the other hand, the common alleles of these SNPs compose the phylogenetically ancestral *1 (GGGCG) haplotype, which was associated with increased susceptibility to RF ($OR = 1.76, p < 0.0001$, **Table 2**).

In contrast, the *c.−1981A* allele was associated with increased susceptibility to valvar stenosis (5/19 or 26.3% vs. 6/89 or 6.7% *A/A* homozygotes and 13/19 or 68.4% vs. 39/89 or 43.8% *A/G* heterozygotes in patients with moderate to severe, vs. light or no valvar stenosis, respectively: $OR = 3.75$ [95%CI = 1.39–10.15], $p = 0.009$). Similarly, the *c.−144A* allele presented an increased susceptibility effect for mitral insufficiency (2/12 or 16.7% vs. 1/75 or 1.3% *A/A* homozygotes and 1/12 or 8.3% vs. 4/75 or 5.3% *A/C* heterozygotes in patients with moderate to severe vs. light or no mitral insufficiency, respectively: $OR = 3.37$ [95%CI = 1.15–9.92], $p = 0.027$). Although no other allele or haplotype were associated either with RHD or other clinical manifestation, this may be due to the relatively small sample size of RHD patients in our setting.

Ficolin-1 Levels

Ficolin-1 serum levels were lower in patients (median: 800.5 ng/mL [324.6–1,715 ng/mL]), compared to controls (1,208 ng/mL [488–2,852 ng/mL, $p < 0.0001$), but did not differ between RHD and RFo patient groups (**Figure 2**).

Patients with the *1 (*GGGCG*) "susceptibility" haplotype presented lower ficolin-1 levels, than those with the *3C2 (*AAGAT*) "protective" haplotype ($p = 0.03$, medians 770.8 and 975.9 ng/mL, respectively) (**Figure 3**).

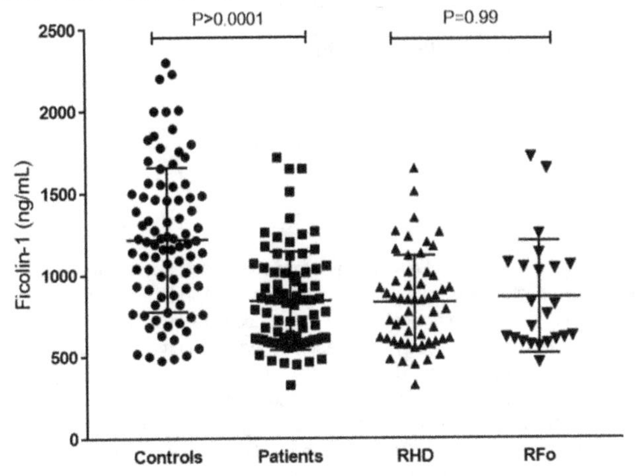

FIGURE 2 | Ficolin-1 serum levels in controls and RF patients. RHD, Rheumatic Heart Disease; RFo, Rheumatic Fever only (not present RHD).

DISCUSSION

The complement system plays an important role both in the defense against GAS infection, as well as in the development of RHD (28, 36, 37). Among studies focusing on complement genetic polymorphisms (30–34), this is the first considering the role of a complement membrane-bound molecule of the lectin pathway in the development of RF and RHD. Our results indicate that *FCN1* polymorphisms may play a dual role in the physiopathology of RF. On one hand, they increase resistance to GAS infection and on the other hand, predispose the patient to RHD symptoms, once the infection is established.

A protective role for *FCN1* promoter variants against RF has been observed (**Figure 4**). Among the investigated *FCN1* alleles, those four occurring within the *3C2 haplotype that were associated with RF protection and ficolin-1 levels have also been associated with higher *FCN1* gene expression (GTEx Portal) and ficolin-1 serum levels in other studies (23, 26, 29). Indeed, it has been suggested that the minor alleles *−542A* and *−144A* may facilitate the binding of transcription factors, causing amplified gene expression (29). Thus, it is conceivable that higher *FCN1* gene and protein expression could increase resistance against GAS infection due to ficolin-1 anti-bacterial properties. In fact ficolin-1 is able to bind sialic acid on Group B *Streptococcus* bacteria (20, 38) as well as GAS's carbohydrate A (GlcNAc) which is a preferable ficolin ligand. GAS recognition by ficolins may culminate in complement activation, despite the described complement evasion mechanisms of the bacteria, e.g., through C5a, as well as C2–C9 cleavage (39). Moreover, it is known that GAS infection occurs through fibronectin binding in the extracellular matrix (39). Fibronectin is also a ligand for ficolin-1 (40), thus competition for fibronectin binding sites may occur. Additionally, ficolin-1 anchors to GPCR43, a G-protein coupled receptor on monocytes. Ficolin-1/GPCR43 activation results in signal transduction through NFkB and interleukin-8 (IL8) gene expression. IL8 is a chemokine that attracts phagocytes to the infection site, enhancing bacterial elimination (20). Taken together, these events corroborate the eventual protective effect of ficolin-1 in the development of RF.

On the other hand, these *FCN1* variants associated with high ficolin-1 expression may contribute to excessive complement activation, leading to chronic inflammation and tissue injury, thereby predisposing the patient to RHD symptoms such as valvar stenosis and mitral insufficiency in the advanced phase of the disease. In addition, exposure to neoepitopes on bacteria-damaged valvar tissue would not only induce autoantibody production, but also promote complement activation with MAC deposition, thereby increasing tissue injury. C9, the last MAC complement, was indeed exclusively found in RHD patients with mitral stenosis, compared to control subjects (13). Thus, in the advanced phase of the disease, high ficolin-1 levels would probably not be beneficial. Even though ficolin-1 levels did not differ between RHD and RFo patients, it is possible that the quantification of ficolin-1 in serum does not reflect the levels of membrane-bound ficolin-1, and that the valvar damage could be instead related to this last ficolin-1 form. Keeping this balance—pathogen elimination vs. host preservation, has proven to be very difficult in circumstances where ineffective pathogen elimination induces chronic persistence of the infection with autoimmune features, as is the case of RF/RHD. This would explain other apparently opposite associations of ficolin-1, reported formerly in leprosy for *−542A*, *−144C*, and *+33T* (26), *−1981A* in rheumatoid arthritis (28) and earlier chronic *Pseudomonas aeruginosa* colonization in cystic fibrosis patients

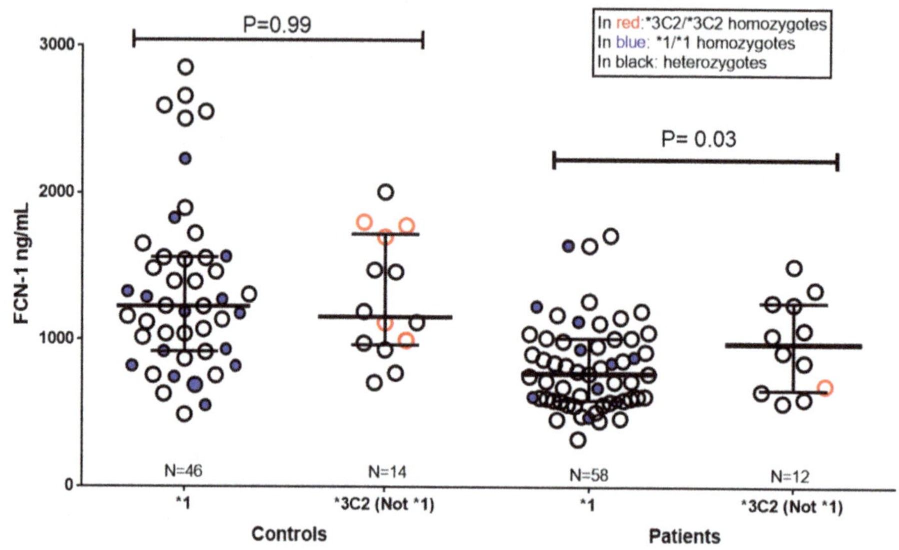

FIGURE 3 | Ficolin-1 serum levels in controls and RF patients, according to *FCN1* genotype. *1: carriers of the **1* "risk" haplotype (*GGGCG*). Not **1/*3C2*: carriers of **3C2* "protective" haplotype (*AAGAT*), but not of the **1* "risk" haplotype. In red: **3C2/*3C2* homozygotes. In blue: **1/*1* homozygotes. Subjects carrying the other FCN1 haplotypes are not represented in the figure (Controls $N = 26$, Patients $N = 8$).

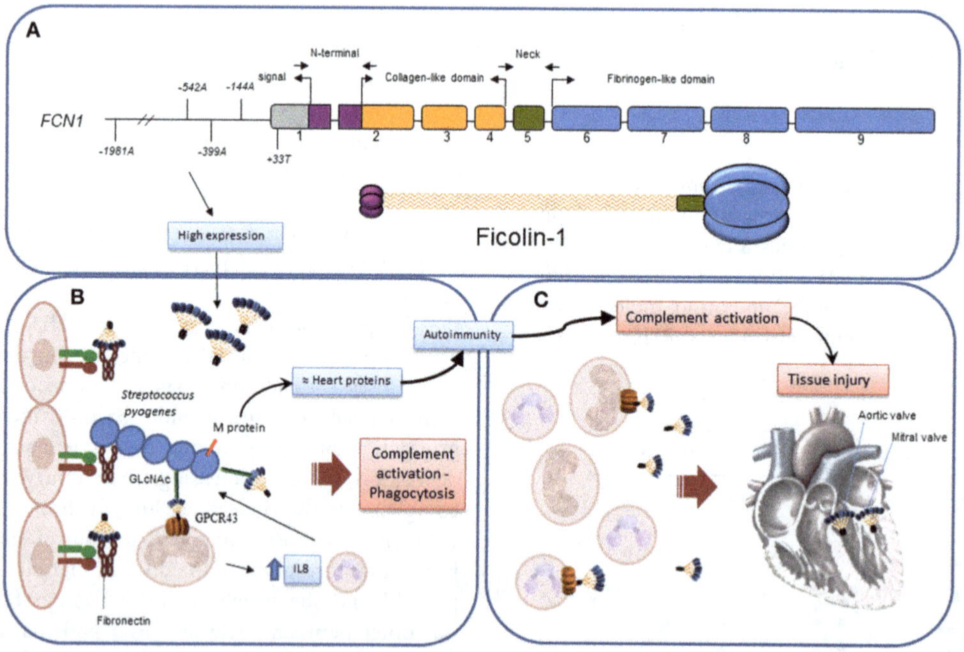

FIGURE 4 | Hypothetical actions of Ficolin-1 in RF/RHD. **(A)** Exon structure and correspondence to domains in the structural trimeric ficolin-1 subunit: gray – untranslated region, purple – N-terminal trimerization domain, orange – collagenous stalk, green – neck region, blue – fibrinogen C-domain. Approximate location of the investigated polymorphisms is given according to number of base pairs, counting from the first transcribed nucleotide. **(B)** Higher ficolin-1 levels, associated with certain *FCN1* alleles in the promoter region, improved resistance against GAS infection, slowing down the process by which autoantibodies are produced due to exposure of neoepitopes in damaged tissue and structural homology of GAS's M protein with myosin/tropomyosin. This may occur through competition for fibronectin binding in the extracellular matrix; recognition of GlcNAc in GAS carbohydrate A by phagocyte membrane-bound ficolin-1 and consequent bacteria internalization; complement activation, despite GAS's abilities to cleave C5a, as well as C2-C9; ficolin-1/GPCR43 activation on monocytes, transducing signals through NFkB and activating interleukin-8 (IL8) gene expression, leading to chemoattraction of more phagocytes to the infection site. **(C)** After established infection, structures on damaged/altered cells recognized by membrane-bound or soluble ficolin-1 mediate complement activation and increases tissue injury, which may become irreversible in the cardiac valves.

(27), as well as ficolin-1 deficiency in a mouse model of collagen Ab-induced arthritis (41).

Lower ficolin-1 levels were found in RF patients, an effect that might purely indicate considerable ficolin-1 consumption in RF. In contrast to our study, ficolin-1 serum levels were higher in patients with vasculitis syndrome or rheumatoid arthritis, than in those with myositis, whereas no difference was observed among patients with systemic lupus erythematosus and Behcet's disease (42). Ficolin-1 levels further correlated with several inflammatory markers, including C-reactive protein (CRP), serum amyloid protein (SAP) and complement factor C3 (42) and strongly associated with the severity of ischemic stroke, in another group (43). Interestingly, part of the benefit of intravenous immunoglobulin (IVIG) therapy relies on ficolin-1 pulldown (reported for Kawasaki disease, the most common form of acquired heart disease in childhood) (44). IVIG therapy has also been proven beneficial for Sydenham's Chorea associated with rheumatic fever (45). Moreover, anti-ficolin-1 mAb ameliorated symptoms of collagen antibody-induced arthritis (CAIA) in animal model (42). Additionally, acute injury leads to higher *FCN1* gene expression, due to specific regulatory proteins such as hypoxia factor HIF-1a (46). This collection of evidence is in line with our results associating high-*FCN1* producing promoter variants with heart damage, in later stages of the disease.

This study has some limitations, especially regarding sample size of individuals with measured ficolin-1 levels which probably affected some of the results. Increased ficolin-1 levels were observed in patients carrying the **3C2* haplotype, however this effect was not evident among controls possibly due to low sample size. In addition we cannot dismiss the possibility that there may be other causal variants responsible for modulating *FCN1* expression, not investigated in this study, such as rs12377780 (in intron 1), rs7857015 (5′ upstream) and rs7858307 (3′UTR) (http://raggr.usc.edu/). Well-designed case control studies including higher number of individuals and different *FCN1* gene polymorphisms are necessary to better define the action of ficolin-1in RF. Concluding, we suggest a role for ficolin-1 in fighting GAS infection, with a possible damaging effect when infection succeeds, due to excessive complement activation. Inhibiting the final steps of complement activation may be a therapeutic clue for preventing valvar damage in patients with RHD.

AUTHOR CONTRIBUTIONS

FA, AB, LG, and IM-R designed the study and analyzed the data. SC performed all the assays, analyzed the data, and performed statistical tests. All of the authors contributed toward manuscript preparation and revision, and provided final approval of the version to be published.

FUNDING

This work was supported by CNPq (Conselho Nacional de Desenvolvimento Científico e Tecnológico), Fundação Araucária and BNDES (The National Bank for Economic and Social Development).

ACKNOWLEDGMENTS

We gratefully acknowledge all the patients for their participation in this study, and the staff of the Molecular Immunology Laboratory of HC/UFPR for their assistance. We are thankful to CAPES and CNPq for research grants to IM-R, and to BNDES (The National Bank for Economic and Social Development) for its research grants to LG.

REFERENCES

1. Steer AC. Historical aspects of rheumatic fever. *J Paediatr Child Health* (2015) 51:21–27. doi: 10.1111/jpc.12808
2. Guilherme L, Kalil J. Rheumatic heart disease: molecules involved in valve tissue inflammation leading to the autoimmune process and Anti-*S. pyogenes* vaccine. *Front Immunol.* (2013) 4:352. doi: 10.3389/fimmu.2013.00352
3. Bono-Neri F. Acute rheumatic fever: global persistence of a preventable disease. *J Pediatr Heal Care* (2017) 31:275–84. doi: 10.1016/j.pedhc.2016.09.001
4. Martin WJ, Steer AC, Smeesters PR, Keeble J, Inouye M, Carapetis J, et al. Post-infectious group A streptococcal autoimmune syndromes and the heart. *Autoimmun Rev.* (2015) 14:710–25. doi: 10.1016/j.autrev.2015.04.005
5. Zühlke LJ, Beaton A, Engel ME, Hugo-Hamman CT, Karthikeyan G, Katzenellenbogen JM, et al. Group A streptococcus, acute rheumatic fever and rheumatic heart disease: epidemiology and clinical considerations. *Curr Treat Options Cardiovasc Med.* (2017) 19:15. doi: 10.1007/s11936-017-0513-y
6. Roberts K, Colquhoun S, Steer A, Reményi B, Carapetis J. Screening for rheumatic heart disease: current approaches and controversies. *Nat Rev Cardiol.* (2013) 10:49–58. doi: 10.1038/nrcardio.2012.157
7. Tian C, Hromatka BS, Kiefer AK, Eriksson N, Noble SM, Tung JY, et al. Genome-wide association and HLA region fine-mapping studies identify susceptibility loci for multiple common infections. *Nat Commun.* (2017) 8:599. doi: 10.1038/s41467-017-00257-5
8. Matsushita M. Ficolins in complement activation. *Mol Immunol.* (2013) 55:22–6. doi: 10.1016/j.molimm.2012.08.017
9. Garred P, Honoré C, Ma YJ, Rørvig S, Cowland J, Borregaard N, et al. The genetics of ficolins. *J Innate Immun.* (2009) 2:3–16. doi: 10.1159/000242419
10. Ermert D, Weckel A, Agarwal V, Frick IM, Björck L, Blom AM. Binding of complement inhibitor C4b-binding protein to a highly virulent *Streptococcus pyogenes* M1 strain is mediated by protein H and enhances adhesion to and invasion of endothelial cells. *J Biol Chem.* (2013) 288:32172–83. doi: 10.1074/jbc.M113.502955
11. Ramasawmy R, Spina GS, Fae KC, Pereira AC, Nisihara R, Messias Reason IJ, et al. Association of mannose-binding lectin gene polymorphism but not of mannose-binding serine protease 2 with chronic severe aortic regurgitation of rheumatic etiology. *Clin Vaccine Immunol.* (2008) 15:932–6. doi: 10.1128/CVI.00324-07
12. Beltrame MH, Catarino SJ, Goeldner I, Boldt ABW, de Messias-Reason IJ. The lectin pathway of complement and rheumatic heart disease. *Front Pediatr.* (2015) 2:148. doi: 10.3389/fped.2014.00148

13. Mukherjee S, Jagadeeshaprasad MG, Banerjee T, Ghosh SK, Biswas M, Dutta S, et al. Proteomic analysis of human plasma in chronic rheumatic mitral stenosis reveals proteins involved in the complement and coagulation cascade. *Clin Proteomics* (2014) 11:1–18. doi: 10.1186/1559-0275-11-35
14. Wu X, Yue Q, Jia W, Zhang J, Ouyang H, Xin D, et al. A novel approach for characterizing variations in serum peptides in rheumatic heart disease. *Indian J Med Res.* (2017) 145:365–72. doi: 10.4103/ijmr.IJMR_1581_14
15. Garred P, Borregaard N. The ficolins. *J Innate Immun.* (2010) 2:1–2. doi: 10.1159/000254982
16. Boldt ABW, Boschmann SE, Catarino SJ, Andrade FA, de Messias-Reason IJ. MASP1 and MASP2. In Choi S, editor. *Encyclopedia of Signaling Molecules.* New York, NY: Springer New York (2016). p.1–18.
17. Vignesh P, Rawat A, Sharma M, Singh S. Complement in autoimmune diseases. *Clin Chim Acta* (2017) 465:123–30. doi: 10.1016/j.cca.2016.12.017
18. Honoré C, Hummelshoj T, Hansen BE, Madsen HO, Eggleton P, Garred P. The innate immune component ficolin 3 (Hakata antigen) mediates the clearance of late apoptotic cells. *Arthritis Rheum.* (2007) 56:1598–607. doi: 10.1002/art.22564
19. Rørvig S, Honore C, Larsson L-I, Ohlsson S, Pedersen CC, Jacobsen LC, et al. Ficolin-1 is present in a highly mobilizable subset of human neutrophil granules and associates with the cell surface after stimulation with fMLP. *J Leukoc Biol.* (2009) 86:1439–49. doi: 10.1189/jlb.1008606
20. Zhang J, Yang L, Ang Z, Yoong SL, Tran TTT, Anand GS, et al. Secreted M-Ficolin anchors onto monocyte transmembrane G protein-coupled receptor 43 and cross talks with plasma C-reactive protein to mediate immune signaling and regulate host defense. *J Immunol.* (2010) 185:6899–910. doi: 10.4049/jimmunol.1001225
21. Kjaer TR, Hansen AG, Sørensen UBS, Nielsen O, Thiel S, Jensenius JC. Investigations on the pattern recognition molecule M-ficolin: quantitative aspects of bacterial binding and leukocyte association. *J Leukoc Biol.* (2011) 90:425–37. doi: 10.1189/jlb.0411201
22. Ren Y, Ding Q, Zhang X. Ficolins and infectious diseases. *Virol Sin.* (2014) 29:25–32. doi: 10.1007/s12250-014-3421-2
23. Ammitzbøll CG, Kjær TR, Steffensen R, Stengaard-Pedersen K, Nielsen HJ, Thiel S, et al. Non-synonymous polymorphisms in the FCN1 gene determine ligand-binding ability and serum levels of M-ficolin. *PLoS ONE* (2012) 7:e50585. doi: 10.1371/journal.pone.0050585
24. Kasperkiewicz K, Eppa Ł, Swierzko AS, Bartłomiejczyk MA, Zuber ZM, Siniewicz-Luzenczyk K, et al. Lectin pathway factors in patients suffering from juvenile idiopathic arthritis. *Immunol Cell Biol.* (2017) 95:666–75. doi: 10.1038/icb.2017.31
25. Addobbati C, de Azevêdo Silva J, Tavares NAC, Monticielo O, Xavier RM, Brenol JCT, et al. Ficolin gene polymorphisms in Systemic Lupus Erythematosus and rheumatoid arthritis. *Ann Hum Genet.* (2016) 80:1–6. doi: 10.1111/ahg.12129
26. Boldt ABW, Sanchez MIN, Stahlke ERS, Steffensen R, Thiel S, Jensenius JC, et al. Susceptibility to leprosy is associated with M-ficolin polymorphisms. *J Clin Immunol.* (2013) 33:210–9. doi: 10.1007/s10875-012-9770-4
27. Haerynck F, Van Steen K, Cattaert T, Loeys B, Van Daele S, Schelstraete P, et al. Polymorphisms in the lectin pathway genes as a possible cause of early chronic Pseudomonas aeruginosa colonization in cystic fibrosis patients. *Hum Immunol.* (2012) 73:1175–83. doi: 10.1016/j.humimm.2012.08.010
28. Vander Cruyssen B, Nuytinck L, Boullart L, Elewaut D, Waegeman W, Van thielen M, et al. Polymorphisms in the ficolin 1 gene (FCN1) are associated with susceptibility to the development of rheumatoid arthritis. *Rheumatology* (2007) 46:1792–5. doi: 10.1093/rheumatology/kem266
29. Munthe-Fog L, Hummelshoj T, Honoré C, Moller ME, Skjoedt MO, Palsgaard I, et al. Variation in FCN1 affects biosynthesis of ficolin-1 and is associated with outcome of systemic inflammation. *Genes Immun.* (2012) 13:515–22. doi: 10.1038/gene.2012.27
30. Schafranski MD, Stier A, Nisihara R, Messias-Reason IJT. Significantly increased levels of mannose-binding lectin (MBL) in rheumatic heart disease: a beneficial role for MBL deficiency. *Clin Exp Immunol.* (2004) 138:521–5. doi: 10.1111/j.1365-2249.2004.02645.x
31. Schafranski MD, Pereira Ferrari L, Scherner D, Torres R, Jensenius JC, de Messias-Reason IJ. High-producing MBL2 genotypes increase the risk of acute and chronic carditis in patients with history of rheumatic fever. *Mol Immunol.* (2008) 45:3827–31. doi: 10.1016/j.molimm.2008.05.013
32. Messias Reason IJ, Schafranski MD, Jensenius JC, Steffensen R. The association between mannose-binding lectin gene polymorphism and rheumatic heart disease. *Hum Immunol.* (2006) 67:991–8. doi: 10.1016/j.humimm.2006.08.296
33. Messias-Reason IJ, Schafranski MD, Kremsner PG, Kun JFJ. Ficolin 2 (FCN2) functional polymorphisms and the risk of rheumatic fever and rheumatic heart disease. *Clin Exp Immunol.* (2009) 157:395–9. doi: 10.1111/j.1365-2249.2009.03975.x
34. Catarino SJDS, Boldt ABW, Beltrame MH, Nisihara RM, Schafranski MD, de Messias-Reason IJ. Association of MASP2 polymorphisms and protein levels with rheumatic fever and rheumatic heart disease. *Hum Immunol.* (2014) 75:1197–202. doi: 10.1016/j.humimm.2014.10.003
35. Carithers LJ, Moore HM. The Genotype-Tissue Expression (GTEx) project. *Biopreserv Biobank* (2015) 13:307–8. doi: 10.1089/bio.2015.29031.hmm
36. Degn SE, Jensenius JC, Thiel S. Disease-causing mutations in genes of the complement system. *Am J Hum Genet.* (2011) 88:689–705. doi: 10.1016/j.ajhg.2011.05.011
37. Thiel S, Kolev M, Degn S, Steffensen R, Hansen AG, Ruseva M, et al. Polymorphisms in mannan-binding lectin (MBL)-associated serine protease 2 affect stability, binding to MBL, and enzymatic activity. *J Immunol.* (2009) 182:2939–47. doi: 10.4049/jimmunol.0802053
38. Ma YJ, Skjoedt M-O, Garred P. Collectin-11/MASP complex formation triggers activation of the lectin complement pathway–the fifth lectin pathway initiation complex. *J Innate Immun.* (2013) 5:242–50. doi: 10.1159/000345356
39. Hamada S, Kawabata S, Nakagawa I. Molecular and genomic characterization of pathogenic traits of group A Streptococcus pyogenes. *Proc Jpn Acad Ser B Phys Biol Sci.* (2015) 91:539–59. doi: 10.2183/pjab.91.539
40. Swierzko AS, Bartlomiejczyk MA, Brzostek A, Lukasiewicz J, Michalski M, Dziadek J, et al. Mycobacyerial antigen 85 complex (Ag85) as a target for ficolins and mannose-binding lectin. *Int J Med Microbiol.* (2016) 306:212–21. doi: 10.1016/j.ijmm.2016.04.004
41. Banda NK, Acharya S, Scheinman RI, Mehta G, Takahashi M, Endo Y, et al. Deconstructing the lectin pathway in the pathogenesis of experimental inflammatory arthritis: essential role of the lectin ficolin B and mannose-binding protein–associated serine protease 2. *J Immunol.* (2017) 199:1835–45. doi: 10.4049/jimmunol.1700119
42. Katayama M, Ota K, Nagi-Miura N, Ohno N, Yabuta N, Nojima H, et al. Ficolin-1 is a promising therapeutic target for autoimmune diseases. *Int Immunol.* (2018)1–10. doi: 10.1093/intimm/dxy056
43. Kouchaki E, Babamohammadi A, Nikoueinejad H, Sehat M. Association of serum levels of Pentraxin-3, M-ficolin, and surfactant protein A with the severity of ischemic stroke complement activators in ischemic stroke. *Iran J Allergy Asthma Immunol.* (2017) 16:140–6.
44. Okuzaki D, Ota K, Takatsuki SI, Akiyoshi Y, Naoi K, Yabuta N, et al. FCN1 (M-ficolin), which directly associates with immunoglobulin G1, is a molecular target of intravenous immunoglobulin therapy for Kawasaki disease. *Sci Rep.* (2017) 7:6–11. doi: 10.1038/s41598-017-11108-0
45. Dean SL, Singer HS. Treatment of sydenham's chorea: a review of the current evidence. *Tremor Other Hyperkinet Mov.* (2017) 7:456. doi: 10.7916/D8W95GJ2
46. Merchant S, Korbelik M. Upregulation of genes for C-reactive protein and related pentraxin/complement proteins in photodynamic therapy-treated human tumor cells: enrolment of PI3K/Akt and AP-1. *Immunobiology* (2013) 218:869–74. doi: 10.1016/j.imbio.2012.10.010

15

Substitution of Mannan-Binding Lectin (MBL)-Deficient Serum with Recombinant MBL Results in the Formation of New MBL/MBL-Accociated Serine Protease Comptexec

Mischa P. Keizer[1,2], Angela Kamp[1], Gerard van Mierlo[1], Taco W. Kuijpers[2,3] and Diana Wouters[1]*

[1] *Department of Immunopathology, Sanquin Blood Supply, Division Research and Landsteiner Laboratory of the Academic Medical Center, University of Amsterdam, Amsterdam, Netherlands,* [2] *Department of Pediatric Hematology, Immunology and Infectious Diseases, Emma Children's Hospital, AMC, University of Amsterdam, Amsterdam, Netherlands,* [3] *Department of Blood Cell Research, Sanquin Blood Supply, Division Research and Landsteiner Laboratory of the AMC, University of Amsterdam, Amsterdam, Netherlands*

Correspondence:
Mischa P. Keizer
m.keizer@sanquin.nl,
smpd.keizer@gmail.com

The lectin pathway (LP) of complement activation depends on the activation of the MBL-associated serine proteases (MASPs) circulating in complex with mannan-binding lectin (MBL). MBL deficiency is the most common complement deficiency and has been associated with several pathological conditions. As we had previously shown, plasma-derived MBL (pdMBL) contains pre-activated MASPs that upon *in vivo* pdMBL substitution results in restoration of MBL concentrations but no LP functionality due to immediate inactivation of pdMBL–MASP complexes upon infusion. In this study, we analyzed MBL-sufficient and -deficient serum by size-exclusion chromatography for complexes of LP activation. In both sera, we identified non-bound free forms of MASP-2 and to lesser extent MASP-1/3. After addition of recombinant MBL (rMBL) to MBL-deficient serum, these free MASPs were much less abundantly present, which is highly suggestive for the formation of high-molecular complexes that could still become activated upon subsequent ligand binding as shown by a restoration of C4-deposition of MBL-deficient serum. Ficolin (FCN)-associated MASPs have been described to redistribute to ligand-bound MBL, hereby forming new MBL/MASP complexes. However, reconstitution of MBL-deficient serum with rMBL did not change the relative size of the FCN molecules suggestive for a limited redistribution in fluid phase of already formed complexes. Our findings demonstrate that rMBL can associate with free non-bound MASPs in fluid phase while preserving full restoration of LP functionality. In contrast to pdMBL products containing pre-activated MASPs which become inactivated almost immediately, these current data provide a rationale for substitution studies using rMBL instead.

Keywords: recombinant MBL, MBL-associated serine protease, redistribution, mannan-binding lectin–MBL-associated serine protease complexes, size-exclusion chromatography

INTRODUCTION

The complement system is an intricate and subtle cascade comprising more than 50 soluble and cell-bound proteins to defend against a wide range of bacterial and fungal pathogens. The complement system has an array of different functions, which includes opsonization and lysis of pathogens, elimination of immune complexes, and stimulation and chemotaxis of leukocytes (1, 2).

In general, the complement system is divided into three activating pathways, which all converge into the so-called terminal pathway. The antibody-dependent classical pathway (CP) is activated upon the binding of C1q to immune complexes. Upon binding of mannan-binding lectin (MBL) (or other collectins such as CL-L1 or CL-K1), or one of the three ficolins (FCNs), to pathogen-specific carbohydrates, the MBL-associated serine proteases (MASPs) are activated resulting in activation of the lectin pathway (LP). The alternative pathway is spontaneously activated on surfaces that lack complement regulatory proteins and can act as an amplification loop for both the CP and the LP. All three activating pathways converge at the level of C3 and can subsequently activate the terminal pathway to form the membrane attack complex for complement-mediated lysis of target cells.

Several LP pattern-recognition molecules (PRMs) have been identified. Most important are MBL and the so-called FCNs (3). In serum, the basic unit of MBL (a trimer of 32 kDa polypeptide chain) oligomerizes to form higher-order molecules ranging from dimers to hexamers (650 kDa) and higher (4, 5). MBL circulates in complex with the inactive zymogens of MASPs (4). The different higher-order oligomeric forms of MBL may have a different composition of MASPs, possibly combining different MASPs in one complex (6, 7). There are two major MASPs: i.e., MASP-2 and MASP-1. The 74-kDa MASP-2 is auto-activated upon ligand binding of the PRMs, and the activation is greatly increased in the presence of 77-kDa MASP-1 (8, 9). MASP-3 is a splice variant of the same *MASP1/3* gene with catalytic activity and has an important role in the activation of factor D (10). Different MASPs can be present within a single oligomeric MBL–MASP complex (6, 8). The role of MASP-1 in the activation of MASP-2 suggests that a heterocomplex of these MASPs with MBL is required for LP activation (8, 9). Alternatively, smaller MBL–MASP complexes could bind in close vicinity to allow cross-activation of MASP-2 by MASP-1 (6).

Mannan-binding lectin deficiency is a common complement deficiency. Depending on the definition up to 20% of the human population is affected, and MBL deficiency has been associated with several diseases (11–13). MBL deficiency in different vulnerable patient groups, including pediatric oncology patients (12), neonates (14), and patients with cystic fibrosis (15), has shown an increased severity and frequency of infections. Earlier MBL-substitution trials with plasma-derived MBL (pdMBL) in MBL-deficient individuals have shown to be safe, without any major adverse event reported (11). Although MBL levels were restored, LP functionality remained unexpectedly low following *in vivo* MBL substitution (16). This was found to be due to immediate interaction of inhibitors, such as C1-inhibitor (C1-INH), in the recipient blood with the pre-activated MBL–MASP complexes in the pdMBL product (17). Substitution with rMBL would restore the C4-deposition of MBL-deficient serum upon substitution (18), without the rapid inactivation seen in pdMBL. For this reason, there is renewed interest in the use of rMBL.

In this study, we analyzed the composition and size of LP-activating complexes in MBL-sufficient, MBL-deficient, and rMBL-reconstituted deficient serum in detail to determine whether rMBL associates with MASPs to act as effective LP-activating complexes upon MBL substitution.

MATERIALS AND METHODS

Reagents

Mouse monoclonal antibodies (mAbs) against MBL (e.g., αMBL-1; murine IgG1) were generated at our department, and the properties have been described before (19–21). mAbs against MASP-1/3 (4H2A9; murine IgG1), MASP-2 (8B5; murine IgG1), FCN-2 (GN4; murine IgG1), and FCN-3 (4H5; murine IgG1) were obtained from Hycult Biotech (Uden, the Netherlands). A second mAb against FCN-3 (334; murine IgG1) was obtained from Enzo Life Sciences (Bruxelles, Belgium). Affinity-purified recombinant human MBL [rMBL at 3.1 mg/ml in 10 mM Tris–HCl with 140 mM NaCl, pH 7.4, and 5 mM EDTA (TBS-E)] (22), recombinant human MASP-1 (rMASP-1 at 0.28 mg/ml), recombinant MASP-2 (rMASP-2) at 3.1 μg/ml (23), and recombinant MASP-3 (0.425 mg/ml), all expressed in HEK cells, and mAbs against MASP-1/3 (4H2A9) and MASP-3 (38:12.3) were a kind gift of Professor J. C. Jensenius (Aarhus University, Aarhus, Denmark). High-performance ELISA buffer (HPE) and poly-HRP-labeled streptavidin (poly-HRP) were obtained from Sanquin (Amsterdam, the Netherlands). 3,5,3′,5′-Tetramethylbenzidine (TMB) was obtained from Merck (Darmstadt, Germany). Mannan and acetylated BSA were obtained from Sigma-Aldrich (St. Louis, MO, USA). Serum from healthy volunteers was obtained with informed consent and prepared as described elsewhere (24). Ethical review and approval were obtained for this study in accordance with the local legislation and institutional requirements (Sanquin Research Medical Ethical Committee). MBL status was determined by genotype and MBL serum levels. All serum aliquots were stored at −80°C until tested.

Monoclonal Anti-MASP-2 Antibody (mAb 12D12) and MASP-Specific ELISAs

Monoclonal antibodies against pdMBL were obtained by a fusion of spleen cells from a mouse immunized with MBL purified from Cohn fraction III (20). We and others have described that during purification of MBL several other proteins are co-purified (17, 25). During selection of the mAbs, several mAbs appeared to be non-responsive to recombinant MBL (rMBL). These mAbs were further characterized for their reactivity toward MASPs. Briefly, 96-well Nunc Maxisorp microtiter plates were coated overnight with 0.5 μg/ml of different recombinant MASPs in PBS (MASP-1 and MASP-2). All following steps were conducted in HPE. The reactivity of biotinylated mAbs obtained from the original immunization, and control (biotinylated) antibodies (αMASP-1 4H2A9 and αMASP-3 38:12.3) were assessed by titration on the plate. After washing, plates were incubated with 0.01% poly-HRP and developed using 0.1 mg/ml TMB in 0.1 M sodium acetate containing 0.03% (v/v) H_2O_2, pH 5.5. Absorbance was measured at 450 nm. In total, 42 non-MBL-binding mAbs were tested for their specificity. mAb 12D12 detected only MASP-2, and not MASP-1 and MASP-3 (Figure S1A in Supplementary Material). As a control for coating the MASPs, we also developed an assay with mAbs against MASP-1/3 (Figure S1B in Supplementary Material).

MBL Serum Levels and Genotyping

Mannan-binding lectin concentration was measured by ELISA as previously described by Brouwer et al. (16). Briefly, mannan was coated to the solid phase, and biotinylated αMBL-1 was used as detection mAb. After washing, plates were incubated with 0.01% poly-HRP and developed as described earlier. Samples were compared with the mean MBL serum level found in a pool of 3,000 healthy control sera (1.5 μg/ml MBL). MBL status was confirmed using genotyping, as described previously by Frakking et al. (26) In short, a TaqMan assay with specific primers and minor groove binding for each SNP were used, hereby directly amplifying, using both forward and reverse allele-specific primers, the coding polymorphisms.

Size-Exclusion Chromatography (SEC)

Size-exclusion chromatography was performed in running buffer [veronal-buffered (VB) saline with added 140 mM NaCl]. MBL-deficient serum was reconstituted with rMBL [final concentration 50 μg/ml and incubated at room temperature (RT) for 60 min and, like MBL-sufficient and MBL-deficient sera, double filtered with a 0.2 μM Whatman filter (GE Healthcare, Buckinghamshire, UK)], before 500 μl sample was applied to 23.5 ml, 10 mm × 300 mm Superdex™ 200 10/300 GL (GE Healthcare, Buckinghamshire, UK) prepacked column equilibrated and eluted with running buffer at a constant 0.5 ml/min flow rate. 500 μl fractions were collected in 96-deep well plates and stored at 4°C until tested. The column was calibrated with GE Filtration Calibration Kits (GE Healthcare, Buckinghamshire, UK) according to the manufacturer's guidelines.

LP Components Detected by ELISA

All incubations were performed in 100 μl volume at RT, all washes in between incubation steps were done with water. Different fractions, obtained from SEC, were incubated at mannan-coated plates, as described earlier, and incubated for 60 min at RT. After washing, different components (MBL, MASP-1/3, and MASP-2) were detected using specific biotinylated mAbs (αMBL-1, αMASP-1/3 4H2A9, and αMASP-2 12D12) by incubation for 1 h at RT. Finally, poly-HRP [0.01% in VB with added 10 mM $CaCl_2$, 2 mM $MgCl_2$, 0.3% (v/v) BSA, and 0.02% (v/v) Tween-20 (VB^{2+} B/T)] was added to each well and incubated for 20 min at RT. Plates were developed as described previously.

To circumvent binding of already preformed MBL/MASP complexes and to detect the presence of MASP-1/3 and MASP-2 in MBL-deficient serum, mannan-coated plates were incubated with a fixed amount of rMBL (0.2 μg/ml). Briefly, different fractions were diluted (1:5) in VB saline with added 10 mM $CaCl_2$, 2 mM $MgCl_2$, 0.3% (v/v), and 0.02% (v/v) Tween-20 (VB^{2+} B/T) and incubated for 1 h at RT. Plates were developed and detected as described earlier. Absorbance was measured at 450 nm and compared with a normal serum pool which was set to 100%.

The functional binding of FCN-1, FCN-2, and FCN-3 was determined by overnight coating with acetylated BSA (5 μg/ml in 0.1 M carbonate buffer, pH 9.6) in 96-well Nunc Maxisorp microtiter plates (Invitrogen, Breda, the Netherlands). After washing, different fractions were diluted 1:50 in VB^{2+} B/T and incubated for 60 min. The binding of FCN was determined by incubation for 60 min at RT with specific biotinylated mAbs: αFCN-1 (AF4209), αFCN-2 (GN4), and αFCN-3 (FCN334) in VB^{2+} B/T. Finally, plates were developed with poly-HRP (0.01% in VB^{2+} B/T) and developed by addition of 0.1 mg/ml TMB I 0.11 M sodium acetate, containing 0.003% (v/v) H_2O_2, pH 5.5. Absorbance was measured at 450 nm and compared with a normal serum pool.

RESULTS

Elution Profile of MBL-Deficient and MBL-Sufficient Serum

Serum of either MBL-sufficient or MBL-deficient donors was fractionated by SEC to determine the elution profile of MBL and the MASPs. MBL serum levels of MBL-deficient donor were below 0.1 μg/ml and confirmed by genotype (HYPD/LXPA). The MBL-sufficient donor had MBL serum levels of 6.4 μg/ml (genotype HYPA/LYQA). MBL-deficient serum was completely restored in LP functionality following *in vitro* substitution with rMBL, indicating the presence of normal levels of LP components (data not shown).

Before fractionation of serum, the column used in the SEC was equilibrated using running buffer and calibrated with low- and high-weight markers (**Figure 1A**). A direct correlation ($r^2 = 0.994$) between elution volume and marker size was calculated (**Figure 1B**), allowing us to correlate the relative size of the protein based on the elution profile.

First, all fractions were incubated on mannan-coated plates, and bound MBL and complexed MASPs were detected. As expected, after fractionation of MBL-deficient serum, no LP components were detected on mannan-coated plates (**Figure 2A**). Fractionation of MBL-sufficient serum showed the presence of MBL and MBL/MASP-2 complexes binding to the mannan-coated plate (**Figure 2B**). Mannan-bound MBL was mainly observed at 550 kDa and around 80 kDa, corresponding to a polymeric and a trimer of the 32-kDa MBL protein. A single peak of complexed MBL/MASP-2, around 430 kDa, was observed, indicating that MASP-2 only associated with higher-order oligomers. We did not find any MASP-1/3 in the higher polymeric forms of MBL being not detected on mannan-coated plates in these experimental conditions.

Redistribution of MASPs

To investigate whether MASP-1/3 and MASP-2 were able to redistribute from serum and associate to mannan-bound rMBL, all fractions were incubated on the mannan coat, which was first saturated with rMBL. Detection with mAb against MASP-1/3 and MASP-2 revealed that both MASP-1/3 and MASP-2 from the MBL-deficient serum were able to associate with mannan-bound rMBL (**Figure 2C**). MASP-1/3 that associated with rMBL on the plate was derived from fractions containing proteins

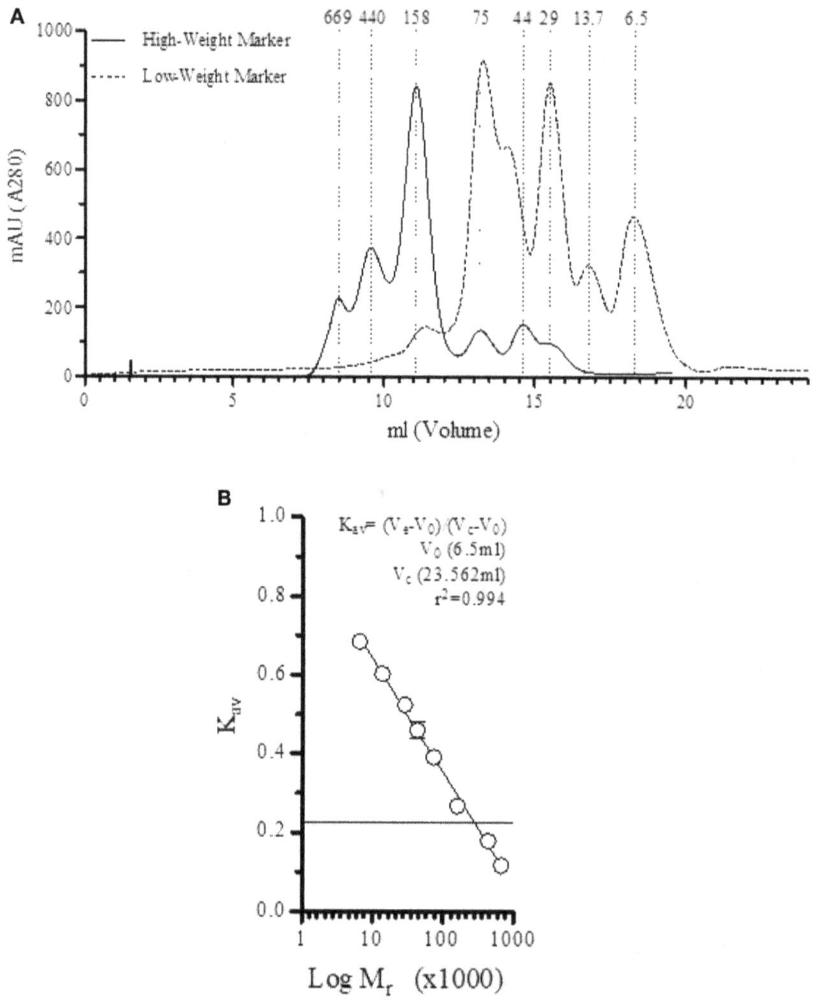

FIGURE 1 | Direct correlation between elution fraction and size. **(A)** Elution profile of low-weight and height-weight markers on the Superdex™ 200 10/300 GL in veronal-buffered saline (1 M NaCl, pH 7.4). **(B)** A strong correlation (r^2 = 0.994) is found between the elution volume and the marker size.

with different molecular sizes, i.e., at around 100–130 and 210–260 kDa. MASP-2 showed a similar elution profile with a peak around 440 kDa. Both MASPs were apparently also present in their monomeric free form, not bound to any collectin including MBL, as indicated by the presence of the protein in fractions corresponding to a molecular size of 70 kDa.

MBL-associated serine protease-2 from the MBL-sufficient serum that associated with rMBL on the plate was derived from fractions containing high-molecular weight proteins (peak around 540 kDa) in which the polymeric MBL was present, and from fractions containing lower molecular weight proteins (65–84 kDa), corresponding to non-complexed monomers of MASP-2. In this serum, MASP-1/3 showed a more diffuse elution pattern with a peak around 430 kDa, which was at a higher molecular weight compared with that in MBL-deficient serum and could correspond to serum fractions containing FCNs. Like MASP-2, MASP-1/3 was also found in a fraction of MBL-sufficient serum with a relative size corresponding to a non-complexed, free monomeric form (**Figure 2D**).

Restoration of MBL-Deficient Serum by rMBL

The addition of rMBL to MBL-deficient serum can completely restore the LP functionality *in vitro* as shown by a recovery of C4-deposition (18). To investigate whether rMBL associates with free MASPs in fluid phase or MASPs that are in complex with other collectins (for instance, FCNs) may redistribute to rMBL, MBL-deficient serum was reconstituted with rMBL and subsequently fractionated. rMBL contains primarily trimeric (225 kDa), tetrameric (300 kDa), and pentameric (375 kDa) oligomers (16, 27). All fractions were incubated on a mannan-coated plate and tested for the presence of MBL–MASP complexes.

Both MBL/MASP-1/3 and MBL/MASP-2 were detected in fractions containing high-molecular weight proteins (**Figure 3A**), indicating that in fluid-phase rMBL associated with MASP-1/3 and MASP-2. MBL/MASP-1/3 complexes were found in a diffuse pattern, but the most prominent peaks were around 350 and 710 kDa. MBL/MASP-2 complexes showed a similar pattern with a main peak around 710 kDa.

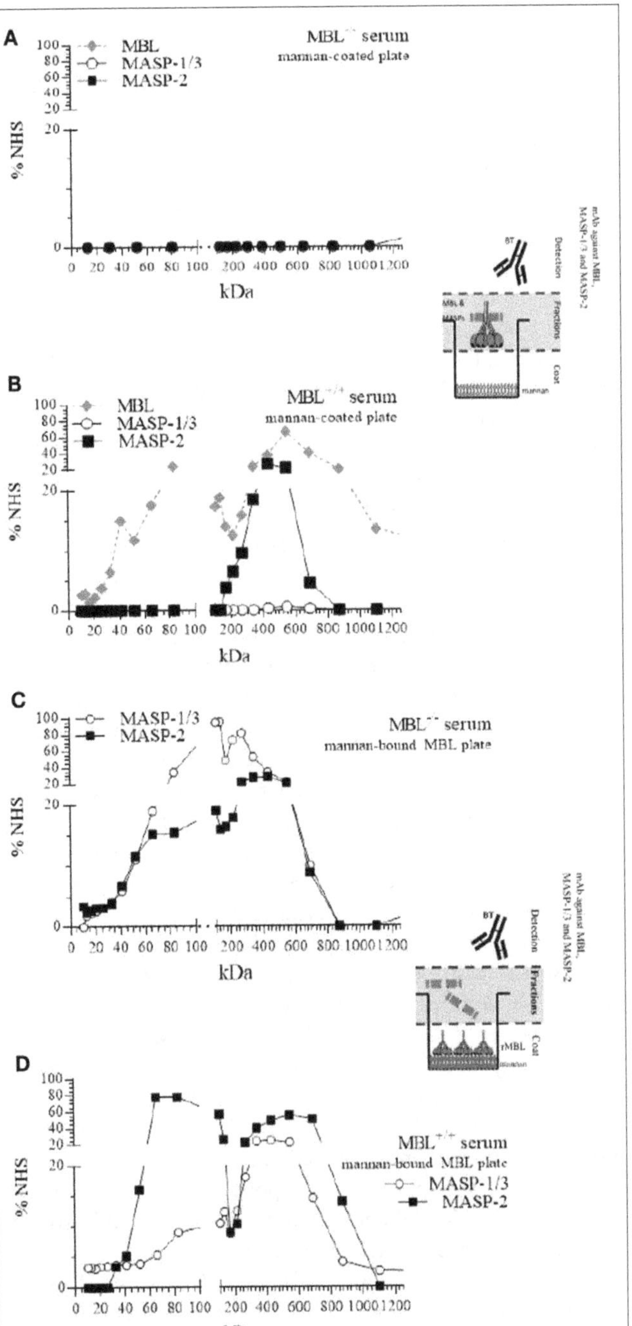

FIGURE 2 | Size-exclusion chromatography (SEC) of mannan-binding lectin (MBL)-deficient and MBL-sufficient serum. SEC of MBL-deficient serum **(A,C)** or MBL-sufficient serum **(B,D)**. Serum was fractionated on a Superdex™ 200 10/300 GL column **(A,C)**. Fractions were tested for the presence of MBL, or MBL–MBL-associated serine protease (MASP)-1/3, MBL–MASP-2 complexes on mannan-coated plates and compared with a pool of normal human sera (NHS). **(B,D)** Mannan-coated plates were pre-incubated with fixed amount of recombinant MBL, and followed by the different fractions of MBL-deficient or MBL-sufficient serum, and the formation of new MBL–MASP-1/3 or MBL–MASP-2 complexes was detected and compared with a pool of NHS.

To determine the origin of the MASPs that associated with rMBL in fluid phase, all fractions were also analyzed on mannan-coated plates saturated with rMBL (**Figure 3B**). Both MASP-1/3

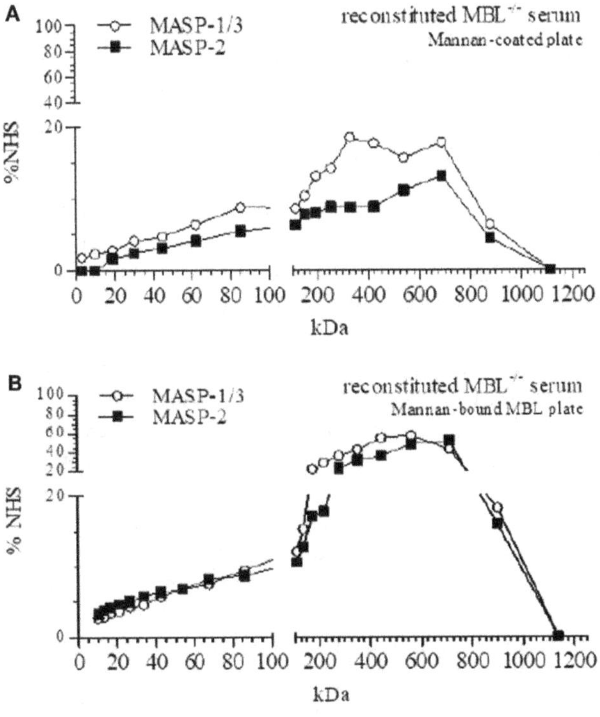

FIGURE 3 | Size-exclusion chromatography (SEC) of mannan-binding lectin (MBL)-reconstituted MBL-deficient serum. SEC of MBL-deficient serum reconstituted to 50 µg/ml MBL. **(A)** Fractions were tested for the presence of MBL–MBL-associated serine protease (MASP)-1/3 and MBL–MASP-2 complexes on mannan-coated plates. **(B)** Mannan-coated plates were pre-incubated with MBL, and followed by the different fractions of reconstituted MBL-deficient serum, and the formation of MBL–MASP-1/3 and MBL–MASP-2 complexes was detected.

and MASP-2 were found in a distinct peak around a relative size of 440–560 kDa for MASP-1/3 and around 560–710 kDa for MASP-2. In contrast to the previously observed double peak for MASP-1/3, we now observed a single peak at a higher molecular weight with a noted absence of the non-complexed form of MASP, suggesting that free soluble MASP-1/3 and MASP-2 associated with rMBL once added. However, our experimental setup was not able to distinguish between heterocomplexes of MASP-1/3 and MASP-2 within a single MBL protein or separate complexes of either MBL-associated MASP-1/3 or MBL-associated MASP-2.

FCN/MASP Complexes

We hypothesized that formation of MBL/MASP complexes more readily happens when MBL is bound to mannan, hereby attracting MASPs from FCN/MASP complexes (**Figure 2**). We therefore investigated the presence of different FCNs in the fractions of MBL-deficient and reconstituted MBL-deficient serum. FCN-1 was not detected in any of the fractions.

The fractions of MBL-deficient serum and reconstituted MBL-deficient serum showed the functional binding of FCN-2 to acetylated BSA as a peak around 540 kDa (**Figure 4A**), which did not alter after rMBL-reconstitution. Similar observations were made for FCN-3 (**Figure 4B**). Neither FCN-2 nor FCN-3 showed a different elution profile after reconstitution with rMBL, suggesting that the detected MASPs, in the mannan-bound MBL assay, are not derived from FCN/MASP complexes but were unbound MASPs (low molecular fraction) that reacted with the ligand-bound MBL.

DISCUSSION

In this study, we investigated the association of rMBL with MASPs in MBL-deficient serum. Our data demonstrated the unexpected presence of free non-complexed MASP-1/3 and MASP-2 that could associate to fluid-phase rMBL when added to MBL-deficient serum.

MBL-associated serine protease-1/3 and MASP-2 can associate with different LP PRMs. It has been hypothesized that MASPs are in equilibrium and can freely associate with the different available PRMs which act as carrier proteins (23, 28). We hypothesized that upon binding of these PRMs to their ligands the equilibrium of MASP binding would shift in favor of the ligand-bound protein, resulting in the formation of PRM/MASP complexes to initiate the complement activation cascade. *In vitro* substitution of MBL-deficient serum with rMBL restored the C4-deposition on mannan-coated plates, indicating the formation of functional rMBL/MASP complexes. Our findings showed the ability of mannan-bound rMBL to form new rMBL/MASP complexes in MBL-deficient serum and MBL-sufficient serum. Both MASP-1/3 and MASP-2 were found to associate with mannan-bound rMBL. The relative size of the newly formed complexes suggested that

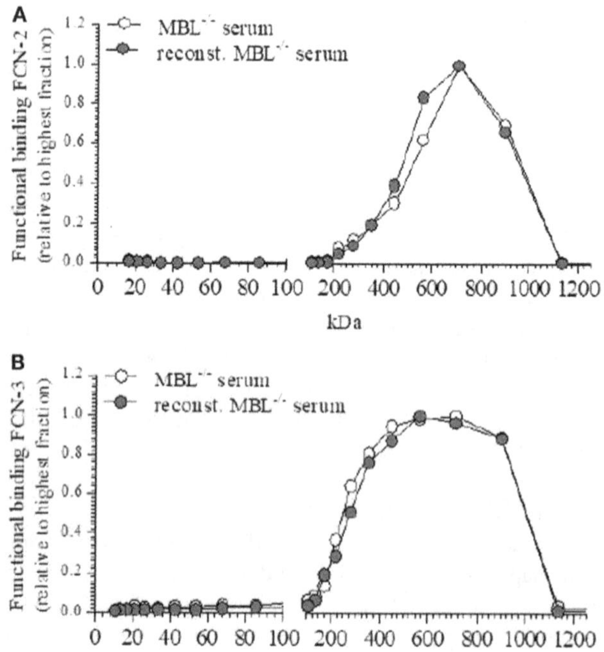

FIGURE 4 | Functional binding of ficolin (FCN)-2 and FCN-3. Effect on the distribution of FCN-2 and FCN-3 after reconstitution to 50 µg/ml mannan-binding lectin (MBL). **(A)** Fractions were tested for the ligand binding of FCN-2 before and after reconstitution. **(B)** Fractions were tested for the ligand binding of FCN-3 before and after reconstitution.

MASPs are present as free non-complexed proteins as well as in a bound form, being associated with different LP complexes. A likely source of these LP complexes would be FCN-2 and FCN-3 in MBL-deficient serum. This is different form previous published reports showing the tendency of MASPs to form a dimeric molecule following analysis of recombinant proteins or complexes (29–31), which could be related to the origin of the proteins analyzed.

The elution profile of MBL-sufficient serum showed immediate similarity with the previously published results of Dahl et al. (4) These authors described different polymeric forms of MBL, ranging from relative sizes of 275 kDa and smaller (MBL-I), to 345–580 kDa (MBL-II), 580–900 kDa (MBL-III), and 900 kDa and above (MBL-IV). Although we were able to detect MASP-1 in unfractionated MBL-sufficient serum, the different fractions obtained from SEC after fractionation showed no detectable signal on mannan-coated plates. We confirmed that MASP-2 primarily associated with MBL-II in MBL-sufficient serum. After reconstitution of MBL-deficient serum, we were able to detect both MASP-1/3 and MASP-2 on mannan and mannan-bound MBL plates primarily in fractions corresponding to higher sizes, between 200 and 900 kDa. This suggests that an association takes place between other LP complexes and rMBL in fluid phase. We were unable to detect the presence of FCN-1 in our fractions, which was to be expected, given the low serum concentration of FCN-1 and further dilution during fractionation (32, 33). In contrast to FCN-1, higher-order oligomers of FCN-2 were detected in fractions corresponding to a relative size of 710 kDa, and FCN-3 oligomers were detected in a broad range of sizes 400–900 kDa. Although Ohashi and Erickson (34) and Munthe-Fog et al. (35) have reported even larger sizes around 800–870 kDa, our column has a lower discriminatory sensitivity for the very high-molecular weights. The distribution patterns of FCN-2 and FCN-3 are similarly between MBL-deficient serum and reconstituted MBL-deficient serum, supporting the hypothesis of MASP-2 preferentially binding to a ligand-bound protein. This is also supported by Megyeri et al. (36) who showed an increased yield of MBL/MASP complexes following addition of recombinant MBL and subsequent purification using mannan-sepharose. The pattern of FCN-2 and FCN-3 appear to correspond to the observed pattern of newly formed MASP complexes on mannan-bound MBL, we were unable to observe a relative change in size.

The presence of a non-complexed form of MASP-2 and MASP-1/3 provides a new mechanism of restoration of the LP activity following MBL reconstitution. This non-complexed free form of MASP-2 and MASP-1/3 could no longer be detected following addition of rMBL to MBL-deficient serum, leading to the formation of a new complex with a larger molecular size indicating a redistribution of MASPs, which was suggested before by Megyeri et al. (36). Whether these different MASPs consist of homodimers or heterodimers before association with oligomeric MBL is still debated (6, 28, 37, 38).

Early MBL substitution studies in MBL-deficient patients have shown the safety of infusion of pdMBL (11), but a limited restoration of the LP functionality was observed despite reaching high plasma MBL levels (16). Analysis of pdMBL showed high levels of associated pre-activated MASP-2 (27), which is rapidly inactivated upon *in vivo* infusion by natural inhibitors such as C1-inhibitor (17). The MBL-associated MASPs in the pdMBL product are rapidly cleared within 24 h after substitution with limited restoration of the LP (16). By contrast, rMBL has been shown to efficiently restore the LP functionality as indicated by C4-deposition both *in vitro* (18) and *in vivo* (36). The potential therapeutic value of MBL replacement depends on the potential to form activating complexes with MASPs that are functional upon ligand binding. Our study showed the presence of a natural non-bound form of MASP-2 in serum to explain the mechanism by which rMBL can restore LP functionality in MBL-deficient patients. These rMBL–MASP complexes are not yet activated, in contrast to the pre-activated MASPs bound to MBL due to affinity chromatography purification (17, 25). Our results indicate that rMBL—upon its formation of functional complexes after infusion—will not be promptly inhibited and cleared as we had previously observed for pdMBL (17). Both the fact that rMBL substitution was well-tolerated in a phase I trial (39) and the presence of non-bound forms of MASPs able to associate with rMBL and restore LP functionality provide a rationale to consider new clinical rMBL substitution studies in carefully selected patients.

AUTHOR CONTRIBUTIONS

Study concept and design; drafting of manuscript: MK, DW, and TK. Acquisition of data: MK, AK, and GM. Statistical analysis of data: MK, AK, and DW. Interpretation of data: MK, AK, DW, and TK. Critical revision of the manuscript for important intellectual content: all the authors.

FUNDING

This study was supported by a grant from KiKa (stichting Kinderen Kankervrij) (project 41).

SUPPLEMENTARY MATERIAL

FIGURE S1 | Specific monoclonal antibody (mAb) against MBL-associated serine □). protease (MASP)-2. Plates were directly coated with recombinant proteins, respectively, rMASP-1 (○), recombinant MASP-2 (rMASP-2) (■), and rMASP-3 (36). Coated proteins were detected using a titration of specific biotinylated mAbs against MASP-1/3 (4H2A9) (36), against MASP-2 (12D12) or against MASP-3 (38:12-3) (**(A)** mAb 12D12 binds only to MASP-2 and does not show cross-reactivity toward the other serine protease. **(B)** mAb 4H2A9 is able to detect both MASP-1 and MASP-3 bound to the plate, by binding to a shared epitope (40).

FIGURE S2 | Reconstitution with recombinant MBL (rMBL) restores lectin pathway functionality. Plates were directly coated with mannan and a serum dilution of reconstituted mannan-binding lectin (MBL)-deficient serum with 50 µg/ml rMBL (●), MBL-deficient serum (○), or MBL-sufficient serum was tested for their C4-converting function.

REFERENCES

1. Walport MJ. Complement. Second of two parts. *N Engl J Med* (2001) 344:1140–4. doi:10.1056/NEJM200104123441506
2. Orsini F, De Blasio D, Zangari R, Zanier ER, De Simoni MG. Versatility of the complement system in neuroinflammation, neurodegeneration and brain homeostasis. *Front Cell Neurosci* (2014) 8:380. doi:10.3389/fncel.2014.00380
3. Troldborg A, Hansen A, Hansen SW, Jensenius JC, Stengaard-Pedersen K, Thiel S. Lectin complement pathway proteins in healthy individuals. *Clin Exp Immunol* (2017) 188(1):138–47. doi:10.1111/cei.12909
4. Dahl MR, Thiel S, Matsushita M, Fujita T, Willis AC, Christensen T, et al. MASP-3 and its association with distinct complexes of the mannan-binding lectin complement activation pathway. *Immunity* (2001) 15:127–35. doi:10.1016/S1074-7613(01)00161-3
5. Jensen PH, Laursen I, Matthiesen F, Hojrup P. Posttranslational modifications in human plasma MBL and human recombinant MBL. *Biochim Biophys Acta* (2007) 1774:335–44. doi:10.1016/j.bbabio.2007.03.004
6. Degn SE, Jensen L, Olszowski T, Jensenius JC, Thiel S. Co-complexes of MASP-1 and MASP-2 associated with the soluble pattern-recognition molecules drive lectin pathway activation in a manner inhibitable by MAp44. *J Immunol* (2013) 191:1334–45. doi:10.4049/jimmunol.1300780
7. Teillet F, Dublet B, Andrieu JP, Gaboriaud C, Arlaud GJ, Thielens NM. The two major oligomeric forms of human mannan-binding lectin: chemical characterization, carbohydrate-binding properties, and interaction with MBL-associated serine proteases. *J Immunol* (2005) 174:2870–7. doi:10.4049/jimmunol.174.5.2870
8. Degn SE, Jensen L, Hansen AG, Duman D, Tekin M, Jensenius JC, et al. Mannan-binding lectin-associated serine protease (MASP)-1 is crucial for lectin pathway activation in human serum, whereas neither MASP-1 nor MASP-3 is required for alternative pathway function. *J Immunol* (2012) 189:3957–69. doi:10.4049/jimmunol.1201736
9. Heja D, Kocsis A, Dobo J, Szilagyi K, Szasz R, Zavodszky P, et al. Revised mechanism of complement lectin-pathway activation revealing the role of serine protease MASP-1 as the exclusive activator of MASP-2. *Proc Natl Acad Sci U S A* (2012) 109:10498–503. doi:10.1073/pnas.1202588109
10. Dobo J, Szakacs D, Oroszlan G, Kortvely E, Kiss B, Boros E, et al. MASP-3 is the exclusive pro-factor D activator in resting blood: the lectin and the alternative complement pathways are fundamentally linked. *Sci Rep* (2016) 6:31877. doi:10.1038/srep31877
11. Keizer MP, Wouters D, Schlapbach LJ, Kuijpers TW. Restoration of MBL-deficiency: redefining the safety, efficacy and viability of MBL-substitution therapy. *Mol Immunol* (2014) 61:174–84. doi:10.1016/j.molimm.2014.06.005
12. Dommett R, Chisholm J, Turner M, Bajaj-Elliott M, Klein NJ. Mannose-binding lectin genotype influences frequency and duration of infectious complications in children with malignancy. *J Pediatr Hematol Oncol* (2013) 35:69–75. doi:10.1097/MPH.0b013e31827076e5
13. Sorensen R, Thiel S, Jensenius JC. Mannan-binding-lectin-associated serine proteases, characteristics and disease associations. *Springer Semin Immunopathol* (2005) 27:299–319. doi:10.1007/s00281-005-0006-z
14. Wahab Mohamed WA, Saeed MA. Mannose-binding lectin serum levels in neonatal sepsis and septic shock. *J Matern Fetal Neonatal Med* (2012) 25:411–4. doi:10.3109/14767058.2011.582903
15. Haerynck F, Van Steen K, Cattaert T, Loeys B, Van Daele S, Schelstraete P, et al. Polymorphisms in the lectin pathway genes as a possible cause of early chronic *Pseudomonas aeruginosa* colonization in cystic fibrosis patients. *Hum Immunol* (2012) 73:1175–83. doi:10.1016/j.humimm.2012.08.010
16. Brouwer N, Frakking FN, van de Wetering MD, van Houdt M, Hart M, Budde K, et al. Mannose-binding lectin (MBL) substitution: recovery of opsonic function in vivo lags behind MBL serum levels. *J Immunol* (2009) 183:3496–504. doi:10.4049/jimmunol.0900445
17. Keizer MP, Kamp AM, Brouwer N, van de Wetering MD, Wouters D, Kuijpers TW. Plasma-derived mannose-binding lectin shows a direct interaction with C1-inhibitor. *Mol Immunol* (2014) 58:187–93. doi:10.1016/j.molimm.2013.11.022
18. Jensenius JC, Jensen PH, McGuire K, Larsen JL, Thiel S. Recombinant mannan-binding lectin (MBL) for therapy. *Biochem Soc Trans* (2003) 31:763–7. doi:10.1042/bst0310763
19. Bos IG, Lubbers YT, Roem D, Abrahams JP, Hack CE, Eldering E. The functional integrity of the serpin domain of C1-inhibitor depends on the unique N-terminal domain, as revealed by a pathological mutant. *J Biol Chem* (2003) 278:29463–70. doi:10.1074/jbc.M302977200

20. Bultink IE, Hamann D, Seelen MA, Hart MH, Dijkmans BA, Daha MR, et al. Deficiency of functional mannose-binding lectin is not associated with infections in patients with systemic lupus erythematosus. *Arthritis Res Ther* (2006) 8:R183. doi:10.1186/ar2095
21. Wolbink GJ, Bollen J, Baars JW, ten Berge RJ, Swaak AJ, Paardekooper J, et al. Application of a monoclonal antibody against a neoepitope on activated C4 in an ELISA for the quantification of complement activation via the classical pathway. *J Immunol Methods* (1993) 163:67–76. doi:10.1016/0022-1759(93)90240-8
22. Vorup-Jensen T, Sorensen ES, Jensen UB, Schwaeble W, Kawasaki T, Ma Y, et al. Recombinant expression of human mannan-binding lectin. *Int Immunopharmacol* (2001) 1:677–87. doi:10.1016/S1567-5769(00)00052-7
23. Thiel S, Kolev M, Degn S, Steffensen R, Hansen AG, Ruseva M, et al. Polymorphisms in mannan-binding lectin (MBL)-associated serine protease 2 affect stability, binding to MBL, and enzymatic activity. *J Immunol* (2009) 182:2939–47. doi:10.4049/jimmunol.0802053
24. Lachmann PJ. Preparing serum for functional complement assays. *J Immunol Methods* (2010) 352:195–7. doi:10.1016/j.jim.2009.11.003
25. Valdimarsson H, Vikingsdottir T, Bang P, Saevarsdottir S, Gudjonsson JE, Oskarsson O, et al. Human plasma-derived mannose-binding lectin: a phase I safety and pharmacokinetic study. *Scand J Immunol* (2004) 59:97–102. doi:10.1111/j.0300-9475.2004.01357.x
26. Frakking FN, van de Wetering MD, Brouwer N, Dolman KM, Geissler J, Lemkes B, et al. The role of mannose-binding lectin (MBL) in paediatric oncology patients with febrile neutropenia. *Eur J Cancer* (2006) 42:909–16. doi:10.1016/j.ejca.2005.10.027
27. Laursen I. Mannan-binding lectin (MBL) production from human plasma. *Biochem Soc Trans* (2003) 31:758–62. doi:10.1042/bst0310758
28. Parej K, Hermann A, Donath N, Zavodszky P, Gal P, Dobo J. Dissociation and re-association studies on the interaction domains of mannan-binding lectin (MBL)-associated serine proteases, MASP-1 and MASP-2, provide evidence for heterodimer formation. *Mol Immunol* (2014) 59:1–9. doi:10.1016/j.molimm.2013.12.003
29. Kjaer TR, Le le TM, Pedersen JS, Sander B, Golas MM, Jensenius JC, et al. Structural insights into the initiating complex of the lectin pathway of complement activation. *Structure* (2015) 23(2):342–51. doi:10.1016/j.str.2014.10.024
30. Wallis R, Dodd RB. Interaction of mannose-binding protein with associated serine proteases: effects of naturally occurring mutations. *J Biol Chem* (2000) 275(4):30962–9. doi:10.1074/jbc.M004030200
31. Thielens NM, Cseh S, Thiel S, Vorup-Jensen T, Rossi V, Jensenius JC, et al. Interaction properties of human mannan-binding lectin (MBL)-associated serine proteases-1 and -2, MBL-associated protein 19, and MBL. *J Immunol* (2001) 166(8):5068–77. doi:10.4049/jimmunol.166.8.5068
32. Troldborg A, Thiel S, Jensen L, Hansen S, Laska MJ, Deleuran B, et al. Collectin liver 1 and collectin kidney 1 and other complement-associated pattern recognition molecules in systemic lupus erythematosus. *Clin Exp Immunol* (2015) 182:132–8. doi:10.1111/cei.12678
33. Sallenbach S, Thiel S, Aebi C, Otth M, Bigler S, Jensenius JC, et al. Serum concentrations of lectin-pathway components in healthy neonates, children and adults: mannan-binding lectin (MBL), M-, L-, and H-ficolin, and MBL-associated serine protease-2 (MASP-2). *Pediatr Allergy Immunol* (2011) 22:424–30. doi:10.1111/j.1399-3038.2010.01104.x
34. Ohashi T, Erickson HP. Two oligomeric forms of plasma ficolin have differential lectin activity. *J Biol Chem* (1997) 272:14220–6. doi:10.1074/jbc.272.22.14220
35. Munthe-Fog L, Hummelshoj T, Hansen BE, Koch C, Madsen HO, Skjodt K, et al. The impact of FCN2 polymorphisms and haplotypes on the ficolin-2 serum levels. *Scand J Immunol* (2007) 65:383–92. doi:10.1111/j.1365-3083.2007.01915.x
36. Megyeri M, Jani PK, Kajdácsi E, Dobó J, Schwaner E, Major B, et al. Serum MASP-1 in complex with MBL activates endothelial cells. *Mol Immunol* (2014) 59(1):39–45. doi:10.1016/j.molimm.2014.01.001
37. Rosbjerg A, Munthe-Fog L, Garred P, Skjoedt MO. Heterocomplex formation between MBL/ficolin/CL-11-associated serine protease-1 and -3 and MBL/ficolin/CL-11-associated protein-1. *J Immunol* (2014) 192:4352–60. doi:10.4049/jimmunol.1303263
38. Kjaer TR, Jensen L, Hansen A, Dani R, Jensenius JC, Dobo J, et al. Oligomerization of mannan-binding lectin dictates binding properties and complement activation. *Scand J Immunol* (2016) 84:12–9. doi:10.1111/sji.12441
39. Petersen KA, Matthiesen F, Agger T, Kongerslev L, Thiel S, Cornelissen K, et al. Phase I safety, tolerability, and pharmacokinetic study of recombinant human mannan-binding lectin. *J Clin Immunol* (2006) 26:465–75. doi:10.1007/s10875-006-9037-z
40. Degn SE, Jensen L, Gal P, Dobo J, Holmvad SH, Jensenius JC, et al. Biological variations of MASP-3 and MAp44, two splice products of the MASP1 gene involved in regulation of the complement system. *J Immunol Methods* (2010) 361:37–50. doi:10.1016/j.jim.2010.07.006

16

Evasion of Classical Complement Pathway Activation on *Plasmodium falciparum*-Infected Erythrocytes Opsonized by PfEMP1-Specific IgG

Mads Delbo Larsen[1,2†], Maria del Pilar Quintana[1], Sisse Bolm Ditlev[1], Rafael Bayarri-Olmos[2], Michael Fokuo Ofori[3], Lars Hviid[1,4‡] and Peter Garred[2*‡]*

[1] Centre for Medical Parasitology, Department of Immunology and Microbiology, Faculty of Health and Medical Sciences, University of Copenhagen, Copenhagen, Denmark, [2] Laboratory of Molecular Medicine, Department of Clinical Immunology, Rigshospitalet, Copenhagen, Denmark, [3] Department of Immunology, Noguchi Memorial Institute of Medical Research, University of Ghana, Accra, Ghana, [4] Centre for Medical Parasitology, Department of Infectious Diseases, Rigshospitalet, Copenhagen, Denmark

***Correspondence:**
Lars Hviid
lhviid@sund.ku.dk
Peter Garred
peter.garred@regionh.dk

†Present Address:
Mads Delbo Larsen,
Department of Experimental Immunohematology, Sanquin Research and Landsteiner Laboratory, Amsterdam UMC, University of Amsterdam, Amsterdam, Netherlands

‡These authors shared senior authorship

Members of the PfEMP1 protein family are expressed on the surface of *P. falciparum*-infected erythrocytes (IEs), where they contribute to the pathogenesis of malaria and are important targets of acquired immunity. Although the PfEMP1-specific antibody response is dominated by the opsonizing and complement-fixing subclasses IgG1 and IgG3, activation of the classical complement pathway by antibody-opsonized IEs does not appear to be a major immune effector mechanism. To study the molecular background for this, we used ELISA and flow cytometry to assess activation of the classical component pathway by recombinant and native PfEMP1 antigen opsonized by polyclonal and monoclonal PfEMP1-specific human IgG. Polyclonal IgG specific for VAR2CSA-type PfEMP1 purified from a pool of human immune plasma efficiently activated the classical complement pathway when bound to recombinant PfEMP1 in ELISA. In contrast, no activation of complement could be detected by flow cytometry when the same IgG preparation was used to opsonize IEs expressing the corresponding native PfEMP1 antigen. After engineering of a VAR2CSA-specific monoclonal antibody to facilitate its on-target hexamerization, complement activation was detectable in an ELISA optimized for uniform orientation of the immobilized antigen. In contrast, the antibody remained unable to activate complement when bound to native VAR2CSA on IEs. Our data suggest that the display of PfEMP1 proteins on IEs is optimized to prevent activation of the classical complement pathway, and thus represents a hitherto unappreciated parasite strategy to evade acquired immunity to malaria.

Keywords: malaria, complement, evasion, PfEMP1, antibodies, knobs

INTRODUCTION

Malaria remains a major health problem with an estimated 219 million cases and 435,000 deaths in 2017 alone (1). The human disease is caused by several protozoan parasites of the genus *Plasmodium*, but *P. falciparum* is responsible for most severe cases and essentially all malaria mortality (2).

The particular virulence of *P. falciparum* is related to the unique ability of this parasite to express members of a family of clonally variant surface antigens called *P. falciparum* erythrocyte membrane protein 1 (PfEMP1) on the surface of the infected erythrocytes (IEs) (3). This enables sequestration of IEs in the microvasculature, mediated by interaction of PfEMP1 with vascular host receptors such as CD36, endothelial protein C receptor (EPCR), and oncofetal chondroitin sulfate (4–7). The ensuing accumulation of IEs in tissues can lead to severe disease, precipitated by excessive inflammation and circulatory dysfunction.

The PfEMP1 antigens are important targets of naturally acquired immunity to *P. falciparum* malaria, and semi-immune individuals living in areas of stable parasite transmission possess a broad repertoire of PfEMP1-specific antibodies, dominated by the opsonizing and complement-fixing subclasses IgG1 and IgG3 (8, 9). It is therefore noteworthy that activation of the classical complement pathway does not appear to play a major role in acquired immunity to IEs, although acquired immunity leads to activation of complement by antibody-opsonized sporozoites and merozoites (10, 11). Indeed, *P. falciparum* has evolved several mechanisms to evade activation of the alternative and classical pathways by hijacking soluble complement regulators to these developmental stages, emphasizing the clinical importance of complement-mediated attack on malaria parasites (12–16). The display of PfEMP1 on the IE surface is normally restricted to electron-dense protrusions known as "knobs" (17). Although knob-less variants can express PfEMP1 and thrive *in vitro*, knob expression is generally thought to be required for *P. falciparum* survival *in vivo*, and the protection from falciparum malaria afforded by several hemoglobinopathies is thought related to abnormal knob formation on IEs (18). Nevertheless, the role of knobs in *P. falciparum* survival remains unclear. In this article, we investigate the hypothesis that the knob restriction of PfEMP1 on the IE surface may have evolved to prevent classical complement activation by preventing on-target hexamerization of IgG (19). We show that although polyclonal, and even monoclonal, IgG can activate the classical complement pathway when bound to surface-bound recombinant PfEMP1, such activation does not occur when the IgG is bound to native PfEMP1 expressed on the IE surface.

MATERIALS AND METHODS

Recombinant Protein Production

The full-length ectodomain of the VAR2CSA-type PfEMP1 IT4VAR04 (FV2) was produced in ExpiCHO-S cells as a recombinant C-terminal histidine-tagged protein, as described elsewhere (20).

A recombinant version of the human monoclonal IgG1 antibody (mAb) PAM1.4 (21), which is specific for a conformational epitope in VAR2CSA-type PfEMP1, was produced as described elsewhere by cloning and inserting the variable domains of the antibody into plasmids encoding the constant regions of the γ_1-chain and the κ-chain (22). This antibody has previously been shown to bind both plastic-immobilized FV2 in ELISA and the corresponding native antigen on the IE surface (20).

We also produced two variants of this antibody (PAM1.4-E345K and PAM1.4-E430G) by introducing single-nucleotide substitutions in the γ_1-chain, using the QuickChange site-directed mutagenesis kit (Agilent) according to manufacturer's instructions. Briefly, mutations were introduced by a PCR reaction of the entire plasmid with a high-fidelity DNA-polymerase and a complementary primer pair with the desired mutation (E345K forward: 5′-CCAAAGGGCAGCCCCGA<u>A</u>AACCACAGGTGTA-3′; E430G forward:5′-CCGTGATGCATG<u>G</u>GCTCTGCACAACCACT-3′; substitutions are underlined). Plasmids were subsequently sequenced to confirm the introduction of the substitutions. All the recombinant antibodies were produced in human embryonic kidney cells (293-F; Gibco) according to manufacturer's instructions. Briefly, the cells were grown to ~1.5 × 10^6 cells/mL, and adjusted to 1 × 10^6 cells/mL 1 h prior to transfection, and co-transfected with heavy- and light chain plasmids (0.5 µg DNA/plasmid/mL culture) and FreeStyle MAX reagent (1 µL/µg DNA). Cultures were incubated for seven days before harvesting the supernatant. The recombinant antibodies were purified using Protein G-coupled agarose beads (Pierce).

IgG Purification From Human Plasma Samples

Total IgG was purified from pools of plasma from ten Ghanaian donors with natural exposure to *P. falciparum* parasites expressing VAR2CSA-type PfEMP1. The samples were collected in a previous study approved by the Institutional Review Board of Noguchi Memorial Institute for Medical Research, University of Ghana (study no. 038/10-11) (23). Samples were collected only after consent had been obtained in writing from each participant. One pool consisted of the ten available samples with the highest reactivities toward FV2, while the other consisted of the ten available samples with the lowest FV2 reactivities. IgG was purified from each pool of plasma using Gammabind G sepharose (GE Healthcare), using standard methodology. Affinity purification on FV2 was not employed, to allow direct comparison of the pools with high and low FV2 reactivity. However, previous studies have shown that PfEMP1 is the dominant IE target antigen of naturally acquired IgG (24).

Classical Complement Pathway Activation ELISA

Flat-bottomed 96-well plates (Nunc) were coated (4°C, overnight in PBS) with FV2 (2 µg/mL), mAbs (PAM1.4; PAM1.4 E345K; PAM1.4 E430G), purified human IgG (Invitrogen), or human serum albumin (HSA; 10 µg/mL; Sigma Aldrich). Wells were blocked with PBS supplemented with TWEEN (0.05%) and BSA (1%) and subsequently incubated (1 h on shaker, as all subsequent

Abbreviations: AU, arbitrary units; BSA, bovine serum albumin; FV2, full-length ectodomain of the VAR2CSA-type PfEMP1 IT4VAR04; HAS, human serum albumin; IE, infected erythrocyte; mAb, monoclonal antibody; NHS, non-immune human serum; PfEMP1, *Plasmodium falciparum* erythrocyte membrane protein-1; TCC, terminal complement complex.

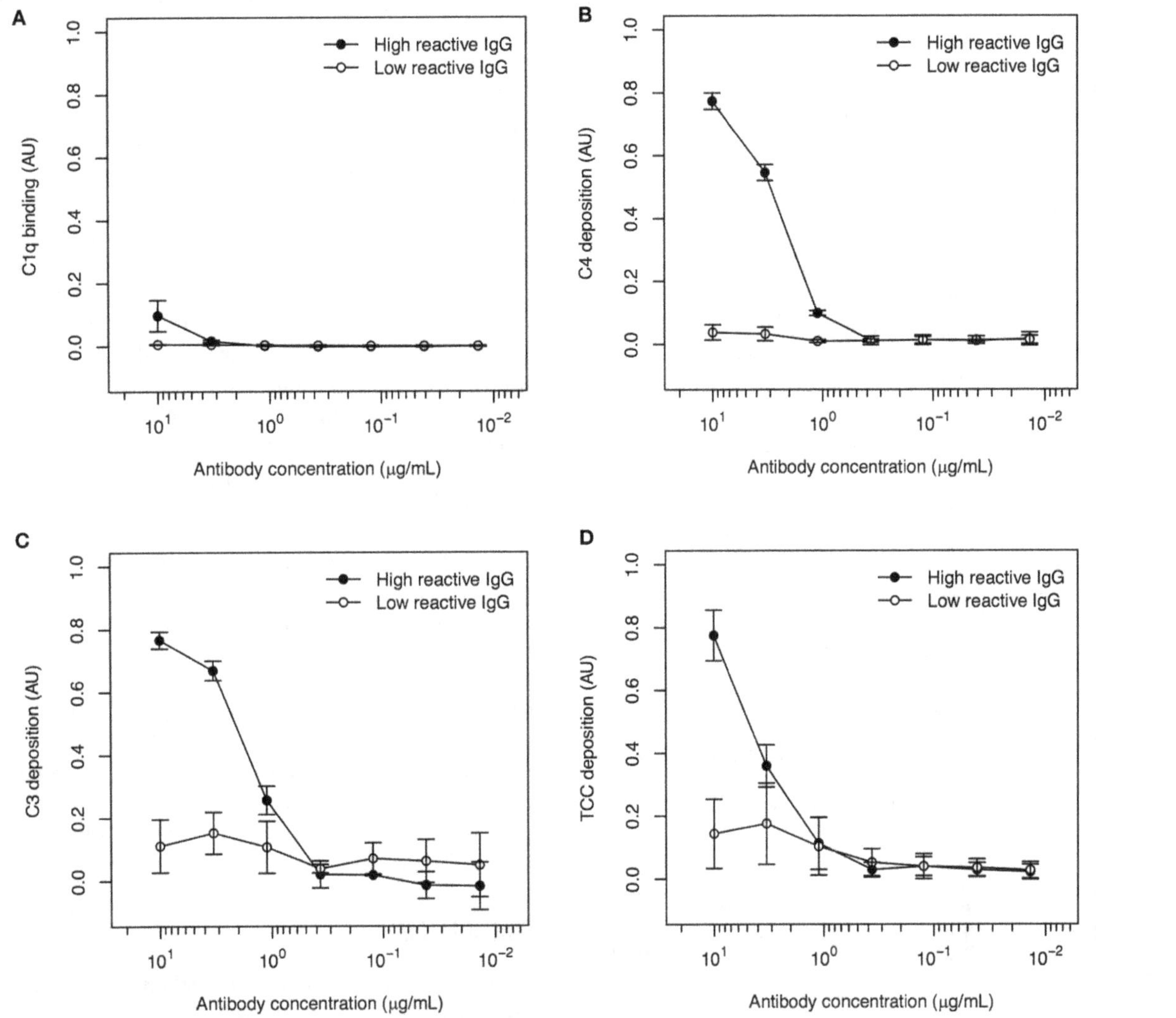

FIGURE 1 | Classical complement pathway activation in ELISA, using IgG with high and low FV2-reactivity and FV2 coated directly to plastic. Binding of C1q **(A)**, deposition of C4 **(B)** and C3 **(C)**, and formation of TCC **(D)** to IgG purified from plasma pools with high (•) and low (○) FV2-reactivity and bound to FV2 immobilized directly on plastic. All data were normalized relative to control wells coated with HSA and incubated with rabbit anti-HSA. Data points representing the means and standard deviations (error bars) of three individual experiment are shown.

steps) with the above-mentioned VAR2CSA-specific mAbs or with control reagents [mAb AB01, specific for a non-VAR2CSA-type PfEMP1 (25) or polyclonal rabbit anti-HSA (Dako)]. In some experiments, 96–well plates pre-coated with nickel, pre-blocked with BSA and coated with FV2 (5 μg/mL) in PBS supplemented with TWEEN (0.05%) were used (Pierce).

After incubation with antibody reagents, the plates were washed four times in Barbital-Tween buffer [sodium barbital (4 mM), NaCl (145 mM), $CaCl_2$ (2.64 mM), $MgCl_2$ (2.12 mM), Tween (0.05%)] and incubated (1 h, 37°C) in the same buffer supplemented with non-immune human serum (NHS; 1%) as source of complement components. After washing as above, bound complement components were detected with polyclonal rabbit anti-human C1q (2 μg/mL; Dako), rabbit anti-human C4c (1 μg/mL; Dako), rabbit anti-human C3c (1 μg/mL; Dako), or monoclonal mouse-anti human-terminal complement complex (TCC; 1 μg/L; clone ae11). All the complement-specific antibody reagents were biotinylated prior to the experiments. After the last washing as above, bound antibody was detected by incubation with streptavidin-conjugated horse radish peroxidase (1:2,000; GE Healthcare), followed by TMB ONE (ECO-TEK). The color reaction was terminated with H_2SO_4 (0.2 M), and quantified at 450 nm. Arbitrary units (AU) were calculated as (OD_{Test} - OD_{Blank}) / ($OD_{Control}$ - OD_{Blank}).

P. falciparum Culture *in vitro* and Selection for Expression of PfEMP1 and Knobs

The *P. falciparum* laboratory isolate IT4/FCR3 was cultured in serum-free medium as described elsewhere (26).

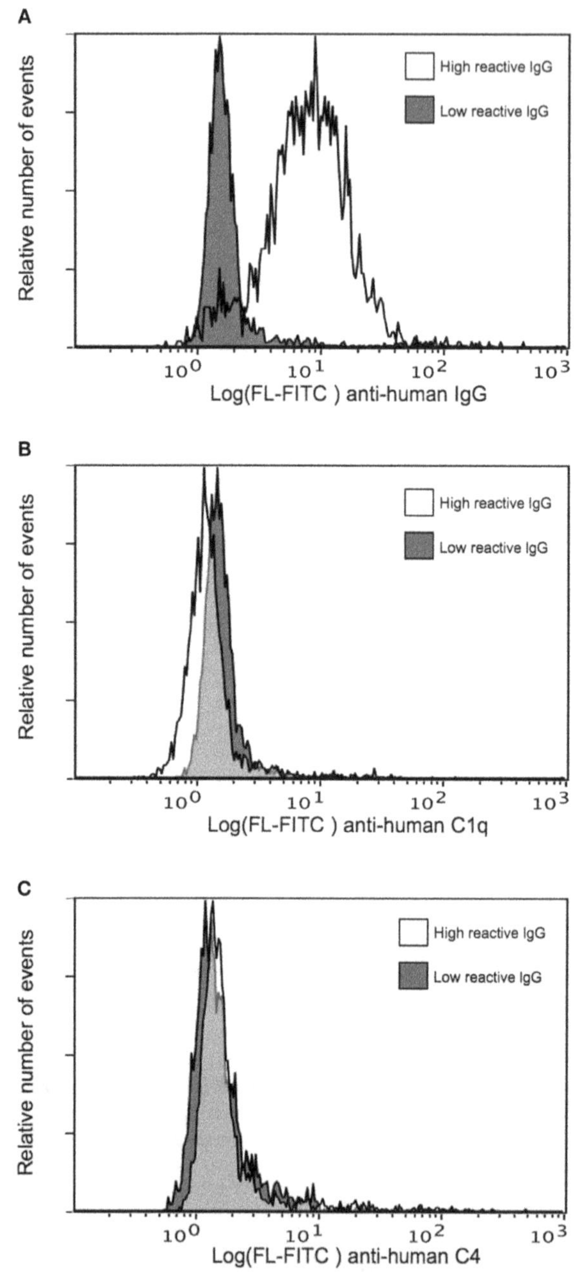

FIGURE 2 | Classical complement pathway activation on IEs, using IgG with high and low FV2 reactivity. Binding of purified immune IgG **(A)** and C1q **(B)**, and deposition of C4 **(C)** to *P. falciparum*-infected erythrocytes selected *in vitro* to express the VAR2CSA-type PfEMP1 IT4VAR04. Representative results of two independent experiments using IgG with high (white) and low (gray) FV2-reactivity are shown.

Parasites were selected by antibody panning and density separation monthly to ensure expression of the VAR2CSA-type PfEMP1 IT4VAR04 and IE surface knobs as described previously (27). Briefly, cultures with primarily late trophozoite-stage IEs were incubated (20 min, 37°C) in culture medium supplemented with gelatin (0.75%) to separate late trophozoite-stage knobby IEs from uninfected erythrocytes and ring-stage IEs. The late trophozoite-stage IEs were then incubated with DynaBeads A (DYNAL) that had been pre-incubated (30 min) with saturating amounts of PAM1.4 antibody. Bound IEs were isolated using a DynaMag (DYNAL).

Classical Complement Activation on IEs

Late trophozoite-stage IEs were purified by magnet-activated cell sorting (Miltenyi Biotec) in PBS supplemented with BSA (1%) (28). The purified IEs (2×10^6 cells/mL) were incubated (30 min, 4°C) with mAbs (10 μg/mL) or purified pooled human IgG (1 mg/mL), followed by incubation (1 h, 37°C) with NHS (1%) and compstatin (6 nM; Tocris) (to inhibit cleavage of C3). As positive and negative controls, type A and 0 erythrocytes were incubated with type 0 NHS and compstatin.

Complement components were detected by incubation (4°C, 30 min) with the same antibodies as above, but at different concentrations (anti-C1q: 30 μg/mL; anti- C4c: 0.5 μg/mL), followed by incubation with FITC-conjugated goat anti-rabbit IgG (1:150; Vector) and ethidium bromide (2 μg/mL; to visualize parasite DNA). Binding of human IgG to the IEs was detected in a similar way, using FITC-conjugated goat anti-human IgG (1:150; Jackson Immuno Research) (28). All incubations, dilutions, and washes were done in PBS supplemented with BSA (1%), except for the incubation with NHS and compstatin, which was done in BSA-supplemented VBS^{++} buffer containing Ca^{2+} and Mg^{2+} (Complement Technology). Samples were run on a Cytomics FC500 flow cytometer (Beckman Coulter). Single ethidium bromide-positive cells were analyzed for complement components and antibody labeling by FlowLogic (Inivai Technologies).

RESULTS

Human Specific IgG Bound to Immobilized Recombinant PfEMP1 Activates the Classical Complement Pathway

To our knowledge, the ability of PfEMP1-specific human IgG to activate the classical complement pathway has not been reported previously. Binding of C1q (**Figure 1A**), deposition of C4 (**Figure 1B**) and C3 (**Figure 1C**), and formation of TCC (**Figure 1D**) were detected in recombinant FV2-ELISA after incubation with human IgG purified from a plasma pool with known high FV2-reactivity, followed by NHS as a source of complement components. When IgG from the pool of low-reactive plasma was used instead of the highly FV2-reactive IgG, no complement deposition was detected (**Figure 1**). We conclude that naturally acquired PfEMP1-reactive IgG is able to activate the classical complement pathway when bound to recombinant FV2 that has been randomly immobilized on plastic.

Human Specific IgG Bound to Native PfEMP1 on Infected Erythrocytes Does Not Activate the Classical Complement Pathway

We next assessed the ability of human IgG purified from the same plasma pools to activate complement when bound to IEs

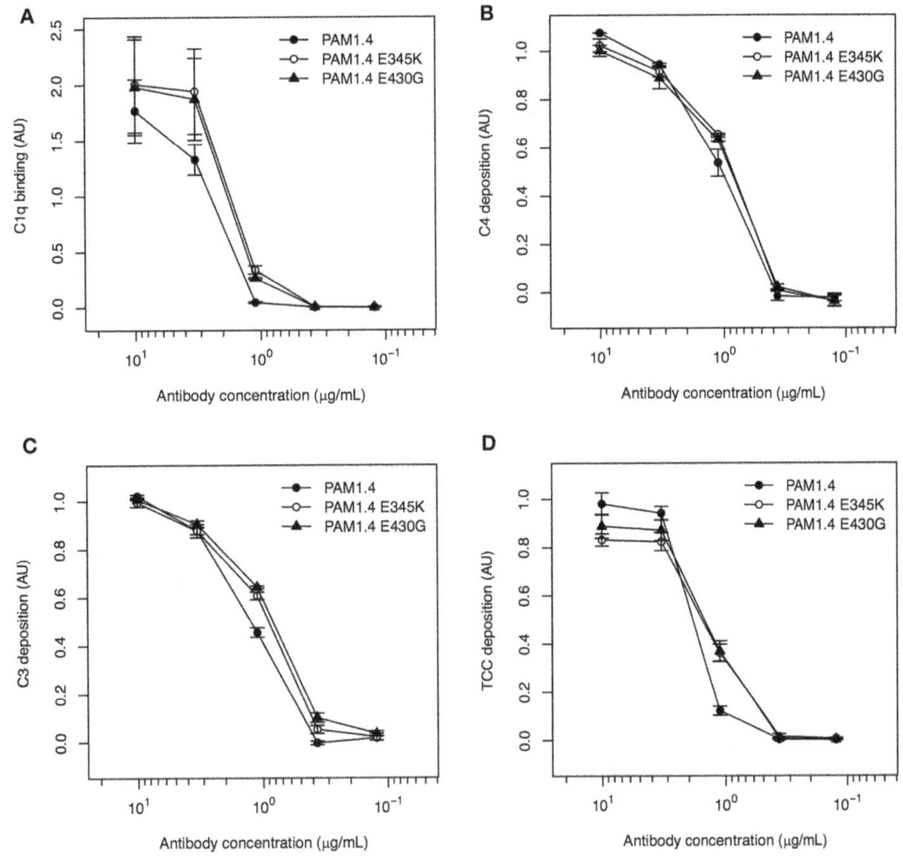

FIGURE 3 | Classical complement pathway activation in ELISA, using FV2-specific monoclonal IgG with and without mutations enhancing on-target hexamerization, coated directly to plastic. Binding of C1q **(A)**, deposition of C4 **(B)** and C3 **(C)**, and formation of TCC **(D)**, using the FV2-specific mAbs PAM1.4 (•), PAM1.4-E345K (○), and PAM1.4-E430G (▲) immobilized directly on plastic. Data representation as in **Figure 1**.

expressing the native PfEMP1 (IT4VAR04) represented by FV2. IgG purified from the highly FV2-reactive pool efficiently labeled the IEs, in contrast to the low FV2-reactivity IgG (**Figure 2A**). However, essentially no binding of C1q (**Figure 2B**) or deposition of C4 (**Figure 2C**) could be detected after incubation of IEs with either IgG preparation. The functionality of the assay was confirmed in experiments using uninfected type A and type 0 erythrocytes incubated with type 0 NHS (**Figure S1**). These findings suggest that the distribution of PfEMP1 on IEs inhibits classical complement activation, possibly due to the clustered, knob-restricted distribution of the antigen.

Activation of Complement by Monoclonal IgG Bound to Immobilized Recombinant PfEMP1 Depends on Antigen Orientation

It was recently reported that complement activation by IgG requires on-target, Fc-dependent hexamerization of the antibody (19). We therefore proceeded to test whether the lack of complement activation by PfEMP1-specific IgG bound to IEs was due to an inability of the antibodies to form hexamers after binding to native PfEMP1 on the IE surface. To do so, we used IEs selected for surface expression of IT4VAR04, and a mAb (PAM1.4) with specificity for VAR2CSA-type PfEMP1 (including IT4VAR04). We also used two variants of this mAb (PAM1.4-E345K and PAM1.4-E430G), where we had introduced mutations in the Fc-region (E345K and E430G, respectively), known to enhance on-target hexamerization of IgG (19, 29).

All three mAbs had similar ability to activate complement when coated directly to ELISA plates, as binding of C1q (**Figure 3A**), as well as deposition of C4 (**Figure 3B**), C3 (**Figure 3C**), and TCC (**Figure 3D**) could be detected in a concentration-dependent manner. This agrees with the observation that enhanced complement activation by hexamerization-improved Fc mutants requires binding of the antibodies to their cognate antigen (29). To confirm this requirement directly, the mAbs were next applied in a setup where the ELISA plates were first coated with FV2 as in the experiments with purified immune IgG above. However, neither PAM1.4 nor the Fc-mutated variants of the mAb activated complement in this setup (**Figure S2**).

In the studies first identifying the complement activation-enhancing mutations, the assays involved cell lines over-expressing the targeted antigen (19, 29). We therefore speculated that the lack of complement activation in our setup with

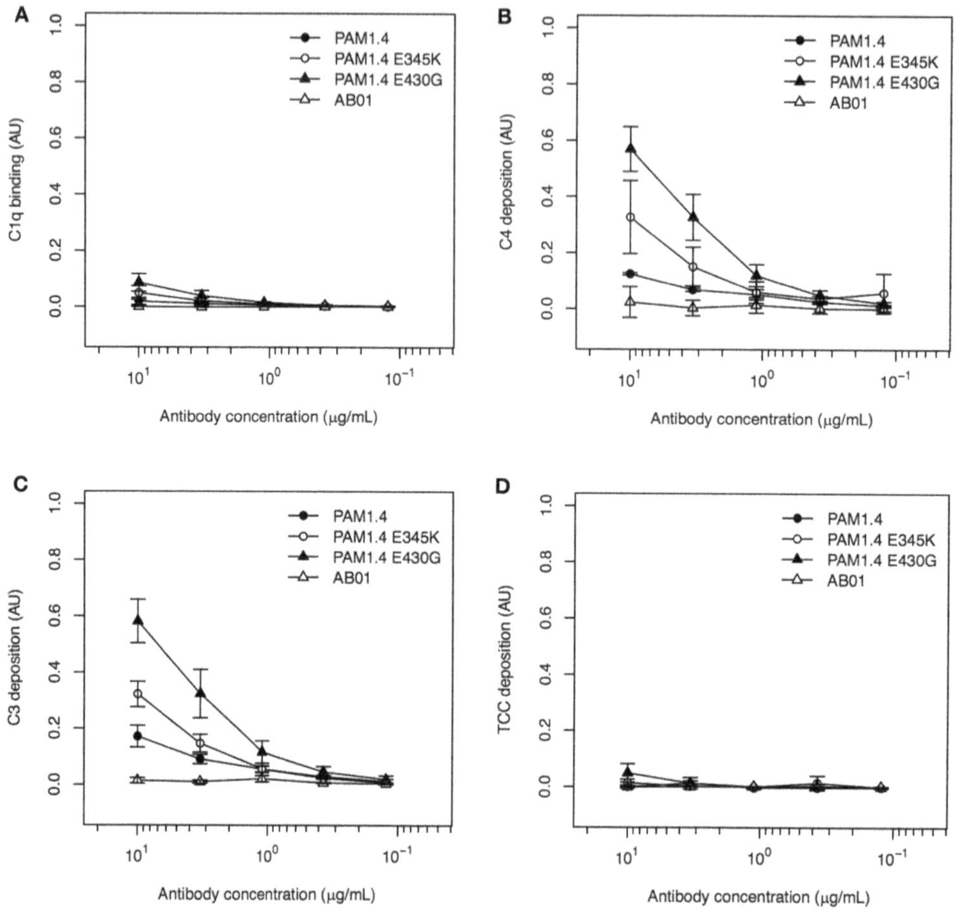

FIGURE 4 | Classical complement pathway activation in ELISA, using FV2-specific monoclonal IgG, bound to plastic coated with FV2 by His-tag::nickel interaction. Binding of C1q **(A)**, deposition of C4 **(B)** and C3 **(C)**, and formation of TCC **(D)** on the FV2-specific mAbs PAM1.4 (•), PAM1.4-E345K (○), and PAM1.4-E430G (▲), and the control mAb AB01 (Δ) in assays employing uniformly oriented FV2 immobilized by interaction between the C-terminal His-tag on FV2 and nickel-coated plastic. Data representation as in **Figure 1**.

recombinant FV2 bound to plastic might be related to the random orientation of the immobilized antigen, in contrast to the usually uniform display of a given antigen on the surface of cells. To approximate such an ordered display, we exploited the fact that our FV2 protein has a C-terminal poly-histidine tag, and immobilized the recombinant protein on ELISA plates pre-coated with nickel. Because the nickel ions bind to the FV2 poly-histidine tags, this should facilitate homogeneous orientation of the antigen similar to the orientation of the native protein on IEs, although the distribution of the FV2 would remain more homogenous than the knob-restricted distribution of native PfEMP1 proteins on IEs. In this setup, binding of C1q (**Figure 4A**), and in particular deposition of C4 (**Figure 4B**) and C3 (**Figure 4C**), could be detected in a concentration-dependent manner for all three mAbs, whereas TCC formation was minimal (**Figure 4D**). Although this might theoretically be due to activation of the alternative pathway by binding of mannan-binding lectin to glycosylation determinants on the recombinant antibodies, this appears unlikely. Firstly, the glycosylation pattern of the cells used to express the recombinant antibodies is very similar to native human IgG (30). Secondly, the hexamerization-enhanced Fc-region mutants, in particular PAM1.4-E430G, were superior to PAM1.4 (if the binding of C4 and C3 were due to activation of the lectin rather than the classical pathway, similar activation by wildtype PAM1.4 and the two hexamerization-enhanced mutants would be expected). When this improved assay was used to test complement activation by purified immune IgG, C4 deposition could be detected with both the high and the low FV2-reactive preparation, although the highly FV2-reactive IgG was superior (**Figure S3**).

Our data confirm that the E345K and E430G mutations in the Fc-region enhance the ability of IgG to activate complement, probably by facilitating on-target hexamerization. Furthermore, the results highlight antigen orientation as an important parameter in *in vitro* assays of classical complement pathway activation.

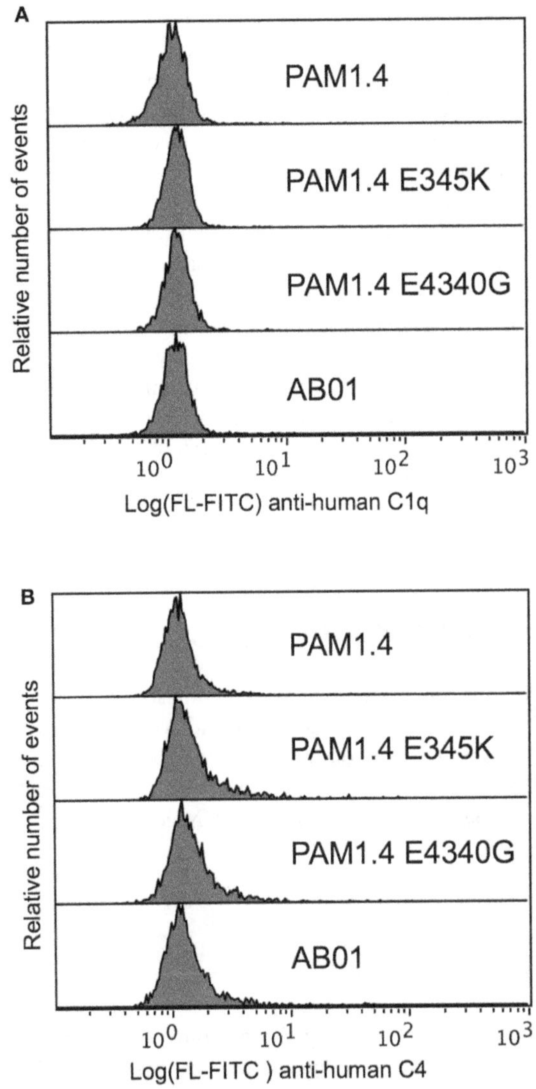

FIGURE 5 | Classical complement pathway activation on IEs, using FV2-specific monoclonal IgG with and without mutations enhancing on-target hexamerization. Binding of C1q **(A)** and deposition of C4 **(B)**, using the FV2-specific mAbs PAM1.4 (Top), PAM1.4-E345K (Second), and PAM1.4-E430G (Third), or the control mAb AB01 (Bottom). Representative results of two independent experiments are shown.

Hexamerization-Enhancing Fc Mutations Do Not Lead to Activation of Complement by Monoclonal PfEMP1-Specific IgG Bound to Infected Erythrocytes

To investigate whether the lack of complement activation on IEs (**Figure 2**) could be overcome by enhancing the antibody capacity for on-target hexamerization, we tested the ability of PAM1.4 and the two Fc mutants to activate complement when bound to IEs. We did not detect C1q binding (**Figure 5A**) or C4 deposition (**Figure 5B**) with any of the mAbs. It thus appears that the distribution of native PfEMP1 prevents hexamerization of monoclonal IgG in a way that could not be overcome by Fc mutations enhancing the ability of PAM1.4 to form hexamers. Although we cannot exclude that other mAbs might be able to form hexamers when bound to PfEMP1 on the IE surface, or that on-target hexamerization might occur with Fc-mutated polyclonal IgG preparations, it seems most likely that PfEMP1 is distributed on the IE surface in a way that prevents the interactions among Fc regions of adjacent IgG molecules that would facilitate binding of C1q and activation of the classical complement pathway.

DISCUSSION

IgG antibodies specific for the asexual parasites multiplying in the blood are a key element in naturally acquired protective immunity to *P. falciparum* malaria (31, 32). Antibodies to antigens on the surface of the IEs – in particular PfEMP1 – are of particular importance in this respect (3). This is probably due to their ability to block the vascular sequestration of IEs, which can otherwise cause inflammation and circulatory dysfunction (33). Unsurprisingly, *P. falciparum* has evolved a range of strategies to avoid PfEMP1-specific immunity, such as antigen polymorphism, clonal antigenic variation, acquisition of soluble host factors etc. (34).

The antibody response to *P. falciparum* asexual blood stage antigens, including the VAR2CSA-type PfEMP1 studied here, is dominated by IgG1 and IgG3 (35). It is therefore likely that phagocytosis of merozoites and IEs opsonized by antibody and complement also contribute significantly to parasite clearance. Although the role of the complement system in *P. falciparum* infections has been the focus of several recent studies, most have focused on the alternative pathway. The ability of IEs (13), merozoites (14), and gametocytes (12) to acquire the soluble complement regulator Factor H to their surface thus clearly suggests that this activation pathway is important in controlling parasitemia, and likely has forced the parasites to evolve strategies to evade this host defense. A very recent study indicates that this host-parasite tug-of-war is even more complicated, and that Factor H-related protein 1 may be involved in a host effort to overcome malaria parasite evasion of complement attack by acquisition of Factor H (36).

The clinical importance of classical complement pathway activation following opsonization by IgG has been less studied, although binding of C1q to IgG-coated merozoites and sporozoites has been associated with protection of malaria in patients from Oceania and Africa (10, 11). In addition, evasion of such immunity by hijacking of C1-inhibitor by merozoites was recently reported (15). The clinical relevance of antibody-dependent complement attack on merozoites may be limited by the fact that this free-living stage is only exposed to antibody and complement for 1-2 min before invading a new erythrocyte. It is questionable whether this is long enough for antibody binding and classical complement attack, as *in vitro* experiments required >2.5 min. before C3 deposition could be demonstrated (15). By then, many merozoites would be expected to have safely reinvaded (37). In the case of sporozoites, the parasite is exposed to antibody and complement for longer (38), and it therefore seems more likely that complement plays a decisive role in the immune response against this developmental stage. However, the intra-erythrocytic parasites should theoretically be vulnerable to classical complement attack for the ~30 of the 48-h asexual life cycle, where they express PfEMP1 on the IE surface to facilitate tissue sequestration and avoidance of destruction in the spleen (39). This notwithstanding, little is known about classical complement attack on IEs, let alone parasite strategies to evade this threat.

Here, we show that human IgG purified from plasma and having high reactivity to PfEMP1 can activate the classical complement pathway in ELISA. However, no complement activation was seen when the same IgG was bound to the corresponding native PfEMP1 on the surface of IEs. The molecular dimensions of IgG and PfEMP1 molecules, combined with estimates of the number of PfEMP1 molecules per IE (40–46) suggest that on-target hexamerization [required for efficient activation of the classical complement cascade by IgG (19)] would occur if the PfEMP1 molecules were evenly distributed over the IE surface. We therefore hypothesized that the lack of activation is related to the knob-restricted expression of PfEMP1 on the IE surface, which prevents on-target hexamerization of IgG molecules bound to PfEMP1 molecules on neighboring knobs, as these are too far apart. The clustered distribution might thus represent a hitherto unidentified strategy by *P. falciparum* to evade acquired, IgG-mediated protective immunity. However, the molecular dimensions of knobs make on-target hexamerization of IgG bound to different PfEMP1 molecules within a given knob theoretically possible. We therefore produced two PfEMP1-specific mAbs with substitutions in the Fc-region that enhance their capacity for on-target hexamerization and complement activation (19, 29). Although we could demonstrate enhanced complement-activating capacity of Fc-mutated mAbs by ELISA, the mutations did not suffice to activate complement following binding of the mAbs to native PfEMP1 on the IE surface. Even with polyclonal immune IgG containing IgG with specificity for the many antibody epitopes that exist in VAR2CSA (21), we did not find evidence of activation of the classical complement cascade at the IE surface. Although the reason for the above observations is not known, the simplest explanation is that PfEMP1 molecules are not evenly distributed, even within the confines of a single knob, but are instead clustered together. Whether this is the case is not currently known, however.

Erythrocytes are inherently susceptible to complement attack, and they therefore possess endogenous membrane-bound complement regulators such as decay-accelerating factor (CD55) and protectin (CD59) to prevent inadvertent phagocytosis and lysis of complement-opsonized erythrocytes. Although CD59 has been reported as the factor preventing complement-mediated lysis of IEs (47), IE lysis is likely to be less important than opsonization for phagocytosis. In this study, we decided to focus on complement components upstream of the erythrocyte membrane-bound complement regulators' point of action, to avoid complications imposed by the need to enzymatically remove membrane-bound regulators.

To conclude, we report that although PfEMP1-specific IgG can activate the classical complement pathway in a system where the antigens are homogeneously distributed, this appears not to happen at the IE surface, where PfEMP1 display is restricted to well-defined knobs. The most parsimonious explanation for this discrepancy is that the focal display of native PfEMP1 interferes with the on-target hexamerization of IgG, which is a requirement for binding of C1q and activation of the classical complement cascade. The knob-restricted display may thus represent a hitherto unrealized strategy of *P. falciparum* to evade acquired protective immunity.

AUTHOR CONTRIBUTIONS

ML, LH, and PG formulated the hypothesis and designed the experiments and analyzed the data and wrote the paper. ML, MQ, SD, and RB-O produced the recombinant proteins. ML carried out all the experiments. MO was responsible for collection of the biological samples. All authors reviewed and edited the manuscript.

FUNDING

This work was supported by grants from the Danish Research Foundation of Independent Research (DFF-4183-00539 and DFF-6110-00489), the Sven Andersen Research Foundation, Novo Nordisk Research Foundation (NNF15OC0017654) and Rigshospitalet (R102-A4174). Sample collection in Ghana was supported by grants from the Consultative Committee for Development Research (DFC-12-081RH) and the Ghana Educational Trust Fund.

ACKNOWLEDGMENTS

We thank all plasma donors, health-care workers, and research staff involved in the field study in Ghana. We thank Maiken Visti and Anne Corfitz for excellent technical assistance.

REFERENCES

1. World Health Organization. *World Malaria Report 2018*. (2018).
2. Cowman AF, Healer J, Marapana D, Marsh K. Malaria: biology and disease. *Cell* (2016) 167:610–24. doi: 10.1016/j.cell.2016.07.055
3. Hviid L, Jensen AT. PfEMP1 - A parasite protein family of key importance in *Plasmodium Falciparum* malaria immunity and pathogenesis. *Adv Parasitol.* (2015) 88:51–84. doi: 10.1016/bs.apar.2015.02.004
4. Baruch DI, Gormley JA, Ma C, Howard RJ, Pasloske BL. *Plasmodium falciparum* erythrocyte membrane protein 1 is a parasitized erythrocyte

receptor for adherence to CD36, thrombospondin, and intercellular adhesion molecule 1. *Proc Natl Acad Sci USA.* (1996) 93:3497–502.

5. Reeder JC, Cowman AF, Davern KM, Beeson JG, Thompson JK, Rogerson SJ, et al. The adhesion of *Plasmodium falciparum*-infected erythrocytes to chondroitin sulfate A is mediated by *P. falciparum* erythrocyte membrane protein 1. *Proc Natl Acad Sci USA.* (1999) 96:5198–202. doi: 10.1073/pnas.96.9.5198
6. Salanti A, Dahlback M, Turner L, Nielsen MA, Barfod L, Magistrado P, et al. Evidence for the involvement of VAR2CSA in pregnancy-associated malaria. *J Exp Med.* (2004) 200:1197–203. doi: 10.1084/jem.20041579
7. Turner L, Lavstsen T, Berger SS, Wang CW, Petersen JE, Avril M, et al. Severe malaria is associated with parasite binding to endothelial protein C receptor. *Nature* (2013) 498:502–5. doi: 10.1038/nature12216
8. Piper KP, Roberts DJ, Day KP. *Plasmodium falciparum*: analysis of the antibody specificity to the surface of the trophozoite-infected erythrocyte. *Exp Parasitol.* (1999) 91:161–9. doi: 10.1006/expr.1998.4368
9. Vigan-Womas I, Lokossou A, Guillotte M, Juillerat A, Bentley G, Garcia A, et al. The humoral response to *Plasmodium falciparum* VarO rosetting variant and its association with protection against malaria in Beninese children. *Malar J.* (2010) 9:267. doi: 10.1186/1475-2875-9-267
10. Boyle MJ, Reiling L, Feng G, Langer C, Osier FH, Aspeling-Jones H, et al. Human antibodies fix complement to inhibit *Plasmodium falciparum* invasion of erythrocytes and are associated with protection against malaria. *Immunity* (2015) 42:580–90. doi: 10.1016/j.immuni.2015.02.012
11. Kurtovic L, Behet MC, Feng G, Reiling L, Chelimo K, Dent AE, et al. Human antibodies activate complement against *Plasmodium falciparum* sporozoites, and are associated with protection against malaria in children. *BMC Med.* (2018) 16:61. doi: 10.1186/s12916-018-1054-2
12. Simon N, Lasonder E, Scheuermayer M, Kuehn A, Tews S, Fischer R, et al. Malaria parasites co-opt human factor H to prevent complement-mediated lysis in the mosquito midgut. *Cell Host Microbe.* (2013) 13:29–41. doi: 10.1016/j.chom.2012.11.013
13. Rosa TF, Flammersfeld A, Ngwa CJ, Kiesow M, Fischer R, Zipfel PF, et al. The *Plasmodium falciparum* blood stages acquire factor H family proteins to evade destruction by human complement. *Cell Microbiol.* (2016) 18:573–90. doi: 10.1111/cmi.12535
14. Kennedy AT, Schmidt CQ, Thompson JK, Weiss GE, Taechalertpaisarn T, Gilson PR, et al. Recruitment of factor H as a novel complement evasion strategy for blood-stage *Plasmodium falciparum* infection. *J Immunol.* (2016) 196:1239–48. doi: 10.4049/jimmunol.1501581
15. Kennedy AT, Wijeyewickrema LC, Huglo A, Lin C, Pike R, Cowman AF, et al. Recruitment of human C1 Esterase Inhibitor controls complement activation on blood stage *Plasmodium falciparum* merozoites. *J Immunol.* (2017) 198:4728–37. doi: 10.4049/jimmunol.1700067
16. Simon N, Friedrich O, Kappes B. Quantification of human complement factor H binding to asexual malaria blood stages by an enzyme-linked immunosorbent assay. *Vaccine* (2018) 36:1545–7. doi: 10.1016/j.vaccine.2018.01.080
17. Horrocks P, Pinches RA, Chakravorty SJ, Papakrivos J, Christodoulou Z, Kyes SA, et al. PfEMP1 expression is reduced on the surface of knobless *Plasmodium falciparum* infected erythrocytes. *J Cell Sci.* (2005) 118:2507–18. doi: 10.1242/jcs.02381
18. Cholera R, Brittain NJ, Gillrie MR, Lopera-Mesa TM, Diakite SA, Arie T, et al. Impaired cytoadherence of *Plasmodium falciparum*-infected erythrocytes containing sickle hemoglobin. *Proc Natl Acad Sci USA.* (2008) 105:991–6. doi: 10.1073/pnas.0711401105
19. Diebolder CA, Beurskens FJ, De Jong RN, Koning RI, Strumane K, Lindorfer MA, et al. Complement is activated by IgG hexamers assembled at the cell surface. *Science* (2014) 343:1260–3. doi: 10.1126/science.1248943
20. Lopez-Perez M, Larsen MD, Bayarri-Olmos R, Ampomah P, Stevenson L, Arevalo-Herrera M, et al. IgG Responses to the *Plasmodium falciparum* antigen VAR2CSA in Colombia are restricted to pregnancy and are not induced by exposure to *Plasmodium vivax. Infect Immun.* (2018) 86:e00136–18. doi: 10.1128/IAI.00136-18
21. Barfod L, Bernasconi NL, Dahlback M, Jarrossay D, Andersen PH, Salanti A, et al. Human pregnancy-associated malaria-specific B cells target polymorphic, conformational epitopes in VAR2CSA. *Mol Microbiol.* (2007) 63:335–47. doi: 10.1111/j.1365-2958.2006.05503.x
22. Tiller T, Meffre E, Yurasov S, Tsuiji M, Nussenzweig MC, Wardemann H. Efficient generation of monoclonal antibodies from single human B cells by single cell RT-PCR and expression vector cloning. *J Immunol Methods* (2008) 329:112–24. doi: 10.1016/j.jim.2007.09.017
23. Ampomah P, Stevenson L, Ofori MF, Barfod L, Hviid L. B-cell responses to pregnancy-restricted and -unrestricted *Plasmodium falciparum* erythrocyte membrane protein 1 antigens in Ghanaian women naturally exposed to malaria parasites. *Infect Immun.* (2014) 82:1860–71. doi: 10.1128/IAI.01514-13
24. Chan JA, Howell KB, Reiling L, Ataide R, Mackintosh CL, Fowkes FJ, et al. Targets of antibodies against *Plasmodium falciparum*-infected erythrocytes in malaria immunity. *J Clin Invest.* (2012) 122:3227–38. doi: 10.1172/JCI62182
25. Barfod L, Dalgaard MB, Pleman ST, Ofori MF, Pleass RJ, Hviid L. Evasion of immunity to *Plasmodium falciparum* malaria by IgM masking of protective IgG epitopes in infected erythrocyte surface-exposed PfEMP1. *Proc Natl Acad Sci USA.* (2011) 108:12485–90. doi: 10.1073/pnas.1103708108
26. Cranmer SL, Magowan C, Liang J, Coppel RL, Cooke BM. An alternative to serum for cultivation of *Plasmodium falciparum in vitro. Trans R Soc Trop Med Hyg.* (1997) 91:363–5. doi: 10.1016/S0035-9203(97)90110-3
27. Staalsoe T, Nielsen MA, Vestergaard LS, Jensen AT, Theander TG, Hviid L. *In vitro* selection of *Plasmodium falciparum* 3D7 for expression of variant surface antigens associated with severe malaria in African children. *Parasite Immunol.* (2003) 25:421–7.doi: 10.1111/j.1365-3024.2003.00652.x
28. Staalsoe T, Giha HA, Dodoo D, Theander TG, Hviid L. Detection of antibodies to variant antigens on *Plasmodium falciparum*-infected erythrocytes by flow cytometry. *Cytometry* (1999) 35:329–36.
29. De Jong RN, Beurskens FJ, Verploegen S, Strumane K, Van Kampen MD, Voorhorst M, et al. A novel platform for the potentiation of therapeutic antibodies based on antigen-dependent formation of IgG hexamers at the cell surface. *PLoS Biol.* (2016) 14:e1002344. doi: 10.1371/journal.pbio.1002344
30. Dekkers G, Plomp R, Koeleman CA, Visser R, Von Horsten HH, Sandig V, et al. Multi-level glyco-engineering techniques to generate IgG with defined Fc-glycans. *Sci Rep.* (2016) 6:36964. doi: 10.1038/srep36964
31. Cohen S, Mcgregor IA, Carrington S. Gammaglobulin and acquired immunity to human malaria. *Nature* (1961) 192:733–7. doi: 10.1038/192733a0
32. Bouharoun-Tayoun H, Attanath P, Sabchareon A, Chongsuphajaisiddhi T, Druilhe P. Antibodies that protect humans against *Plasmodium falciparum* blood stages do not on their own inhibit parasite growth and invasion *in vitro*, but act in cooperation with monocytes. *J Exp Med.* (1990) 172:1633–41. doi: 10.1084/jem.172.6.1633
33. Storm J, Craig AG. Pathogenesis of cerebral malaria - inflammation and cytoadherence. *Front Cell Infect Microbiol.* (2014) 4:100. doi: 10.3389/fcimb.2014.00100
34. Yam XY, Preiser PR. Host immune evasion strategies of malaria blood stage parasite. *Mol Biosyst.* (2017) 13:2498–508. doi: 10.1039/c7mb00502d
35. Megnekou R, Staalsoe T, Taylor DW, Leke R, Hviid L. Effects of pregnancy and intensity of *Plasmodium falciparum* transmission on immunoglobulin G subclass responses to variant surface antigens. *Infect Immun.* (2005) 73:4112–8. doi: 10.1128/IAI.73.7.4112-4118.2005
36. Reiss T, Rosa TFA, Blaesius K, Bobbert RP, Zipfel PF, Skerka C, et al. FHR-1 binding impairs Factor H-mediated complement evasion by the malaria parasite *Plasmodium falciparum. J Immunol.* (2018) 201:3497–502. doi: 10.4049/jimmunol.1800662
37. Weiss GE, Crabb BS, Gilson PR. Overlaying molecular and temporal aspects of malaria parasite invasion. *Trends Parasitol.* (2016) 32:284–95. doi: 10.1016/j.pt.2015.12.007
38. Sidjanski S, Vanderberg JP. Delayed migration of *Plasmodium* sporozoites from the mosquito bite site to the blood. *Am J Trop Med Hyg.* (1997) 57:426–9. doi: 10.4269/ajtmh.1997.57.426
39. David PH, Hommel M, Miller LH, Udeinya IJ, Oligino LD. Parasite sequestration in *Plasmodium falciparum* malaria: spleen and antibody modulation of cytoadherence of infected erythrocytes. *Proc Natl Acad Sci USA.* (1983) 80:5075–9. doi: 10.1073/pnas.80.16.5075
40. Nagao E, Kaneko O, Dvorak JA. *Plasmodium falciparum*-infected erythrocytes: qualitative and quantitative analyses of parasite-induced knobs by atomic force microscopy. *J Struct Biol.* (2000) 130:34–44. doi: 10.1006/jsbi.2000.4236

41. Joergensen LM, Salanti A, Dobrilovic T, Barfod L, Hassenkam T, Theander TG, et al. The kinetics of antibody binding to *Plasmodium falciparum* VAR2CSA PfEMP1 antigen and modelling of PfEMP1 antigen packing on the membrane knobs. *Malar J.* (2010) 9:100. doi: 10.1186/1475-2875-9-100
42. Clausen TM, Christoffersen S, Dahlback M, Langkilde AE, Jensen KE, Resende M, et al. Structural and functional insight into how the *Plasmodium falciparum* VAR2CSA protein mediates binding to chondroitin sulfate A in placental malaria. *J Biol Chem.* (2012) 287:23332–45. doi: 10.1074/jbc.M112.348839
43. Quadt KA, Barfod L, Andersen D, Bruun J, Gyan B, Hassenkam T, et al. The density of knobs on *Plasmodium falciparum*-infected erythrocytes depends on developmental age and varies among isolates. *PLoS ONE* (2012) 7:e45658. doi: 10.1371/journal.pone.0045658
44. Xu X, Efremov AK, Li A, Lai L, Dao M, Lim CT, et al. Probing the cytoadherence of malaria infected red blood cells under flow. *PLoS ONE* (2013) 8:e64763. doi: 10.1371/journal.pone.0064763
45. Stevenson L, Huda P, Jeppesen A, Laursen E, Rowe JA, Craig A, et al. Investigating the function of F_C-specific binding of IgM to *Plasmodium falciparum* erythrocyte membrane protein 1 mediating erythrocyte rosetting. *Cell Microbiol.* (2015) 17:819–31. doi: 10.1111/cmi.12403
46. Subramani R, Quadt K, Jeppesen AE, Hempel C, Petersen JE, Hassenkam T, et al. *Plasmodium falciparum*-infected erythrocyte knob density is linked to the PfEMP1 variant expressed. *mBio* (2015) 6:e01456–15. doi: 10.1128/mBio.01456-15
47. Wiesner J, Jomaa H, Wilhelm M, Tony HP, Kremsner PG, Horrocks P, et al. Host cell factor CD59 restricts complement lysis of *Plasmodium falciparum*-infected erythrocytes. *Eur J Immunol.* (1997) 27:2708–13. doi: 10.1002/eji.1830271034

17

Chimeric Proteins Containing MAP-1 and Functional Domains of C4b-Binding Protein Reveal Strong Complement Inhibitory Capacities

Cecilie E. Hertz[1†], Rafael Bayarri-Olmos[1†], Nikolaj Kirketerp-Møller[1], Sander van Putten[2], Katrine Pilely[1], Mikkel-Ole Skjoedt[1] and Peter Garred[1]*

[1] Laboratory of Molecular Medicine, Department of Clinical Immunology Section, Rigshospitalet, Faculty of Health and Medical Sciences, University of Copenhagen, Copenhagen, Denmark, [2] Finsen Laboratory, Rigshospitalet, Biotech Research and Innovation Center (BRIC), Faculty of Health and Medical Sciences, University of Copenhagen, Copenhagen, Denmark

***Correspondence:**
Rafael Bayarri-Olmos
rafael.bayarri.olmos@regionh.dk

†These authors have contributed equally to this work and are joint first authors

The complement system is a tightly regulated network of proteins involved in defense against pathogens, inflammatory processes, and coordination of the innate and adaptive immune responses. Dysregulation of the complement cascade is associated with many inflammatory disorders. Thus, inhibition of the complement system has emerged as an option for treatment of a range of different inflammatory diseases. MAP-1 is a pattern recognition molecule (PRM)-associated inhibitor of the lectin pathway of the complement system, whereas C4b-binding protein (C4BP) regulates both the classical and lectin pathways. In this study we generated chimeric proteins consisting of MAP-1 and the first five domains of human C4BP ($C4BP^{1-5}$) in order to develop a targeted inhibitor acting at different levels of the complement cascade. Two different constructs were designed and expressed in CHO cells where MAP-1 was fused with $C4BP^{1-5}$ in either the C- or N-terminus. The functionality of the chimeric proteins was assessed using different *in vitro* complement activation assays. Both chimeric proteins displayed the characteristic Ca^{2+}-dependent dimerization and binding to PRMs of native MAP-1, as well as the co-factor activity of native C4BP. In ELISA-based complement activation assays they could effectively inhibit the lectin and classical pathways. Notably, MAP-1:$C4BP^{1-5}$ was five times more effective than rMAP-1 and $rC4BP^{1-5}$ applied at the same time, emphasizing the advantage of a single inhibitor containing both functional domains. The MAP-1/C4BP chimeras exert unique complement inhibitory properties and represent a novel therapeutic approach targeting both upstream and central complement activation.

Keywords: complement activation, lectin pathway, classical pathway, MAP-1, C4BP, complement inhibition, chimeric protein

INTRODUCTION

The complement system constitutes a central effector arm of the vertebrate immune system occupying a pivotal position as an early danger sensor and mediator of immunological and inflammatory processes (1, 2). Complement is activated via three distinct pathways, i.e., the classical (CP) the lectin (LP) and the alternative pathway (AP) that converge on the generation and deposition of opsonins, release of anaphylatoxins, and generation of the terminal complement complex (TCC) which all together help coordinating the cellular and humoral immune responses (3–6).

Initiation of CP is mediated mainly by the binding of C1q to immune-complexes, but also to conserved pathogen-specific structures, altered self-antigens or interaction with the pentraxins (7) and leads to the activation of the serine proteases C1r and C1s (8, 9). The LP is initiated by two groups of pattern recognition molecules (PRM): c-type lectins, such as mannose-binding lectin (MBL), collectin-10 (CL-10, CL-L1), and collectin-11 (CL-11, CL-K1) and ficolins, i.e., ficolin-1 (M-ficolin), ficolin-2 (L-ficolin), and ficolin-3 (H-ficolin or Hakata antigen). Binding of PRMs to ligands activates the MBL-associated serine proteases (MASPs), causing cleavage and activation of C2 and C4 (10). The AP is constantly "probing" surfaces in a non-specific fashion by means of a constitutive low level of spontaneous hydrolysis of C3 into the C3b analog C3(H_2O) (11). Maybe more importantly, C3b generated from any of the three pathways is amplified via the AP. In fact, AP amplification may account for up to 90% of the total complement activation independently of the triggering pathway (7, 12). Whether the AP can be activated via a similar PRM-dependent mechanism involving properdin remains controversial (13, 14).

Complement is much more than a pathogen-sensing system, with ties spanning into coagulation, inflammation and embryonic development (2). In order to carry out its diverse functions it relies on a delicate balance between activation and inhibition by means of a set of membrane-bound and soluble regulatory proteins (15), the latter including the LP inhibitor MBL/ficolin/CL-associated protein 1 (MAP-1, also named MAp44), and the LP and CP regulators C4b-binding protein (C4BP) and C1 inhibitor (a protease inhibitor of the serpin super family that inactivates C1r, C1s, MASP-1, and MASP-2) (16).

Two genes encode all five naturally-occurring MASP isoforms in mammals (17): three proenzymes (i.e., MASP-1, -2, and -3) and the two non-proteolytic proteins sMAP (MAp19) and MAP-1. The proteolytic MASPs consist of a heavy chain—comprised of two CUB domains separated by an epidermal growth factor (EGF) domain, and two complement control protein/short consensus repeats (CCP/SCR) modules—and a light chain composed of the serine protease domain. MAP-1 differs from the proteolytic MASPs in that it lacks the second SCR and SP domain and thus it cannot activate complement. MAP-1 competes with the MASPs in binding to recognition molecules of the LP leading to decreased complement activation. This has been demonstrated *in vitro* (18–20), and in multiple *in vivo* disease models (21, 22).

C4BP is a soluble protein encoded in the regulator of complement activation (RCA) gene locus of chromosome 1 (23) and possesses a unique structure among the RCA proteins in being a polymer composed of several CCP containing polypeptides. The most abundant isoform in the circulation is composed of seven identical α-chains (75 kDa each) and one β-chain (45 kDa) linked together by a central core and found in a high affinity complex with the anticoagulant vitamin K-dependent protein S (24, 25). The complement regulatory functions of C4BP are located within the first CCP domains of the α-chains. C4BP binds to the negatively-charged surface of C4b via the first three CCP domains of the α-chain preventing the assembly of the classical and lectin pathways C3 convertases (26, 27). Additionally, C4BP acts as a cofactor in the complement factor I (fI)-mediated proteolytic inactivation of both soluble and membrane bound C4b (28–30). By binding to C3b via the first 4 CCP domains of the α-chain, C4BP also participates in the fI-dependent C3b degradation to iC3b in the fluid phase (31). Although it is difficult to speculate upon the genuine physiological role of the inhibitory function of C4BP since no C4BP deficiency has been diagnosed in humans (32), C4BP injected peritoneally has been shown to alleviate inflammation and tissue damage in collagen- and collagen antibody-induced arthritis mouse models (33).

Since the US Food and Drug Administration approval of the first complement-specific drug in 2007 (34), rational modulation of the complement cascade using complement inhibitors has gradually demonstrated its potential as a drug discovery strategy and therapeutic treatment (35). Especially recombinant chimeric proteins targeting different levels of the cascade are of great interest in complement-mediated therapy and have previously been created with success (36, 37). Here we aimed to create a dual inhibitor with the ability to target initial activation by both the lectin and classical pathways by combining full length MAP-1 with the first five N-terminal CCP domains of the α-chain of C4BP. This could provide a unique platform for a novel class of complement inhibitor and thus contribute to the emerging field of complement therapeutics.

MATERIALS AND METHODS

Buffers

The following buffers were used: PBS (0.2 M Na_2HPO_4, 35 mM K_2HPO_4, 0.15 M NaCl, 15 mM KCl), PBS/NaCl (0.2 M Na_2HPO_4, 35 mM K_2HPO_4, 0.5 M NaCl, 15 mM KCl), TBS/Ca^{2+} and TBS/Tw/Ca^{2+} (20 mM Tris-HCl, 150 mM NaCl, 5 mM $CaCl_2$, with/without 0.05% Tween-20), TBS/EDTA and TBS/Tw/EDTA (20 mM Tris-HCl, 150 mM NaCl, 10 mM EDTA, with/without 0.05% Tween), VBS/Tw and sample buffer (4 mM $C_8H_{11}N_2NaO_3$, 145 mM NaCl, 2.6 mM $CaCl_2$, 2 mM $MgCl_2$, with 0.05% Tween-20 or 0.5% BSA respectively).

Design of Chimeric Proteins and Transfection

The coding sequences for MAP-1 (NM_001031849.2) and C4BP (NM_000715.3) were optimized for expression in Chinese hamster ovarian (CHO) cells in terms of codon adaptation index, mRNA stability, GC content, removal of cryptic splice sites, and repeats, 5' UTR, and signal peptide. All DNA manipulations were performed in Visual Gene Developer (38). MAP-1:$C4BP^{1-5}$ comprises the coding sequence of MAP-1 followed by the first five CCP domains of the α-chain of C4BP ($C4BP^{1-5}$). The reverse construct $C4BP^{1-5}$:MAP-1 was designed with the coding

Abbreviations: CP, LP, AP, Classical, lectin, and alternative pathway; PRM, Pattern recognition molecule; IC50, Half maximal inhibitory concentration; Kd, half maximal binding concentration; SEM, Standard error of the mean; PTEC, Proximal tubular epithelial cells.

sequence of $C4BP^{1-5}$ located in the N-terminus of MAP-1 and separated by a flexible glycine serine linker $(G_4S)_3$. A control construct consisting of $C4BP^{1-5}$ alone was designed with a C-terminal hexa histidine-tag. In all cases, the signal peptide of MAP-1 was used to ensure secretion. The chimeric constructs were cloned into the pcDNA5/FRT vector and transfected into Flp-in CHO cells (both from Invitrogen, Thermo Fisher Scientific, USA) according to the manufacturer's instructions. Positive transfectants were selected for Hygromycin resistance in complete medium with Ham's F-12 Nutrient Mix, 10% fetal calf serum, 2 mM L-Glutamine, 1% Penicillin-Streptomycin (Sigma-Aldrich, USA), and 500 mM of Hygromycin B (all from Gibco, Thermo Fisher Scientific unless otherwise stated), and maintained at 37°C in a humidified atmosphere with 5% CO_2.

Purification of Recombinant Proteins

The chimeric constructs were purified by immunoaffinity chromatography using the monoclonal antibody (mAb) anti-MAP-1 20C4 (39) coupled to cyanogen bromide-activated-sepharose 4B (Sigma-Aldrich). Briefly, filtered cell culture supernatants were applied to the column and washed in PBS/NaCl. Bound protein was eluted with 0.5% (w/v) citric acid (pH 2.5) and neutralized with 1 M Tris-HCl (pH 9). Elution fractions were applied on a NuPAGE bis-tris 4–12% polyacrylamide gel (Invitrogen), followed by a direct protein stain with Instant Blue (Expedeon LTD, UK) to assess the purity. The concentration of the chimeric proteins was interpolated by ELISA using rMAP-1 as standard. $rC4BP^{1-5}$ was purified with a HisTrap excel column (GE Healthcare, Denmark) according to the manufacturer's instructions.

SDS-Page and Western Immunoblotting

SDS-PAGE was performed using NuPAGE bis-tris 4–12% gels with or without reducing agent and blotted onto Hybond™-ECL nitrocellulose membranes (GE Healthcare) according to the manufacter's instructions. The membranes were probed with 0.5 μg/ml anti-MAP-1 20C4 or 0.3 μg/ml anti-human C4BP polyclonal antibody (pAb; Abnova, 722-D01P, Taiwan) overnight, followed by 1 h incubation with 0.4 μg/ml rabbit anti-mouse-HRP pAb (Dako, P0260, Denmark) or a 1:4000 dilution of donkey anti-rabbit-HRP pAb (GE Healthcare, NA934V) for MAP-1 and C4BP, respectively. The membranes were developed with SuperSignal WestFemto (Thermo Fisher Scientific) and analyzed with Microchemi (Bio-imaging systems, Israel).

Fluid Phase C4BP Cofactor Assay

The cofactor activity of C4BP, MAP-1:$C4BP^{1-5}$, and $C4BP^{1-5}$:MAP-1 was assessed with an established fluid phase cofactor activity assay (40, 41) measuring the fI-cofactor activity of C4BP in the proteolytic inactivation of C4b and C3b. Briefly, C4b and C3b were incubated with fI, complement factor H (fH), and equimolar concentrations of full length C4BP (all from Complement Technology Inc., USA), recombinant MAP-1 (rMAP-1, produced in house), MAP-1:$C4BP^{1-5}$, or $C4BP^{1-5}$:MAP-1 for 2 h at 37°C. The reactions were stopped with LDS sample buffer and reducing agent (both from Invitrogen). Samples were subjected to electrophoresis and immunoblotting as described above. Cleavage of C3b was visualized by incubation with 1.6 μg/ml rabbit anti-human C3d pAb (Dako, A006302) followed by donkey anti rabbit-HRP (GE Healthcare, NA934V) in a 1:5000 dilution. C4b cleavage was assessed by incubation with 0.3 μg/ml mouse anti-human C4d mAb (Thermo Fischer Scientific) and 0.4 μg/ml rabbit anti mouse-HRP (Dako). Membranes were developed as described previously.

Size Exclusion Chromatography (SEC)

The chimeric proteins (50 μg) were applied to a Superdex 200 HR 10/30 column (GE Healthcare) with a flow rate of 0.5 ml/min in TBS/Ca^{2+} or TBS/EDTA. The eluate was collected in 1 ml fractions and analyzed by ELISA (see below).

ELISA

Assessment of Ca^{2+}-Dependent Dimerization by Sandwich ELISA Following SEC

Microtiter wells (MaxiSorp plate; Thermo Fisher Scientific) were coated with anti-C4BP pAb (2 μg/ml) in PBS overnight at 4°C. SEC fractions were applied in a two-fold dilution starting at 1:20 and incubated for 2 h. Biotinylated 8B3 mAb (2 μg/ml), recognizing the common heavy chain of MASP-1, MASP-3 and MAP-1 (39), was used as detection antibody for 2 h. Streptavidin-HRP conjugate (Sigma Aldrich, RPN1231V) (1:2000) was added for 1 h and the plates were developed with substrate solution TMB One (Kem Em Tek, Denmark). The reaction was stopped with 0.2 M H_2SO_4 and the absorbance was measured at 450 nm using an ELx80 absorbance reader (BioTek, USA).

Binding of Chimeric Proteins to Ligand-Bound MBL and CL-11

Microtiter wells were coated with 10 μg/ml mannan (Sigma Aldrich) in PBS overnight at 4°C followed by incubation with recombinant MBL or recombinant CL-11 (rMBL and rCL-11 produced in house; 2 μg/ml) (42). Serial dilutions of MAP-1:$C4BP^{1-5}$, $C4BP^{1-5}$:MAP-1, rMAP-1, and $rC4BP^{1-5}$ in TBS/Tween/Ca^{2+} or TBS/Tween/EDTA starting at 13.5 nM were allowed to complex with rMBL for 2 h. Detection and development were done as described above. Binding of rMBL and rCL-11 to mannan was confirmed using biotinylated anti-MBL Hyb-131-1 mAb and anti-CL-11 Hyb-15 mAb (2 μg/ml), respectively.

Complement Activation Assays

Inhibition of complement activation via the LP was determined by an established ELISA-based assay (42) using specific antibodies to detect the activated and deposited products of C4, C3, and TCC. The chimeric proteins ability to inhibit complement was tested in MBL defect serum (43) and normal human serum (NHS). Mannan (10 μg/ml) was immobilized onto microtiter plates and incubated in PBS overnight at 4°C followed by incubation with 2 μg/ml rMBL for 1.5 h. Serial dilutions of rMAP-1, $C4BP^{1-5}$:MAP-1, and MAP-1:$C4BP^{1-5}$ starting at 667 nM were incubated with mannan/rMBL complexes for 1 h prior to addition of 2% MBL defect serum. When using NHS as a complement source, serial dilutions of $C4BP^{1-5}$:MAP-1, MAP-1:$C4BP^{1-5}$, MAP-1, and purified C4BP, starting at 667 nM, were added to round bottom non-absorbent titration plates (Thermo Fisher Scientific) with 2% NHS. The serum-protein mix was incubated 30 min at 4°C, transferred to mannan (10 µg/ml) coated plates and incubated for 45 min at 37°C. Detection of deposition fragments was quantified with 2 µg/ml biotinylated mouse mAbs anti-human C4 (Anti-C4) (Bioporto Diagnostics, Denmark, Hyb 162-02), 2 µg/ml anti-human C3bc BH6 (44), and 1 µg/ml anti-human C5b-9 (anti-TCC; Bioporto, Dia 011-01) incubated for 2 h. Finally, Streptavidin-HRP conjugate was added in a 1:2000 dilution for 1 h. Unless otherwise specified, all washes and incubation steps were done with VBS/Tw. Development was performed with substrate solution TMB One. Data are represented as inhibition (%), calculated as $[(OD_{inhibitor} - OD_{background})/(OD_{noinhibitor} - OD_{background})]100$.

Total Complement Screen

The Wieslab^{TM} Complement System Screenkit COMPL 300 (Euro diagnostica, Sweden) (45), a standardized immunoassay for measuring TCC formation by all three complement pathways, was used to assess the inhibitory capabilities of the chimeric proteins beyond the LP. MAP-1:$C4BP^{1-5}$, $C4BP^{1-5}$:MAP-1, rMAP-1, r$C4BP^{1-5}$, and rMAP-1 plus r$C4BP^{1-5}$ (starting at 667 nM for LP and CP, and at 2667 nM for AP) were applied in a two-fold dilution in non-absorbent titration plates in the respective buffers for each pathway provided with the kit. NHS in a 1:100 dilution for the CP and LP and a 1:20 for the AP was co-incubated with the inhibitors for 30 min at 4°C. Protein/serum mixes were transferred to pre-coated 96-well microtiter plates and incubated 1 h at 37°C. Following incubation the samples were analyzed with the Wieslab Complement System Screenkit according to the instruction from the manufacturer. Data are represented as described in the previous paragraph without background subtraction.

Flow Cytometry

Complement activation on kidney cells was studied by flow cytometry using HK-2 cells (ATCC, CRL-2190), an immortalized human proximal tubular epithelial cell (PTEC) line reported to be a suitable alternative to freshly isolated PTCs (46). Cells were cultured in Keratinocyte Serum Free Medium supplemented with bovine pituitary extract, human recombinant epidermal growth factor (all from Gibco) and 0.5% Penicillin-Streptomycin (Sigma-Aldrich). On the day of the experiments, the cells were detached with TryPLE Express Enzyme, washed with pre-warmed Hank's balanced salt solution (both from Gibco) with calcium and magnesium, and transferred to polystyrene round bottom tubes (Corning, USA). Data was collected using a Gallios flow cytometer and analyzed by the Kaluza software 1.2 (both from Beckman Coulter, USA). Values are reported as median fluorescence intensities (MFI). To ensure analysis of single cells, a forward scatter area vs. height gate was defined upon a uniform gated population on the forward vs. side scatter (see **Supplementary Figure 1**). A total of 10,000 events were recorded per experimental condition.

Binding of MBL to Kidney Cells

HK-2 cells (1.0×10^5 cells/test) were incubated with serial dilutions of rMBL for 30 min at 4°C in sample buffer with or without EDTA. Prior to the addition of the detection antibody, the cells were fixed in a 1% solution of paraformaldehyde (Sigma Aldrich) for 10 min. Bound rMBL was detected using anti-human MBL Hyb 131-11 mAb (2 µg/ml) for 30 min plus goat anti-mouse PE conjugate (Sigma, P9670) in a 1:20 dilution for 20 min in the dark. The cells were washed with sample buffer at $300 \times g$ for 5 min in between steps and all manipulations were performed at 4°C.

Complement Deposition on Kidney Cells

HK-2 cells (1.0×10^5 cells/test) were incubated with rMBL for 30 min, followed by 10% MBL defect serum for 1 h. The cells were fixed with 1% paraformaldehyde for 10 min. Surface-bound C4 was measured with biotinylated anti-human C4c pAb (2 µg/ml) (Dako, Q036905) for 30 min followed by Streptavidin APC conjugate (1:400) (Invitrogen, SA1005) for 20 min in the dark. To study the impact of the chimeric inhibitors on C4 deposition, serial dilutions of MAP-1:$C4BP^{1-5}$, and $C4BP^{1-5}$:MAP-1, rMAP-1, and $C4BP^{1-5}$ (200 nM) were allowed to react with 10% MBL defect serum for 20 min prior to incubating with the rMBL-bound HK-2 cells for 1 h. After fixing the cells C4 deposition was measured as described previously. All washes and incubation steps were done in sample buffer at 4°C.

Statistics

All statistical analyses were performed in GraphPad Prism software 7.02 (GraphPad, USA). Kd values (i.e., ligand concentration required to achieve half of the maximum binding) were calculated using the equation specific binding with Hill slope after subtracting the background OD and constraining the Bmax (maximum number of binding sites) to a value shared between all inhibitors (**Figure 3**). The half maximal inhibitory concentration (IC50) was calculated using a global nonlinear regression with the equation inhibitor concentration vs. response constraining the top and bottom parameters to equal 100 and 0 respectively (**Figures 4**, **5**, **8**). The significance of inhibitory differences was analyzed using one-way ANOVA with Tukey's corrections for multiple comparisons on the best-fit IC50 values from data sets with an acceptable goodness-of-fit (adjusted R-squared > 0.8). Significance of the binding of rMBL and MBL-dependent C4 deposition on the surface of HK-2 cells was assessed using a two-tailed *t*-test, while inhibition was analyzed using multiple unpaired *t*-tests with the Holm-Sidak correction for multiple comparisons. Data are represented as mean ± SEM of three independent experiments.

RESULTS

Production and Purification of Chimeric Proteins

We designed two differently-oriented chimeric inhibitors: MAP-1:$C4BP^{1-5}$, with the first five CCP domains of the α-chain of C4BP (alias $C4BP^{1-5}$) located in the C-terminus of MAP-1; and $C4BP^{1-5}$:MAP-1, where $C4BP^{1-5}$ was placed in the

N-terminus of MAP-1 via a flexible glycine-serine linker. A control protein, C4BP$^{1-5}$ without MAP-1, was designed with a terminal hexa His-tag (**Figure 1A**). All three constructs were cloned into a pcDNA5/FRT plasmid and transfected into Flp-In CHO cells. MAP-1-containing chimeric proteins were purified by antibody affinity chromatography and C4BP1-5 was purified via immobilized metal ion affinity chromatography on a HisTrap excel column. Under reducing conditions, the chimeric proteins

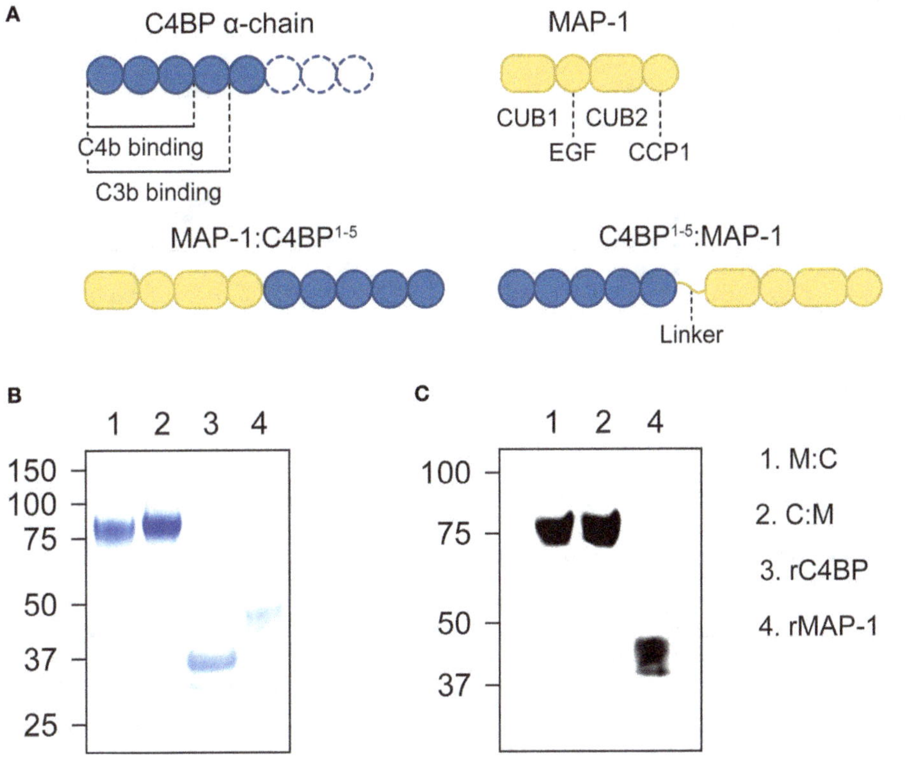

FIGURE 1 | Recombinant constructs and purified proteins. **(A)** Diagram of the domain distribution of MAP-1, C4BP α-chain and the recombinant proteins. **(B)** Instant blue stain of purified MAP-1:C4BP$^{1-5}$, C4BP$^{1-5}$:MAP-1, and C4BP$^{1-5}$via affinity chromatography. **(C)** The identity of the protein bands was confirmed by Western blotting using anti-MAP-1 mAb and rMAP-1 as positive control.

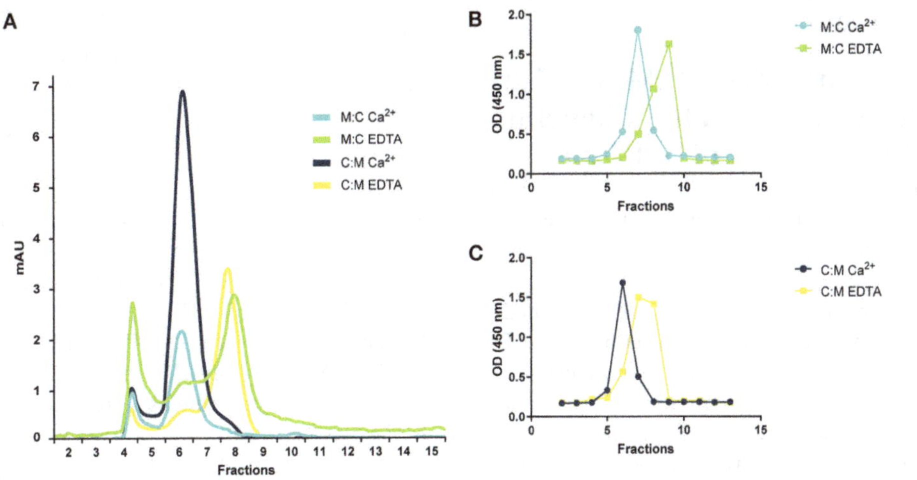

FIGURE 2 | Gel filtration chromatography of chimeric proteins. **(A)** Gel filtration profile of MAP-1:C4BP$^{1-5}$ (M:C) and C4BP$^{1-5}$:MAP-1 (C:M) under physiological calcium conditions or 10 mM EDTA. The identity of the gel filtration profiles was confirmed by analyzing the elution fractions of M:C **(B)** or C:M **(C)** by sandwich ELISA using anti-C4BP as capture antibody and anti-MASP-1/-3/MAP-1 as detection. Relative abundance of the chimeric proteins in the elution fractions following gel filtration under calcium conditions or EDTA is expressed as OD. mAU, milli absorption units.

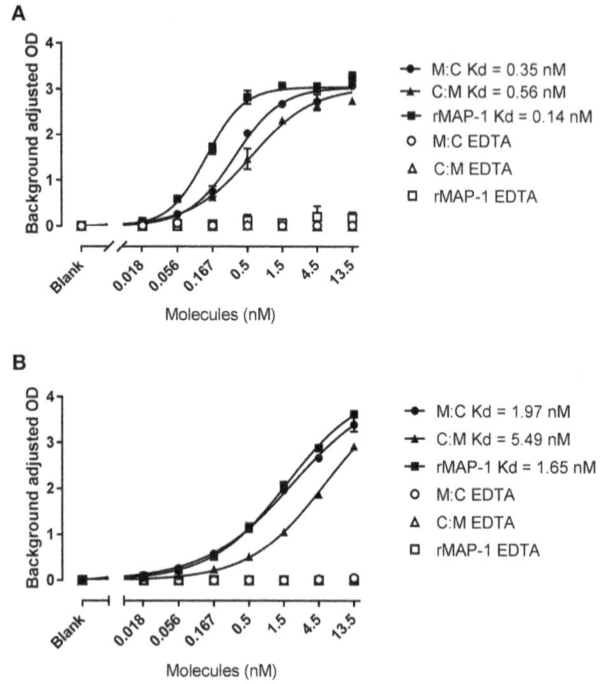

FIGURE 3 | MAP-1:C4BP$^{1-5}$ (M:C), C4BP$^{1-5}$:MAP-1 (C:M) and MAP-1 binding to MBL **(A)** and CL-11 **(B)**. rMBL and rCL-11 were immobilized onto mannan-coated plates. Recombinant proteins were applied in a two-fold dilution in the presence of calcium or EDTA. Binding was determined using an anti-MAP-1 mAb. Connecting lines display nonlinear fitting using the equation specific binding with hill slope. Results are representative of three independent experiments and error bars represent minimum and maximum values of triplicate measurements.

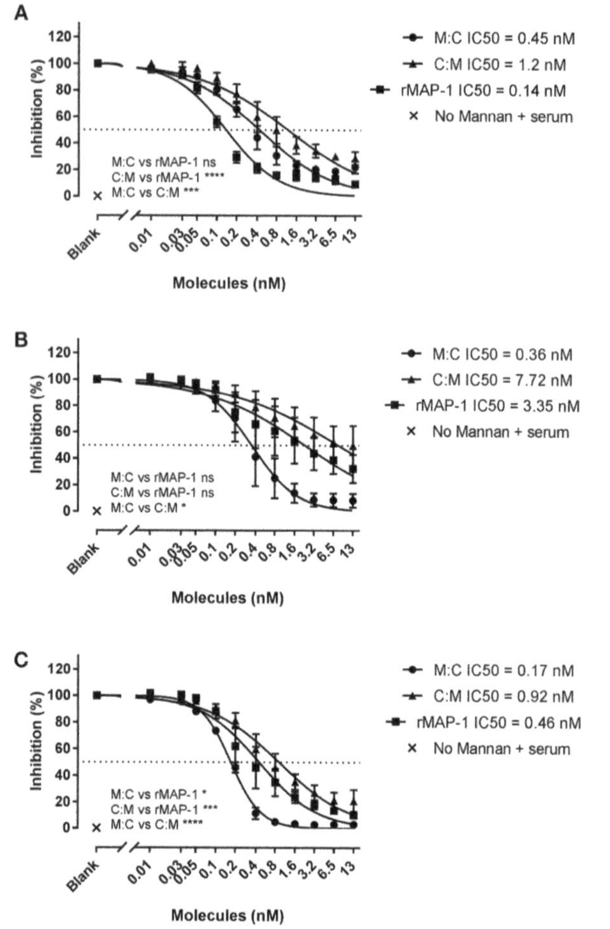

FIGURE 4 | Chimeric and rMAP-1 complement inhibition after pre-incubation on rMBL/mannan. Serial dilutions of MAP-1:C4BP$^{1-5}$ (M:C), C4BP$^{1-5}$:MAP-1 (C:M), and rMAP-1 were allowed to form complexes with mannan-bound rMBL prior to addition of MBL-defect serum as a source of complement. Detection of C4 **(A)**, C3 **(B)**, and TCC **(C)** deposition was quantified using anti-C4, anti-C3, and anti-TCC mouse mAbs. Connecting lines are four parameters nonlinear fitting using the equation inhibitor concentration vs. slope. Data are reported as $[(OD_{inhibitor}-OD_{background})/(OD_{noinhibitor}-OD_{background})]100$. Error bars represent the SEM of three independent experiments, and the dashed line the 50% inhibition level. $^{*}P < 0.05$; $^{***}P < 0.001$; $^{****}P < 0.0001$.

migrated as a single band with an apparent molecular weight of ~80 kDa, equivalent to the sum of rMAP-1 and rC4BP$^{1-5}$ molecular weights (i.e., ~44 kDa and ~37 kDa respectively; **Figure 1B**). The identity of the protein bands was confirmed by Western blotting (**Figure 1C**).

MAP-1:C4BP$^{1-5}$ and C4BP$^{1-5}$:MAP-1 Form Dimers and Associate With the Collectins of the LP in the Presence of Calcium

The MASPs are known to form head-to-tail dimers via the interaction of the CUB1 and EGF domains and to associate with the recognition molecules of the LP in a Ca^{2+}-dependent manner (18, 47, 48). To study the effect of calcium in the dimerization of our recombinant inhibitors, we performed gel filtration with and without EDTA, a Ca^{2+}-chelating agent. Both chimeric proteins eluted in a single overlapping peak in fractions 6–8 under physiological calcium concentrations. In the presence of EDTA, the previous peak was drastically reduced and a new one appeared in fractions 7–9 indicating that both are capable of assembling into dimers stabilized by Ca^{2+} (**Figure 2**).

Both chimeric proteins and MAP-1 were able to bind to rMBL and rCL-11 in a dose-dependent manner with equivalent dose-response curves in the presence of Ca^{2+} (**Figure 3**). On rMBL, MAP-1:C4BP$^{1-5}$ and C4BP$^{1-5}$:MAP-1 exhibited a similar Kd of 0.35 and 0.56 nM respectively, slightly lower affinity than rMAP-1 at the given conditions (0.14 nM; **Figure 3A**). The same tendency, albeit with weaker interactions, was observed with rCL-11 (**Figure 3B**): rMAP-1 displayed the lowest Kd (1.65 nM), followed by MAP-1:C4BP$^{1-5}$ (1.97 nM) and lastly C4BP$^{1-5}$:MAP-1 (5.49 nM). As expected, no binding could be detected when the proteins were incubated in the presence of EDTA.

Inhibition of LP Activation With MBL Defect Serum and NHS

To study the effect of the chimeric constructs on LP-mediated complement activation we used mannan-bound rMBL as the activating PRM. MAP-1:C4BP$^{1-5}$ and C4BP$^{1-5}$:MAP-1

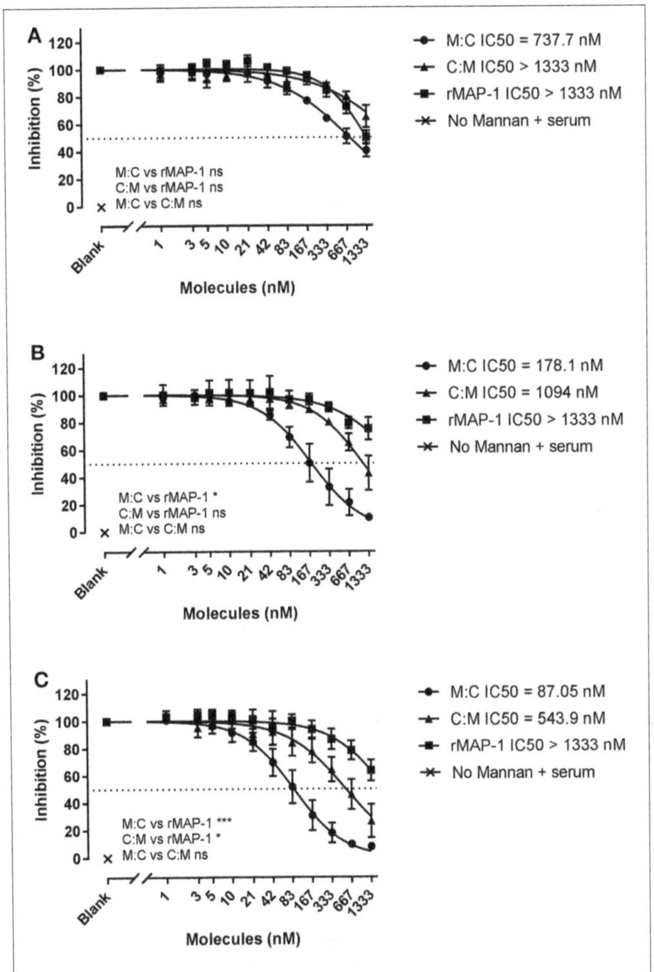

FIGURE 5 | Chimeric and rMAP-1 complement inhibition after co-incubation with NHS. Serial dilutions of MAP-1:C4BP$^{1-5}$ (M:C), C4BP$^{1-5}$:MAP-1 (C:M), and rMAP-1 were co-incubated with 2% NHS in non-adsorbent titration plates for 30 min prior to addition to mannan-bound rMBL. Detection of deposition of C4 **(A)**, C3 **(B)**, and TCC **(C)** was determined as described before. Connecting lines are four parameters nonlinear fitting using the equation inhibitor concentration vs. slope. Dashed line Data are reported as $[(OD_{inhibitor} - OD_{background})/(OD_{noinhibitor} - OD_{background})]100$. Error bars represent the SEM of three independent experiments, and the dashed line the 50% inhibition level. $^{*}P < 0.05$; $^{***}P < 0.001$.

exhibited a strong dose-dependent inhibition on C4, C3, and TCC level when they were allowed to form complexes with rMBL prior to the addition of 2% MBL defect serum as complement source (**Figure 4**). rMAP-1 was the most effective at the C4 level: IC50 MAP-1 (0.14 nM) vs. IC50 MAP-1:C4BP$^{1-5}$ (0.45 nM), non-significant; IC50 MAP-1 (0.14 nM) vs. IC50 C4BP$^{1-5}$:MAP-1 (1.2 nM), $P < 0.0001$. Nonetheless, MAP-1:C4BP$^{1-5}$ outperformed the rest when measuring C3 (IC50 MAP-1:C4BP$^{1-5}$ = 0.36 nM vs. 7.72 nM C4BP$^{1-5}$:MAP-1, $P < 0.05$, and 3.35 nM MAP-1, non-significant) and TCC deposition (IC50 MAP-1:C4BP^{1-}5 = 0.17 nM vs. 0.92 nM C4BP$^{1-5}$:MAP-1, $P < 0.0001$, and 0.46 nM MAP-1, $P < 0.05$).

Next, we tested the inhibitors by directly incubating them with 2% NHS in non-adsorbent titration plates before applying the inhibitor/serum mix to mannan (**Figure 5**). Under these conditions, both chimeric inhibitors demonstrated higher inhibition than rMAP-1 alone in the later steps of the complement cascade (i.e., C3 and TCC formation). MAP-1:C4BP$^{1-5}$ exhibited a more pronounced inhibition of C4 (non-significant tendency), C3 ($P < 0.05$), and TCC deposition ($P < 0.001$). The other construct appeared to be less active but still outperformed rMAP-1 at the C3 (non-significant trend) and TCC levels ($P < 0.05$). No complement deposition was observed when MBL defect serum was incubated without rMBL (**Figure 4**) or with rMBL but no mannan (**Figure 5**).

C4BP Cofactor Activity in FI-Mediated Cleavage of Soluble C4b/C3b

It has previously been reported that C4BP can act as a cofactor in the fI-mediated proteolytic inactivation of C3b and C4b (29, 31, 49). Hence we examined whether our chimeric proteins retained the fI cofactor activity of native C4BP.

When C4b was incubated with fI in combination with native full length C4BP or one of the two chimeric proteins, the α-chain of C4b was cleaved and a band corresponding to the smaller cleavage product C4d appeared (**Figure 6A**). As expected no full cofactor activity was observed for MAP-1 but the cleavage product iC4b was observed when MAP-1 was in combination with FI and C4b. Similarly, a low level proteolysis of C3b into iC3b could be observed in the presence of fI and MAP-1. Both are probably artifacts from the elevated fI concentrations used in the assays. No C4b proteolysis was apparent in the absence of cofactors or fI, with the notable exception of purified native C4BP. When C4b was incubated with C4BP alone a cleavage of the α-chain and generation of the iC4b was observed, hinting at a possible contamination of the purified C4BP. We performed a new immunoblotting with C4BP alone and in combination with fI or C4b. The iC4b band was visible in all wells, suggesting that iC4b had been co-purified with C4BP (data not shown).

A cleavage of the C3b α-chain band was observed together with the appearance of a band corresponding to iC3b when C3b was subjected to fI in combination with C4BP or one of the two chimeric proteins (**Figure 6B**). Full cleavage of C3b to C3dg could only be archived when fH was applied in combination with C3b and fI. As expected no cofactor activity was observed for MAP-1.

Reduction of MBL-Dependent C4 Deposition in Kidney Proximal Tubular Epithelial Cells

The complement system, and in particular MBL, has been documented as one of the key mediators of kidney injury following renal ischemia (50–53). Proximal tubular epithelial cells (PTECs), responsible for many regulatory and endocrine functions, are especially vulnerable to complement-mediated tissue damage (51). After demonstrating the efficacy of our chimeric inhibitors in the previous ELISA-based assays, we tested whether we could quench complement activation on PTECs. A dose-dependent MBL binding was observed when human PTECs were incubated with increasing concentrations of rMBL (**Figure 7A**). Binding could be neutralized with the

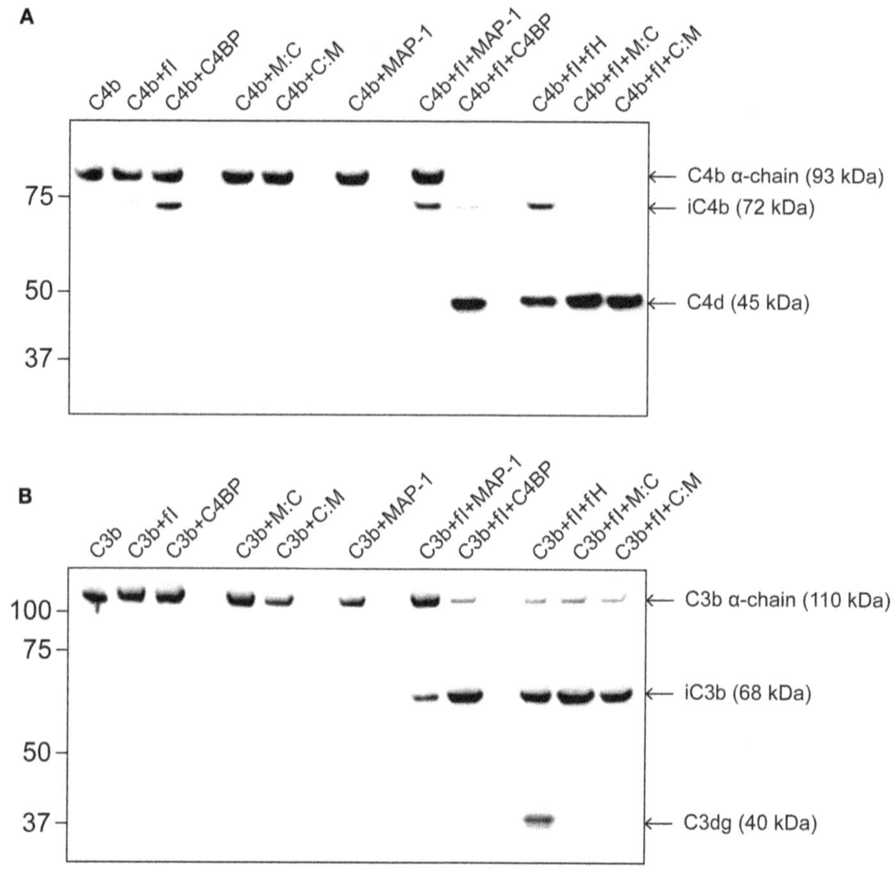

FIGURE 6 | Cofactor activity in factor I-mediated C4b and C3b cleavage. Purified C3b or C4b was incubated with fI and different cofactors for 2 h at 37°C. The reactions were stopped with LDS buffer and subjected to western blotting under reducing conditions using C4d and C3d antibodies. **(A)** Incubation of C4b with fI in the presence of C4BP, fH or C4BP-containing chimeric proteins resulted in the generation of a band corresponding to the inactive degradation products iC4b and C4d. **(B)** Incubation of C3b with fI in the presence of C4BP, fH or C4BP-containing chimeric proteins results in the generation of the 68 kDa degradation fragment. M:C, MAP-1:C4BP$^{1-5}$; C:M, C4BP$^{1-5}$:MAP-1. The blots are representative of three independent experiments.

addition of EDTA in the sample buffer, suggesting a classical c-type lectin interaction. Addition of 10% MBL defect serum to MBL-bound PTECs led to C4 deposition on the cell surface (**Figure 7B**) that was significantly reduced when rMAP-1 or the MAP-1-containing chimeras were incubated in a concentration of 200 nM with serum prior to addition to the MBL-bound cells as compared to the no inhibitor control (**Figure 7C**). Equimolar concentrations of rC4BP$^{1-5}$ alone showed no significant reduction of C4 deposition.

Total Complement Screen

We further assessed the ability of the chimeric inhibitors to regulate all three complement pathways using the commercial total complement screen assay Wielisa (45) (**Figure 8**). In agreement with the above results MAP-1:C4BP$^{1-5}$ was the most effective construct, significantly outperforming all other inhibitors in the LP (**Figure 8A**) and CP (**Figure 8B**) activation assays, while C4BP$^{1-5}$:MAP-1 demonstrated a more modest activity. The combination of rC4BP$^{1-5}$ and rMAP-1 displayed an inhibitory potential comparable to C4BP$^{1-5}$:MAP-1, and 5 to 10 times lower than MAP-1:C4BP$^{1-5}$. In the AP however (**Figure 8C**), MAP-1:C4BP$^{1-5}$ had only a minor effect, with an IC50 value comparable to rC4BP$^{1-5}$ (alone or in combination with rMAP-1). Inhibitors whose dose-response curves had a fitting with an adjusted R-square value < 0.8 were excluded for the analysis—such as rMAP-1 (**Figures 8A,B**) and all inhibitors besides MAP-1:C4BP$^{1-5}$ in the AP activation assay (**Figure 8C**).

DISCUSSION

The unique position of the complement system as an early danger sensor and conductor of downstream humoral and cellular responses makes complement modulation an attractive pharmacological target (36, 54). Rational engineering of existing complement regulators and novel recombinant inhibitors targeting complement on different levels has proven to be a successful strategy, such as mini-fH (41) and chimeric regulators composed of the N-terminal domains of fH merged with CRIg (55) or soluble CR2 (40). Complement factor H is the main soluble regulator of the AP and with CRIg being a C3 regulator

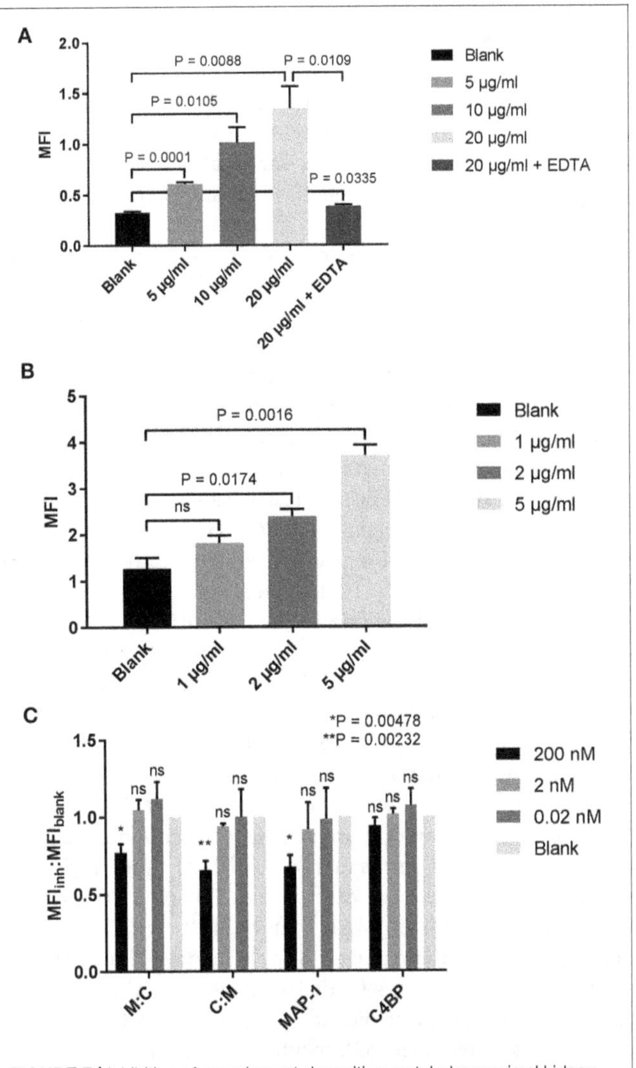

FIGURE 7 | Inhibition of complement deposition on tubular proximal kidney epithelial cells. **(A)** HK-2 cells were incubated with increasing concentrations of rMBL at 4°C and bound MBL was determined using an anti-MBL mAb. **(B)** Binding of MBL results in the deposition of C4. HK-2 cells were incubated with rMBL followed by 10% MBL defect serum for 1 h at 4°C. Bound C4 was determined using an anti-C4c pAb. **(C)** rMBL-mediated C4 deposition after MAP-1:C4BP$^{1-5}$ (M:C), C4BP$^{1-5}$:MAP-1 (C:M), rMAP-1 or full length C4BP co-incubation with 10% MBL defect serum. Inhibition is reported as the ratio of the MFI of the inhibitor to the MFI of the bank (MFI_{inh}:MFI_{blank}). Significance was tested for each concentration of the inhibitors compared to the blank. Data are reported as the mean ± SEM of three independent experiments.

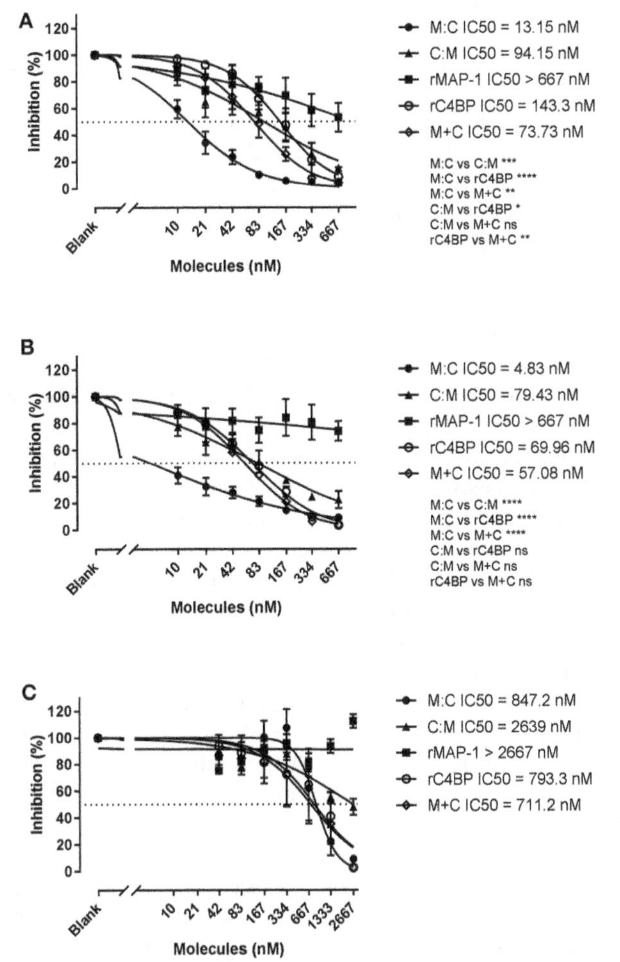

FIGURE 8 | Wielisa total complement screen. Serial dilutions of MAP-1:C4BP$^{1-5}$ (M:C), C4BP$^{1-5}$:MAP-1 (C:M), rMAP-1, rC4BP$^{1-5}$, and rMAP-1 and rC4BP$^{1-5}$ together (M+C) were incubated with NHS and subsequently the protein/serum mix was applied to pre-coated Wielisa plates. Complement activation was quantified using an anti-TCC mAb. **(A)** Lectin pathway activation on mannan-coated plates. **(B)** Classical pathway activation on IgM-coated plates. **(C)** Alternative activation on LPS-coated plates. Connecting lines are nonlinear fitting using the equation inhibitor concentration vs. slope. Values represent OD readings normalized to the OD of the wells without inhibitor times 100. Significance was tested for best-fit IC50 values of data sets with an adjusted R-squared > 0.8. Error bars represent the SEM of three independent experiments, and the dashed line the 50% inhibition level. $^{*}P < 0.05$; $^{**}P < 0.01$; $^{***}P < 0.001$; $^{****}P < 0.0001$.

and CR2 an inhibitor of C3 deposition all these molecules affect exclusively the alternative amplification loop. However, increasing understanding of the involvement of complement in highly diverse clinical conditions suggests a different approach with complement-targeted drugs interfering at various stages of the cascade (35). Our group has previously tested this strategy by combining full length MAP-1 with the first five CCPs of fH, generating a chimeric protein with the potential to target initial recognition and at the same time down-regulate AP amplification (37). We wanted to investigate this approach further and designed two differently-oriented proteins by genetic engineering; MAP-1:C4BP$^{1-5}$, with the sequence of human C4BP$^{1-5}$ fused directly downstream of full length human MAP-1, and C4BP$^{1-5}$:MAP-1, where C4BP$^{1-5}$ was located in the N-terminus and connected to MAP-1 via a flexible glycine-serine linker. In theory, combining two existing complement inhibitors could result in a synergistic effect, giving rise to unique complement-regulatory and anti-inflammatory properties. Furthermore, we hypothesize that the ability of targeting both CP and LP activation may be especially beneficial in multifactorial pathologies where both pathways are involved in driving tissue damage, such as ischemia/reperfusion injuries (56).

MAP-1 forms head-to-tail homodimers (18) stabilized by calcium, that upon complex formation with collectins and ficolins downregulate LP activation (18, 57, 58). MAP-1:C4BP$^{1-5}$, C4BP$^{1-5}$:MAP-1, and rMAP-1 displayed comparable Kd values to rMBL (0.35, 0.56, 0.14 nM respectively) and rCL-11 (1.97, 5.49, and 1.65 nM respectively) in a solid-phase ELISA setup. Hill slopes values above 1 indicate a multivalent binding to MBL. The lower hill slope values observed with rCL-11 may be a consequence of its limited oligomerization and reflect the reduced number of collagen-stalks available for complexation with the inhibitors. Addition of the calcium-chelating agent EDTA completely inhibited binding. This clearly indicates that the interaction of the chimeras with the PRMs is mediated through their MAP-1 part in a calcium-dependent manner. No binding was observed with rC4BP$^{1-5}$ (data not shown).

To investigate the dimerization in detail both chimeras were subjected to SEC in the presence of physiological calcium concentrations or EDTA. We found that both constructs eluted as a single peak in the presence of calcium, whereas when exposed to EDTA-containing buffers the chimeras were separated into monomers leading to a shift in their spectrophotogram profiles toward a lower estimated molecular size. The identity of the peaks was confirmed using a specific ELISA capturing C4BP and detecting MAP-1. These results demonstrate that the constructs maintain the calcium-dependent dimerization of native MAP-1 that is critical for its role as an LP inhibitor.

Our group and others have previously demonstrated that rMAP-1 alone and as part of chimeric constructs inhibits LP activation *in vitro* (18, 20, 21, 37, 39). Here we tested the ability of the chimeric proteins to regulate LP activation in different functional ELISAs. First we incubated the chimeric proteins, rMAP-1, and C4BP$^{1-5}$ with MBL bound to mannan-coated plates, and subsequently added 2% MBL defect serum as complement source. While rMAP-1 alone seemed more effective at inhibiting C4 deposition, MAP-1: C4BP$^{1-5}$ clearly outperformed rMAP-1 on the C3 and TCC levels. C4BP$^{1-5}$:MAP-1 was the least effective regulator of the three. If C4 regulation is solely dependent on MAP-1, then differences on C4 inhibition could be explained by their different binding affinities toward MBL. In a more physiologically-relevant ELISA setup the proteins were co-incubated with 2% NHS, thus allowing direct competition between the inhibitors and intrinsic MASPs for binding to MBL. Again, incubation with MAP-1:C4BP$^{1-5}$ caused a significant inhibition resulting in the almost complete absence of C3, and TCC deposition. While C4BP$^{1-5}$:MAP-1 failed to provide the same inhibition as MAP-1:C4BP$^{1-5}$, it was still more effective than rMAP-1 alone. The difference in inhibition levels of rMAP-1 observed in the two experimental setups is in agreement with other studies (18, 37) and could be attributed to competition with the MASPs on MBL binding. This phenomenon supports our explanation that rMAP-1 occupies MASPs-binding sites at the MBL molecules when pre-incubated (20), that would result in either a lower concentration of catalytically-active MASPs or/and a decreased intercomplex activation by spacing out MBL/MASPs complexes (59). When added simultaneously with serum, rMAP-1 may not be capable of displacing already formed MBL/MASPs complexes (at least under our experimental conditions).

It has been reported that the domains CCP1-4 of the α-chain are critical for the fI cofactor activity of C4BP in the fI-mediated C4b (28–30) and C3b proteolytic inactivation (31). Thereby we expected that the chimeric proteins will manifest intact fI cofactor activity. We showed that C4BP$^{1-5}$-containing constructs were as efficient as full length native C4BP in a fluid phase C3b/C4b degradation assay. Moreover it appears that C4BP is a more effective cofactor in the cleavage of C4b compared to C3b in agreement with a previous study (49).

We next looked for a pathological condition where complement injury was triggered by an initial recognition by the LP. MBL has been documented to be directly involved in kidney damage following renal ischemia (53). We used immortalized human PTECs to test whether we could quench the exacerbated complement activation observed on the tubular epithelium, known to be especially vulnerable to complement attack after reperfusion (51). In agreement with the literature rMBL was capable of binding to the cell surface in a calcium-dependent manner, suggesting a traditional c-type lectin interaction (60). Binding to PTECs led to the deposition of C4 activation fragments. As seen on ELISA, the chimeras and rMAP-1 presented comparable regulatory effects (even when using a five times lower serum dilution than in ELISA). This to a degree limited inhibition can be expected assuming that trace amounts of PRM/MASPs complexes are sufficient to cause detectable C4 deposition, which in turn is mainly mediated by the MAP-1 part while the effect on the late cascade (i.e., C3 and TCC) depends on the combination of MAP-1 and C4BP. No C3 or TCC deposition was observed (see **Supplementary Figure 2**). The assay was performed at 4°C, that while it allowed the cleavage and deposition of C4, it did not result in the assembly of the downstream convertases [62]. Incubation of MBL-bound cells at 37°C led to the disappearance of C4 and MBL surface stain (data not shown). It has been reported that binding of MBL to PTEC causes its internalization followed by complement-independent cell death (60). Thus, this assay may have some inherited limitations to study downstream complement deposition, but is suitable to study the initial inhibiting effect of PRM binding inhibitors.

Finally, we tested the regulatory effect of the chimeric proteins in all three complement pathways using Wielisa, a platform for standardized complement activity measurements. In agreement with our previous results, MAP-1:C4BP$^{1-5}$ demonstrated a strong dose-dependent inhibition of TCC deposition in the LP (IC50 = 13.15 nM). Remarkably, it was also an efficient CP inhibitor (IC50 = 4.83 nM), outperforming rMAP-1 and C4BP$^{1-5}$ alone or in combination. C4BP$^{1-5}$:MAP-1 inhibited the LP and CP to a lesser extent than MAP-1:C4BP$^{1-5}$ equivalent to rMAP-1 and rC4BP$^{1-5}$ added at the same time. The equivalent regulatory effects of the chimeras in the LP and CP, together with the moderate activity of rMAP-1 in the LP, suggests that the observed LP-downregulation is mainly driven by the C4BP part, reflecting a limitation of the assay as a model for LP-mediated activation. Thus, in a physiological setting where both functional domains of the chimeras would be involved, we may observe a more pronounced inhibition [as shown for rMAP-1 (21)]. It should be noted that even though MAP-1 only associates with the PRMs of the LP and not the CP, MAP-1-containing chimeras were more effective than C4BP$^{1-5}$ alone in both CP and LP. This implies that the combination of two regulators within a single molecule—in the right configuration—enables the enhanced functionality of the constructs, and not just displays the function of "free" MAP-1 or C4BP. In the AP activation assay MAP-1:C4BP$^{1-5}$ showed only a minor effect—around 100 to 400-fold lower than in the LP and CP—that was directly comparable to rC4BP$^{1-5}$ (alone or in combination with rMAP-1), suggesting that AP activity is solely mediated by the C4BP part. It is important to highlight that the above-described experiments were performed using diluted serum as a source of complement. Experiments using animal models would be necessary to demonstrate that the chimeric proteins are effective complement inhibitors under physiological conditions.

The mechanism behind the observed differences in inhibitory properties between MAP-1:C4BP$^{1-5}$ and C4BP$^{1-5}$:MAP-1 remain unclear, although it could be explained by their quaternary structure. Dimerization of C4BP$^{1-5}$:MAP-1 could result in MAP-1 bending away from C4BP$^{1-5}$ via the flexible region in the CUB2/EGF region and the artificial linker between C4BP$^{1-5}$ and MAP-1. This contorted folding could give rise to a dimer with impaired ability to reach C4b/C3b and possibly also hindering the complex formation with MBL. On the other hand, MAP-1:C4BP$^{1-5}$ may fold into an elongated dimer with C4BP$^{1-5}$ pointing outwards from a MAP-1 dimer core bound to the collagen-like stalks of the PRMs similar to how the serine domain in the MASPs is assumed to protrude when bound to MBL. This conformation would enable both C4BP$^{1-5}$ monomers to interact with deposited C4b/C3b in the vicinity of the PRM binding site. We propose that the MAP-1 fragment may "dock" the chimeric inhibitor to the PRMs directing the multifunctional soluble inhibitor C4BP to the activating surface, thus increasing the efficacy. While data presented by our group in the present and past reports (37) provide a solid support for our hypothesis, conclusive evidence will require precise structural determination techniques, such as circular dichroism, multi-angle light scattering, small-angle x-ray scattering, or x-ray crystallography.

In conclusion, we have successfully developed a novel complement inhibitor that harnesses the multifaceted functionality of the fluid phase CP and LP regulator C4BP, and directs it to danger foci by the specific association to PRMs mediated by MAP-1. The combination of MAP-1 fused to C4BP$^{1-5}$ presents unique complement regulatory properties *in vitro* and represents a potential novel therapeutic approach by targeting both upstream and central complement activation.

AUTHOR CONTRIBUTIONS

CH, RB-O, NK-M, M-OS, and SvP performed the experiments. KP optimized the ELISA-based inhibition assays. RB-O, M-OS, and PG designed the study. CH, RB-O, PG wrote the manuscript. All authors critically reviewed the manuscript.

FUNDING

The Danish Research Foundation of Independent Research (DFF-6110-00489), the Sven Andersen Research Foundation, and Novo Nordisk Research Foundation.

ACKNOWLEDGMENTS

The authors would like to thank Ms Jytte Bryde Clausen and Mrs. Jesper Andresen for excellent technical assistance.

SUPPLEMENTARY MATERIAL

Supplementary Figure 1 | Gating strategy. HK-2 cells were defined as a uniform population on the forward scatter (FS INT) vs. side scatter (SS INT) plot, and single cells were selected gating on the forward scatter area or integral values (FS INT) vs. forward scatter height or peak (FS PEAK).

Supplementary Figure 2 | MBL-dependent complement deposition on HK-2 cells. Cells were incubated with rMBL for 30 min at 4°C prior to addition of 10% MBL defect serum for 1 h at 4°C. Deposition of C4 **(A)**, C3 **(B)**, and TCC **(C)**. Cells incubated with no MBL, or with MBL but no serum were used as controls. X-Med, median fluorescence intensity.

REFERENCES

1. Merle NS, Church SE, Fremeaux-Bacchi V, Roumenina LT. Complement system part I - molecular mechanisms of activation and regulation. *Front Immunol.* (2015) 6:1–30. doi: 10.3389/fimmu.2015.00262
2. Ricklin D, Hajishengallis G, Yang K, Lambris JD. Complement: a key system for immune surveillance and homeostasis. *Nat Immunol.* (2010) 11:785–97. doi: 10.1038/ni.1923
3. Kersse K, Bertrand MJM, Lamkanfi M, Vandenabeele P. NOD-like receptors and the innate immune system: coping with danger, damage and death. *Cytokine Growth Factor Rev.* (2011) 22:257–76. doi: 10.1016/j.cytogfr.2011.09.003
4. Doyle SL, O'Neill LAJ. Toll-like receptors: from the discovery of NFkB to new insights into transcriptional regulations in innate immunity. *Biochem Pharmacol.* (2006) 72:1102–13. doi: 10.1016/j.bcp.2006.07.010
5. Chaplin DD. Overview of the immune response. *J Allergy Clin Immunol.* (2010) 125:S3–23. doi: 10.1016/j.jaci.2009.12.980
6. Noris M, Remuzzi G. Overview of complement activation and regulation. *Semin Nephrol.* (2013) 33:479–92. doi: 10.1016/j.semnephrol.2013.08.001
7. Wallis R, Mitchell DA, Schmid R, Schwaeble WJ, Keeble AH. Paths reunited: initiation of the classical and lectin pathways of complement activation. *Immunobiology* (2010) 215:1–11. doi: 10.1016/j.imbio.2009.08.006
8. Kishorea U, Rohit Ghaib, Trevor J. Greenhoughc, Shrivec AK, Bonifatid DM et al. Structural and functional anatomy of the globular domain of complement protein C1q. *Immunol Lett.* (2004) 100:113–28. doi: 10.1016/j.imlet.2004.06.015
9. Gaboriaud C, Frachet P, Thielens NM, Arlaud GJ. The human C1q globular domain: Structure and recognition of non-immune self ligands. *Front Immunol.* (2012) 2:1–8. doi: 10.3389/fimmu.2011.00092

10. Garred P, Genster N, Pilely K, Bayarri-Olmos R, Rosbjerg A, Ma YJ, et al. A journey through the lectin pathway of complement-MBL and beyond. *Immunol Rev.* (2016) 274:74–97. doi: 10.1111/imr.12468
11. Bexborn F, Andersson PO, Chen H, Nilsson B, Ekdahl KN. The tick-over theory revisited: Formation and regulation of the soluble alternative complement C3 convertase (C3(H2O)Bb). *Mol Immunol.* (2008) 45:2370–9. doi: 10.1016/j.molimm.2007.11.003
12. Harboe M, Mollnes TE. The alternative complement pathway revisited. *J Cell Mol Med.* (2008) 12:1074–84. doi: 10.1111/j.1582-4934.2008.00350.x
13. Spitzer D, Mitchell LM, Atkinson JP, Hourcade DE. Properdin can initiate complement activation by binding specific target surfaces and providing a platform for de novo convertase assembly. *J Immunol.* (2007) 179:2600–8. doi: 10.4049/jimmunol.179.4.2600
14. Harboe M, Johnson C, Nymo S, Ekholt K, Schjalm C, Lindstad JK, et al. Properdin binding to complement activating surfaces depends on initial C3b deposition. *Proc Natl Acad Sci USA.* (2017) 114:E534–9. doi: 10.1073/pnas.1612385114
15. Zipfel PF, Skerka C. Complement regulators and inhibitory proteins. *Nat Rev Immunol.* (2009) 9:729–40. doi: 10.1038/nri2620
16. Roy D, Steyer GJ, Gargesha M, Stone ME, Wilson L, Davis AE, et al. Biological activities Of C1 inhibitor. *Mol Immunol.* (2008) 45:4057–63. doi: 10.1016/j.molimm.2008.06.028
17. Keizer MP, Wouters D, Schlapbach LJ, Kuijpers TW. Restoration of MBL-deficiency: redefining the safety, efficacy and viability of MBL-substitution therapy. *Mol Immunol.* (2014) 61:174–84. doi: 10.1016/j.molimm.2014.06.005
18. Skjoedt M, Roversi P, Hummelshøj T, Palarasah Y, Rosbjerg A, Johnson S, et al. Crystal structure and functional characterization of the complement regulator mannose-binding lectin (MBL). *J Biol Chem.* (2012) 287:32913–21. doi: 10.1074/jbc.M112.386680
19. Skjoedt MO, Hummelshoj T, Palarasah Y, Hein E, Munthe-Fog L, Koch C, et al. Serum concentration and interaction properties of MBL/ficolin associated protein-1. *Immunobiology.* (2011) 216:625–32. doi: 10.1016/j.imbio.2010.09.011
20. Degn SE, Hansen AG, Steffensen R, Jacobsen C, Jensenius JC, Thiel S, et al. MAp44, a human protein associated with pattern recognition molecules of the complement system and regulating the lectin pathway of complement activation. *J Immunol.* (2009) 183:7371–8. doi: 10.4049/jimmunol.0902388
21. Pavlov VI, Skjoedt MO, Tan YS, Rosbjerg A, Garred P, Stahl GL. Endogenous and natural complement inhibitor attenuates myocardial injury and arterial thrombogenesis. *Circulation* (2012) 126:2227–35. doi: 10.1161/CIRCULATIONAHA.112.123968
22. Banda NK, Mehta G, Kjaer TR, Takahashi M, Schaack J, Morrison TE, et al. Essential role for the lectin pathway in collagen antibody-induced arthritis revealed through use of adenovirus programming complement inhibitor MAp44 expression. *J Immunol.* (2014) 193:2455–68. doi: 10.4049/jimmunol.1400752
23. Oshiumi H, Shida K, Goitsuka R, Kimura Y, Katoh J, Ohba S, et al. Regulator of complement activation (RCA) locus in chicken: identification of chicken RCA gene cluster and functional RCA proteins. *J Immunol.* (2005) 175:1724–34. doi: 10.4049/jimmunol.175.3.1724
24. Dahlbäck B, Smith CA, Müller-Eberhard HJ. Visualization of human C4b-binding protein and its complexes with vitamin K-dependent protein S and complement protein C4b. *Proc Natl Acad Sci USA.* (1983) 80:3461–5.
25. Hillarp A, Dahlbäck B. Cloning of cDNA coding for the beta chain of human complement component C4b-binding protein: sequence homology with the alpha chain. *Proc Natl Acad Sci USA.* (1990) 87:1183–7.
26. Gigli I, Fujita T, Nussenzweig V, Gigli, I, Fujita, T, Nussenzweig V. Modulation of the classical pathway C3 convertase by plasma proteins C4 binding protein and C3b inactivator. *Proc Natl Acad Sci USA.* (1979) 76(3 Pt 1):6596–600. doi: 10.1073/pnas.76.12.6596
27. Suankratay C, Mold C, Zhang Y, Lint TF, Gewurz H. Mechanism of complement-dependent haemolysis via the lectin pathway: role of the complement regulatory proteins. *Clin Exp Immunol.* (1999) 117:442–8. doi: 10.1046/j.1365-2249.1999.00998.x
28. Fujita T, Gigli I, Nussenzweig V. Human C4-binding protein. II. Role in proteolysis of C4b by C3b-inactivator. *J Exp Med.* (1978) 148:1044–51. doi: 10.1084/jem.148.4.1044
29. Scharfstein BYJ, Ferreira A, Gigli I. Human C4-binding protein. i isolation and characterization. *J Exp Med.* (1978) 148:207–22.
30. Nagasawa S, Ichihara C, Stroud RM. Cleavage of C4b by C3b inactivator: production of a nicked form of C4b, C4b', as an intermediate cleavage product of C4b by C3b inactivator. *J Immunol.* (1980) 125:578–82.
31. Blom AM, Kask L, Dahlbäck B. CCP1 - 4 of the C4b-binding protein alpha-chain are required for factor I mediated cleavage of complement factor C3b. *Mol Immunol.* (2003) 39:547–56.
32. Ermert D, Blom AM. C4b-binding protein: the good, the bad and the deadly. Novel functions of an old friend. *Immunol Lett.* (2016) 169:82–92. doi: 10.1016/j.imlet.2015.11.014
33. Blom AM, Nandakumar KS, Holmdahl R. C4b-binding protein (C4BP) inhibits development of experimental arthritis in mice. *Ann Rheum Dis.* (2009) 68:136–42. doi: 10.1136/ard.2007.085753
34. *US Food and Drug Administration. FDA Approves First-of-Its-Kind Drug to Treat Rare Blood Disorder* [Internet]. Rockville, MD, USA; Available online at: http://www.fda.gov/bbs/topics/NEWS/2007/NEW01589.html
35. Ricklin D, Lambris JD. New milestones ahead in complement-targeted therapy. *Semin Immunol.* (2016) 28:208–22. doi: 10.1016/j.smim.2016.06.001
36. Ricklin D, Lambris JD. Complement in immune and inflammatory disorders: therapeutic interventions. *J Immunol Ref J Immunol.* (2013) 190:3839–47. doi: 10.4049/jimmunol.1203200
37. Nordmaj MA, Munthe-Fog L, Hein E, Skjoedt MO, Garred P. Genetically engineered fusion of MAP-1 and factor H domains 1-5 generates a potent dual upstream inhibitor of both the lectin and alternative complement pathways. *FASEB J.* (2015) 29:4945–55. doi: 10.1096/fj.15-277103
38. Jung S-K, McDonald K. Visual gene developer: a fully programmable bioinformatics software for synthetic gene optimization. *BMC Bioinformatics* (2011) 12:340. doi: 10.1186/1471-2105-12-340
39. Skjoedt MO, Hummelshoj T, Palarasah Y, Honore C, Koch C, Skjodt K, et al. A novel mannose-binding lectin/ficolin-associated protein is highly expressed in heart and skeletal muscle tissues and inhibits complement activation. *J Biol Chem.* (2010) 285:8234–43. doi: 10.1074/jbc.M109.065805
40. Hebecker M, Alba-Dominguez M, Roumenina LT, Reuter S, Hyvarinen S, Dragon-Durey M-A, et al. An engineered construct combining complement regulatory and surface-recognition domains represents a minimal-size functional factor H. *J Immunol.* (2013) 191:912–21. doi: 10.4049/jimmunol.1300269
41. Schmidt CQ, Bai H, Lin Z, Risitano AM, Barlow PN, Ricklin D, et al. Rational engineering of a minimized immune inhibitor with unique triple-targeting properties. *J Immunol.* (2013) 190:5712–21. doi: 10.4049/jimmunol.1203548
42. Skjoedt MO, Palarasah Y, Munthe-Fog L, Jie Ma Y, Weiss G, Skjodt K, et al. MBL-associated serine protease-3 circulates in high serum concentrations predominantly in complex with Ficolin-3 and regulates Ficolin-3 mediated complement activation. *Immunobiology* (2010) 215:921–31. doi: 10.1016/j.imbio.2009.10.006
43. Garred P, Larsen F, Madsen HO, Koch C. Mannose-binding lectin deficiency—revisited. *Mol Immunol.* (2003) 40:73–84. doi: 10.1016/S0161-5890(03)00104-4
44. Garred P, Mollnes TE, Lea T, Fischer E. Characterization of a monoclonal antibody MoAb bH6 reacting with a neoepitope of human C3 expressed on C3b, iC3b, and C3c. *Scand J Immunol.* (1988) 27:319–27.
45. Seelen MA, Roos A, Wieslander J, Mollnes TE, Sjöholm AG, Wurzner R, et al. Functional analysis of the classical, alternative, and MBL pathways of the complement system: standardization and validation of a simple ELISA. *J Immunol Methods* (2005) 296:187–98. doi: 10.1016/j.jim.2004.11.016
46. Ryan MJ, Johnson G, Kirk J, Fuerstenberg SM, Zager RA, Torok-Storb B. HK-2: an immortalized proximal tubule epithelial cell line from normal adult human kidney. *Kidney Int.* (1994) 45:48–57. doi: 10.1038/ki.1994.6
47. Teillet F, Gaboriaud C, Lacroix M, Martin L, Arlaud GJ, Thielens NM. Crystal structure of the CUB1-EGF-CUB2 domain of human MASP-1/3 and identification of its interaction sites with mannan-binding lectin and ficolins. *J Biol Chem.* (2008) 283:25715–24. doi: 10.1074/jbc.M803551200
48. Thielens NM, Cseh S, Thiel S, Vorup-Jensen T, Rossi V, Jensenius JC, et al. Interaction properties of human mannan-binding lectin (MBL)-associated serine proteases-1 and–2, MBL-associated protein 19, and MBL. *J Immunol.* (2001) 166:5068–77. doi: 10.4049/jimmunol.166.8.5068

49. Seya T, Nakamura K, Masaki T, Ichihara-Itoh C, Matsumoto M, Nagasawa S. Human factor H and C4b-binding protein serve as factor I-cofactors both encompassing inactivation of C3b and C4b. *Mol Immunol.* (1995) 32:355–60. doi: 10.1016/0161-5890(94)00157-V
50. Thurman JM, Ljubanovic D, Edelstein CL, Gilkeson GS, Holers VM. Lack of a functional alternative complement pathway ameliorates ischemic acute renal failure in mice. *J Immunol.* (2003) 170:1517–23. doi: 10.4049/jimmunol.170.3.1517
51. Zhou W, Farrar CA, Abe K, Pratt JR, Marsh JE, Wang Y, et al. Predominant role for C5b-9 in renal ischemia/reperfusion injury. *J Clin Invest.* (2000) 105:1363–71. doi: 10.1172/JCI8621
52. Thurman JM. Triggers of inflammation after renal ischemia/reperfusion. *Clin Immunol.* (2007) 123:7–13. doi: 10.1016/j.clim.2006.09.008
53. Moller-Kristensen M, Wang W, Ruseva M, Thiel S, Nielsen S, Takahashi K, et al. Mannan-binding lectin recognizes structures on ischaemic reperfused mouse kidneys and is implicated in tissue injury. *Scand J Immunol.* (2005) 61:426–34. doi: 10.1111/j.1365-3083.2005.01591.x
54. Morgan BP, Harris CL. Complement, a target for therapy in inflammatory and degenerative diseases. *Nat Rev Drug Discov.* (2015) 14:857–77. doi: 10.1038/nrd4657
55. Qiao Q, Teng X, Wang N, Lu R, Guo L, Zhang X, et al. A novel CRIg-targeted complement inhibitor protects cells from complement damage. *FASEB J.* (2014) 28:4986–99. doi: 10.1096/fj.14-258046
56. Chen G, Chen S, Chen X. Role of complement and perspectives for intervention in transplantation. *Immunobiology* (2013) 218:817–27. doi: 10.1016/j.imbio.2012.09.002
57. Wallis R. Interactions between mannose-binding lectin and MASPs during complement activation by the lectin pathway. *Immunobiology* (2007) 212:289–99. doi: 10.1016/j.imbio.2006.11.004
58. Hansen S, Selman L, Palaniyar N, Ziegler K, Brandt J, Kliem A, et al. Collectin 11 (CL-11, CL-K1) is a MASP-1/3-associated plasma collectin with microbial-binding activity. *J Immunol.* (2010) 185:6096–104. doi: 10.4049/jimmunol.1002185
59. Van Der Pol P, Schlagwein N, Van Gijlswijk DJ, Berger SP, Roos A, Bajema IM, et al. Mannan-binding lectin mediates renal ischemia/reperfusion injury independent of complement activation. *Am J Transplant.* (2012) 12:877–87. doi: 10.1111/j.1600-6143.2011.03887.x
60. Wahrmann M, Exner M, Regele H, Derfler K, Körmöczi GF, Lhotta K, et al. Flow cytometry based detection of HLA alloantibody mediated classical complement activation. *J Immunol Methods* (2003) 275:149–60. doi: 10.1016/S0022-1759(03)00012-7

18

Complement Activation in Inflammatory Skin Diseases

Jenny Giang[1], Marc A. J. Seelen[2], Martijn B. A. van Doorn[3], Robert Rissmann[4], Errol P. Prens[3] and Jeffrey Damman[1]*

[1] Department of Pathology, Erasmus Medical Center Rotterdam, Rotterdam, Netherlands, [2] Department of Nephrology, University Medical Center Groningen, Groningen, Netherlands, [3] Department of Dermatology, Erasmus Medical Center Rotterdam, Rotterdam, Netherlands, [4] Center for Human Drug Research, Leiden, Netherlands

*Correspondence:
Jeffrey Damman
j.damman@erasmusmc.nl

The complement system is a fundamental part of the innate immune system, playing a crucial role in host defense against various pathogens, such as bacteria, viruses, and fungi. Activation of complement results in production of several molecules mediating chemotaxis, opsonization, and mast cell degranulation, which can contribute to the elimination of pathogenic organisms and inflammation. Furthermore, the complement system also has regulating properties in inflammatory and immune responses. Complement activity in diseases is rather complex and may involve both aberrant expression of complement and genetic deficiencies of complement components or regulators. The skin represents an active immune organ with complex interactions between cellular components and various mediators. Complement involvement has been associated with several skin diseases, such as psoriasis, lupus erythematosus, cutaneous vasculitis, urticaria, and bullous dermatoses. Several triggers including auto-antibodies and micro-organisms can activate complement, while on the other hand complement deficiencies can contribute to impaired immune complex clearance, leading to disease. This review provides an overview of the role of complement in inflammatory skin diseases and discusses complement factors as potential new targets for therapeutic intervention.

Keywords: complement, dermatology, skin diseases, innate immunity, psoriasis, hidradenitis suppurativa, lupus erythematosus, bullous pemphigoid

INTRODUCTION

The Complement System

The complement system consists of a network of more than 50 different plasma and membrane-associated proteins. It is a part of the innate immune system and plays a key role in host defense against pathogens as well as in tissue homeostasis. The complement system can be activated through three distinct pathways: the classical, lectin, and alternative pathway (**Figure 1**). Classical pathway activation occurs after binding of the first component C1q to antibody-antigen complexes, cell particles, or certain acute phase proteins such as C-reactive protein or serum amyloid P. Once the complement activation cascade is initiated, the attached serine proteases C1r and C1s become activated. This is followed by cleavage of, respectively, C4 and C2, leading to the formation of a C3 convertase (C4b2a) that can activate C3 (1). The lectin pathway is activated when mannan binding lectin (MBL), ficolins, and/or collectins interact with carbohydrate structures predominantly present on invading pathogens. Consequently, this activates MBL-associated serine proteases 1 and 2 (MASP1 and MASP2), subsequently cleaving C4 and C2. The classical and lectin pathways generate

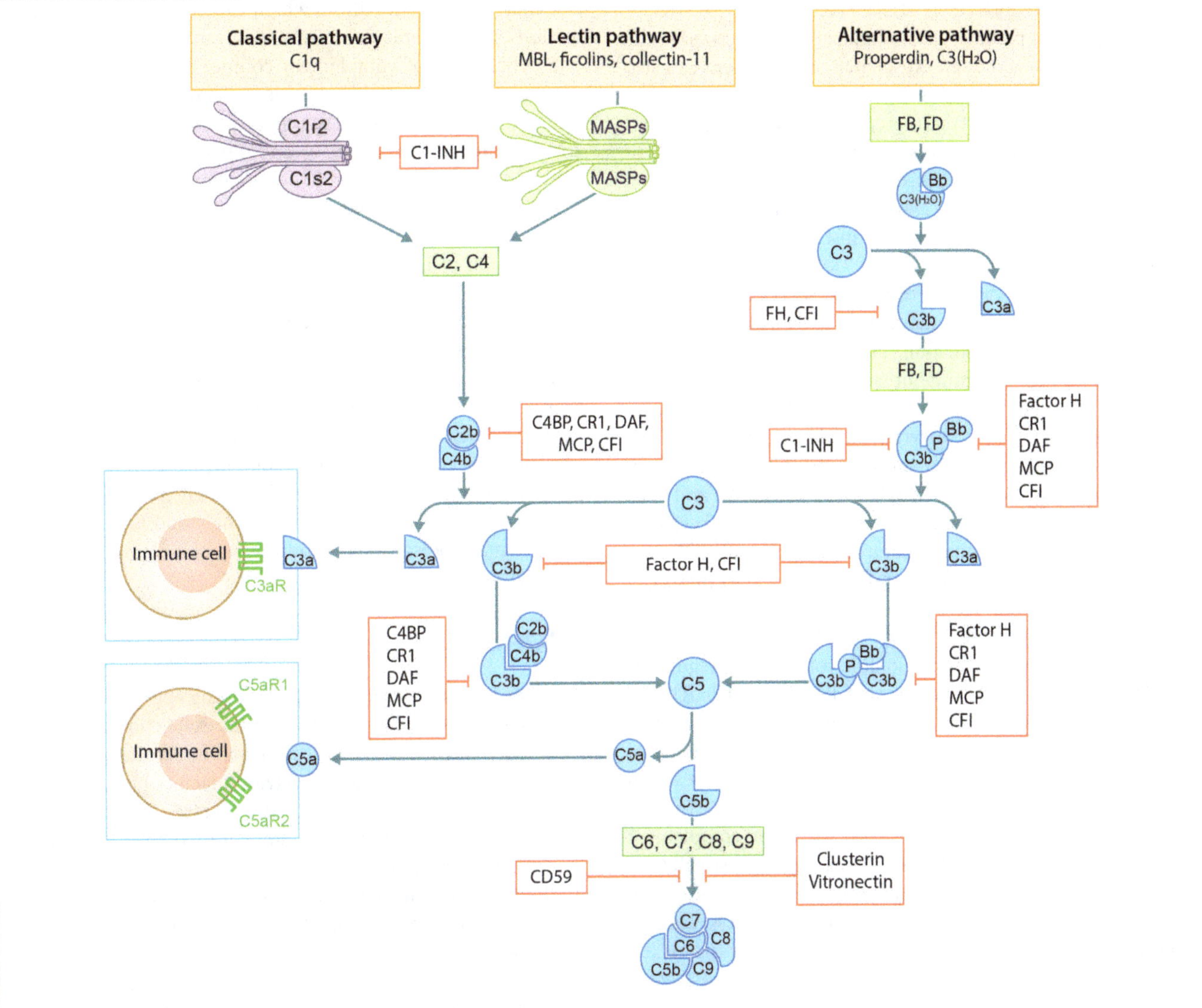

FIGURE 1 | Schematic overview of the complement system: activation and regulation.

the shared C3 convertase C4b2a, which in turn generates the opsonin C3b and anaphylatoxin C3a through cleavage of native C3. In contrast to the classical and lectin pathways, the alternative pathway is activated by low grade spontaneous hydrolysis of systemic native C3 ("C3 tickover") or *via* properdin binding to certain cell surfaces (e.g., bacteria). Hydrolyzed C3 [C3(H_2O)] can associate with Factor B (FB), which is subsequently activated by Factor D. This results in the formation of a C3 convertase (C3$H_2$0Bb) that can finally cleave C3. This fluid phase C3 convertase cleaves C3 to generate C3a and C3b. C3b can covalently bind to nearby structures and provides the basis for generation of the surface bound C3 convertase C3bBb. Alternative pathway activation can also be initiated as an amplification loop when C3b, generated by either one of the three pathways, is deposited on the triggered surface and binds to FB, which also results in the formation of the surface bound C3 convertase C3bBb. C3 convertases can be stabilized by factor P (properdin). C3b, generated by the classical, lectin, or alternative pathway, combines with the C3 convertases to form the C5 convertases (C4b2aC3b and C3bBbC3b), initiating the terminal complement cascade. C5 convertases cleave C5 into C5b and anaphylatoxin C5a, eventually resulting in the assembly of C5b-9 by combining C5b with C6-C9. C5b-9 can form channels into the cell membrane causing cell lysis. In addition to the capacity to generate C5b-9, complement split products iC3b and C3dg are known to have immunomodulating functions (1–3).

Several soluble and cell-bound regulators are capable of mediating complement regulation on different levels of the complement cascade to limit damage to self-cells (**Figure 1**). C1-esterase inhibitor (C1-INH), C4b binding protein (C4BP), FH, FI, vitronectin, and clusterin are the soluble regulators. However, if complement components still manage to deposit on the cell membrane, inactivation of complement can be achieved by cell-bound regulators. These include decay-accelerating factor (DAF/CD55), membrane cofactor protein (MCP/CD46), complement receptor-1 (CR1), and CD59 (protectin) (4).

Complement System and the Skin

Plasma complement proteins are predominantly synthesized in the liver by hepatocytes, although extrahepatic complement can also be produced by other cell types such as endothelial cells, epithelial cells, and immune cells. Furthermore, complement receptors and membrane regulators can also be synthesized by other types of cells, such as leukocytes, fibroblasts, adipocytes, and endothelial cells (5). An important role of extrahepatic synthesized complement components is the protection against micro-organisms and inflammation at tissue or organ level.

The skin is the body's largest organ that serves as an immune and physical barrier against pathogenic organisms, irritant, xenobiotics, allergens, UV-irradiation, and mechanical injury. The epidermis is an active immune organ equipped with immune-competent cells, including Langerhans cells, keratinocytes, dendritic epidermal T-lymphocytes, and melanocytes, of which the keratinocyte is the predominant cell type. The dermis harbors many immune cells such as dermal dendritic cells (DC) and mast cells. Multiple reports have demonstrated that human keratinocytes are able to produce several complement proteins including complement components C3, C4, and FB of which synthesis can be regulated and enhanced by interleukin- 1α (IL-1α), interferon-γ (IFN-γ), and tumor necrosis factor-α (TNF-α). Furthermore, keratinocytes can also synthesize soluble complement regulators such FH and FI, complement receptors CR1, cC1qR, C5aR1, and CR2 and cell-bound complement regulator proteins MCP, DAF, and CD59. Importantly, IFN-γ can enhance the production of FH and FI locally, thereby preventing epidermal damage which could be caused by locally produced C3, C4, and FB (6, 7). Besides keratinocytes, also melanocytes express cell-bound complement regulator proteins DAF, MCP, and CD59, making these cells less vulnerable to autologous complement attack. For example in vitiligo, melanocytes and keratinocytes seem to express less cell-bound regulators, which adds to the cells susceptibility to lysis (8). Langerhans cells and DC are the antigen-presenting cells, which have the capacity to initiate primary immune responses. Human DCs are able to produce most of the complement components and are also qualified to identify soluble and cell-bound complement effector molecules. Interestingly, the functional development of DCs depends on complement production and activation. Hence, T-cell differentiation can be indirectly determined by complement, in particular the anaphylatoxins C3a and C5a (5).

The skin is colonized by a diversity of microbes including commensals and potential pathogens. The skin plays an important role in restraining the invasion of opportunistic or pathogenic organisms. The complement system may partly impact this microbial ecosystem by regulating complement C5aR1 signaling. Inhibition of C5aR1 signaling results in lower microbial diversity, making the skin less resistant to pathogenic organisms (2). Moreover, inhibiting C5aR1 signaling also decreases expression of various chemokines, cytokines, anti-microbial peptides, and pattern recognition receptors (2). In particular, downregulation of IL-12 by complement might impact the differentiation and development of T cells (9).

Overall, the complement system forms an important bridge between the innate and adaptive immune system. Complement activation products are known to mediate chemotaxis, opsonization, and mast cell degranulation, which can contribute to the elimination of pathogenic organisms. Aberrant expression and genetic deficiencies of complement components or regulators are associated with certain skin diseases. Complement activation in different skin diseases has experienced a first period of high-level attention already in the 1970s and 1980s. However, in the following decades the interest in complement has declined, paralleling intensified research into lymphocyte function, adaptive immunity, and immunogenetic associations in skin diseases. The introduction of immunosuppressive agents targeting the adaptive immune system, for example, cyclosporine in the treatment of psoriasis, shifted the interest from innate to adaptive. A second "wave of attention" in complement occurred after the development and introduction of several new complement inhibiting agents. These complement inhibitors are now effectively being used in clinical practise in several diseases, for example, in the treatment of renal disease. The main purpose of this review is to provide an overview of the role of complement in inflammatory skin diseases and to discuss the rationale and potential targets for pharmacological intervention using complement inhibiting therapeutics.

PSORIASIS

Psoriasis is a chronic skin disease, affecting approximately 2–4% of the Western population. Although the exact etiology of psoriasis remains unclear, it is considered a multifactorial disease with genetic, environmental, and behavioral factors playing a role in the pathogenesis and course of the disease. Psoriasis vulgaris (plaque psoriasis) is the most common form of the disease (affecting 70% of the patients) and usually presents as symmetrical erythematous papules or plaques covered with thick silvery scales located on the extensor side of the elbows and knees, scalp, and lumbosacral area. The scales are a consequence of a hyperproliferative epidermis, which is reflected on histology by parakeratosis, alternating regular hyperplasia with elongation of the rete ridges, loss or absence of the granular layer, and dilated capillaries of the papillary dermis (**Figure 2**). In addition, the epidermis may show transepidermal migration of neutrophils, and to a lesser extent lymphocytes, to the corneal layer that results in the formation of Munro microabscesses (10, 11). A Munro microabscess is a collection of neutrophils in the stratum corneum and can be considered as one of the characteristic histological findings of psoriasis. Inflammation in the dermis is characterized by a superficial perivascular infiltrate of lymphocytes.

Already in the 1970s and 1980s, several research groups have examined the scale extracts from psoriatic lesions, unraveling the underlying mechanisms of transepidermal leukocyte migration, and Munro microabscess formation. It was found that psoriatic scales exhibit chemotactic and chemokinetic properties compared with scales from non-psoriatic patients (12, 13). Subsequently, the presence of C3a in the extracts of psoriatic scales was demonstrated (14). Deposition of C3b in the presence of immunoglobulins in stratum corneum of skin biopsies from psoriasis patients suggested activation of the classical pathway of complement (15). Furthermore, also C5a was found in psoriatic leukotactic factor (PLF) and appeared to be the most potent

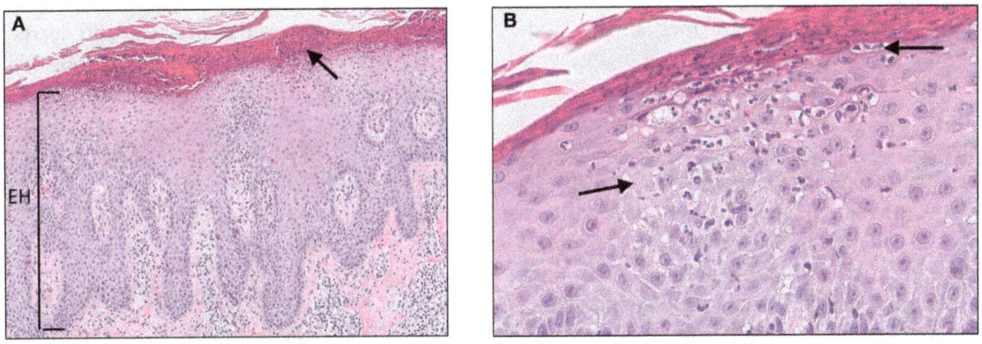

FIGURE 2 | Psoriasis vulgaris. Confluent parakeratosis, psoriasiform epidermal hyperplasia [**(A)**, EH], hypogranulosis, and influx of numerous neutrophils in the corneal layer [**(A)**, arrow]. **(B)** Transepidermal migration of neutrophils from the dermis to the corneal layer (arrows).

chemotactic factor in psoriatic scales. Several subsequent studies were able to confirm these findings by monitoring elevated levels of anaphylatoxins (C3a, C4a, C5a, C5a des-Arg) in scales of psoriatic lesions (16–19). Deposition of complement and the presence of complement activation products in psoriatic scales might be explained by locally produced and activated complement. In addition, systemic derived complement components and/or systemic complement activation could also be an important source of complement deposition in psoriasis.

Regarding systemic complement activation, sera, and plasma from psoriasis patients showed elevated levels of complement components, complement split products, and regulator proteins including FB, Bb, C3, C3a, C3b, C4, C4a, C4d, C5b-9, C1-INH, C4BP, FH, and FI. These results suggest involvement of both classical and alternative pathways in systemic complement activation (20–24). Marley et al. demonstrated low-circulating properdin levels in psoriatic patients, also indicating alternative pathway activation (25). Ohkohchi et al. found that, although circulating levels of classical complement pathway regulators C1-INH and C4BP were slightly increased, marked increase of alternative pathway regulator proteins were found and associated with disease activity and skin involvement (23). Altogether, these findings support a prominent role for systemic alternative pathway activation in psoriasis. However, the most convincing and controlled study was performed by Fleming et al., taking into account and excluding confounders that could potentially bias results from the previously described studies. These included discrepancy in the involved pathways, infection, and different types of psoriasis. It was found that circulating C5b-9 levels did not correlate with the extent and disease activity. More importantly, the absence of specific associated components, such as the immune complexes C1r-C1s-C1-INH and C3bBbP, in the plasma of psoriasis patients with elevated C5b-9 levels is a direct evidence that systemic complement is not activated in psoriasis (20).

Thus, previously cited literature shows that local complement is activated in psoriatic scales but systemic complement is unlikely to be activated in psoriasis. Therefore, it is reasonable to assume that complement activation products in the circulation originate from spillover of local products into the circulation (26). Important questions in this respect are: what are the triggers for local complement activation and what is the overall contribution of complement activation in the pathogenesis of psoriasis.

There are several hypotheses that might explain the activation of complement and the inherent generation of C5a in psoriatic scales. Firstly, natural auto-antibodies are directed against carbohydrate antigens in the stratum corneum and this results in IgG, C3b, and/or C4b deposition, reflecting classical pathway activation (27, 28). However, one study provided evidence that IgG and C3b binding to stratum corneum also occurred in other parakeratotic lesions such as verruca vulgaris and lichen simplex chronicus. Yet these parakeratotic lesions do not evolve into psoriatic lesions, suggesting that immunoglobulin binding and complement activation within the lesional stratum corneum might not be a consequential pathogenic event in psoriasis (15). Secondly, complement is activated independent of immunoglobulins *via* direct cleavage of C5 by serine proteinases present in the stratum corneum or *via* alternative pathway activation. The alternative pathway can be activated when serum comes in direct contact with the stratum corneum after traumatic injury (29, 30). Thirdly, complement is activated by microbial products, which is supported by the fact that infections can trigger the exacerbation of psoriasis in a much higher number of patients than was previously believed (26, 31). Lastly, complement is activated in the dermis, pervades into the epidermis, causing neutrophils to migrate, and damage epidermal cells (32). Although previously cited studies have shown local complement activation in psoriatic scales, one should argue what is the source of complement in the upper epidermis. In the literature, there have been several reports of keratinocytes being a rich source of producing complement components including C3, FB, FH, and FI. Regarding the terminal complement components (C5–C9), a study revealed keratinocytes to express and release C7 and C9 (33). Moreover, both TNF-α and IFN-γ have been shown to augment the production of C3 by keratinocytes (34). Although systemic complement *activation* is unlikely to play a role in psoriasis as previously described, circulating complement components could also be a rich source for local activation.

Whatever the cause of complement activation in psoriasis might be, it is interesting to speculate about the concept that complement might be one of the initiating factors in the pathogenesis of psoriasis. Psoriasis is regarded as an auto-immune disease and therefore therapy in psoriasis has mainly focused on targeting the adaptive immune system. Clinical and mechanistic studies are generally conducted in patients with stable plaque type psoriasis (psoriasis vulgaris), characterized by an adaptive T-cell predominant phenotype. However, to study the pathogenesis of psoriasis, one has to take into account the stage, activity, and type of psoriasis. Early psoriatic lesions are characterized clinically by pinpoint papules, papulopustular lesions or as pustular psoriasis. Histologically, early psoriatic lesion show influx of neutrophils in the dermal papillae, transepidermal migration of neutrophils (squirting papillae), dermal capillary activation, tortuous dilatation, and angiogenesis (35–37). Importantly, this stage is characterized by predominance of neutrophils, in particular in pustular psoriasis. The pathogenesis is auto-inflammatory and driven by innate immune activation, in contrast to lymphocyte predominant auto-immune activation in stable plaque type psoriasis. In the complex immunopathology of psoriasis, it is thought that during innate immune activation, plasmacytoid dendritic cells (pDCs) are activated together with IL-1β and TNF-α producing keratinocytes in response to dendritic Toll-like receptor activation by DNA (LL-37). In this initiating phase, neutrophil recruitment has mainly been attributed to the release of IL-1β and TNF-α. However, anaphylatoxin C5a is the most potent chemo-attractant for various inflammatory cells including neutrophils, monocytes, and macrophages. It was hypothesized that in the earliest psoriatic neutrophil predominant lesions, complement is activated in the stratum corneum, C5a is released which can activate immune cells and keratinocytes. C5a can migrate to the dermal microvasculature, activating endothelial cells, and mast cell degranulation, which results in capillary tortuous dilatation, so characteristic for (early) psoriasis. To investigate this hypothesis, Tagami et al. analyzed the effect of intradermal PLF (mainly consisting of C5a) injections in guinea pigs. Light microscopy of skin biopsies revealed features reminiscent of actual psoriasis lesions and comparable with injection of C5a *in vivo* in healthy human volunteers (38). These histological features included dense infiltration of neutrophils in the dermis followed by increased epidermopoiesis, epidermal proliferation, and degeneration. In contrast, PLF/C5a did not induce proliferation or influenced the viability of cultured human epidermal cells (32). These results suggest that PLF/C5a requires specific circumstances necessary to exert its effect on skin, most probably the presence of neutrophils from the circulation. Altogether, besides IL-1β and TNF-α, C5a is likely to play a role in the early neutrophil predominant and auto-inflammatory phase of psoriasis. Following auto-inflammatory initiation, the response is shifted toward auto-immune activation including activation of the IL-23/IL-17 axis characteristic for stable plaque-type psoriasis. However, more and more evidence points toward bimodal immune activation in psoriasis. Alternating waves of auto-inflammatory bursts of neutrophils coexist with T-cell driven auto-immune activation (37). Complement might be one of these factors linking innate auto-inflammatory and adaptive auto-immune responses in psoriasis. Two recent studies have provided evidence supporting this theory. Treatment of mice with siRNA targeting C3 reduced skin disease in a mouse model of psoriasis (39). Furthermore, using the imiquimod-induced model of psoriasis, it was found that C3 deficient mice showed significantly reduced levels of IL-1β, TNF-α, IL-17a, and IL-23 in the skin and draining lymph nodes and decreased infiltration of neutrophils (40). These studies clearly show a link between complement activation and activation of IL-23/IL-17 axis of adaptive immunity. Clinical studies targeting complement activation might investigate whether flares of psoriasis can be prevented by targeting innate immunity instead of treating adaptive immune activation in well-established psoriatic plaques.

ACNE VULGARIS AND HIDRADENITIS SUPPURATIVA (HS)

Acne Vulgaris

Acne vulgaris is a common cutaneous disorder and its pathogenesis is multifactorial including genetic, infectious, and hormonal factors. The distribution of the skin lesions in acne vulgaris reflects that of sebaceous glands. Patients present with comedones predominantly on the face, nose, forehead, and chest (sebaceous areas). Light microscopy reveals open and closed comedones, which are a result of excessive sebum secretion, hyperkeratosis of the sebaceous duct, and follicular infundibulum, subsequently followed by hair follicle dilatation. Excessive dilatation of the follicular infundibulum eventually results in rupture of the epithelial layer. Besides distension, epithelial damage is also attributed to overgrowth of *Propionibacterium acnes* (*P. acnes*) in the hair follicle lumen. *P. acnes* is an anaerobic bacterium and a habitual follicular resident. Although data exist implicating *P. acnes* in the initiation of follicular distension and obstruction, the bacterium is primarily involved in the subsequent inflammatory response of the hair follicle. Once ruptured, secondary inflammatory changes occur, such as granulomatous inflammation in response to epithelial fragments, and chronic-active inflammation (41, 42).

Today, it is still not known what is the sequence of events that is responsible for evolution of a non-inflamed into an inflamed acne lesion. Evidence exists that complement activation could be one of the primary triggers in this inflammatory response in acne. In 1966, Puhvel et al. revealed that high levels of complement fixing antibodies are present in patients with severe acne compared with patients with mild or no acne (43). Scott et al. analyzed non-inflamed (white- and black heads) and inflamed (papules and nodules) acne lesions. The most frequent finding was perivascular granular and/or linear pilosebaceous basement membrane zone (of affected units) deposition of C3b in both non- and inflamed acne lesions (44). Similar findings were reported by Dahl et al. in early acne lesions (12). In non-inflamed acne lesions, C3b deposition preceded influx of mononuclear cells while inflamed lesions showed both C3b deposition as well as mononuclear inflammation. Kligman et al. observed that microscopic hair follicle rupture precedes clinical inflammation. In uninvolved skin of patients with acne sometimes microcomedones are seen with early inflammatory changes, with migration of neutrophils into intact follicular epithelium. In a later stage, the follicular epithelium becomes spongiotic and small foci of neutrophils can be found in the hair follicle lumen (45). These findings suggest that in the early stages of acne chemotactic factors are released from the intact hair follicle to recruit neutrophils. Complement activation products, in particular C5a, is the most likely factor involved in the chemokinesis of neutrophils that initiates the conversion of a non-inflamed into an inflamed lesion. Interestingly, C3b deposition was almost exclusively found without concurrent immunoglobulin or C1q deposition, suggesting that the alternative pathway might be primarily involved in the development of acne vulgaris. A candidate triggering factor for complement activation might be *P. acnes*, since bacteria are well known to activate complement. It has been shown that both the alternative and classical complement pathways can be activated in normal human serum upon interaction with comedonal contents as well as *P. acnes* (46–49). Another possibility is the direct activation of the alternative pathway by the stratum corneum (30). Both Dahl et al. and Scott et al. only found isolated granular C3b deposition or granular C3b with immunoglobulin deposition along the dermo-epidermal junction in a few biopsies. This could hypothetically represent immune complex formation with *P. acnes* and possibly subsequent classical pathway activation (12, 44). Whatever the trigger or route of complement activation might be, C5a is released acting as a potent chemokinetic factor in the recruitment of neutrophils. Therefore, it is plausible to hypothesize that the increased influx of neutrophils in acne vulgaris is, at least in part, dependent on complement activation and may therefore be amenable to complement inhibiting therapies.

Hidradenitis Suppurativa

Hidradenitis suppurativa (synonym: acne inversa) is a severe inflammatory follicular skin disease causing severe patient discomfort and psychosocial burden. HS is a common, yet unrecognized and underdiagnosed disease with a prevalence of 1–4% of the European population. Patients present in the acute stage with painful inflamed nodules (boils) in the inverse apocrine bearing regions of the body such as the groin and axilla. In a late stage, sinus tract formation occurs with formation of abscesses and scarring. Importantly, systemic therapy with immunosuppressive agents (systemic corticosteroids, dapsone, and cyclosporin) has been investigated in the past decade and has shown limited efficacy.

Although the exact pathogenesis of HS still has yet to be unraveled, different theories have been proposed during the last decade. In general, it is believed that HS is a multifactorial disease in which genetic, environmental factors (such as smoking, microbial colonization, and obesity) and the immune system interact. Follicular occlusion is thought to be the primary event in HS and is caused by follicular infundibular epithelial hyperplasia and hyperkeratosis. It is hypothesized that this could be a result of microbial overgrowth due to a deficient follicular skin immune system or, in contrast, an overactive immune system that reacts to normal skin flora. Eventually, follicular plugging and occlusion will result in hair follicle rupture. Upon rupture, classical histological features are observed as seen in a ruptured epidermal cyst or comedone such as granulomatous inflammation on keratin fibers and chronic inflammation (**Figure 3**). Although such material is rapidly cleared in ruptured epidermal/acne cysts, the inflammatory response in HS persists, leading to chronicity with formation of sinus tracts and scarring (50–52).

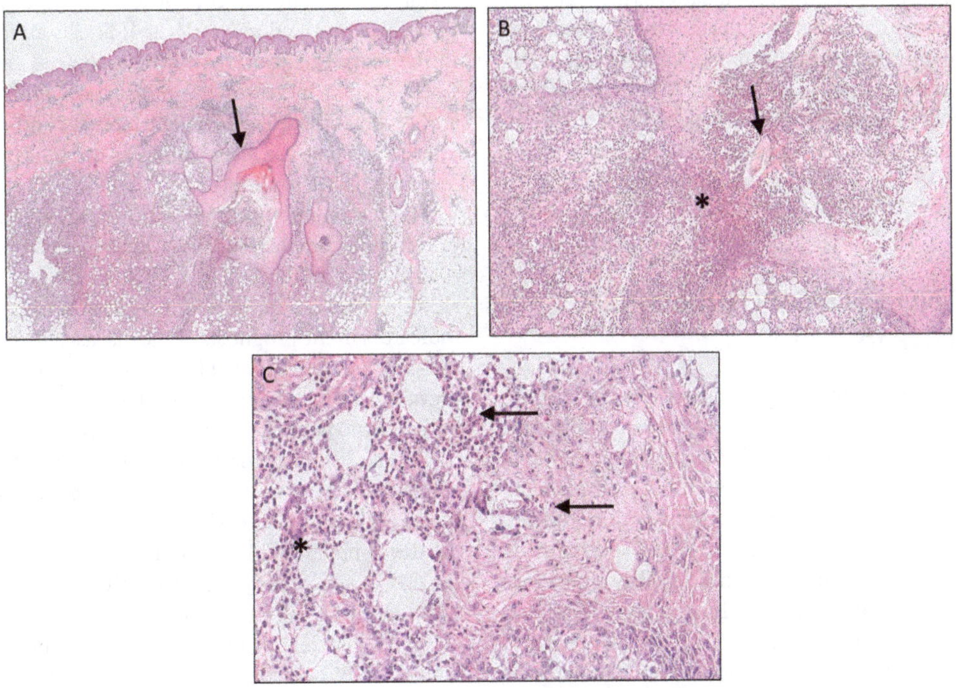

FIGURE 3 | Hidradenitis suppurativa. Sinus tracts [**(A)**, arrow], active inflammation, and rupture [**(B)**, asterisks] of the follicular epithelium with "floating" hair fragments [**(B)**, arrow]. Subsequently, a secondary inflammatory response is induced with influx of numerous neutrophils [**(C)**, arrows] and granulomatous foreign body reaction with giant cells [**(C)**, asterisks].

Although "HS" is a misnomer since involvement of sweat glands is not a central event in the pathogenesis of HS, HS is indeed characterized by suppuration with deep abscess formation. Although not classified as a neutrophilic dermatosis, influx of numerous neutrophils is a characteristic histological feature of HS. However, it is uncertain whether this is an early or late event in the pathogenesis of this disease. The inflammatory response in HS is characterized by increased levels of IL-1β and TNF-α, both in (peri)lesional skin biopsies as well as circulating levels in HS patients (53). The important role of these cytokines is illustrated with the clinical improvement observed after treatment with TNF-α antagonists infliximab and adalimumab (54). Recruitment of neutrophils has been mainly attributed to TNF-α and IL-1β, however, the role of complement activation has only recently been studied. Blok et al. found induction of complement pathway genes in lesional HS skin biopsies, indicating involvement of the complement system in this disease (55). An open label phase 2 study is currently underway with the C5a inhibitor IFX-1 in patients with moderate to severe HS (NCT 03001622). Recent results from this study demonstrated systemic complement activation in HS patients reflected by increased circulating levels of C5a and C5b-9 (56). Furthermore, increased C5a serum levels in HS patients were able to activate neutrophils, thereby contributing to HS symptoms. Up to 83%, HS clinical response rate was achieved at the endpoint of anti-C5a treatment in this phase 2 clinical study. Thus, targeting the C5a–C5aR axis may represent a promising therapeutic strategy for HS patients, most probably *via* inhibition of systemic neutrophil activation. Besides systemic activation, also local complement could potentially be activated in HS since commensal follicular skin bacteria, similar to acne vulgaris, might function as pathogen-associated molecular patterns that can activate classical and alternative complement pathways. Furthermore and in a later stage after hair follicle rupture, cellular fragments might function as danger-associated molecular patterns, which can also activate complement. Whether complement activation, and aberrant immune activation in general in HS, is a primary or secondary event to an initial hair follicle process remains to be investigated.

SYSTEMIC AND CUTANEOUS LUPUS ERYTHEMATOSUS (LE)

Lupus erythematosus is a heterogeneous auto-immune disease, which is characterized by the presence of elevated immune complexes, high titers of auto-antibodies against nuclear and cytoplasmic components and consumption of complement components. Deposition of immune complexes within various organs causes tissue damage, producing a broad spectrum of clinical manifestations ranging from systemic to solely cutaneous lesions. Epidemiological studies have estimated the prevalence of systemic LE (SLE) to be around 0.2–0.7% occurring predominantly in patients older than 40 years of age, with a female/male ratio of 9:1 (57). The cause of SLE is multifactorial with genetic, environmental, and hormonal contributions, also integrated in the American College of Rheumatology (ACR) guideline for SLE. This guideline requires at least four of the 11 clinical and laboratory components to be present before diagnosing SLE. Whereas the revised classification Systemic Lupus International Collaborating Clinics requires four components with one clinical and one immunologic item (58). Studies have shown that skin involvement will eventually develop in about 70% of patients with SLE, although primary cutaneous LE (CLE) mainly develops in the absence of systemic features. The probability of progression from CLE to SLE is approximately 20% (59). There are a few subsets in which CLE can be classified: acute LE, subacute (SCLE), and chronic cutaneous LE (CCLE), of which CCLE can be further subdivided into discoid LE, LE profundus, LE tumidus, chilblain lupus, and bullous LE (60).

Literature over the years suggests that the pathogenesis of SLE and CLE might share common features, along with the developmental consequences of genetic, environmental factors, and immune dysregulation. Several haplotypes and certain alleles of the major histocompatibility complex (MHC) have shown association with different subtypes of CLE. From a mechanistic point of view, MHC polymorphisms may lead to an increase of auto-reactive T-lymphocytes mediated by a selection error in the thymus (61). Furthermore, a panel of single nucleotide polymorphisms (SNPs) has been shown to be associated with CLE, including TYK2, IRF5, and CTLA4. These polymorphisms may have an influence on the IFN cytokine signaling (62).

A well-known trigger of CLE is ultraviolet light (UVL), also one of the ACR criteria of SLE, included as photosensitivity. Firstly, UVL can penetrate through different layers of the skin, causing acute inflammation as well as damage to the DNA, thereby inducing keratinocyte apoptosis (63). Accumulation of apoptotic material due to decreased clearance can result in the formation of immune complexes, which in turn can enhance the IFN-α production by pDCs. IFN-α is an important cytokine in the recruitment of Th1 and cytotoxic T cells (62). Secondly, UVL directly increases the production of TNF-α, interferons, and several interleukins of keratinocytes and dermal fibroblasts. These cytokines are responsible for the infiltration of leukocytes in skin biopsies of CLE (61).

Numerous auto-antibodies, resulting from impaired clearance of immune complexes, can be found in patients with CLE. The role of auto-antibodies in CLE is not completely understood, although some auto-antibodies have been found to be useful indicators in the prognosis of the disease. Patients with anti-RNP, anti-Sm, and anti-aPL antibodies are closely associated with high prevalence of malar rash, while patients with only anti-Ro/SSA antibodies demonstrated to have an increased risk for nephritis (62).

Besides genetic variation in certain MHC class I and II alleles, congenital deficiencies of classical complement pathway components C1q, C1r, C1s, C4, and C2 are strongly associated with the development of SLE (62). In addition, a homozygous SNP of the C1QA gene appears to be highly associated with SCLE (64). Boeckler et al. were the first to demonstrate a high prevalence of partial deficiency of C2, C4 and combined C2/C4 in patients with CLE (65). Furthermore, C4 copy number variation of *C4A* and *C4B genes* is also associated with the risk of SLE (extensively reviewed elsewhere) (66). Two concepts could potentially explain the development of SLE in patients deficient in classical pathway components. Firstly, early classical pathway components are involved in the induction of immune tolerance in germinal centers of lymph nodes. It is well known that CD35/CR1 and CD21/CR2 on follicular DC bind and present complement factors to virgin B-cells in order to differentiate self from non-self B-cells. More specifically, it was demonstrated that CD21, CD35, or C4 deficient mice resulted in high levels of anti-nuclear antibodies and severe lupus-like disease (67). Therefore, complement deficiency results in the breach of self-tolerance and subsequently the development of SLE. Secondly, complement deficiency results to the inability of efficiently clearing apoptotic cells/debris and could render them to become auto-antigens, induce auto-antibody formation and thereby SLE. Most research has been performed on the latter concept, in particular the role of C1q deficiency in LE. There are three sets of findings that link C1q to the development of SLE. Firstly, congenital C1q deficiency is the strongest genetic risk factor known for the development of SLE (68). Secondly and paradoxically, circulating levels of C1q are strongly decreased in SLE as a result of classical complement activation. Thirdly, anti-C1q antibodies can be found in approximately 33% of the patients with SLE and usually coincides with classical pathway activation (69, 70).

One of the main functions of C1q is to act as an opsonin to stimulate removal of apoptotic cell fragments. C1q can directly bind to the surface of apoptotic keratinocytes through its globular heads, which results in the formation of C3 convertases. This is followed by cleavage of C3 and the release anaphylatoxin C3a and the opsonin C3b which results in the clearance of apoptotic cells by phagocytosis (71). Furthermore, the collagenous region of C1q can bind to the calreticulin/CD91 complex, which is expressed on the surface of phagocytes. This binding enhances phagocytosis, leading to ingestion of C1q coated apoptotic cells (72). C1q deficiency therefore directly interferes with the clearance of apoptotic cell debris. Although this is interesting from a mechanistic point of view, most SLE patients are C1q sufficient and therefore other mechanisms underlie the impaired clearance of apoptotic debris in SLE. Impaired clearance of apoptotic cells could lead to secondary necrosis, causing disintegration, and high expression of potential auto-antigens on the surface of apoptotic bodies and blebs (73). This induces the production of auto-antibodies against these "lupus auto-antigens" by B-cells. In turn, auto-antibody-antigen complexes bind C1q thereby activating the classical pathway of complement (74). Together with classical pathway activation as a result of C1q bound to apoptotic blebs, this explains the paradox that SLE patient show strong ongoing complement activation with low and sometimes undetectable serum complement levels (secondary hypocomplementemia). Furthermore, it is thought that prolonged exposure of C1q bound to the surface of apoptotic blebs could become antigenic due to impaired clearance that consequently induces production of auto-antibodies to C1q (75). Recent studies have demonstrated that anti-C1q specifically interacts with C1q bound to early apoptotic cells and not to C1q bound to immunoglobulins or immune complexes. Antigen-C1q-anti-C1q complexes induce classical pathway activation also causing secondary hypocomplementemia. Besides, this results in interference of the uptake of apoptotic cells and impaired C1q-dependent phagocytosis (76, 77).

The deposition of auto-antibody-antigen complexes can be visualized in skin biopsies by immunofluorescence in the so-called "lupus band test," demonstrable as granular or linear deposits of IgG, C3b and occasionally IgA and IgM along the dermo-epidermal junction. The lupus band test can be applied to differentiate SLE from CLE and also as a prognostic parameter for patients with LE. A positive reaction can be observed in both lesional as well as non-lesional skin in SLE. However, in CLE only lesional skin shows a positive lupus band test. More importantly, sun-exposed skin biopsies of healthy individuals may also exhibit a positive lupus band test; therefore, it is essential to perform direct immunofluoresence on sun-protected skin (78). Interestingly, also MBL deposition was recently found in lesional skin of patients with SLE, indicating involvement of the lectin pathway (79).

Lastly, there seems to be no clear difference in the role of complement between SLE and CLE. The complement system, especially C1q, appears to play a crucial role in the pathogenesis of SLE and CLE. The absence of functional C1q can lead to impaired clearance of apoptotic cells, resulting in expression of auto-antigens, and induction of auto-antibody generation. Furthermore, C1q can eventually bind to these surface blebs stimulating the production of auto-antibodies to C1q itself. Despite the increased knowledge concerning the pathogenesis of SLE, it remains a complex disease in which multiple mechanisms are of significance.

CUTANEOUS SMALL VESSEL VASCULITIS (CSVV)

Cutaneous small vessel vasculitis is defined as inflammation of the postcapillary venules in the skin. CSVV without presence of systemic vasculitis is currently named as single organ CSVV, according to the updated Chapel Hill Nomenclature for Vasculitis (80). There are also other subtypes of CSVV with systemic involvement such as anti-neutrophil cytoplasmic antibodies (ANCA)-associated vasculitis and cryoglobulinemic vasculitis. CSVV is the most common type of vasculitis with an incidence of 15 per million. The majority of the patients are adults with a slight preference for females (81). Over the years, numerous studies have revealed multiple factors taking part in the development of CSVV. The disease seems to be associated with drugs, infections, and systemic disorders such as SLE, RA, or malignancy. However, in many patients there is no identifiable cause and in these cases CSVV is then considered as a primary idiopathic entity (82, 83).

The classical presentation of CSVV usually occurs 7–14 days after exposure to a triggering agent. Palpable purpura are the hallmark of CSVV, and appear as red-purple discolorations on the skin varying from 2 to 5 mm in size. However, CSVV presents as many clinical variants, depending on the severity and duration of the disease including urticaria, pustules, erosions, and ulcers (81).

The histopathologic pattern observed in CSVV is leukocytoclastic vasculitis (LCV), which is characterized by a superficial infiltrate surrounding the postcapillary venules predominantly composed of neutrophils, leukocytoclasis, endothelial swelling, extravasation of erythrocytes, and eventually fibrinoid necrosis (**Figure 4**) (82). Moreover, the presence of eosinophils can be an indicator of drug-induced CSVV.

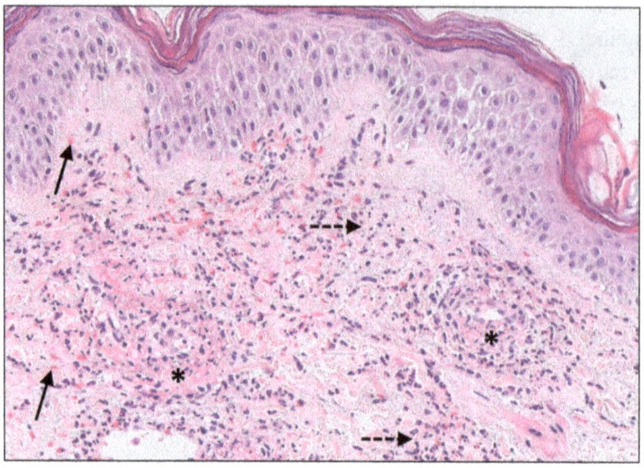

FIGURE 4 | Small vessel leucocytoclastic vasculitis. The section shows all features of leucocytoclastic vasculitis. A mixed inflammatory cell population surrounding the postcapillary venules of the superficial dermis. The infiltrate consists of neutrophils with nuclear dust (dashed arrows) and shows high affinity for the vessels. Features of vascular injury are shown including fibrinoid necrosis (asterisks) and erytrocyt extravasation (solid arrows).

Accumulating evidence has indicated that the complement system plays a significant role in the pathogenesis of CSVV. Immunofluorescence studies have supported this hypothesis by demonstrating deposits of immunoglobulins of IgM- and IgG classes, C3c and fibrinogen in, and around dermal vessel walls in LCV. Grunwald et al. demonstrate these immunoreactants in skin biopsies of early, mature, and healing stages of vasculitis (84). Detection of vascular IgA deposition is defined for Henoch–Schonlein purpura (85). Vascular immunoglobulin and complement were also detected in non-lesional skin, suggesting that deposition of these immunoreactants is a primary event, and not secondary to endothelial damage (81). In addition, Dauchel and colleagues reported that C3d and C5b-9 were significantly increased in plasma of patients with LCV compared with controls, whereas C3, C1q, C2, C4, and FB were within normal ranges. These findings indicate local as well as systemic complement activation in patients with LCV. Moreover, the increased level of C3d and C5b-9 has been shown to correlate with vasculitis activity. Interestingly, circulating C3d and C5b-9 levels did correlate with disease activity but not with the intensity of perivascular cutaneous depositions, suggesting that C3d and C5b-9 plasma levels are caused by systemic complement activation instead of passive diffusion from cutaneous lesions into the circulation (86).

The most widely accepted concept of the pathogenesis is deposition of immune complexes in postcapillary venules, with inflammation occurring after complement activation. As mentioned previously, multiple etiologies can trigger the formation of circulating immune complexes. These consist of foreign antigens and antibodies in slight excess of antigen, and therefore easily get trapped and subsequently deposited in small vessels. These immune complexes lead to activation of the complement cascade *via* the classical pathway. Among the activated complement products, C5a and C5b-9 seem to be mainly responsible for the endothelial damage observed in CSVV (82, 83). C5a induces activation of neutrophils and upregulation of several adhesion molecules (E-selectin, ICAM-1, and V-CAM) on the surface of endothelial cells, allowing neutrophils, and other inflammatory cells to migrate from the circulation into the site of inflammation (87). Activated neutrophils can secrete reactive oxygen species and also dysregulate the expression of serine proteinases elastase and cathepsin G, which eventually leads to endothelium damage (88). Additionally, decreased tissue plasminogen activator (t-PA) in response to released cytokines due to vascular damage leads to abnormal fibrinolysis and may eventually result in fibrin deposition as reflected on histology (89). Under physiologic conditions, various regulators secreted or/and expressed by endothelial cells maintain control of complement activation. These include C1-INH, FH, FI, vitronectin, clusterin, and CD55/DAF (90). Interestingly, Boom et al. observed that DAF expression on endothelial cells of cutaneous vasculitis was almost completely absent, while DAF expression on intraluminal erythrocytes was unaffected. Expression of DAF on the surface can restrain assembly of the terminal cascade by binding to C3b, and thereby interfering with the C5 convertases. The authors suggest that the absence of DAF might be the consequence of local downregulation of DAF synthesis and might play an important role in the pathogenesis of CSVV (91). However, there is only sparse literature available about potent downregulators of DAF.

In aggregate, the complement system appears to be associated with the development of CSVV. The interaction between complement components and activation products, and the endothelial cells seem to play an essential role in the pro-inflammatory response seen in CSVV. Activation of classical pathway of complement has been recognized in CSVV, regarding to the immune complex-mediated process. In particular, the effects of C5a and MAC on endothelial cells and neutrophils may eventually lead to structural and functional damage of the endothelium resulting in CSVV.

URTICARIA AND URTICARIAL VASCULITIS (UV)

Urticaria

Urticaria is widely held to be one of the most common skin diseases, affecting up to approximately 20% of the population during lifetime. Urticarial lesions are characteristically pruritic, edematous, erythematous papules, or wheals often with pale centers, which can merge into larger plaques and usually resolve within 24 h. Urticaria consists of a wide spectrum ranging from localized wheals to widespread recurrent wheals with angioedema. Coexisting episodes of angioedema appear to be present in approximately 40% of patients with urticaria (92). Angioedema can be characterized as edema in the deep dermal layer and subcutaneous or submucosal tissues. Acute urticaria is defined by disease duration of less than 6 weeks, whereas recurrent urticarial lesions persisting for a period beyond 6 weeks is defined as chronic urticaria (CU). CU can be further divided into chronic inducible urticaria and chronic spontaneous urticaria (CSU). Inducible urticaria is caused by a response to external triggers, including cold, heat, allergens, sunlight, sweat, and pressure (92).

CSU is mainly idiopathic, although researchers have identified a subpopulation with an auto-immune etiology. The histopathology of an urticarial lesion mostly involves changes in the upper dermis, consisting of mild dermal edema, and sparse perivascular and interstitial mixed inflammatory infiltrate composed of a variable number of lymphocytes, monocytes, mast cells, eosinophils, and neutrophils (**Figure 5**) (93). The pathophysiological events in the formation of wheals involve activation of dermal mast cells and basophils by various triggers, including anaphylatoxins C3a and C5a, and also physical stimuli. It is well established that binding of antigen to antigen-specific IgE on mast cells and basophils activates and degranulates these inflammatory cells (type 1 hypersensitivity reaction). The most important active substance in urticaria is histamine. Histamine induces vasodilation, increases vascular permeability, and stimulation of sensory nerve endings leading to pain or itching. Other important mediators such as TNF-α, leukotrienes, platelet-activator, and prostaglandin D2 may also promote an inflammatory response (94). The exact trigger or cause of histamine release has not been identified in most patients with CSU. Evidence of an auto-immune etiology in approximately 45% of patients has been presented. Patients with CSU have shown to possess circulating IgG auto-antibodies directed against the α subunit of IgE (anti-FcεR1α) and IgE receptor in their sera, corresponding to a type 2 hypersensitivity reaction (95). Additionally, increased frequency of thyroid dysfunction and thyroid auto-antibodies (anti-microsomal peroxidase and anti-thyroidglobulin) are found in patients with CSU (96).

IgG auto-antibodies bound to IgE or IgE receptor on mast cells results in the activation of complement *via* the classical pathway followed by generation of C5a and C5b-9. Subsequently, C5a can mediate mast cell activation *via* C5aR1 ligation with subsequent degranulation and release of mediators, resulting in urticarial wheals (97, 98). Accumulated evidence has shown that complement is involved in degranulation of mast cells and basophils in some patients with CSU (97). Firstly, one study demonstrated that heat inactivation of serum complement of patients with CU, decreased the capacity of serum to release histamine from basophils (99). Ferrer and colleagues found that unless serum containing C2 and C5 was added to IgG derived from CU sera, histamine is not released from mast cells, implicating that activation of the classical complement pathway is required for mast cell degranulation (100). In parallel with early studies, the presence of complement, especially C5a, had a role in augmenting IgG-dependent histamine release from basophils (101). Although the immune reaction in urticaria is regarded as a type 1 and type 2 hypersensitivity reaction, also local complement deposition can be found in about one-third of chronic urticarial lesions without signs of systemic activation, suggesting a type 3 hypersensitivity reaction as well (102–105).

Urticarial Vasculitis

Urticarial vasculitis is a relatively uncommon disease with an estimated prevalence of 5%, occurring more often in women. Clinical cutaneous manifestations of UV consist of erythematous urticarial papules and plaques that last 24–72 h with a tendency to heal with purpura or hyperpigmentation. Patients with UV can be classified as normocomplementemic UV (NUV) or hypocomplementemic UV (HUV) depending on serum complement levels. Although NUV is mostly idiopathic, HUV is associated with a more severe form of disease and can indicate an underlying disease like SLE or hypocomplementemic urticarial vasculitis syndrome (HUVS) (106). HUVS is characterized by urticaria with hypocomplementemia, arthralgia/arthritis, glomerulonephritis, recurrent abdominal pain, and obstructive lung disease (107). According to retrospective observations, there seems to be no transition among UV subtypes (108). Histopathologically, lesions of UV reveal combined features of urticaria with superimposed vascular damage. In contrast to LCV, vascular damage in UV is more subtle with endothelial activation, sparse karyorrhexis, and focal fibrinoid necrosis present in only the minority of cases (109).

Various reports support the hypothesis that UV is an immune complex-mediated disease. Deposits of immunoglobulins, complement, and/or fibrinogen in the vessel walls are often observed by immunofluorescence in patients with UV. Additionally, immune complexes are also regularly detected in the blood circulation of patients with UV. There are numerous etiologies that can trigger the formation of immune complexes in UV, including auto-antibodies, infections, and medications. Formation of immune complexes leads to activation of the complement cascade *via* the classical pathway and subsequently generation of C3a, C5a, and C5b-9.

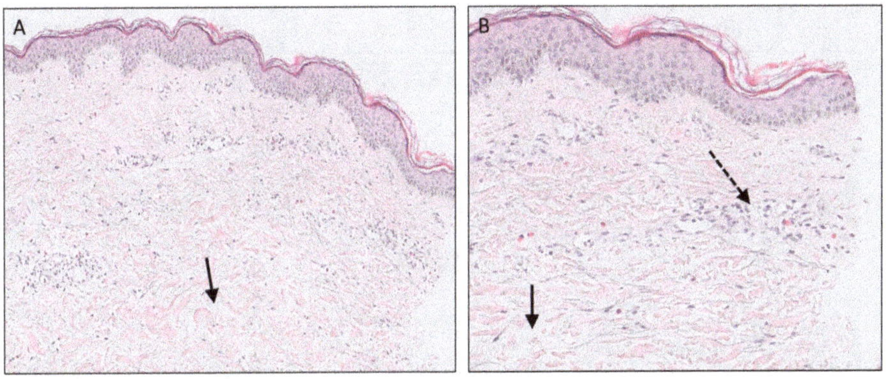

FIGURE 5 | Urticaria. Dermal edema [solid arrows in **(A,B)**] and a sparse superficial predominantly perivascular and interstitial infiltrate of lymphocytes and eosinophils without signs of vasculitis (dashed arrow).

Release of C5a can lead to a chain of events, including activation of neutrophils, mast cell degranulation, and eosinophil degranulation, which in turn can result in endothelial damage (106).

Wisnieski et al. were the first to suggest that the pathogenesis of HUVS might involve abnormal genetic background (110). Subsequently, one study found that genetic mutations in the DNASE1L3 gene are associated with a familial form of HUVS and SLE. The protein encoded by this gene functions as endonuclease, which is possibly responsible for the removal of DNA during apoptosis (111). This finding supports the link between SLE and HUVS. Another similar feature in both diseases is the presence of auto-antibodies against C1q that can be detected in 100% of the patients with HUVS and in approximately one-third of the patients with SLE (69, 108). Anti-C1q antibodies bind to the collagenous region of C1q and usually coincide with decreased levels of classical pathway complement components as a result of complement activation. Additionally, decreased levels of CH50, C2, and C4 were also found in patients with HUVS (106). These findings implicate that complement might contribute to the pathogenesis of HUVS.

To summarize, UV consist of a wide spectrum of cutaneous, systemic features ranging from urticaria with mild vasculitis to systemic vasculitis combined with hypocomplementemia. Classical activation of complement is involved in the pathogenesis of UV and HUVS.

BULLOUS PEMPHIGOID (BP)

In this section, we will review the role of complement in the most common auto-immune bullous dermatosis, BP. Although complement has also been shown to be involved in the pathogenesis of other auto-immune bullous dermatoses, such as mucous membrane pemphigoid, epidermolysis bullosa acquisita, dermatitis herpetiformis, and bullous systemic LE, the reader is referred elsewhere to more detailed publications on this topic (112–114).

Bullous pemphigoid is the most frequently encountered acquired auto-immune blistering disease most commonly affecting the elderly. Clinically, patients present with tense pruritic dome-shaped fluid filled blisters measuring up to several centimeters in diameter. The most commonly recognized BP antigens are BP180 (BPAG2) and BP230 (BPAG1) and less frequently, antibodies can be found against plectins and LAD1. Most antibodies in BP are directed against the NC16A domain of BP180, which is a major non-collagenous extracellular antigenic site. Separation in BP occurs at the level of the lamina lucida. A skin biopsy from an established blister reveals a subepidermal blister, often accompanied by a superficial dermal infiltrate of lymphocytes, eosinophils, neutrophils, mast cells, and monocytes/macrophages (**Figure 6**). These inflammatory cells are also found in the blister fluid in the cell-rich variant of BP. Immunofluorescence demonstrates specific linear IgG and/or C3b deposition along the basement membrane zone. Although deposition of complement fragments such as C3c and C1q is routinely used for diagnostic reasons, activation of the complement system has also been shown to play a crucial role in the development of disease.

Complement components and activation fragments including C1q, C3, C3c, C3d, C4, C4d, C5, C5b-9, FB, FH, and properdin have been found at the basement membrane zone and blister fluid in BP. These findings indicate involvement of both classical and alternative pathways in the pathogenesis of BP (115–117).

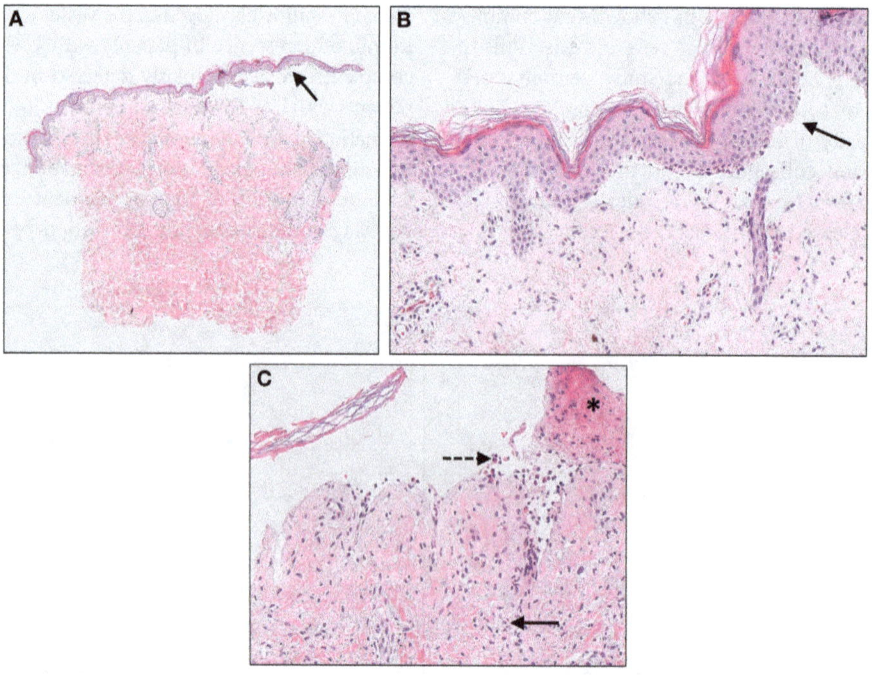

FIGURE 6 | Bullous pemphigoid. Subepidermal blistering [solid arrows in **(A,B)**] and influx of inflammatory cells including eosinophils and neutrophils in the dermis [solid arrow **(C)**] and blister cavity [dashed arrows **(C)**]. In **(C)** also deposition of fibrin is noted (asterisks).

Recently, complement split products C3d and C4d have been shown to be deposited along the basement membrane zone in formalin fixed paraffin embedded tissue and might be a potential substitute for direct immunofluorescence in the near future (118–122).

Liu et al. developed an experimental mouse model of BP using a rabbit antibody against murine BP180NC14A, a homolog of human BP180NC16A, which is, however, very poorly conserved in murine protein. This antibody was passively transferred in neonatal mice and developed a subepidermal blistering disease closely mimicking clinical BP. This experimental model of BP has demonstrated a critical role for complement activation in BP. Mice deficient of C5 or depleted of complement by cobra venom factor showed no clinical or histological evidence of BP in contrast to wild-type (WT) or complement sufficient mice. Also, injection of F(ab')2 fragments prepared from the pathogenic rabbit anti-murine BP180 did not show induction of BP, indicating a crucial role for the IgG Fc portion in BP. It is the Fc portion of antibody that expresses antigen-binding sites for C1q, thereby initiating classical complement activation (123). Using the same BP model, C4 deficient and WT mice pretreated with anti-mC1q were resistant to develop BP, also strongly indicating a crucial role for classical complement activation in BP. However, FB deficient mice developed delayed and less intense blisters, indicating that also the alternative pathway is involved in BP, probably acting in concert with classical pathway activation *via* the amplification loop (124, 125). The complement-mediated development of BP appeared to be dependent on mast cells and neutrophils. Mice depleted of circulating neutrophils did not develop BP after injection of anti-mBP180. Reconstitution with C5a or injection with neutrophil chemokine IL-8 in C5 deficient mice regained susceptibility to BP (126). These findings indicate that neutrophil recruitment in BP is C5a dependent. However, mice deficient in mast cells or C5aR1 deficient mast cells failed to develop BP, despite the activation of complement and in the presence of neutrophils. The passive transfer model exhibits extensive mast cell degranulation, preceding neutrophil infiltration, and subepidermal blistering. It was found that complement-dependent chemokinesis of neutrophils is, at least in part, dependent on mast cell degranulation *via* C5aR1 (124, 127).

Although interesting, it is questionable whether this mice model can be easily translated to the human situation since BP180NC14a is poorly preserved in mice. Therefore, a humanized mice model was developed in which mouse BP180NC14A was replaced with the homologous human BP180NC16A epitope cluster region. Mice injected with anti-human BP180NC16A subsequently development BP (128). A similar model was developed by Nishie et al. introducing the human COL17 cDNA transgene into Col17-null mice (129). Importantly, the previous findings of complement-dependent development of BP were confirmed (128).

Notably, although complement plays an important role in the pathogenesis of BP, more and more evidence emerges that also complement-independent mechanisms exist. Several groups have shown direct pathogenic effects of auto-antibodies leading to depletion of COL17 in keratinocytes and contributing to skin fragility in a complement-independent manner (130–132).

Most of the previously cited studies were performed in animal or *in vitro* models, making interpretation of the data limited. However, in a large cohort ($n = 300$) patient study, Romeijn et al. have shown that in the majority of BP skin biopsies, complement deposition could be demonstrated. More interestingly, deposition of complement was related to clinical and serological disease activity strengthening the crucial role of complement in this disease (133).

COMPLEMENT INHIBITING STRATEGIES IN SKIN DISEASES

For years, many attempts in producing complement-specific drugs have been made with limited success. The main challenge in creating complement-specific drugs has been to discover the balance between sufficient blocking of complement activity in order to prevent local tissue damage and preserving the protection of this system. As outlined in the current review, clinical and experimental studies have demonstrated variable roles of complement in the pathogenesis of skin diseases. The findings and proposed triggers for complement activation in different skin diseases are summarized in **Table 1**. With the impending recognition of neutrophil driven auto-inflammatory diseases, IL-1β and TNF-α inhibitors have now been proven beneficial for the treatment of specific auto-inflammatory diseases such as the use of adalimumab in the treatment of HS (54). The successful use of these agents is primarily based on the inhibition of neutrophil chemotaxis. As described previously, C5a acts as a potent recruiter of neutrophils by binding to C5aR1 expressed primarily by neutrophils. Moreover, C5a can trigger increased vascular permeability on endothelial cells and activate the adaptive immune system. Therapeutic intervention in C5a–C5aR axis could therefore be a promising target for the treatment of neutrophil driven skin diseases such as psoriasis and HS as well as other neutrophilic dermatoses. Selective neutralization of the C5a–C5aR interaction offers opportunities to inhibit complement activation without interfering with membrane attack complex formation and thereby the defensive potential of complement. A decade ago, C5aR antagonist PMX53 has already been evaluated and trialed in psoriasis with initial encouraging results. Orally administered cyclic peptidomimetic PMX-53 was tested in a phase 1b/2a trial in 10 patients with psoriasis and positive results in many disease measures were obtained. However, unfortunately, this drug has a very short half-life of only 70 min which severely limits its use in clinical practice (134). Besides psoriasis, intervention in C5a–C5aR axis has very recently been shown to beneficial in the treatment of HS. Blockade of C5a by an anti-C5a antibody demonstrated up to 83% HS clinical response rate at the endpoint of anti-C5a treatment in a phase 2 clinical study, indicating the importance of complement in this disease (NCT03001622). Furthermore, a promising new therapeutic agent is a small molecule C5aR inhibitor CCX168 (Avacopan). The drug can be orally administered, shows a relatively long half-life, has shown limited side effects and promising results in other neutrophil driven diseases, for example, in ANCA-associated vasculitis (135). These therapeutic agents are preferred over the use of Eculizumab (Soliris) which is a recombinant humanized

TABLE 1 | Overview of complement in skin diseases and the proposed triggers of complement activation.

Skin disease	Species	System	Findings related to complement	Proposed triggers of complement activation and/or results	Reference
Psoriasis	Human	Scale extracts	Elevated: C3a, C4a, C5a, C5a-des-Arg	1. Natural anti-SC antibodies 2. C5 cleavage by serine proteases in SC 3. Microbial products 4. Alternative pathway activation after trauma	Tagami et al. (14, 32) Ohkohchi et al. (17) Schröder et al. (18) Takematsu et al. (19) Mrowietz et al. (16)
	Human	Skin biopsies	Deposition: C3b	IgG, IgM, IgG deposition	Weiss et al. (15)
	Human	Serum	Elevated: FB, Bb, C3, C3a, C3b, C4, C4a, C4d, C5b-9, C1-INH, C4bBp, FH, FI Decreased: properdin Normal: C3bBb, C1s-C1-INH	Systemic complement is not activated based on normal circulating C3bBb and C1s-C1-INH complexes (20)	Fleming et al. (20) Kapp et al. (21) Ohkohchi et al. (22, 23) Rosenberg et al. (24) Marley et al. (25)
	Mice	IMQ psoriasis model, C3−/−	Elevated: C3 gene expression in WT mice after IMQ treatment	Trigger: unknown Results: protection against development of psoriatic phenotype in C3−/− mice	Giacomassi et al. (40)
Acne vulgaris	Human	Skin biopsies	C3b deposition	1. *P. Acnes* 2. Natural anti-SC antibodies 3. Immune complexes	Scott et al. (44) Dahl et al. (12)
HS	Human	Skin biopsies	Gene induction of complement pathways	Trigger: unknown	Blok et al. (55)
	Human	Serum	Elevated: C5a, C5b-9	PAMPs and DAMPS	Kanni et al. (56)
LE	Human	Genome	Congenital deficiency of C1q, C1r, C1s, C4, C2. C4 copy number variation	1. Breach of self-tolerance and auto-antibody formation 2. Inefficient clearing of apoptotic cells/debris	Racila et al. (64) Boeckler et al. (65) Chen JY et al. (66)
	Human	Serum	Elevated: anti-C1q auto-antibodies	Immune complexes, (anti-C1q) auto-antibodies	Prodeus et al. (67) Antes et al. (69) Hoekzema et al. (70)
CSVV	Human	Skin biopsies	C3c deposition in vessel wall	Immune complexes	Grunwald et al. (84)
	Human	Serum	Elevated: C3d, C5b-9	Immune complexes	Dauchel et al. (86)
CU	Human	Serum	Complement-dependent histamine release from basophils and mast cells	Type 2 hypersensitivity reaction: auto-antibodies against IgE-FcεR1α and IgE receptor	Zweiman et al. (99) Ferrer et al. (100)
UV	Human	Serum	Elevated: Anti-C1q auto-antibodies Hypocomplementemia	(Anti-C1q) auto-antibodies, immune complexes	Wisnieski et al. (108)
BP	Human	Skin biopsies Blister fluid	Deposition: Linear basement membrane deposition of C1q, C3b, C3c, C3d, C4, C4d, C5, C5b-9, FB, FH, properdin	Anti-BP180 and BP230 auto-antibodies	Dahl et al. (115) Jordon et al. (116, 117) Chandler et al. (118) Kassaby et al. (119) Magro et al. (120) Pfaltz et al. (121) Villani et al. (122)
	Mice	C4−/− C5−/− FB−/− Anti-mC1q CVF depletion	Linear basement membrane C3 deposition in WT animals	Mechanism: anti-BP180 and BP230 auto-antibodies →classical pathway activation, alternative pathway activation (amplification loop) Results in complement −/− mice: protection against development of BP	Liu et al. (123) Heimbach et al. (124) Nelson et al. (125) Liu et al. (128) Nishie et al. (129)

SC, stratum corneum; IMQ, imiquimod; HS, hidradenitis suppurativa; PAMPs, pathogen-associated molecular patterns; DAMPs, danger-associated molecular patterns; LE, lupus erythematosus; CSVV, cutaneous small vessel vasculitis; CU, chronic urticaria; UV, urticarial vasculitis; BP, bullous pemphigoid.

monoclonal antibody directed against C5. Eculizumab intercepts the complement cascade at the terminal effector pathway by binding tightly to C5 and preventing cleavage to C5b. Consequently, this suppresses the formation of the C5b-9, increasing susceptibility to infection (136).

Besides therapeutic intervention in C5a–C5aR axis in autoinflammatory diseases, intervention in complement activation is likely to be beneficial in BP. This review discussed several experimental mouse studies of BP that demonstrated a crucial role of complement activation in this auto-immune bullous disease.

Noteworthy, currently two trials with complement inhibitors are ongoing in BP: TNT-009 is a monoclonal antibody against C1s (NCT02502903) while coversin targets C5 and leukotriene B4 (http://adisinsight.springer.com/trials/700284185).

Altogether, intervention in C5a–C5aR axis and the inherent inhibition of neutrophil recruitment might be the most interesting treatment for complement-mediated inflammatory skin diseases.

CONCLUSION

The complement system represents far more than the originally thought function as a non-specific defense mechanism against micro-organisms. By virtue of extensive murine model studies and genome-wide association studies, our knowledge regarding the functions and hidden connections of complement has greatly expanded. Besides the protective role of complement, improper regulated activation of complement can lead to extensive tissue damage. Local and systemic complement activation has been demonstrated in several skin diseases; however, whether complement activation has pathogenic significance in different skin diseases remains to be investigated. Although not all triggers of complement activation are fully elucidated in different skin diseases, antibody, and immune complex deposition play an important role in (classical) complement activation. However, earlier and more recent experimental studies using mice deficient in complement components have shown involvement of complement in the pathogenesis of BP and experimental psoriasis. Furthermore, preliminary results of a phase IIa clinical study in HS shows promising results using a monoclonal anti-C5a antibody. These result indicate that complement mediates, at least in part, inflammatory skin diseases, in particular neutrophil driven diseases. Therefore, inhibition of neutrophil recruitment through intervention in the C5a–C5aR axis might be the most interesting target of intervention in inflammatory skin diseases.

AUTHOR CONTRIBUTIONS

JG, MS, RR and JD wrote the article. MV, EP, and JD edited and approved the final manuscript.

REFERENCES

1. Walport MJ. Complement. First of two parts. *N Engl J Med* (2001) 344(14):1058–66. doi:10.1056/NEJM200104053441406
2. Chehoud C, Rafail S, Tyldsley AS, Seykora JT, Lambris JD, Grice EA. Complement modulates the cutaneous microbiome and inflammatory milieu. *Proc Natl Acad Sci U S A* (2013) 110(37):15061–6. doi:10.1073/pnas.1307855110
3. Walport MJ. Complement. Second of two parts. *N Engl J Med* (2001) 344(15):1140–4. doi:10.1056/NEJM200104123441506
4. Meri S, Jarva H. Complement regulation. *Vox Sang* (1998) 74(Suppl 2): 291–302. doi:10.1111/j.1423-0410.1998.tb05434.x
5. Li K, Fazekasova H, Wang N, Sagoo P, Peng Q, Khamri W, et al. Expression of complement components, receptors and regulators by human dendritic cells. *Mol Immunol* (2011) 48(9–10):1121–7. doi:10.1016/j.molimm.2011.02.003
6. Timar KK, Junnikkala S, Dallos A, Jarva H, Bhuiyan ZA, Meri S, et al. Human keratinocytes produce the complement inhibitor factor I: synthesis is regulated by interferon-gamma. *Mol Immunol* (2007) 44(11):2943–9. doi:10.1016/j.molimm.2007.01.007
7. Timar KK, Pasch MC, van den Bosch NH, Jarva H, Junnikkala S, Meri S, et al. Human keratinocytes produce the complement inhibitor factor H: synthesis is regulated by interferon-gamma. *Mol Immunol* (2006) 43(4):317–25. doi:10.1016/j.molimm.2005.02.009
8. van den Wijngaard RM, Asghar SS, Pijnenborg AC, Tigges AJ, Westerhof W, Das PK. Aberrant expression of complement regulatory proteins, membrane cofactor protein and decay accelerating factor, in the involved epidermis of patients with vitiligo. *Br J Dermatol* (2002) 146(1):80–7. doi:10.1046/j.1365-2133.2002.04604.x
9. Hajishengallis G, Lambris JD. Crosstalk pathways between toll-like receptors and the complement system. *Trends Immunol* (2010) 31(4):154–63. doi:10.1016/j.it.2010.01.002
10. Braun-Falco O, Christophers E. Structural aspects of initial psoriatic lesions. *Arch Dermatol Forsch* (1974) 251(2):95–110. doi:10.1007/BF00560390
11. Nestle FO, Kaplan DH, Barker J. Psoriasis. *N Engl J Med* (2009) 361(5): 496–509. doi:10.1056/NEJMra0804595
12. Dahl MV, Lindroos WE, Nelson RD. Chemokinetic and chemotactic factors in psoriasis scale extracts. *J Invest Dermatol* (1978) 71(6):402–6. doi:10.1111/1523-1747.ep12558281
13. Tagami H, Ofuji S. Leukotactic properties of soluble substances in psoriasis scale. *Br J Dermatol* (1976) 95(1):1–8. doi:10.1111/j.1365-2133.1976.tb15529.x
14. Tagami H, Ofuji S. Demonstration of C3 cleavage product in leukotactic substances of scale extract from pustular psoriasis. *Br J Dermatol* (1977) 96(1):94–5. doi:10.1111/j.1365-2133.1977.tb05194.x
15. Weiss VC, van Den Broek H, Barrett S, West DP. Immunopathology of psoriasis: a comparison with other parakeratotic lesions. *J Invest Dermatol* (1982) 78(3):256–60. doi:10.1111/1523-1747.ep12506623
16. Mrowietz U, Koch WA, Zhu K, Wiedow O, Bartels J, Christophers E, et al. Psoriasis scales contain C5a as the predominant chemotaxin for monocyte-derived dendritic cells. *Exp Dermatol* (2001) 10(4):238–45. doi:10.1034/j.1600-0625.2001.100403.x
17. Ohkohchi K, Takematsu H, Tagami H. Determination of anaphylatoxin concentrations in suction blisters in patients with psoriasis. *J Invest Dermatol* (1986) 87(1):65–7. doi:10.1111/1523-1747.ep12523572
18. Schröder J-M, Christophers E. Transient absence of C5a-specific neutrophil function in inflammatory disorders of the skin. *J Invest Dermatol* (1985) 85(3):194–8. doi:10.1111/1523-1747.ep12276664
19. Takematsu H, Ohkohchi K, Tagami H. Demonstration of anaphylatoxins C3a, C4a and C5a in the scales of psoriasis and inflammatory pustular dermatoses. *Br J Dermatol* (1986) 114(1):1–6. doi:10.1111/j.1365-2133.1986.tb02773.x
20. Fleming CJ, Holme ER, Mackie RM. Systemic complement activation in psoriasis vulgaris. *Clin Exp Dermatol* (1996) 21(6):415–8. doi:10.1111/j.1365-2230.1996.tb00144.x
21. Kapp A, Wokalek H, Schopf E. Involvement of complement in psoriasis and atopic dermatitis – measurement of C3a and C5a, C3, C4 and C1 inactivator. *Arch Dermatol Res* (1985) 277(5):359–61. doi:10.1007/BF00509233
22. Ohkohchi K, Takematsu H, Tagami H. Increased anaphylatoxins (C3a and C4a) in psoriatic sera. *Br J Dermatol* (1985) 113(2):189–96. doi:10.1111/j.1365-2133.1985.tb02064.x
23. Ohkohchi K, Torinuki W, Tagami H. Increased plasma concentrations of complement modulating proteins (C1 inhibitor, C4-binding protein, factor H and factor I) in psoriasis. *Tohoku J Exp Med* (1988) 154(4):315–21. doi:10.1620/tjem.154.315
24. Rosenberg EW, Noah PW, Wyatt RJ, Jones RM, Kolb WP. Complement activation in psoriasis. *Clin Exp Dermatol* (1990) 15(1):16–20. doi:10.1111/j.1365-2230.1990.tb02011.x
25. Marley WM, Belew PW, Rosenberg EW, Urmson JR, Stitzel AE, Spitzer RE. Abnormalities in the alternative pathway of complement in psoriasis. *Clin Exp Dermatol* (1982) 7(4):387–96. doi:10.1111/j.1365-2230.1982.tb02446.x
26. Pasch M, Bos JD, Asghar SS. Activation of complement in psoriasis. *Clin Exp Dermatol* (1998) 23(4):189–90. doi:10.1046/j.1365-2230.1998.00360.x
27. Beutner EH, Grover RK, Plunkett RW, Lewis ME. Comparisons of pathologic and normal skin reactive autoantibodies and the interference phenomenon. *Clin Dermatol* (2012) 30(4):447–9. doi:10.1016/j.clindermatol.2012.03.001
28. Jablonska S, Chorzelski TP, Beutner EH, Maciejowska E, Jarzabek C, Rzesa G. Autoimmunity in psoriasis. Relation of disease activity and forms

of psoriasis to immunofluorescence findings. *Arch Dermatol Res* (1978) 261(2):135–46. doi:10.1007/BF00447158
29. Lazarus GS, Yost FJ Jr, Thomas CA. Polymorphonuclear leukocytes: possible mechanism of accumulation in psoriasis. *Science* (1977) 198(4322):1162–3. doi:10.1126/science.929193
30. Terui T, Kato T, Tagami H. Stratum corneum activation of complement through the antibody-independent alternative pathway. *J Invest Dermatol* (1989) 92(4):593–7. doi:10.1111/1523-1747.ep12709634
31. Valdimarsson H, Sigmundsdottir H, Jonsdottir I. Is psoriasis induced by streptococcal superantigens and maintained by M-protein-specific T cells that cross-react with keratin? *Clin Exp Immunol* (1997) 107(Suppl 1): 21–4.
32. Tagami H, Kitano Y, Suehisa S, Oku T, Yamada M. Psoriatic leukotactic factor. Further physicochemical characterization and effect on the epidermal cells. *Arch Dermatol Res* (1982) 272(3–4):201–13. doi:10.1007/BF00509048
33. Timar KK, Dallos A, Kiss M, Husz S, Bos JD, Asghar SS. Expression of terminal complement components by human keratinocytes. *Mol Immunol* (2007) 44(10):2578–86. doi:10.1016/j.molimm.2006.12.014
34. Terui T, Ishii K, Ozawa M, Tabata N, Kato T, Tagami H. C3 production of cultured human epidermal keratinocytes in enhanced by IFNγ and TNFα through different pathways. *J Invest Dermatol* (1997) 108(1):62–7. doi:10.1111/1523-1747.ep12285633
35. Ragaz A, Ackerman AB. Evolution, maturation, and regression of lesions of psoriasis. New observations and correlation of clinical and histologic findings. *Am J Dermatopathol* (1979) 1(3):199–214. doi:10.1097/00000372-197900130-00002
36. Telner P, Fekete Z. The capillary responses in psoriatic skin*. *J Invest Dermatol* (1961) 36(3):225–30. doi:10.1038/jid.1961.36
37. Christophers E, Metzler G, Rocken M. Bimodal immune activation in psoriasis. *Br J Dermatol* (2014) 170(1):59–65. doi:10.1111/bjd.12631
38. Yancey KB, Hammer CH, Harvath L, Renfer L, Frank MM, Lawley TJ. Studies of human C5a as a mediator of inflammation in normal human skin. *J Clin Invest* (1985) 75(2):486–95. doi:10.1172/JCI111724
39. Schonthaler HB, Guinea-Viniegra J, Wculek SK, Ruppen I, Ximenez-Embun P, Guio-Carrion A, et al. S100A8-S100A9 protein complex mediates psoriasis by regulating the expression of complement factor C3. *Immunity* (2013) 39(6):1171–81. doi:10.1016/j.immuni.2013.11.011
40. Giacomassi C, Buang N, Ling GS, Crawford G, Cook HT, Scott D, et al. Complement C3 exacerbates imiquimod-induced skin inflammation and psoriasiform dermatitis. *J Invest Dermatol* (2017) 137(3):760–3. doi:10.1016/j.jid.2016.11.011
41. Burkhart CG, Burkhart CN, Lehmann PF. Acne: a review of immunologic and microbiologic factors. *Postgrad Med J* (1999) 75(884):328–31. doi:10.1136/pgmj.75.884.328
42. Webster GF. Inflammation in acne vulgaris. *J Am Acad Dermatol* (1995) 33 (2 Pt 1):247–53. doi:10.1016/0190-9622(95)90243-0
43. Puhvel SM, Hoffman IK, Sternberg TH. *Corynebacterium acnes*. Presence of complement fixing antibodies to *Corynebacterium acnes* in the sera of patients with acne vulgaris. *Arch Dermatol* (1966) 93(3):364–6. doi:10.1001/archderm.1966.01600210100020
44. Scott DG, Cunliffe WJ, Gowland G. Activation of complement-a mechanism for the inflammation in acne. *Br J Dermatol* (1979) 101(3):315–20. doi:10.1111/j.1365-2133.1979.tb05625.x
45. Kligman AM. An overview of acne. *J Invest Dermatol* (1974) 62(3):268–87. doi:10.1111/1523-1747.ep12676801
46. Leeming JP, Ingham E, Cunliffe WJ. The microbial content and complement C3 cleaving capacity of comedones in acne vulgaris. *Acta Derm Venereol* (1988) 68(6):468–73.
47. Massey A, Mowbray JF, Noble WC. Complement activation by *Corynebacterium acnes*. *Br J Dermatol* (1978) 98(5):583–4. doi:10.1111/j.1365-2133.1978.tb01947.x
48. Webster GF, Leyden JJ, Nilsson UR. Complement activation in acne vulgaris: consumption of complement by comedones. *Infect Immun* (1979) 26(1):183–6.
49. Webster GF, Leyden JJ, Norman ME, Nilsson UR. Complement activation in acne vulgaris: in vitro studies with *Propionibacterium acnes* and *Propionibacterium granulosum*. *Infect Immun* (1978) 22(2):523–9.
50. Napolitano M, Megna M, Timoshchuk EA, Patruno C, Balato N, Fabbrocini G, et al. Hidradenitis suppurativa: from pathogenesis to diagnosis and treatment. *Clin Cosmet Investig Dermatol* (2017) 10:105–15. doi:10.2147/CCID.S111019
51. Nazary M, van der Zee HH, Prens EP, Folkerts G, Boer J. Pathogenesis and pharmacotherapy of hidradenitis suppurativa. *Eur J Pharmacol* (2011) 672(1–3):1–8. doi:10.1016/j.ejphar.2011.08.047
52. van der Zee HH, Laman JD, Boer J, Prens EP. Hidradenitis suppurativa: viewpoint on clinical phenotyping, pathogenesis and novel treatments. *Exp Dermatol* (2012) 21(10):735–9. doi:10.1111/j.1600-0625.2012.01552.x
53. van der Zee HH, de Ruiter L, van den Broecke DG, Dik WA, Laman JD, Prens EP. Elevated levels of tumour necrosis factor (TNF)-alpha, interleukin (IL)-1beta and IL-10 in hidradenitis suppurativa skin: a rationale for targeting TNF-alpha and IL-1beta. *Br J Dermatol* (2011) 164(6):1292–8. doi:10.1111/j.1365-2133.2011.10254.x
54. Kimball AB, Okun MM, Williams DA, Gottlieb AB, Papp KA, Zouboulis CC, et al. Two phase 3 trials of adalimumab for hidradenitis suppurativa. *N Engl J Med* (2016) 375(5):422–34. doi:10.1056/NEJMoa1504370
55. Blok JL, Li K, Brodmerkel C, Jonkman MF, Horvath B. Gene expression profiling of skin and blood in hidradenitis suppurativa. *Br J Dermatol* (2016) 174(6):1392–4. doi:10.1111/bjd.14371
56. Kanni T, Zenker O, Habel M, Riedemann N, Giamarellos-Bourboulis EJ. Complement activation in hidradenitis suppurativa: a new pathway of pathogenesis? *Br J Dermatol* (2018). doi:10.1111/bjd.16428
57. Pons-Estel GJ, Alarcon GS, Scofield L, Reinlib L, Cooper GS. Understanding the epidemiology and progression of systemic lupus erythematosus. *Semin Arthritis Rheum* (2010) 39(4):257–68. doi:10.1016/j.semarthrit.2008.10.007
58. Yu C, Gershwin ME, Chang C. Diagnostic criteria for systemic lupus erythematosus: a critical review. *J Autoimmun* (2014) 4(8–49):10–3. doi:10.1016/j.jaut.2014.01.004
59. Gronhagen CM, Fored CM, Granath F, Nyberg F. Cutaneous lupus erythematosus and the association with systemic lupus erythematosus: a population-based cohort of 1088 patients in Sweden. *Br J Dermatol* (2011) 164(6):1335–41. doi:10.1111/j.1365-2133.2011.10272.x
60. Zhang YP, Wu J, Han YF, Shi ZR, Wang L. Pathogenesis of cutaneous lupus erythema associated with and without systemic lupus erythema. *Autoimmun Rev* (2017) 16(7):735–42. doi:10.1016/j.autrev.2017.05.009
61. Hejazi EZ, Werth VP. Cutaneous lupus erythematosus: an update on pathogenesis, diagnosis and treatment. *Am J Clin Dermatol* (2016) 17(2):135–46. doi:10.1007/s40257-016-0173-9
62. Achtman JC, Werth VP. Pathophysiology of cutaneous lupus erythematosus. *Arthritis Res Ther* (2015) 17:182. doi:10.1186/s13075-015-0706-2
63. D'Orazio J, Jarrett S, Amaro-Ortiz A, Scott T. UV radiation and the skin. *Int J Mol Sci* (2013) 14(6):12222–48. doi:10.3390/ijms140612222
64. Racila DM, Sontheimer CJ, Sheffield A, Wisnieski JJ, Racila E, Sontheimer RD. Homozygous single nucleotide polymorphism of the complement C1QA gene is associated with decreased levels of C1q in patients with subacute cutaneous lupus erythematosus. *Lupus* (2003) 12(2):124–32. doi:10.1191/0961203303lu329oa
65. Boeckler P, Milea M, Meyer A, Uring-Lambert B, Heid E, Hauptmann G, et al. The combination of complement deficiency and cigarette smoking as risk factor for cutaneous lupus erythematosus in men; a focus on combined C2/C4 deficiency. *Br J Dermatol* (2005) 152(2):265–70. doi:10.1111/j.1365-2133.2004.06308.x
66. Chen JY, Wu YL, Mok MY, Wu YJ, Lintner KE, Wang CM, et al. Effects of complement C4 gene copy number variations, size dichotomy, and C4A deficiency on genetic risk and clinical presentation of systemic lupus erythematosus in East Asian populations. *Arthritis Rheumatol* (2016) 68(6):1442–53. doi:10.1002/art.39589
67. Prodeus AP, Goerg S, Shen LM, Pozdnyakova OO, Chu L, Alicot EM, et al. A critical role for complement in maintenance of self-tolerance. *Immunity* (1998) 9(5):721–31. doi:10.1016/S1074-7613(00)80669-X
68. Pickering MC, Botto M, Taylor PR, Lachmann PJ, Walport MJ. Systemic lupus erythematosus, complement deficiency, and apoptosis. *Adv Immunol* (2000) 76:227–324. doi:10.1016/S0065-2776(01)76021-X
69. Antes U, Heinz HP, Loos M. Evidence for the presence of autoantibodies to the collagen-like portion of C1q in systemic lupus erythematosus. *Arthritis Rheum* (1988) 31(4):457–64. doi:10.1002/art.1780310401
70. Hoekzema R, Swaak AJ, Brouwer MC, van Rooijen A, Nieuwenhuys EJ, Hack CE. Significance of low molecular weight C1q in systemic lupus erythematosus. *Ann Rheum Dis* (1990) 49(9):698–704. doi:10.1136/ard.49.9.698

71. Korb LC, Ahearn JM. C1q binds directly and specifically to surface blebs of apoptotic human keratinocytes: complement deficiency and systemic lupus erythematosus revisited. *J Immunol* (1997) 158(10):4525–8.
72. Martin M, Blom AM. Complement in removal of the dead – balancing inflammation. *Immunol Rev* (2016) 274(1):218–32. doi:10.1111/imr.12462
73. Casciola-Rosen LA, Anhalt G, Rosen A. Autoantigens targeted in systemic lupus erythematosus are clustered in two populations of surface structures on apoptotic keratinocytes. *J Exp Med* (1994) 179(4):1317–30. doi:10.1084/jem.179.4.1317
74. Botto M, Walport MJ. C1q, autoimmunity and apoptosis. *Immunobiology* (2002) 205(4–5):395–406. doi:10.1078/0171-2985-00141
75. Schaller M, Bigler C, Danner D, Ditzel HJ, Trendelenburg M. Autoantibodies against C1q in systemic lupus erythematosus are antigen-driven. *J Immunol* (2009) 183(12):8225–31. doi:10.4049/jimmunol.0902642
76. Bigler C, Schaller M, Perahud I, Osthoff M, Trendelenburg M. Autoantibodies against complement C1q specifically target C1q bound on early apoptotic cells. *J Immunol* (2009) 183(5):3512–21. doi:10.4049/jimmunol.0803573
77. Thanei S, Trendelenburg M. Anti-C1q autoantibodies from systemic lupus erythematosus patients induce a proinflammatory phenotype in macrophages. *J Immunol* (2016) 196(5):2063–74. doi:10.4049/jimmunol.1501659
78. Reich A, Marcinow K, Bialynicki-Birula R. The lupus band test in systemic lupus erythematosus patients. *Ther Clin Risk Manag* (2011) 7:27–32. doi:10.2147/TCRM.S10145
79. Wallim LR, Nisihara R, Skare T, Mocelin V, Messias-Reason IJ. Mannose binding lectin deposition in skin of lupus erythematosus patients: a case series. *Hum Immunol* (2014) 75(7):629–32. doi:10.1016/j.humimm.2014.04.015
80. Jennette JC, Falk RJ, Bacon PA, Basu N, Cid MC, Ferrario F, et al. 2012 revised international Chapel Hill consensus conference nomenclature of vasculitides. *Arthritis Rheum* (2013) 65(1):1–11. doi:10.1002/art.37715
81. Carlson JA, Ng BT, Chen KR. Cutaneous vasculitis update: diagnostic criteria, classification, epidemiology, etiology, pathogenesis, evaluation and prognosis. *Am J Dermatopathol* (2005) 27(6):504–28. doi:10.1097/01.dad.0000181109.54532.c5
82. Lotti T, Ghersetich I, Comacchi C, Jorizzo JL. Cutaneous small-vessel vasculitis. *J Am Acad Dermatol* (1998) 39(5 Pt 1):667–87; quiz 88–90. doi:10.1016/S0190-9622(98)70039-8
83. Sais G, Vidaller A, Jucgla A, Servitje O, Condom E, Peyri J. Prognostic factors in leukocytoclastic vasculitis: a clinicopathologic study of 160 patients. *Arch Dermatol* (1998) 134(3):309–15. doi:10.1001/archderm.134.3.309
84. Grunwald MH, Avinoach I, Amichai B, Halevy S. Leukocytoclastic vasculitis – correlation between different histologic stages and direct immunofluorescence results. *Int J Dermatol* (1997) 36(5):349–52. doi:10.1111/j.1365-4362.1997.tb03094.x
85. Russell JP, Gibson LE. Primary cutaneous small vessel vasculitis: approach to diagnosis and treatment. *Int J Dermatol* (2006) 45(1):3–13. doi:10.1111/j.1365-4632.2005.02898.x
86. Dauchel H, Joly P, Delpech A, Thomine E, Sauger F, Le Loet X, et al. Local and systemic activation of the whole complement cascade in human leukocytoclastic cutaneous vasculitis; C3d,g and terminal complement complex as sensitive markers. *Clin Exp Immunol* (1993) 92(2):274–83. doi:10.1111/j.1365-2249.1993.tb03392.x
87. Albrecht EA, Chinnaiyan AM, Varambally S, Kumar-Sinha C, Barrette TR, Sarma JV, et al. C5a-induced gene expression in human umbilical vein endothelial cells. *Am J Pathol* (2004) 164(3):849–59. doi:10.1016/S0002-9440(10)63173-2
88. Owen CA, Campbell MA, Sannes PL, Boukedes SS, Campbell EJ. Cell surface-bound elastase and cathepsin G on human neutrophils: a novel, non-oxidative mechanism by which neutrophils focus and preserve catalytic activity of serine proteinases. *J Cell Biol* (1995) 131(3):775–89. doi:10.1083/jcb.131.3.775
89. Jordan JM, Allen NB, Pizzo SV. Defective release of tissue plasminogen activator in systemic and cutaneous vasculitis. *Am J Med* (1987) 82(3):397–400. doi:10.1016/0002-9343(87)90436-0
90. Fischetti F, Tedesco F. Cross-talk between the complement system and endothelial cells in physiologic conditions and in vascular diseases. *Autoimmunity* (2006) 39(5):417–28. doi:10.1080/08916930600739712
91. Boom BW, Mommaas AM, Daha MR, Vermeer BJ. Decreased expression of decay-accelerating factor on endothelial cells of immune complex-mediated vasculitic skin lesions. *J Dermatol Sci* (1991) 2(4):308–15. doi:10.1016/0923-1811(91)90055-3
92. Greaves M. Chronic urticaria. *J Allergy Clin Immunol* (2000) 105(4):664–72. doi:10.1067/mai.2000.105706
93. Kaplan AP. Chronic urticaria: pathogenesis and treatment. *J Allergy Clin Immunol* (2004) 114(3):465–74; quiz 75. doi:10.1016/j.jaci.2004.02.049
94. Grattan CEH, Sabroe RA, Greaves MW. Chronic urticaria. *J Am Acad Dermatol* (2002) 46(5):645–60. doi:10.1067/mjd.2002.122759
95. Kaplan AP. Clinical practice. Chronic urticaria and angioedema. *N Engl J Med* (2002) 346(3):175–9. doi:10.1056/NEJMcp011186
96. Kolkhir P, Metz M, Altrichter S, Maurer M. Comorbidity of chronic spontaneous urticaria and autoimmune thyroid diseases: a systematic review. *Allergy* (2017) 72(10):1440–60. doi:10.1111/all.13182
97. Marsland AM. Autoimmunity and complement in the pathogenesis of chronic urticaria. *Curr Allergy Asthma Rep* (2006) 6(4):265–9. doi:10.1007/s11882-006-0058-8
98. Radonjic-Hoesli S, Hofmeier KS, Micaletto S, Schmid-Grendelmeier P, Bircher A, Simon D. Urticaria and angioedema: an update on classification and pathogenesis. *Clin Rev Allergy Immunol* (2018) 54(1):88–101. doi:10.1007/s12016-017-8628-1
99. Zweiman B, Valenzano M, Atkins PC, Tanus T, Getsy JA. Characteristics of histamine-releasing activity in the sera of patients with chronic idiopathic urticaria. *J Allergy Clin Immunol* (1996) 98(1):89–98. doi:10.1016/S0091-6749(96)70230-0
100. Ferrer M, Nakazawa K, Kaplan AP. Complement dependence of histamine release in chronic urticaria. *J Allergy Clin Immunol* (1999) 104(1):169–72. doi:10.1016/S0091-6749(99)70129-6
101. Kikuchi Y, Kaplan AP. A role for C5a in augmenting IgG-dependent histamine release from basophils in chronic urticaria. *J Allergy ClinImmunol* (2002) 109(1):114–8. doi:10.1067/mai.2002.120954
102. Monroe EW. Urticaria and urticarial vasculitis. *Med Clin North Am* (1980) 64(5):867–83. doi:10.1016/S0025-7125(16)31571-1
103. Natbony SF, Phillips ME, Elias JM, Godfrey HP, Kaplan AP. Histologic studies of chronic idiopathic urticaria. *J Allergy Clin Immunol* (1983) 71(2):177–83. doi:10.1016/0091-6749(83)90096-9
104. Sugita Y, Morita E, Kawamoto H, Horiuchi K, Yamada S, Koro O, et al. Correlation between deposition of immuno-components and infiltration pattern of polymorphonuclear leukocytes in the lesions of chronic urticaria. *J Dermatol* (2000) 27(3):157–62. doi:10.1111/j.1346-8138.2000.tb02142.x
105. Synkowski DR, Levine MI, Rabin BS, Yunis EJ. Urticaria. An immunofluorescence and histopathology study. *Arch Dermatol* (1979) 115(10):1192–4. doi:10.1001/archderm.115.10.1192
106. Davis MD, Brewer JD. Urticarial vasculitis and hypocomplementemic urticarial vasculitis syndrome. *Immunol Allergy Clin North Am* (2004) 24(2):183–213, vi. doi:10.1016/j.iac.2004.01.007
107. McDuffie FC, Sams WM Jr, Maldonado JE, Andreini PH, Conn DL, Samayoa EA. Hypocomplementemia with cutaneous vasculitis and arthritis. Possible immune complex syndrome. *Mayo Clin Proc* (1973) 48(5):340–8.
108. Wisnieski JJ. Urticarial vasculitis. *Curr Opin Rheumatol* (2000) 12(1):24–31. doi:10.1097/00002281-200001000-00005
109. Mehregan DR, Hall MJ, Gibson LE. Urticarial vasculitis: a histopathologic and clinical review of 72 cases. *J Am Acad Dermatol* (1992) 26(3 Pt 2):441–8. doi:10.1016/0190-9622(92)70069-R
110. Wisnieski JJ, Emancipator SN, Korman NJ, Lass JH, Zaim TM, McFadden ER. Hypocomplementemic urticarial vasculitis syndrome in identical twins. *Arthritis Rheum* (1994) 37(7):1105–11. doi:10.1002/art.1780370718
111. Ozcakar ZB, Foster J II, Diaz-Horta O, Kasapcopur O, Fan YS, Yalcinkaya F, et al. DNASE1L3 mutations in hypocomplementemic urticarial vasculitis syndrome. *Arthritis Rheum* (2013) 65(8):2183–9. doi:10.1002/art.38010
112. Lessey E, Li N, Diaz L, Liu Z. Complement and cutaneous autoimmune blistering diseases. *Immunol Res* (2008) 41(3):223–32. doi:10.1007/s12026-008-8028-y
113. Preisz K, Sardy M, Horvath A, Karpati S. Immunoglobulin, complement and epidermal transglutaminase deposition in the cutaneous vessels in dermatitis herpetiformis. *J Eur Acad Dermatol Venereol* (2005) 19(1):74–9. doi:10.1111/j.1468-3083.2004.01132.x
114. Seah PP, Fry L, Mazaheri MR, Mowbray JF, Hoffbrand AV, Holborow EJ. Alternate-pathway complement fixation by IgA in the skin in

dermatitis herpetiformis. *Lancet* (1973) 2(7822):175–7. doi:10.1016/S0140-6736(73)93006-7

115. Dahl MV, Falk RJ, Carpenter R, Michael AF. Deposition of the membrane attack complex of complement in bullous pemphigoid. *J Invest Dermatol* (1984) 82(2):132–5. doi:10.1111/1523-1747.ep12259679
116. Jordon RE, Day NK, Sams WM Jr, Good RA. The complement system in bullous pemphigoid. I. Complement and component levels in sera and blister fluids. *J Clin Invest* (1973) 52(5):1207–14. doi:10.1172/JCI107288
117. Jordon RE, Kawana S, Fritz KA. Immunopathologic mechanisms in pemphigus and bullous pemphigoid. *J Invest Dermatol* (1985) 85(1 Suppl):72s–8s. doi:10.1111/1523-1747.ep12275497
118. Chandler W, Zone J, Florell S. C4d immunohistochemical stain is a sensitive method to confirm immunoreactant deposition in formalin-fixed paraffin-embedded tissue in bullous pemphigoid. *J Cutan Pathol* (2009) 36(6):655–9. doi:10.1111/j.1600-0560.2008.01129.x
119. Kassaby SS, Hicks A, Leicht S, Youngberg GA. Bullous pemphigoid: use of C4d immunofluorescent staining in a case with repeated negative conventional direct immunofluorescence studies. *Am J Dermatopathol* (2017) 39:932–4. doi:10.1097/DAD.0000000000000943
120. Magro CM, Dyrsen ME. The use of C3d and C4d immunohistochemistry on formalin-fixed tissue as a diagnostic adjunct in the assessment of inflammatory skin disease. *J Am Acad Dermatol* (2008) 59(5):822–33. doi:10.1016/j.jaad.2008.06.022
121. Pfaltz K, Mertz K, Rose C, Scheidegger P, Pfaltz M, Kempf W. C3d immunohistochemistry on formalin-fixed tissue is a valuable tool in the diagnosis of bullous pemphigoid of the skin. *J Cutan Pathol* (2010) 37(6):654–8. doi:10.1111/j.1600-0560.2009.01450.x
122. Villani AP, Chouvet B, Kanitakis J. Application of C4d immunohistochemistry on routinely processed tissue sections for the diagnosis of autoimmune bullous dermatoses. *Am J Dermatopathol* (2016) 38(3):186–8. doi:10.1097/DAD.0000000000000333
123. Liu Z, Giudice GJ, Swartz SJ, Fairley JA, Till GO, Troy JL, et al. The role of complement in experimental bullous pemphigoid. *J Clin Invest* (1995) 95(4):1539–44. doi:10.1172/JCI117826
124. Heimbach L, Li Z, Berkowitz P, Zhao M, Li N, Rubenstein DS, et al. The C5a receptor on mast cells is critical for the autoimmune skin-blistering disease bullous pemphigoid. *J Biol Chem* (2011) 286(17):15003–9. doi:10.1074/jbc.M111.221036
125. Nelson KC, Zhao M, Schroeder PR, Li N, Wetsel RA, Diaz LA, et al. Role of different pathways of the complement cascade in experimental bullous pemphigoid. *J Clin Invest* (2006) 116(11):2892–900. doi:10.1172/JCI17891
126. Liu Z, Giudice GJ, Zhou X, Swartz SJ, Troy JL, Fairley JA, et al. A major role for neutrophils in experimental bullous pemphigoid. *J Clin Invest* (1997) 100(5):1256–63. doi:10.1172/JCI119639
127. Chen R, Ning G, Zhao M-L, Fleming MG, Diaz LA, Werb Z, et al. Mast cells play a key role in neutrophil recruitment in experimental bullous pemphigoid. *J Clin Invest* (2001) 108(8):1151–8. doi:10.1172/JCI11494
128. Liu Z, Sui W, Zhao M, Li Z, Li N, Thresher R, et al. Subepidermal blistering induced by human autoantibodies to BP180 requires innate immune players in a humanized bullous pemphigoid mouse model. *J Autoimmun* (2008) 31(4):331–8. doi:10.1016/j.jaut.2008.08.009
129. Nishie W, Sawamura D, Goto M, Ito K, Shibaki A, McMillan JR, et al. Humanization of autoantigen. *Nat Med* (2007) 13(3):378–83. doi:10.1038/nm1496
130. Iwata H, Kamio N, Aoyama Y, Yamamoto Y, Hirako Y, Owaribe K, et al. IgG from patients with bullous pemphigoid depletes cultured keratinocytes of the 180-kDa bullous pemphigoid antigen (type XVII collagen) and weakens cell attachment. *J Invest Dermatol* (2009) 129(4):919–26. doi:10.1038/jid.2008.305
131. Natsuga K, Nishie W, Shinkuma S, Ujiie H, Nishimura M, Sawamura D, et al. Antibodies to pathogenic epitopes on type XVII collagen cause skin fragility in a complement-dependent and -independent manner. *J Immunol* (2012) 188(11):5792–9. doi:10.4049/jimmunol.1003402
132. Ujiie H, Sasaoka T, Izumi K, Nishie W, Shinkuma S, Natsuga K, et al. Bullous pemphigoid autoantibodies directly induce blister formation without complement activation. *J Immunol* (2014) 193(9):4415–28. doi:10.4049/jimmunol.1400095
133. Romeijn TR, Jonkman MF, Knoppers C, Pas HH, Diercks GF. Complement in bullous pemphigoid: results from a large observational study. *Br J Dermatol* (2017) 176(2):517–9. doi:10.1111/bjd.14822
134. Kohl J. Drug evaluation: the C5a receptor antagonist PMX-53. *Curr Opin Mol Ther* (2006) 8(6):529–38.
135. Jayne DRW, Bruchfeld AN, Harper L, Schaier M, Venning MC, Hamilton P, et al. Randomized trial of C5a receptor inhibitor avacopan in ANCA-associated vasculitis. *J Am Soc Nephrol* (2017) 28(9):2756–67. doi:10.1681/ASN.2016111179
136. Ricklin D, Lambris JD. Complement-targeted therapeutics. *Nat Biotechnol* (2007) 25(11):1265–75. doi:10.1038/nbt1342

19

Therapeutic Lessons to be Learned from the Role of Complement Regulators as Double-Edged Sword in Health and Disease

Esther C. W. de Boer[1,2], *Anouk G. van Mourik*[1] *and Ilse Jongerius*[1,2*]

[1] *Sanquin Research, Department of Immunopathology, and Landsteiner Laboratory, Amsterdam University Medical Centre, Amsterdam Infection and Immunity Institute, Amsterdam, Netherlands,* [2] *Department of Pediatric Immunology, Rheumatology, and Infectious Diseases, Emma Children's Hospital, Amsterdam University Medical Centre, Amsterdam, Netherlands*

***Correspondence:**
Ilse Jongerius
i.jongerius@sanquin.nl

The complement system is an important part of the innate immune system, providing a strong defense against pathogens and removing apoptotic cells and immune complexes. Due to its strength, it is important that healthy human cells are protected against damage induced by the complement system. To be protected from complement, each cell type relies on a specific combination of both soluble and membrane-bound regulators. Their importance is indicated by the amount of pathologies associated with abnormalities in these complement regulators. Here, we will discuss the current knowledge on complement regulatory protein polymorphisms and expression levels together with their link to disease. These diseases often result in red blood cell destruction or occur in the eye, kidney or brain, which are tissues known for aberrant complement activity or regulation. In addition, complement regulators have also been associated with different types of cancer, although their mechanisms here have not been elucidated yet. In most of these pathologies, treatments are limited and do not prevent the complement system from attacking host cells, but rather fight the consequences of the complement-mediated damage, using for example blood transfusions in anemic patients. Currently only few drugs targeting the complement system are used in the clinic. With further demand for therapeutics rising linked to the wide range of complement-mediated disease we should broaden our horizon towards treatments that can actually protect the host cells against complement. Here, we will discuss the latest insights on how complement regulators can benefit therapeutics. Such therapeutics are currently being developed extensively, and can be categorized into full-length complement regulators, engineered complement system regulators and antibodies targeting complement regulators. In conclusion, this review provides an overview of the complement regulatory proteins and their links to disease, together with their potential in the development of novel therapeutics.

Keywords: complement, complement regulators, complement therapeutics, complement antibodies, complement-mediated disease

INTRODUCTION

The Complement System

Upon its discovery at the end of the 19th century, the complement system was considered to consist of only one component. Nowadays it is known that the complement system is a complex part of the innate immune system, consisting of a large number of proteins and associated regulators (1, 2). In order to respond quickly to pathogens, the components of the complement system are present in plasma and thus are readily available throughout the body (3, 4). Three different pathways can initiate complement activity: the classical pathway (CP), the lectin pathway (LP) and the alternative pathway (AP). Activation of these pathways takes place *via* antibody-binding, recognition of specific sugar patterns or spontaneous C3 hydrolysis, all resulting in formation of a C3 convertase. C3 convertases cleave C3, resulting in opsonization of pathogens and formation of C5 convertases. With C5 convertases the terminal pathway is initiated which will result in chemotaxis and formation of the membrane attack complex (MAC) (3).

Although all three complement pathways result in the formation of a C3 convertase, their initiation and intermediate steps differ (**Figure 1**). The CP is mainly initiated by antibody binding to target cells. The C1 complex consists of C1q, C1r and C1s. C1q is the pattern recognition molecule, and upon surface binding of C1q, the protease C1r is activated, cleaving and activating C1s. C1s can then cleave C2 and C4, which leads to the formation of C3 convertase C4bC2a (3, 5, 6). The LP is activated in a similar way, with ficolin and mannose-binding lectin (MBL) acting as pattern recognition molecules. These molecules recognize microbial carbohydrate structures. Upon recognition, the MBL-associated serine proteases (MASPs), can cleave C2 and C4, to form the C4bC2a C3 convertase (5–7). Lastly, the AP is activated by C3b coming from the other two pathways. In addition, constant background spontaneous hydrolysis of C3 results in formation of $C3(H_2O)$ which also serves as a platform for the AP. C3b or $C3(H_2O)$ will bind Factor

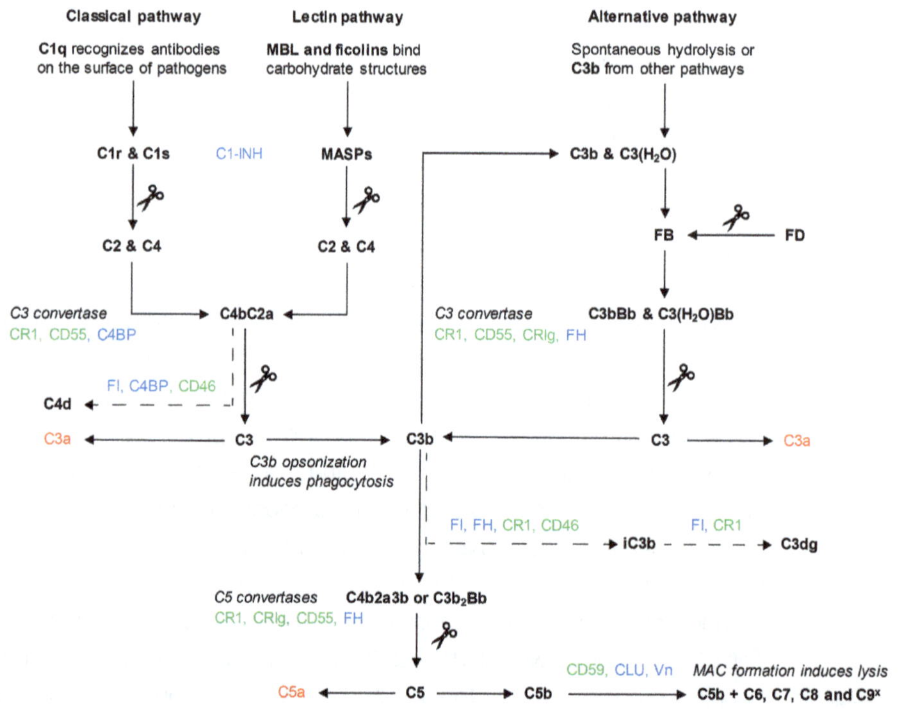

FIGURE 1 | The complement system. Three pathways can lead to complement activation: the classical pathway (CP), the lectin pathway (LP) and the alternative pathway (AP). Activation of the CP (left) starts with binding of C1q to target cells, often *via* antibodies. Binding of C1q leads to cleavage of C1r, which in turn cleaves C1s. The proteolytic activity of C1s results in the cleavage of C2 and C4. These components form the C3 convertase of the CP, C4bC2a. Activation of the LP (middle) starts with the binding of MBL or ficolins to carbohydrate structures on target cell surfaces. As a result, the proteases of the LP, MASPs, cleave C2 and C4, also leading to the formation of C4bC2a. The AP pathway (right) is activated by spontaneous hydrolysis of C3, which leads to the formation of $C3(H_2O)$, or by C3b from the CP or LP. After assembly of C3b, FB binds to C3b or $C3(H_2O)$ and is cleaved by protease FD. This results in the formation of the C3 convertases of the AP, C3bBb or $C3(H_2O)Bb$. C3 convertases of the CP/LP and the AP cleave C3 into C3b and C3a. Usage of C3b in the AP causes an amplification loop, which can amplify the CP and LP. In addition, C3b deposition leads to formation of two C5 convertases: C4b2aC3b (CP/LP) or $C3b_2Bb$ (AP). C5 convertases cleave C5 in C5a and C5b. C5b is used for the formation of the MAC which is formed after assembly of C6, C7, C8 and multiple C9 molecules ($C9^x$). The MAC is inserted into the membrane to induce lysis. C3a and C5a (depicted in red) are anaphylatoxins important for chemotaxis and the initiation of inflammation. Complement components are depicted in bold, scissors indicate cleavage. Complement regulators can be divided in two groups: soluble (depicted in blue) and membrane-bound (depicted in green). These regulators prevent complement activation by targeting the complement pathway in different places, as depicted here. The inactivating breakdown pathways of C3b and C4b respectively by complement regulators are indicated here with a dotted arrow, showing the different breakdown products.

B (FB), which is cleaved by the protease Factor D (FD), leading to the formation of C3bBb, another C3 convertase (5, 8). The AP mechanisms enable it to work as an amplification loop for the CP and LP (9, 10).

After the formation of a C3 convertase, the three pathways all continue with the terminal complement pathway. The C3 convertases cleave C3 into C3a and C3b, which leads to the formation of two different C5 convertases: C4b2a3b and $C3b_2Bb$. The C5 convertase cleaves C5, after which C5b associates with C6 and C7 and inserts itself into the cell membrane. Upon binding of C8 and several C9 units, a lytic pore is formed: the MAC (5). Whilst the main cleavage products of complement ensure the downstream continuation of the pathway, the smaller cleavage products C3a and C5a are anaphylatoxins (3). Anaphylatoxins act as chemoattractant for immune cells and are important mediators in inflammation (11).

Next to its well-known role, it has become evident that intracellular complement plays an important role in homeostasis [reviewed in (12, 13)]. It has been shown that complement proteins are expressed by a large variety of cells that secrete these proteins into the local environment when needed. Recent studies also indicate that T cells not only express C3 but actually need intracellular C3 activation fragments for their survival (12, 13). Next, complement receptor CD46, described in more detail below, has also been identified as an important player in T cell homeostasis (14). Taken together, the complement system is well-orchestrated and highly effective in clearing invading pathogens. In addition, this system also plays an important role in activation of the adaptive immune system (11) and important for T cell homeostasis.

Complement Regulators

The complement system is key in eradicating pathogens, but also plays an important role in clearance of for instance apoptotic or tumor cells. Due to the strength and omnipresence of the complement system regulation of this system is key to prevent damage to host cells (5, 15). However, complement dysregulation can be beneficial in certain circumstances. In retinitis pigmentosa complement overactivation on the levels of C3 results in enhanced phagocytic clearance of apoptotic photoreceptors by microglia resulting in limiting photoreceptor loss (16). In addition, the positive effect of complement activation on human cells was also shown for neuronal development (17). To ensure proper regulation of complement on host cells where needed, and to distinguish these from pathogens, complement regulators are in place. Most of these regulators of complement activity are encoded at the same locus on chromosome 1q32 and are formed by repeated complement control protein (CCP) domains (18). Up to date, a variety of soluble and membrane-bound complement regulators has been identified, which will be described here.

The soluble complement regulators can be found in plasma: Factor I (FI), Factor H (FH), C1-inhibitor (C1-INH), C4b binding protein (C4BP), clusterin (CLU) and vitronectin (Vn) (19, 20). FI is a protease specific for C3b and C4b, that can cleave these proteins in presence of a co-factor, forming their inactive counterparts iC3b and C4d. These co-factors are C4BP, FH and the membrane-bound complement receptor 1 (CR1) and CD46. By acting on C3b and C4b, FI can regulate all the complement pathways (21). Two soluble regulators act exclusively on the CP and LP: C4BP and C1-INH. C4BP prevents the formation of C3 convertase in the LP and CP, by binding to C4b. After C4BP binding of C4b, FI cleaves and inactivates C4b to C4d (19, 22). C1-INH has several roles in the suppression of inflammation and vascular permeability, but in the complement system it blocks the proteolytic activity of C1s, C1r and MASPs (23, 24). As a result, cleavage of C2 and C4 is inhibited resulting in less formation of the C3 convertase, C4bC2a.

FH is a regulator of the AP, next to its co-factor activity for FI. FH binds to sialic acid residues on host cells and to C3b, regulating the formation of C3bBb. FH can remove Bb from C3b, reversing convertase formation (25, 26). FH also has an alternative splice variant, Factor H-like 1 (FHL-1). FHL-1 consists of the first 7 CCP domains and is thereby able to fulfill the AP regulatory capacity similar to FH. However, as FHL-1 lacks the sialic acid residue binding domains of FH (CCP 19-20) its fails to distinguish effectively between host and foreign surfaces (27). FHL-1 CCP domain 7 is able to bind to sulphated glycosaminoglycans (GAGs) therefore, it is postulated that FHL-1 is mainly important in controlling the AP in local tissues such as the such as for example in the eye (28) Next to FH and FHL-1, humans also have five different Factor H-related proteins (FHR), which have arisen from duplication events of the *CFH* gene (29). These molecules share some domains with FH, but lack the complement inhibiting domains. Currently, there is no consensus on the precise function of these molecules *in vivo*, which is why they will not be discussed in detail here (30–32).

The last soluble complement regulators are CLU and Vn, both acting on the terminal complement pathway, inhibiting MAC formation. CLU binds to C7 to prevent membrane attachment, and can also bind C8 and C9 to prevent C9 assembly. Vn prevents the insertion of the MAC into the membrane by binding at the membrane-binding site of C5b-7 (19). Apart from their function as complement regulators, CLU and Vn have a range of cellular functions in lipid transport and cell adhesion respectively (22).

Next to the soluble complement regulators, five different membrane-bound regulators have been discovered that play an important role in regulation: CR1 (also known as CD35), membrane co-factor protein (CD46), decay accelerating factor (DAF, also known as CD55), CD59 and complement receptor immunoglobin (CRIg) (22). CR1 is a transmembrane protein that acts as a cofactor for FI and is a receptor for C3b, iC3b and C4b, inducing decay of C3 and C5 convertases (33). In this way, CR1 inhibits the CP, LP and AP. CR1 also plays a role in other immune functions, such as B and T cell regulation and phagocytosis and particle binding (34, 35). The other membrane-bound co-factor for FI is CD46, a transmembrane glycoprotein. Like CR1 it binds to the C3 and C4 fragments, but it does not have any decay activity, as opposed to CR1 (36, 37). CRIg is another transmembrane protein and an inhibitor of the AP. It is suggested to bind C3b, preventing C3bBb from cleaving C5. Unlike the other membrane-bound regulators that are widely expressed, CRIg is only present on a subset of cells: specific macrophages and dendritic cells (38, 39). Lastly, two other membrane-bound complement regulators are glycosylphosphatidylinositol- (GPI) anchored proteins CD55 and CD59 (3). CD55 accelerates the decay of the C3 convertases (22, 40). CD59, on the other hand, prevents the formation of the MAC by binding to C9 and preventing MAC insertion into the membrane (22, 40).

As the complement system needs to be regulated so tightly by a large number of proteins, it is to be expected that abnormalities in the complement system or the complement regulators are associated with a range of diseases. For many of these diseases, no adequate therapeutics are currently available, which is unsurprising considering that only two complement therapeutics are currently approved: anti-C5 antibodies (eculizumab and ravulizumab) and C1-INH (41, 42). Here, we will first describe the pathologies that complement regulators are involved in. Then, we will explore how the complement regulators can be used as potential therapeutics for these and other pathologies, and discuss relevant therapeutics currently in development. Altogether, this will give an insight in the significance and broad therapeutic applications for complement regulatory proteins.

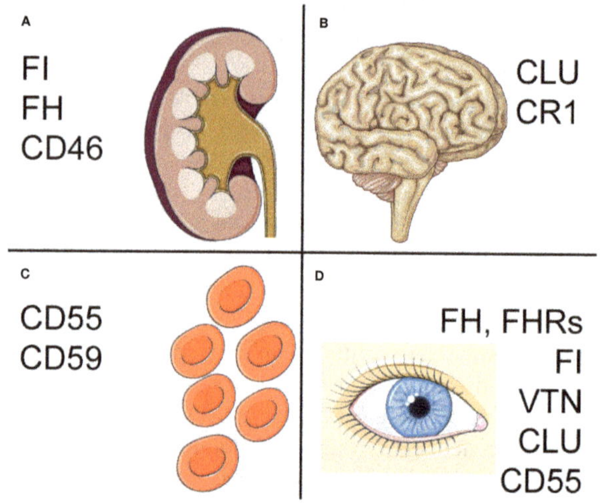

FIGURE 2 | Complement regulators associated with pathologies. Overview of the major pathologies associated with complement regulators and polymorphisms or deficiencies associated with disease. **(A)** In the kidney, mutations in *CFH*, *CFI* and *CD46* are associated with aHUS, C3 glomerulopathy and IgA nephropathy. **(B)** Polymorphisms in *CLU* and *CR1* have been found to increase risk of AD. One of these *CLU* polymorphisms is also a risk factor for PD. **(C)** On erythrocytes, deficiencies of CD55 and CD59 on blood cells contribute to PNH, with isolated CD59-deficiency also associating with chronic hemolysis. **(D)** *CFH*, *CFI* and *VTN*, as well as a *CFHR1-3* deletion have been associated with AMD. A *CLU* polymorphism was found in pseudoexfoliation syndrome and Fuchs' endothelial dystrophy. Lastly, a *CD55* polymorphism is a risk factor for pathological myopia. Figure designed using Servier Medical Art.

THE ROLE OF COMPLEMENT REGULATORS IN PATHOLOGIES

As described above, different cell types and tissues rely on different combinations of complement regulators and abnormalities in complement regulators are associated with a variety of pathologies (22). Amongst these are for example several red blood cell (RBC) mediated diseases, but also different cancerous malignancies and neurological diseases. The pathologies have been linked to both genetic and acquired abnormalities in complement regulators. Here, we will describe the different ways in which complement regulators have been linked to pathologies and focus on the diseases that are most well-studied. The most important polymorphisms and deficiencies are described in **Figure 2**. An overview of other diseases that have been linked to complement regulators, but are not discussed in detail here, are presented in **Table 1**.

The Role of Complement Regulators in Anemic Pathologies

Many of the diseases in which aberrant complement regulation plays a role affect RBCs, which leads to hemolysis and anemia. As RBCs are continuously exposed to the complement system in the blood it is to be expected that they are highly vulnerable to complement-mediated lysis when their complement regulatory proteins are affected (54). The most well-described example of this is paroxysmal nocturnal hemoglobinuria (PNH). PNH is characterized by intra- and extravascular hemolysis and venous thrombosis, caused by the complement system. The disease arises from acquired somatic mutations in *PIGA* in hematopoietic stem cells, which encodes for phosphatidylinositol N-acetylglucosaminyltransferase subunit A, an essential enzyme in the synthesis of GPI-anchored proteins. As a consequence, GPI-anchored proteins are not present on cells arising from these stem cells, such as RBCs, platelets and neutrophils. Amongst these proteins are complement regulators CD55 and CD59, which cause the increased sensitivity to complement-mediated hemolysis (55–57).

Currently, the only treatments approved for PNH are eculizumab and ravulizumab, both C5 monoclonal antibodies, inhibiting C5a generation and formation of the MAC. Eculizumab is able to reduce intravascular hemolysis, fatigue and transfusion requirements in PNH patients, although responses are variable between patients (58–60). The variability of responses can in some cases be explained by a C5 mutation that prevents eculizumab binding (61). However, the main variation arises from the fact that eculizumab does not prevent C3b deposition on RBCs. Opsonization by C3b induces removal of the RBCs by phagocytosis, which leads to an increase in extravascular hemolysis as shown in PNH patients receiving eculizumab treatment (62). Susceptibility to extravascular hemolysis upon eculizumab treatment has been linked to a CR1 polymorphism. Decreased CR1 on the RBC surface would lead to a decrease in C3b decay and thus for increased opsonization that can induce extravascular hemolysis. *CR1* has

TABLE 1 | Additional pathologies where complement regulators were identified to play a role, that were not described in the text.

Pathology	Regulator	Association	Observations	Ref.
Allergic respiratory disease	CD55	Polymorphism	A CD55 SNP linked to decreased transcriptional activity, was associated with susceptibility to pollen and mite-induced respiratory allergies and enhanced specific IgE responses.	(43)
Geographic atrophy	CD46	Protein levels	Retinal pigment epithelial CD46 expression is altered early on in geographic atrophy development.	(44)
Traumatic brain injury	CR1 and CD59	Protein levels	CR1 and CD59 were significantly reduced in the first week after acute brain injury.	(45)
Recurrent miscarriages	C4BP	Polymorphism	C4BP mutations, of which some affecting expression level and FI co-factor activity, were found in women with recurrent miscarriages.	(46)
Cardiovascular disease	CR1	Polymorphism	CR1 polymorphisms are associated with increased risk of coronary artery disease.	(47)
	FH	Polymorphism	The FH Y402H polymorphism in FH was suggested to determine myocardial infarction susceptibility.	(48)
Sudden sensorineural hearing loss	FH	Polymorphism	The FH Y402H polymorphism has been associated with risk of sudden sensorineural hearing loss.	(49)
Idiopathic pulmonary fibrosis	CR1	Polymorphism	A CR1 polymorphism was associated with development of idiopathic pulmonary fibrosis.	(50)
Preeclampsia	CD46 and FH	Polymorphism	Two fetal CD46 SNPs were associated with preeclampsia, where placentas have increased complement deposition. An interaction with maternal FH and a C3 SNP might play a role as well.	(51)
Rheumatic disease	CD55 and CD59	Deficiency	CD55 and/or CD59 erythrocytes are present in a majority of patients with rheumatic disease.	(52)
Schizofrenia	Clusterin	Polymorphism	A clusterin polymorphism was associated with schizophrenia in Chinese patients with family history of disease.	(53)

two co-dominant alleles that lead to either high (H) or low (L) expression of the regulator respectively. It has been shown that PNH patients with a H/L or L/L genotype have a lower expression of CR1 and require more transfusions (63). Although it has been shown that compstatin is a highly effective inhibitor of C3 that can prevent extravascular hemolysis (64, 65), it is not FDA approved yet (66).

Next to the combined CD55- and CD59 deficiency in PNH, a few isolated CD55- and CD59 deficiencies have been described. Isolated genetic CD59-deficiencies have been associated with chronic hemolysis like PNH, as well as with other symptoms such as neuronal damage and recurrent strokes (67, 68). Interestingly, RBCs specific isolated deficiencies of CD55 do not seem to induce hemolysis. A small group of patients has been found to have CD55-deficient RBCs, named the Inab phenotype. These individuals do not have any specific complaints and have a variety of CD55 silencing mutations (69, 70). Although *in vitro* research showed an increase in C3b deposition on the RBCs of this phenotype compared to healthy cells, an increase in hemolysis was not found (71). Not all of these patients are however fully deficient in CD55, which *in vivo* might prevent some complement-mediated activity on RBCs. Furthermore, a CD55 loss-of-function mutation causes an autosomal recessive disorder characterized by hyperactivation of complement, angiopathic thrombosis, and protein-losing enteropathy (CHAPLE) syndrome. Here, the lack of CD55 leads to overactivation of the complement system, which leads to gut inflammation induced by anaphylatoxins in these patients (72–74). Interestingly, again increased hemolysis was not reported in any of the CD55-deficient patients, which could be an indication that CD59 is more important in complement regulation on RBCs. The important role of CD59 is further illustrated by the fact that CD59-deficient RBCs are highly sensitive to complement-mediated lysis. However, RBCs of a PNH patient showed the highest sensitivity for complement mediated lysis compared to the RBCs with a single complement regulator deficiency (75).

Hereditary hemolytic anemias are a group of anemias that share the common feature of decreased RBC survival leading to anemia, which is caused by inherited disorders in certain membranes, enzymes or hemoglobin. Examples are hereditary spherocytis, caused by membrane protein deficiencies, congenital microcytosis, caused by defects in hemoglobin (76) and sickle cells disease, caused by a hemoglobin mutation inducing deformation of affected RBCs under stress conditions, that leads to anemia in homozygous patients (77). The expression of membrane-bound complement regulators CD55 and CD59 in patients with hereditary spherocytis and congenital microcytosis has been investigated. FACS analysis showed a decrease in CD55 expression on erythrocytes of both patient groups compared to controls. However, immunoblot showed a less clear difference. CD59 was unaffected in both patient groups indicating that the decrease in CD55 expression is not caused by a *PIGA* mutation, similar to PNH patients, as a GPI anchor defect would affect both CD55 and CD59. It remains debatable whether low CD55 expression contributes to the anemia in these patients as a correlation between the expression of CD55 and severity of the anemia was not found and the effect on complement-mediated RBCs destruction was not studied (78). Like in the before mentioned anemias, differential expression of CD55 and CD59 on erythrocytes was also found in sickle cell disease patients. Although these patients expressed decreased CD55 and CD59 expression on RBCs, this could not be linked to disease severity, suggesting that these regulators do not play a significant role in the pathophysiology of hemolysis in sickle cell disease (79). Recent research does however suggest a role for complement activation in sickle cell disease pathophysiology, where overactivation of complement has been found on sickle cell erythrocytes compared to healthy erythrocytes (80). Altogether, these studies indicate directions for future research into the mechanistic role of complement regulators and complement activity in hereditary hemolytic anemias to determine the exact role of complement regulators in these pathologies.

The Involvement of Complement Regulators in Renal Disease

Complement is differentially regulated in the kidney compared to other tissues. The glomerular basement membrane is very sensitive to complement damage and relies completely on soluble complement regulators, as it is directly exposed to blood and the complement system, unlike most other basement membranes (81, 82). It is therefore understandable that different kidney pathologies have been associated with anomalies in soluble complement regulators, which results in overactivation of the complement system (83).

Atypical hemolytic uremic syndrome (aHUS) is a kidney disease that can have serious complications, with a mortality rate of 25% without eculizumab treatment (84). Characterized by microangiopathic hemolysis, thrombocytopenia and renal failure, it is caused by disbalance between regulation and activation of the AP. This disbalance is caused by decreased activity of complement regulators, or increased activity of complement proteins. Many aHUS cases have an identified genetic basis. Mutations linked to aHUS have been identified in several complement-related proteins, of which mutations in FH, FI, CD46 and C3 are found in approximately half of the patients. These mutations often lead to altered function or expression (85–87). More rarely, mutations in C2 and FB are found in aHUS patients (83, 88). In around 10% of the patients, autoantibodies against FH have been found. Most of the FH mutations as well as the FH autoantibodies target FH CCP 20. As FH CCP 19-20 is most important for FH binding to GAGs predominantly expressed in the glomeruli basement membrane, it might not come as a surprise that exactly these mutations and antibodies are linked to aHUS (89–91). Current treatment of aHUS consists of either plasma infusion or exchange, or eculizumab. Plasma infusion and exchange can replenish complement regulators in the blood of the patient and is especially beneficial in patients with FH and FI mutations (92). Eculizumab is now the preferred treatment, as it prevents complement-mediated damage as described above for PNH and is more safe than plasma transfusions (84).

Next to aHUS patients, C3 glomerulopathy patients suffer from dysregulation of the AP as well. In contrast to aHUS patients, these patients are characterized by C3 deposits in glomeruli, which leads to disruption of kidney function, but the disease is not associated with thrombocytopenia, anemia, or other systemic involvement (93). The pathophysiology of disease is not always clear, but in some cases it is known to be caused by autoantibody formation against C3bBb, which stabilizes the convertase and thus increases its activity, or by mutations in C3 or the complement regulatory proteins FH or FI (94–96). Another kidney disease where an FH polymorphism increases susceptibility is IgA nephropathy, a form of glomerulonephritis where C3 depositions are found on affected kidney tissue, together with IgA. The FH polymorphism identified for IgA nephropathy has not been linked to aHUS. A meta-analysis showed significant association between this minor allele and IgA nephropathy risk (97). This strengthens the hypothesis that IgA nephropathy is caused by overactivation of complement, although no functional implications of this specific polymorphism have been described.

Lastly, chronic kidney disease (CKD) is a condition where decreased kidney condition takes place over a longer period of time, regardless of the underlying cause. Although the pathologies mentioned above can cause CKD, the majority of cases is caused by diabetes and hypertension (98). Anemia is found in almost half of the CKD patients, being more prevalent in end-stage disease (99). A study of anemic CKD patients investigated CD55 and CD59 expression and showed that patients had an altered expression of CD55 and CD59 on RBCs, with more CD55- and CD59-deficient RBCs in patients than in healthy controls. CD55- and CD59-deficiency would make RBCs more susceptible to complement-mediated hemolysis. Increased hemolysis was confirmed in patients with high levels of CD55- and CD59 deficient RBCs. The underlying cause of CKD in these patients was not reported, making it difficult to speculate on the mechanisms involved (100). Furthermore, *VTN* has been shown to be upregulated in chronic kidney disease. This is possibly related to the fact that it functions as a ligand for the urokinase-type plasminogen activator receptor. This receptor is not found on healthy kidney cells, only getting expressed in diseased kidney cells, where it is involved in cell recruitment and migration (101). Up to date, no studies have been conducted that assess the role of Vn on complement regulation in CKD.

Complement Regulators in Diseases Affecting the Eye

Complement activation in the eye is highly reliant on local production of complement proteins, due to its anatomical characteristics (102). The inner part of the eye is shielded off by a sheet of extracellular matrix called the Bruch's membrane. Like the glomerular basement membrane in the kidney, it is directly exposed to circulation and thus to complement activity, making it vulnerable to dysfunctional complement regulators (103). Bruch's membrane is impermeable to larger proteins, these thus need to be locally produced. This also holds for the larger proteins of the complement cascade, such as C3b, FH, FB, and FI. It has been shown that FHL-1, a truncated splice variant of FH, is small enough to diffuse over Bruch's membrane and could thus play an important role in the eye (28). The importance of complement in the eye has been illustrated in age-related macular degeneration (AMD). As one of the leading causes of blindness AMD is affecting more than 5% of the elderly above 75 years old, for which the role of complement in disease has been widely studied.

AMD is marked by progressive destruction of the macula, as the retinal pigment epithelial cells that normally maintain retinal homeostasis are unable to do so. Currently, AMD is considered to be caused by a combination of genetic and environmental risk factors. Different complement genes have been associated with AMD, which can altogether account for 40–60% of the heritability of the disease. Amongst these genes are *CFH, CFI* and *VTN* which indicates that a dysregulation of complement activation is at play here.

Several mutations were found for *CFH*, amongst which the common Y402H variant, and were all associated with decreased protein expression or functionality of FH and FHL-1 (104, 105). Similarly, the *CFI* mutations found were associated with decreased serum levels of FI, although the effect of these polymorphisms on FI production within the eye is not known (106). For the *VTN* polymorphism identified no functional consequences have been described yet (107). Lastly, serum levels of FHR-4 were increased in AMD patients compared to healthy controls, while complete *CFHR1* and *CFHR3* deletion has been described to be protective against AMD (32, 108). While FHR-3 is locally produced in the retina, FHR-4 expression has not been demonstrated here yet (109, 110). It has been suggested that FHR-4 might inhibit FHL-1 functioning in AMD, as competition assays showed that FHR-4 outcompetes FHL-1 in C3b binding (32).

Pseudoexfoliation syndrome is a pathology characterized by the deposition of abnormal fibrillar extracellular material in both non-ocular and ocular tissue, which can lead to glaucoma (111, 112). CLU is reduced at both mRNA and protein levels in several parts of the eyes of pseudoexfoliation syndrome patients compared to healthy controls (113). Under stress conditions CLU would be conventionally expected to be increased: amongst its biological functions are its role as an extracellular chaperone, which inhibits stress-induced precipitation and the aggregation of misfolded proteins (114). Thus, its downregulation here could be a contributing factor to the accumulation of fibrillar extracellular material (113). A polymorphism in *CLU* might contribute to genetic risk of pseudoexfoliation syndrome, but was not relevant when the age of controls was corrected for, and was not significant in logistic regression. Thus, common genetic variation in the CLU gene does not seem to play a major role (115). Next to the involvement of CLU in pseudoexfoliation syndrome, C3 was found to be significantly upregulated in aqueous humor in eyes of patients with pseudoexfoliation syndrome indicating an important role for complement activation during this disease (112). The mechanisms behind the role of complement in pseudoexfolation syndrome have not been elucidated yet, calling for more research to indicate whether other complement regulators might be implicated in its development.

Furthermore, a *CLU* polymorphism was associated with Fuchs' endothelial dystrophy, which is a degenerative disease of the corneal endothelium. This polymorphism results in overexpression of CLU in the corneal endothelial cells of these patients. It was hypothesized by the authors that this specific polymorphism in the *CLU* gene might affect its secretion by corneal endothelial cells, which would expose these cells to physiological stress (116). Lastly, a polymorphism in CD55 was repeatedly associated with the risk of development of myopia. Myopia, more commonly known as nearsightedness, is the leading cause of vision loss in young people, stemming from excessive axial elongation of the eye (117, 118). The effect of this polymorphism on CD55 function or expression has not been described yet. Complement activity as measured by C3, C4 and CH50 activity in serum is increased in pathological myopia patients, which could be an indication that dysregulation of complement is at play here (119). However, as measurements of complement activity in serum are not proper indications of complement activity in the eye, care should be taken in concluding complement plays a role in myopia patients, for which further research is needed.

Taken together, there are multiple strong links between mutations in complement regulatory proteins and pathology in eye diseases. Studying complement activation and regulation within the eye is difficult, limiting our current knowledge. Although some *in vitro* models have been developed, the current *in vivo* models are still insufficient to mimic complement activity in the human eye (102, 105, 120, 121). Knowledge considering the effect of the currently identified polymorphisms in the eye, could improve our understanding of the pathology and aid in the development of therapeutics.

Complement Regulators in Neurological Disease

The blood–brain barrier is largely impermeable for plasma proteins, like the complement proteins. As only a fraction of complement proteins passes the blood–brain barrier and there is minimal local production, the healthy brain expresses low levels of complement proteins. In diseased brain however, the blood–brain barrier can get disrupted and local production can be increased, contributing to a rise in complement activity. If complement is activated in the brain, the brain's glia cells and neurons have a low tolerance for it, due to low levels of complement regulators (122). The role of complement in diseases of the central nervous system has become more apparent in recent years. It has been shown to play a role in brain development, acute brain trauma and neurogenerative disease (123). Here, we discuss the links between complement regulators and Alzheimer's disease (AD) or Parkinson's disease (PD) as the role of regulators here has been most well-studied and the diseases largely impact global health.

AD is a common neurodegenerative disease, with almost 30 million cases worldwide in 2019, that leads to loss of cognitive function, caused by neuropathologic lesions in the brain (124). These lesions can be caused by amyloid plaques or neurofibrillary degeneration. Complement has been shown to contribute to the inflammation of the brain that occurs in AD, and to be activated in and around the amyloid plaques (122). The overactivation of complement contributes to disease progression, resulting in synapse loss and neurodegeneration (125). The evidence for the association of complement regulatory genes with AD has been given multiple times. Polymorphisms in both *CR1* and *CLU* have been repeatedly demonstrated to increase risk of AD (126–129). *CLU* has been shown to be upregulated in the AD brain, as well as to play a role in the clearance of β amyloid, which is the major component of the amyloid plaques (124). How this upregulation of *CLU* in the AD brain affects local complement activation has not been investigated. The functionality behind *CR1* polymorphisms in AD have not been fully elucidated either. One of the risk-increasing *CR1* polymorphisms results in a single amino acid change that has been associated with mildly increased sCR1 levels and binding affinity for C1q (130). The other is an intronic mutation associated with increased length of the final protein by duplication, resulting in more C3b binding sites which could increase CR1 effectivity (122, 131). However, this variant is also associated with decreased expression levels. Overall, it seems that AD patients with the long CR1 isoform show an progressively decreased expression of CR1 on cells, thus reducing the total effectiveness of CR1 (132). Future research should indicate what the effects of the found *CR1* and *CLU* polymorphisms are on protein levels and functionality within the brain.

PD is another common neurodegenerative disease, which is also characterized by protein depositions in the brain. Research on the brains of PD patients has repeatedly shown complement activation in affected tissues (133, 134), and the dysregulated complement system has been suggested to play a role in pathology of PD (123). This was reason to investigate the abovementioned found polymorphisms for AD in PD. Only one of the *CLU* polymorphisms found for AD also showed to be a risk factor for the development of PD (135). However, levels of CLU in cerebrospinal fluid and plasma were not found to differ between patients and healthy controls. A correlation between CLU levels and amyloid- ß42, T-tau and P-tau levels was found, which are proteins that play a role in both AD and PD. Altogether these results suggest a direct interaction between amyloid- ß42, tau and CLU (136). It might not be surprising to see that CLU is associated with several neurological diseases, as it has been implicated in neuronal synapse function (53). Further research should indicate whether CLU also contributes *via* its role as complement regulatory protein in this system.

Complement Regulators in Oncology

The complement system has become strongly implicated in different types of cancer in recent years, but its role in oncology has not been well defined (137). In fact, the role of complement in carcinogenesis, has been described as a dual-edged sword (138). The dual mechanism of complement in carcinogenesis could be similar to that of inflammation, in which complement is a large contributing factor. Initially, acute inflammation can cause early detection and clearance of malignant cells, but chronic inflammation might also contribute to the spread of malignant cells (139). Specifically, the anaphylatoxins C3a and C5a have been described to contribute to an inflammatory tumor microenvironment. Their production upon local activity of the CP and AP on the tumor creates an environment that favors tumor growth and metastatic spread, contributing to tumor progression (137, 139–141). This role for C3a and C5a has been shown in different cancer types, in the form of promoting angiogenesis, inhibiting anti-tumor immune responses and by triggering tumorigenic, survival and anti-apoptotic pathways in tumor cells (141).

Although the importance of complement in cancer has been demonstrated, its function and overall effect have not been fully elucidated. The currently available literature on complement regulators in cancer specifically is limited and sometimes contradictory. This could in part be explained by the fact that only few human studies are available, with most of the data stemming from animal models or *in vitro* studies (137). In addition, complement regulators do not only have impact on the complement system, but also play an important role in the adaptive immune system by regulating and activating T-cells (142), making studies regarding their role extremely difficult. In general, it is believed that high expression of complement regulatory proteins is linked to worse clinical outcome (142). Here, we will give a brief overview of the currently available human studies of complement regulators in cancer.

Colon cancer is the second-most lethal cancer in the world (143). Although no complement regulator polymorphisms for risk of colon cancer have been identified, CD46, CD55, and CD59 were all upregulated in colon cancer compared to adjacent healthy tissue (144, 145), with CD55 and CD59 expression correlating with tumor stage and differentiation level (146). In addition, patients with an increased CD55 expression in their tumor tissue had a worse 7-year survival rate, with tumors with high levels of CD55 more aggressive than tumors with low CD55-levels (147). Patients with colorectal cancer also showed increased soluble CD55 in stool specimens compared to healthy controls and to patients with other gastrointestinal disease. Whether the soluble CD55 was secreted as such, or whether it arose from cleaved membrane-bound CD55, was unclear (148). These studies combined suggest that the increased expression of complement regulators protects malignant colorectal cells from being attacked by the human immune system, especially for CD55. A mouse xenograft study has shown that a blocking CD55-antibody inhibits tumor growth and increases survival of mice. *In vitro*, the combination of a blocking CD55-antibody with regular chemotherapy has a synergistic effect (149). This therapeutic effect suggests a clinical relevance for CD55 in colon cancer.

Another common and deadly cancer type is non-small cell lung cancer (NSCLC). NSCLC has been associated with the complement system in multiple ways, but the precise mechanisms in place have not been elucidated yet (150). On the genetic level, both a CD55 and a CR1 polymorphism have been associated with risk of NSCLC development (138, 151). The CD55 polymorphism found in NSCLC is associated with decreased transcriptional activity of CD55. This was a surprising finding, as complement regulation was initially expected to be increased on malignant cells, protecting them from detection by the complement system (151, 152). There might be a differential effect of CD55 between healthy and cancer cells at play here, as CD55 in NSCLC is not only down-regulated, but also sialylated. Possibly, sialylated CD55 can execute its function longer than regular CD55, as it has a high resistance against proteolysis and can thus be retained on the cell surface for a longer time (153). Another explanation could be that NSCLC tissue does not require complement regulation as much, as the bulky tissue formation ensures that not all cells are exposed to the alveolar cavity, and thus to complement activity (153). The CR1 polymorphism found in NSCLC was not further functionally described. Furthermore, at the protein level *in vivo* xenograft study in mice showed that FH expression is critical for NSCLC tumor growth. Whilst NSCLC cells *in vitro* were shown to be insensitive to complement-mediated lysis, even largely when FH was blocked, blocking FH *in vivo* significantly decreased xenograft size (154).

Apart from the solid tumors described above, some research is available that links different types of leukemia and lymphoma to complement regulators. In a group of leukemia patients, comprised of patients with acute myeloid leukemia, acute lymphoblastic leukemia and chronic lymphocytic leukemia, soluble CR1 was found in high concentrations, regardless of specific leukemia type (155). The soluble CR1 originates from cleaved and shed membrane-bound CR1. This soluble CR1 maintains its complement regulatory activity, allowing for complement regulation in serum. Although it seems unlikely that this would lead to reduced overall complement activity in plasma *in vivo*, it could be that soluble CR1 shedding leads to local down-regulation of complement activity at sites of tumor infiltration, which could aid the malignant cells locally (155). This regulating characteristic of soluble CR1 has also been demonstrated in other studies, and soluble CR1 is now used to therapeutic advantage in complement-mediated diseases (156–158) as discussed below. The effects found for soluble complement regulators could be caused by their effects on the tumor microenvironment. The tumor microenvironment is the total of cancer cells, stromal cells and extracellular components around the tumor, where complement has been shown to play a regulatory role to which soluble regulators might contribute (159, 160).

The last type of tumor to be described here is non-Hodgkin's lymphoma. Non-Hodgkin's lymphoma is the most common type of lymphoma, with around half a million new cases a year and diffuse large B cell lymphoma and follicular lymphoma as its most common subtypes (161). In follicular lymphoma, a CD46 polymorphism is associated with decreased event-free survival, while the CD55 and FH polymorphisms are associated with increased event free survival. In diffuse large B cell lymphoma, a possible association with increased event-free survival was found for a *CLU* polymorphism (162). Unfortunately, there are no studies available linking any of these polymorphisms to expression levels or functionality of the protein, and there is no consensus on the role of complement in these diseases. A more recent study acknowledged that the role of complement in lymphoma is complex, but could indicate FHR-3 as a biomarker for the response to specific immunotherapies (163).

In conclusion, both solid malignancies and blood cancers have been associated with complement regulators. Here, we have described a selection of cancer types related to complement regulators, based on the extent to which they have been studied in humans. Based on this research, it is not possible to be conclusive on the role of complement regulators in cancer. The current indications of the many polymorphisms in complement regulators involved in cancer, can be used as directions for future research into the mechanisms and purposes of complement regulation in cancer.

Overall, we have demonstrated the broad range of diseases in which complement plays a role, giving examples from RBCs, the eyes, kidney, brain and oncology. In addition, **Table 1** shows other pathologies found linked to complement regulators in the current research. Altogether, the great amount of pathologies linking to dysfunction of complement regulators implies that future therapeutics based on complement regulators could potentially be applied widely. Next, we will explore the potential of such therapeutics currently available and under development.

FUTURE POTENTIAL OF UTILIZING COMPLEMENT REGULATORS IN THERAPEUTICS

As discussed above, a broad range of pathologies arises from dysfunction of complement regulation, leading to overactivation of the complement system on healthy cells, or insufficient complement activation on malignant cells (22, 137). Currently, only two therapeutics are approved to target the complement system, eculizumab/ravulizumab and C1-INH, which is insufficient to treat the wide range of complement-related pathologies. Other complement-targeting therapeutics are currently in development, such as compstatin, and FB and FD inhibitors (42, 164). The clinical success of these drugs has been limited to this date. The anti-C5 antibody eculizumab, as mentioned previously, is currently approved for diseases such as PNH and aHUS. When effective, eculizumab treatment increases patients' life expectancy to that of healthy person (165, 166). However, the drug is not effective in all patients (165, 166). Around 15% of aHUS patients do not respond to treatment, as well as 3% of PNH patients, with 30% of treated patients still requiring regular blood transfusions (61, 167, 168). In AMD, a phase III trial with eculizumab and a similar trial with an anti-FD antibody did not show a slowing effect on geographic atrophy development (169, 170). Together, this data indicates that although the fact that complement plays an important role in AMD, complement modulation seems a challenging and uncertain therapeutic option. Lastly, compstatin is a small cyclic peptide that binds C3 and inhibits convertase formation and C3 cleavage, of which two analogs have been clinically evaluated: AMY-101 and APL-2. To this date, AMY-101 has only been tested in a phase I trial, with phase II trials still expected to start (66). APL-2, a compstatin variant with an increased half-life due to adapted pegylation, has been successfully tested in PNH patients in phase I studies, with a phase III study on its way (66, 83).

Finding targets for complement therapeutics is not easy, as it is often unclear which of the many complement components is involved in the pathology of disease and the functions of the system are broad, meaning that side-effects of drugs interfering with the complement system are likely to occur. Furthermore, the plasma concentrations and turnover rate of the complement proteins are high and their production occurs at different sites in the body which can complicate drug delivery (4). The field of complement therapeutics has been evolving to solve these challenges, looking at complement regulators to prevent side-effects of targeting complement systemically. Here, we discuss therapeutics based on complement regulators currently in the pipeline, and future possibilities to use the mechanisms of complement regulators in therapeutics (**Figure 3**).

Plasma-Derived and Recombinant Full-Length Complement Regulators

Full-length complement regulators can be therapeutically used to aid patients with deficiencies functional defects in their regulators. The best example of this approach is the use of C1-INH in hereditary angioedema. Hereditary angioedema is caused by a genetic C1-INH deficiency which can result in life-threatening edema from excessive bradykinin release (171, 172). The plasma-derived C1-INH can prevent angioedema attacks completely, providing a safe treatment option with no significant side effects (171, 173). Additionally, C1-INH has been recombinantly produced from the milk of transgenic New Zealand white rabbits (174). The recombinant and plasma-derived C1-INH did show comparable activity in hereditary angioedema, but the half-life of recombinant C1-INH was much shorter (171). This might pose a problem when using recombinant C1-INH for complement mediated diseases such as ischemia–reperfusion injury, acute myocardial infarction, autoimmune hemolytic anemia and renal transplantation (175–178).

Another complement regulator for which both a plasma-derived and a recombinant variant is in development is FH. As described, mutations of FH are clearly linked to development of complement-mediated renal diseases. As described above for aHUS, patients with functional FH mutations can be treated with plasma infusions. However, plasma infusions are not without risks, as they can lead to allergic reactions or fluid overload (179). Plasma-derived or recombinant FH could potentially be more purposeful in supplementing mutated non-functional FH. FH-deficient mice, mimicking C3 glomerulopathy, have been treated with human plasma-derived FH, resulting in a reduction in complement activity and C3 deposition on the glomerular basement membrane (180–182). Recombinant FH has been produced in insect cells, the yeast *Pichia pastoris*, mammalian HEK and COS7 cell lines (91, 183, 184). Although the produced proteins were biologically active, success was limited by low yield and aberrant glycosylation patterns. Currently, the most

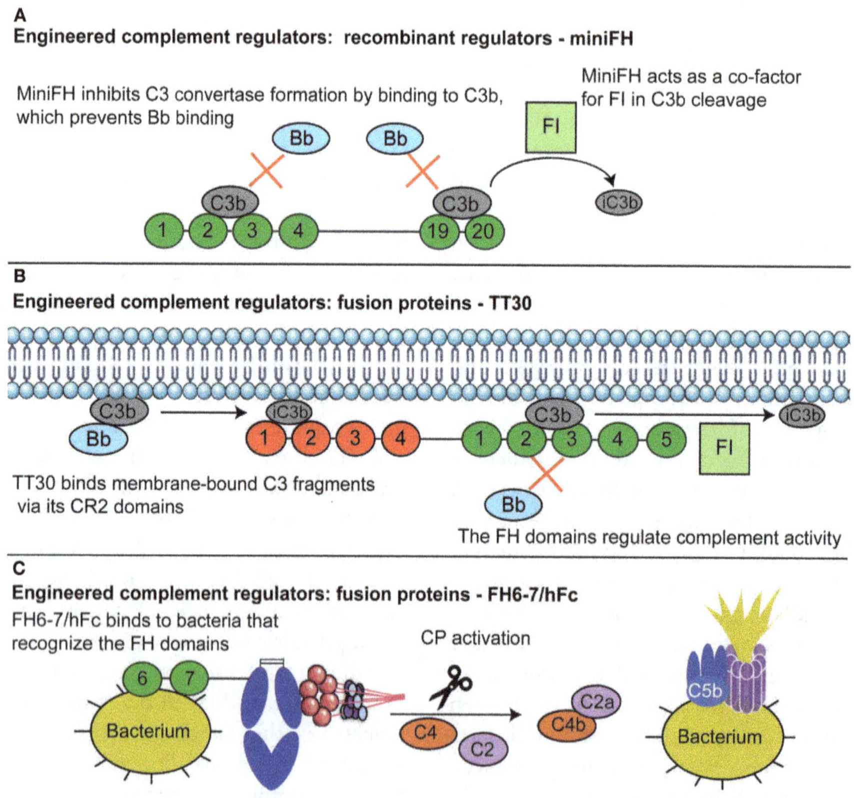

FIGURE 3 | Therapeutics based of complement regulators. **(A)** MiniFH has been designed from FH CCPs 1-4 and 19-20 to open up an extra C3b binding domain. This means it can bind two C3b molecules simultaneously, where regular FH can only bind one. MiniFH inhibits C3bBb formation and exert FI co-factor activity. **(B)** TT30 is a fusion protein of the first 4 domains of CR2 and the first 5 domains of FH. The CR2 domains recognize tissue-bound C3 fragments, while the FH domains regulate complement activity. Thus, the protein is targeted towards tissues where complement is already activated, where the FH domains can then exert complement regulatory activity. **(C)** FH6-7/hFc contains FH CCP 6 and 7, and the Fc part of an antibody. Certain bacteria bind FH *via* CCP FH6-7, normally to evade the complement system. These CCPs are utilized here to target these bacteria, upon which the hFc induces CP activation by C1q binding resulting in complement activation *via* the CP finally resulting in opsonization and lysis of bacteria. Figure designed using Servier Medical Art.

successful production of recombinant FH with full human glycosylation pattern has been achieved in the moss *Physcomitrella patens* (FHmoss) (185, 186). FHmoss has full biological activity and was shown to reduce complement activation and hemolysis in aHUS patient sera. Experiments in FH-deficient mice treated with FHmoss showed a reduction of glomerular C3 accumulation and AP activity. These experiments also showed that FHmoss is cleared from the circulation faster than plasma-derived FH and could not be detected anymore in plasma after 6 h, which is a potential obstacle for the clinical use of FHmoss (185). The success of the *P. patens* system has been further illustrated by the production of MFHR1, which is a recombinant regulator with domains from FH and FHR-1. This is a biologically stable protein that has an even stronger *in vitro* regulatory activity on the AP than FH (187).

Next to the fluid-phase regulators C1-INH and FH, recombinant soluble variants of membrane-bound regulators have been developed. While soluble CR1 (sCR1), CD46, CD55 and CD59 were all produced and tested successfully *in vitro* (188–190), only sCR1 has progressed to clinical trials (158). With regards to sCR1, two highly similar recombinant molecules have been designed (TP10 and TP20). Both are effective inhibitors of C3 and C5 convertases and were shown to prevent complement-mediated tissue damage in different animal models of vascular injury (158, 191). TP20 is a derivative of TP10 that contains Sialyl-Lewis X tetrasaccharide (sLe^x) groups to target it towards the endothelium *via* binding of E- and P-selectin receptors. This modification has made it more effective in *in vivo* models of cardiovascular and lung disease than TP10 (191, 192). Recently, TP10 has been clinically evaluated in several indications requiring cardiopulmonary bypass, as complement activity has been shown to play a role in the inflammatory response after acute myocardial infarction. Intravenous administration of TP10 reduced complications and mortality in male patients undergoing cardiopulmonary bypass, but not in female patients, although this gender difference was not caused by the complement suppressing effects of sCR1 (156). In lung transplantations, TP10 administration led to a shorter intubation time, although other clinical outcomes were not affected by TP10 (156). Taken together, use of full length complement regulators seems an efficient strategy. Use of plasma-derived proteins is limited due to the availability of plasma, while recombinant proteins struggle with a short half-life. In addition to the proteins described here, we could imagine the use of full length FI to be further explored, as it has been shown that plasma infusions are also successful in aHUS patients suffering from a mutation in FI (92, 193).

Engineered Complement Regulators

Apart from the variety of full-length complement regulators researched for therapeutic usage, engineered complement regulators are also under development. These proteins are recombinant complement regulators, but rather than being designed to mimic the human regulator as closely as possible, they are adapted to enhance their therapeutic effects (194). For FH, two engineered variants have been designed: miniFH and midiFH. MiniFH contains CCP 1-4 and 19-20 of FH, whilst midiFH is its duplicated variant, coupling two miniFH molecules with a short linker (**Figure 3A**). MiniFH was designed specifically to enhance C3b binding activity, as the CCPs masking the C-terminal C3b binding domain in full-length FH are deleted. Both proteins are more effective in decay accelerating activity than FH and FHL-1, but less effective in FI co-factor activity (195, 196). MidiFH outcompetes miniFH in the inhibition of AP activation, which can probably be explained by its extra C3b binding sites (195). Engineered variants of FH could be relevant in the treatment of PNH as *in vitro* studies already showed that both miniFH and midiFH are effective in protecting PNH erythrocytes from complement-mediated lysis (195, 197). The efficacy of miniFH could even be improved by introducing the dimerization domain of FHRs in the protein, which lead to the formation of homodimers and prolonged its half-life. These homomeric miniFHs have been tested *in vivo* in FH-deficient mice, where they showed a reduction in glomerular accumulation of C3 (198). Taken together, engineered complement regulators such a miniFH show promising results both *in vitro* as well as *in vivo*. To date, Amyndas has engineered a mini FH for which phase-1 clinical studies for treatment of AMD are planned (42).

A different approach to engineered complement regulators is the design of fusion proteins to optimally utilize their regulatory activity. Currently, fusion proteins have been described containing (parts of) CR1, CD55, CD46, and FH to target the AP, CP and/or the LP. Mirococept is a fusion molecule containing the first three CR1 SCRs, containing the complement regulatory activity, followed by an amphiphilic peptide that increases its affinity for cell surfaces. *In vitro*, Mirococept can inhibit C3 and C5 convertase activity similar to CR1 (199). Mirococept is also beneficial *in vivo*, which was demonstrated using rat models for intestinal ischaemia and reperfusion injury and for kidney transplantation (199, 200). Mirococept was shown to be safe in a phase I clinical trial, with a phase II clinical trial in kidney transplantations currently underway (201). To the best of our knowledge, the results of this trial have not been published yet (202).

TT30 is an FH and CR2 fusion protein that has been designed to selectively inhibit the AP locally at activation sites in order to minimize the risk of infection or autoimmune disease which could increase upon systemic complement inhibition (**Figure 3B**) (203). To this end CR2 domains were used, as CR2 only binds to the tissue-bound C3b breakdown products iC3b, C3dg, and C3d, thereby specifically acting at sites of complement activation on tissue. TT30 contains the first four CCPs of CR2, which bind to the C3b breakdown products, and the first five domains of FH, which regulate AP activity. *In vitro*, TT30 is effective in both inhibiting the C3 and C5 convertase. Next, subcutaneous administration of TT30 in cynomolgus monkeys showed almost complete inhibition of the AP, lasting up to 24 h, and partial inhibition of the CP (203).

The above-mentioned fusion proteins utilize CR1 and CR2, which mainly target the AP. Although the role of the AP has been well described in diseases as PNH and aHUS, it is not the only complement pathway to think of when aiming to target the complement system with therapeutics. Recently, fusion proteins to target the LP were developed and suggested to have potential in the treatment of ischemia–reperfusion injury and delayed kidney graft function (204). These proteins consist of the first domains of CR1, CD55 or FH with MAP-1 or sMAP in order to inhibit LP activation at the C3 level and prevent MAC formation. MAP-1 and sMAP are alternative splice variants of MASP-1 and MASP-3 respectively, lacking the proteolytic site, thus binding to the pattern recognition molecules of the LP without inducing subsequent C2 and C4 cleavage (7, 205). MAP-1:CD55$^{1\text{-}4}$ and MAP-1:CD35$^{1\text{-}3}$ effectively inhibit the LP in *in vitro* assays that measured deposition of C3, C4, and MAC on mannan. The effects of MAP-1:CD55$^{1\text{-}4}$ were stronger, especially at the terminal pathway level. The root of this difference could not be pinpointed, although it was suggested to be caused by the absence of certain CD35 domains in MAP-1:CD35$^{1\text{-}3}$ that are normally involved in its co-factor activity (205). A different study fused full-length murine MAP-1, murine sMAP or human sMAP to the same FH domains. The murine MAP-1 FH fusion protein, MAp44-FH, showed only limited activity both *in vitro* and *in vivo*, while the murine sMAP-FH inhibited the activity of both the AP and LP. Human sMAP-FH showed an inhibitory effect on the AP and LP in human serum as well, which was stronger than the effect of the sMAP or FH domains separately (206). The stronger effect of sMAP-FH than of MAp44-FH could possibly be explained by their competition with MASPs to form complexes with the pattern recognition molecules. sMAP competes with MASP-2 for binding, while MAp44 competes with MASP-1 and -3. MASP-1 is 13.6 times more abundant in serum than MASP-2, which results in MASP-1 outcompeting MAp44-FH in serum at the studied concentrations, which were constant between MAp44-FH and sMAP-FH (206). To conclude, several LP inhibiting complement regulators have been engineered, of which the FH domain also targets the AP. The AP and LP both contribute to diseases as AMD and ischemia–reperfusion injuries, were MAP-1:CD55$^{1\text{-}4}$, MAP-1:CD35$^{1\text{-}3}$, and sMAP-FH could potentially aid in the treatment of such pathologies.

The last fusion protein composed of two different complement regulators to be described here is decay-cofactor protein (DCP), a fusion product of CD55 and CD46 (207) that was designed to target both the AP and CP. Different CCPs of CD55 and CD46 were combined into fusion proteins that would retain their inhibitory effect on CP and AP activation. A fusion protein of CD55 CCP2-3 and CD46 CCP3-4 showed the largest inhibitory activity *in vitro*, upon which DCP with maximal inhibitory effect was achieved by selecting the most effective mutant (207). Although successful inhibition of the AP and CP could be achieved *in vitro*, this protein has to this date not been tested *in vivo*.

Next to the fusions of complement proteins with the regulators, other fusion proteins contain (parts of) antibodies. Three different types of regulators fuse parts of antibodies with a complement regulator, which have been developed to target myasthenia gravis, the AP in several pathologies or bacterial infections respectively. Firstly, the fusion protein designed to treat myasthenia gravis contains CD55 and an antibody fragment. Myasthenia gravis is an autoantibody-mediated disease, where damage to neurons at the neuromuscular junction is enhanced by complement activity (208). The fusion protein to treat this disease consists of an scFv antibody fragment targeting the nicotine acetylcholine receptor, that did not affect ion channel function, and CD55, which would regulate complement activation on the neuron surface. This fusion protein induced a reduction in complement activation *in vitro* and reduced clinical severity *in vivo* (208, 209). Secondly, a fusion protein of CRIg and Fc of a murine IgG1 (CRIg-Fc) is a soluble version of CRIg and was designed to inhibit the AP selectively by binding to cells opsonized with antibodies and inhibiting C3 convertase (210, 211). Successful reduction of inflammation was shown *in vivo* in mouse models of experimental arthritis, ischemia/reperfusion injury and FH-deficient mice that mimick C3 glomerulopathy (210, 212, 213).

While most engineered proteins focus on inhibiting complement-mediated diseases, complement regulators can also be used in a different way. A fusion protein consisting of FH CCP 6 -7 and the Fc region of a human IgG is designed to treat bacterial infections by activating the complement system (**Figure 3C**). This protein makes clever use of the fact that pathogenic bacteria often bind to FH CCP 6-7 in order to evade the complement system (19). In addition, the Fc domain would then be able to initiate the CP by binding to C1q, which can in turn lead to C3b deposition and phagocytosis (214). This protein has been effective in enhancing complement-mediated killing *in vivo* for *Streptococcus pyogenes*, *Haemophilus influenzae* and *Neisseria meningitidis* (214–216). The increased killing of *S. pyogenes* upon FH6-7/hFC administration demonstrate that the protein can induce opsonophagocytosis, as this Gram-positive pathogen cannot be lysed by the MAC. Furthermore, FH6-7/hFc was also shown to outcompete FH for *S. pyogenes* binding, resulting in reduced complement evasion by the pathogen. This shows that the activating effect of FH6-7/hFC on the complement system is two-fold: it reduces complement evasion by outcompeting FH for binding, and it initiates more complement activation by binding to C1q (215).

Altogether, the engineered complement regulators are designed to enhance therapeutic efficacy of the regulators with two main aims. The engineered regulators are either designed to increase the regulatory power of the original protein, or they are designed to be targeted to a specific tissue and prevent systemic effects. These engineered regulators have shown promising results in a range of *in vivo* studies, although most have not been evaluated clinically to this date.

Potentiating and Inhibiting Complement Regulation Using Antibodies

Next to the use of plasma-derived and full-length regulators and the development of engineered therapeutics, we here discuss the therapeutic use of antibodies. While those antibodies are mainly used in development of cancer therapeutics, as will be described below, we have recently developed an antibody that could be used to treat complement-mediated aHUS. The anti-FH antibodies anti-FH.07 and FH07.1 are designed to potentiate the regulatory function of FH. The antibodies bind to FH domain 18, and enhance its activity specifically on human cells. Hence, these antibodies have the potential as a therapeutic in aHUS, especially in patients that suffer from FH dysfunction. This could be an alternative to eculizumab, which has the disadvantage of inhibiting complement activity against pathogens as well. This antibody can restore FH activity in aHUS patient sera (217). In addition, we recently showed that this potentiating antibody not only potentiates wild type FH, but also four common aHUS mutated FHs *in vitro* (218).

Most antibodies that are currently developed to target complement regulators are used to target these in cancer. As discussed above, complement regulatory proteins are often highly expressed on tumor cells and have been described to compromise the efficiency of antibody-based immunotherapies. This has raised the interests in finding blocking antibodies for the complement regulators. The effects of these antibodies can be twofold: either, complement regulators can be targeted with immunotherapy, as they are specifically upregulated in certain tumor cells, or, they can be targeted to block their function and make the tumor cells more susceptible to complement-mediated killing (**Figure 4**) (149, 154, 219, 220). However, targeting complement regulators with antibodies is not without risk. As described in the previous section, different membrane-bound regulators seem to be differentially expressed on tumor cells, but where some studies show upregulation of complement regulators, others do not. This means that usage of these antibodies would require a personalized medicine approach, in which the tumor is first extensively characterized before a drug is selected for a specific patient. More importantly, the regulators are also expressed on many other cell types throughout the body. Several studies have shown successful usage of neutralizing CD55 or CD59 antibodies in colon cancer or NSCLC, but these were investigated in cell lines or in mouse xenograft models. Here, antibodies directed against the human regulators would give rise to only very limited off-target effects, as the antibodies will only minimally recognize the mouse homologs (149, 221, 222). In addition to complement regulatory inhibiting antibodies, oligonucleotides such as anti-sense phosphorothioate oligonucleotides (S-ODNs) and small interfering RNAs (siRNAs) have been designed to silence to complement regulators. Successful silencing has been shown *in vitro*, but further developments with regards to their stability and targeting *in vivo* are still required (219, 220)

The prevention of healthy host cell targeting by these complement regulator-targeted antibodies and oligonucleotides is one of the main challenges in developing such therapeutics, as inhibiting complement regulators on healthy cells is undesirable. By administering antibodies that solely target complement regulators, a dangerous situation could arise where healthy cells expressing complement regulators are also targeted by the antibody. This poses a serious challenge for this therapeutic approach, as all healthy cells express complement regulators and most complement regulators are expressed by a majority of cells. Several possibilities are under investigation to circumvent this problem, such as bispecific antibodies or a biotin–avidin system, or circumventing the usage of antibodies altogether (220). Firstly, the bispecific antibodies are composed of Fabs of two different monoclonal antibodies: one that recognizes a complement regulator, and another that targets a tumor-specific antigen. These showed to be promising in animal models, but have not been clinically tested yet (220, 223, 224). Another possible strategy is to use a biotin–avidin system, which combines biotin-labeled mini-antibodies against CD55 and CD59 with biotin-rituximab, which targets CD20, and avidin. The mini-antibodies do not work independently, but only when combined with biotin-rituximab *via* avidin. This was shown to be effective in an *in vivo* model of B-cell lymphoma (225).

Summarizing, one potentiating antibody for a complement regulator has been successfully produced, targeting FH. The development of complement regulator inhibiting antibodies to be used as a cancer therapeutic is however still in its infancy. Several practical challenges remain to be overcome in order to test these antibodies in the clinic.

DISCUSSION

In conclusion, this review described the wide range of human pathologies involving complement regulators. Most of the pathologies identified affect tissues where complement or complement regulation is organized in a different way than in the rest of the body, such as the kidney, eyes and brain (28, 81, 122). The role of complement regulators in cancer was also discussed, however, there is no consensus yet on the role of complement itself in cancer (137–139) and the current evidence does not allow us to make a general statement about the role of complement regulators in cancer, which seems to differ per cancer type.

All in all, a diverse group of complement regulatory therapeutics is currently in development (4, 42, 164). There are however still challenges to overcome before these therapeutics can be used in the clinic. Although the effects of plasma-derived and recombinant molecules are highly similar, with recombinant molecules easier to produce, a shortcoming of the recombinant regulators is that their half-life is often much shorter (171, 185), which might hinder their clinical applications. In addition, the targeting or inhibiting of complement regulatory proteins in cancer is still in its infancy. Although some promising results have been shown *in vitro* and *in vivo* (149, 154, 219–221), current knowledge on expression and role of the regulators in different tumor types is lacking, which should be further clarified to develop future therapeutics. However, other drugs have found clever ways to ensure specificity of the complement regulatory effect, as has been described for the fusion proteins. The therapeutics described here have not been clinically evaluated, with the exception of recombinant soluble CR1, which would be interesting possibilities for future research (156). Their clinical success remains to be seen, as for most pathologies described in this paper targeting the complement system has not yet been proven a successful strategy. An interesting point of contention is whether this lack of success can be contributed to the specific

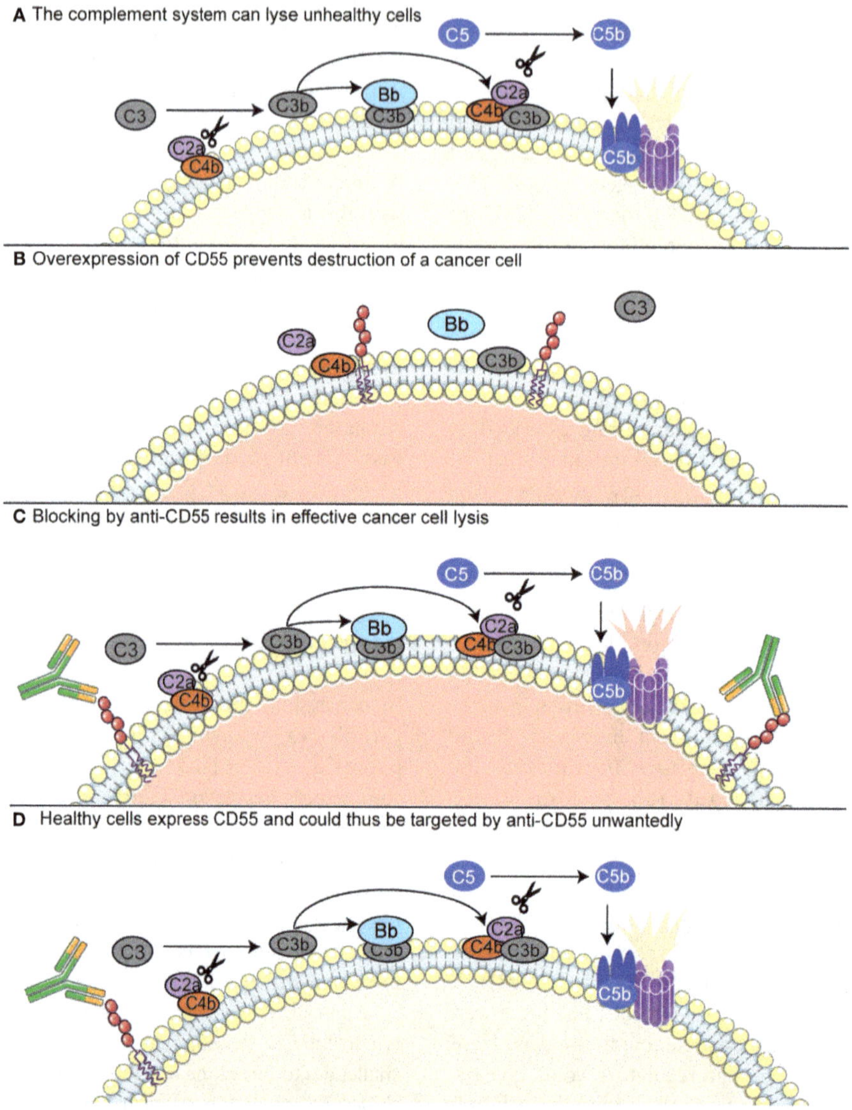

FIGURE 4 | Antibodies targeting complement regulators. Antibodies targeting complement regulators can be used as immunotherapy in cancer, as some cancer types upregulate these regulators. CD55 has been shown to be overexpressed in NSCLC and colon cancer. **(A)** The complement system contributes to killing of unhealthy cells, such as cancer cells, both *via* lysis by the MAC and opsonization inducing phagocytosis (not depicted here). For MAC-mediated lysis, the complement system depends on C5 convertase (CP convertase depicted here) formation. **(B)** Cancer cells overexpressing CD55 are protected from the complement system, as CD55 has a decay accelerating activity on the C3 convertases. **(C)** An anti-CD55 antibody targets the CD55-overexpressing cancer cells and inhibits the complement regulatory activity of CD55. Thus, the cancer cells are resensitized to the complement system. **(D)** Healthy cells, conventionally expressing CD55, can also be targeted by anti-CD55 and lysed unwantedly. Figure designed using Servier Medical Art.

complement modulators used in previous studies, for example in AMD, or whether a different treatment strategy should be pursued altogether.

The current research also indicates some starting points for the development of future therapeutics, if the abovementioned limitations with regards to specificity and half-time can be overcome. One clear shortcoming of the currently available therapeutics, is that there is no possibility to target the complement system at the C3 level specifically on the target tissue. As has been described above, there is a clear need for this in specific groups of PNH patients, that suffer from extravascular hemolysis under eculizumab treatment. Potentially, treatments based on complement regulatory proteins that target C3, could be a solution there, as for example FH-CR2, miniFH and anti-FH07 (197, 218). Next, the successful *in vivo* tests of FH-IgG chimeric proteins in bacterial infections, indicate that there might lie success in similar approaches using C4BP, C1-INH or Vn, which all are used by bacteria in complement evasion mechanisms (19). Lastly, future research could focus at the development of plasma-purified complement regulators other than C1-INH. Successful plasma-purification could especially be useful for FH and FI, of which mutations have been shown to affect several eye and kidney diseases and of which recombinant variants have not yet been successfully tested in a clinical setting (106, 226).

To conclude, we have described the significant role of complement regulators in a broad range of diseases. Currently, there are many therapeutics under development that use complement regulators, ranging from full-length and engineered regulators to antibodies targeting complement regulators. Altogether, the current research shows several promising directions for future clinical studies and applications of complement therapeutics based on regulators.

AUTHOR CONTRIBUTIONS

All authors contributed to the article and approved the submitted version.

FUNDING

This work is part of the research programme Aspasia with project number 015.014.069, which is (partly) financed by the Netherlands Organisation for Scientific Research (NWO).

REFERENCES

1. Ehrnthaller C, Ignatius A, Gebhard F, Huber-Lang M. New insights of an old defense system: Structure, function, and clinical relevance of the complement system. *Mol Med* (2011) 17(3–4):317–29. doi: 10.2119/molmed.2010.00149
2. Nesargikar P, Spiller B, Chavez R. The complement system: History, pathways, cascade and inhibitors. *Eur J Microbiol Immunol* (2012) 2 (2):103–11. doi: 10.1556/EuJMI.2.2012.2.2
3. Merle NS, Church SE, Fremeaux-Bacchi V, Roumenina LT. Complement system part I - molecular mechanisms of activation and regulation. *Front Immunol* (2015) 6:1–30. doi: 10.3389/fimmu.2015.00262
4. Harris CL. Expanding horizons in complement drug discovery: challenges and emerging strategies. *Semin Immunopathol* (2017) 40(1):125–40. doi: 10.1007/s00281-017-0655-8
5. Ricklin D, Hajishengallis G, Yang K, Lambris JD. Complement: A key system for immune surveillance and homeostasis. *Nat Immunol* (2010) 11 (9):785–97. doi: 10.1038/ni.1923
6. Mathern DR, Heeger PS. Molecules great and small: The complement system. *Clin J Am Soc Nephrol* (2015) 10(9):1636–50. doi: 10.2215/CJN.06230614
7. Garred P, Genster N, Pilely K, Bayarri-Olmos R, Rosbjerg A, Ma YJ, et al. A journey through the lectin pathway of complement—MBL and beyond. *Immunol Rev* (2016) 274(1):74–97. doi: 10.1111/imr.12468
8. Bexborn F, Andersson PO, Chen H, Nilsson B, Ekdahl KN. The tick-over theory revisited: Formation and regulation of the soluble alternative complement C3 convertase (C3(H2O)Bb). *Mol Immunol* (2008) 45 (8):2370–9. doi: 10.1016/j.molimm.2007.11.003
9. Harboe M, Ulvund G, Vien L, Fung M, Mollnes TE. The quantitative role of alternative pathway amplification in classical pathway induced terminal complement activation. *Clin Exp Immunol* (2004) 138(3):439–46. doi: 10.1111/j.1365-2249.2004.02627.x
10. Harboe M, Garred P, Karlstrøm E, Lindstad JK, Stahl GL, Mollnes TE. The down-stream effects of mannan-induced lectin complement pathway activation depend quantitatively on alternative pathway amplification. *Mol Immunol* (2009) 47(2–3):373–80. doi: 10.1016/j.molimm.2009.09.005
11. Merle NS, Noe R, Halbwachs-Mecarelli L, Fremeaux-Bacchi V, Roumenina LT. Complement system part II: Role in immunity. *Front Immunol* (2015) 6 (MAY):1–26. doi: 10.3389/fimmu.2015.00257
12. West EE, Kunz N, Kemper C. Complement and human T cell metabolism: location, location, location. *Immunol Rev* (2020) 295(1):68–81. doi: 10.1111/imr.12852
13. West EE, Kemper C. Complement and T Cell Metabolism: Food for Thought. *Immunometabolism* (2019) 1(T Cell Metabolic Reprogramming): e190006. doi: 10.1111/imr.12852
14. Liszewski MK, Kolev M, Le Friec G, Leung M, Bertram PG, Fara AF, et al. Intracellular Complement Activation Sustains T Cell Homeostasis and Mediates Effector Differentiation. *Immunity* (2013) 39(6):1143–57. doi: 10.1016/j.immuni.2013.10.018
15. Trouw LA, Blom AM, Gasque P. Role of complement and complement regulators in the removal of apoptotic cells. *Mol Immunol* (2008) 45:1199–207. doi: 10.1016/j.molimm.2007.09.008
16. Silverman SM, Ma W, Wang X, Zhao L, Wong WT. C3- And CR3-dependent microglial clearance protects photoreceptors in retinitis pigmentosa. *J Exp Med* (2019) 216(8):1925–43. doi: 10.1084/jem.20190009
17. Veerhuis R, Nielsen HM, Tenner AJ. Complement in the brain. *Mol Immunol* (2011) 48(14):1592–603. doi: 10.1016/j.molimm.2011.04.003
18. Ojha H, Ghosh P, Singh Panwar H, Shende R, Gondane A, Mande SC, et al. Spatially conserved motifs in complement control protein domains determine functionality in regulators of complement activation-family proteins. *Commun Biol* (2019) 2(1):1–12. doi: 10.1038/s42003-019-0529-9
19. Hovingh ES, van den Broek B, Jongerius I. Hijacking complement regulatory proteins for bacterial immune evasion. *Front Microbiol* (2016) 7(DEC):1–20. doi: 10.3389/fmicb.2016.02004
20. Ermert D, Ram S, Laabei M. The hijackers guide to escaping complement: Lessons learned from pathogens. *Mol Immunol* (2019) 114:49–61. doi: 10.1016/j.molimm.2019.07.018
21. Nilsson SC, Sim RB, Lea SM, Fremeaux-Bacchi V, Blom AM. Complement factor I in health and disease. *Mol Immunol* (2011) 48:1611–20. doi: 10.1016/j.molimm.2011.04.004
22. Zipfel PF, Skerka C. Complement regulators and inhibitory proteins. *Nat Rev Immunol* (2009) 9(10):729–40. doi: 10.1038/nri2620
23. Davis AE, Mejia P, Lu F. Biological activities of C1 inhibitor. *Mol Immunol* (2008) 45:4057–63. doi: 10.1016/j.molimm.2008.06.028
24. Zeerleder S. C1-inhibitor: More than a serine protease inhibitor. *Semin Thromb Hemost* (2011) 37(4):362–74. doi: 10.1055/s-0031-1276585
25. Blaum BS, Hannan JP, Herbert AP, Kavanagh D, Uhrín D, Stehle T. Structural basis for sialic acid-mediated self-recognition by complement factor H. *Nat Chem Biol* (2015) 11(1):77–82. doi: 10.1038/nchembio.1696
26. Parente R, Clark SJ, Inforzato A, Day AJ. Complement factor H in host defense and immune evasion. *Cell Mol Life Sci* (2017) 74:1605–24. doi: 10.1007/s00018-016-2418-4
27. Dopler A, Guntau L, Harder MJ, Palmer A, Höchsmann B, Schrezenmeier H, et al. Self versus Nonself Discrimination by the Soluble Complement Regulators Factor H and FHL-1. *J Immunol* (2019) 202(7):2082–94. doi: 10.4049/jimmunol.1801545
28. Clark SJ, Schmidt CQ, White AM, Hakobyan S, Morgan BP, Bishop PN. Identification of Factor H-like Protein 1 as the Predominant Complement Regulator in Bruch's Membrane: Implications for Age-Related Macular Degeneration. *J Immunol* (2014) 193(10):4962–70. doi: 10.4049/jimmunol.1401613
29. Skerka C, Chen Q, Fremeaux-Bacchi V, Roumenina LT. Complement factor H related proteins (CFHRs). *Mol Immunol [Internet]* (2013) 56(3):170–80. doi: 10.1016/j.molimm.2013.06.001
30. Józsi M. Factor H family proteins in complement evasion of microorganisms. *Front Immunol* (2017) 8:1–8. doi: 10.3389/fimmu.2017.00571
31. Józsi M, Tortajada A, Uzonyi B, Goicoechea de Jorge E, Rodríguez de Córdoba S. Factor H-related proteins determine complement-activating surfaces. *Trends Immunol* (2015) 36:374–84. doi: 10.1016/j.it.2015.04.008
32. Cipriani V, Lorés-Motta L, He F, Fathalla D, Tilakaratna V, McHarg S, et al. Increased circulating levels of Factor H-Related Protein 4 are strongly associated with age-related macular degeneration. *Nat Commun* (2020) 11 (1):1–15. doi: 10.1038/s41467-020-14499-3

33. Java A, Liszewski MK, Hourcade DE, Zhang F, Atkinson JP. Role of complement receptor 1 (CR1; CD35) on epithelial cells: A model for understanding complement-mediated damage in the kidney. *Mol Immunol* (2015) 67(2):584–95. doi: 10.1016/j.molimm.2015.07.016
34. Khera R, Das N. Complement Receptor 1: Disease associations and therapeutic implications. *Mol Immunol* (2009) 46:761–72. doi: 10.1016/j.molimm.2008.09.026
35. Ernst JD. Macrophage Receptors for Mycobacterium tuberculosis. *Infect Immun* (1998) 66(4):1277–81. doi: 10.1128/IAI.66.4.1277-1281.1998
36. Liszewski MK, Kemper C. Complement in Motion: The Evolution of CD46 from a Complement Regulator to an Orchestrator of Normal Cell Physiology. *J Immunol* (2019) 203(1):3–5. doi: 10.4049/jimmunol.1900527
37. Ni Choileain S, Astier AL. CD46 processing: A means of expression. *Immunobiology* (2012) 217:169–75. doi: 10.1016/j.imbio.2011.06.003
38. Small AG, Al-Baghdadi M, Quach A, Hii C, Ferrante A. Complement receptor immunoglobulin: a control point in infection and immunity, inflammation and cancer. *Swiss Med Wkly* (2016) 146(April):w14301. doi: 10.4414/smw.2016.14301
39. He JQ, Wiesmann C, van Lookeren Campagne M. A role of macrophage complement receptor CRIg in immune clearance and inflammation. *Mol Immunol* (2008) 45(16):4041–7. doi: 10.1016/j.molimm.2008.07.011
40. Kim DD, Song WC. Membrane complement regulatory proteins. *Clin Immunol* (2006) 118(2–3):127–36. doi: 10.1016/j.clim.2005.10.014
41. Zelek WM, Xie L, Morgan BP, Harris CL. Compendium of current complement therapeutics. *Mol Immunol* (2019) 114(July):341–52. doi: 10.1016/j.molimm.2019.07.030
42. Harris CL, Pouw RB, Kavanagh D, Sun R, Ricklin D. Developments in anti-complement therapy; from disease to clinical trial. *Mol Immunol* (2018) 102 (May):89–119. doi: 10.1016/j.molimm.2018.06.008
43. Kawai T, Takeshita S, Imoto Y, Matsumoto Y, Sakashita M, Suzuki D, et al. Associations between decay-accelerating factor polymorphisms and allergic respiratory diseases. *Clin Exp Allergy* (2009) 39(10):1508–14. doi: 10.1111/j.1365-2222.2009.03316.x
44. Vogt SD, Curcio CA, Wang L, Li CM, McGwin G, Medeiros NE, et al. Retinal pigment epithelial expression of complement regulator CD46 is altered early in the course of geographic atrophy. *Exp Eye Res* (2011) 93 (4):413–23. doi: 10.1016/j.exer.2011.06.002
45. Goetzl EJ, Yaffe K, Peltz CB, Ledreux A, Gorgens K, Davidson B, et al. Traumatic brain injury increases plasma astrocyte-derived exosome levels of neurotoxic complement proteins. *FASEB J* (2020) 34(2):3359–66. doi: 10.1096/fj.201902842R
46. Mohlin FC, Mercier E, Fremeaux-Bacchi V, Liszewski MK, Atkinson JP, Gris JC, et al. Analysis of genes coding for CD46, CD55, and C4b-binding protein in patients with idiopathic, recurrent, spontaneous pregnancy loss. *Eur J Immunol* (2013) 43(6):1617–29. doi: 10.1002/eji.201243196
47. de Vries MA, Trompet S, Mooijaart SP, Smit RAJ, Böhringer S, Castro Cabezas M, et al. Complement receptor 1 gene polymorphisms are associated with cardiovascular risk. *Atherosclerosis* (2017) 257:16–21. doi: 10.1016/j.atherosclerosis.2016.12.017
48. Kardys I, Klaver CCW, Despriet DDG, Bergen AAB, Uitterlinden AG, Hofman A, et al. A Common Polymorphism in the Complement Factor H Gene Is Associated With Increased Risk of Myocardial Infarction. The Rotterdam Study. *J Am Coll Cardiol* (2006) 47(8):1568–75. doi: 10.1016/j.jacc.2005.11.076
49. Nishio N, Teranishi M, Uchida Y, Sugiura S, Ando F, Shimokata H, et al. Contribution of complement factor H Y402H polymorphism to sudden sensorineural hearing loss risk and possible interaction with diabetes. *Gene* (2012) 499(1):226–30. doi: 10.1016/j.gene.2012.02.027
50. Zorzetto M, Ferrarotti I, Trisolini R, Agli LL, Scabini R, Novo M, et al. Complement receptor 1 gene polymorphisms are associated with idiopathic pulmonary fibrosis. *Am J Respir Crit Care Med* (2003) 168(3):330–4. doi: 10.1164/rccm.200302-221OC
51. Banadakoppa M, Balakrishnan M, Yallampalli C. Common variants of fetal and maternal complement genes in preeclampsia: pregnancy specific complotype. *Sci Rep* (2020) 10(1):1–9. doi: 10.1038/s41598-020-60539-9
52. Asimakopoulos JV, Terpos E, Papageorgiou L, Kampouropoulou O, Christoulas D, Giakoumis A, et al. The presence of CD55- and/or CD59-deficient erythrocytic populations in patients with rheumatic diseases reflects an immunemediated bone-marrow derived phenomenon. *Med Sci Monit* (2014) 20:123–39. doi: 10.12659/MSM.889727
53. Zhou Y, Wang J, Wang K, Li S, Song X, Ye Y, et al. Association analysis between the rs11136000 single nucleotide polymorphism in clusterin gene, rs3851179 single nucleotide polymorphism in clathrin assembly lymphoid myeloid protein gene and the patients with schizophrenia in the Chinese population. *DNA Cell Biol* (2010) 29(12):745–51. doi: 10.1089/dna.2010.1075
54. Flegel WA. Pathogenesis and mechanisms of antibody-mediated hemolysis. *Transfusion* (2015) 55(July):S47–58. doi: 10.1111/trf.13147
55. Rosti V. The molecular basis of paroxysmal nocturnal hemoglobinuria. *Hametologica* (2000) 85:82–7. doi: 10.3324/%25x
56. Takeda J, Miyata T, Kawagoe K, Iida Y, Endo Y, Fujita T, et al. Deficiency of the GPI anchor caused by a somatic mutation of the PIG-A gene in paroxysmal nocturnal hemoglobinuria. *Cell* (1993) 73(4):703–11. doi: 10.1016/0092-8674(93)90250-T
57. Lee SCW, Abdel-Wahab O. The mutational landscape of paroxysmal nocturnal hemoglobinuria revealed: New insights into clonal dominance. *J Clin Invest* (2014) 124(10):4227–30. doi: 10.1172/JCI77984
58. Brodsky RA, Young NS, Antonioli E, Risitano AM, Schrezenmeier H, Gaya A, et al. Multicenter phase 3 study of eculizumab for the treatment of PNH. *Blood* (2008) 111(4):1840–7. doi: 10.1182/blood-2007-06-094136
59. Hillmen P, Young NS, Schubert J, Brodsky RA, Socié G, Muus P, et al. The complement inhibitor eculizumab in paroxysmal nocturnal hemoglobinuria. *N Engl J Med* (2006) 355(12):1233–43. doi: 10.1056/NEJMoa061648
60. Socié G, Caby-Tosi MP, Marantz JL, Cole A, Bedrosian CL, Gasteyger C, et al. Eculizumab in paroxysmal nocturnal haemoglobinuria and atypical haemolytic uraemic syndrome: 10-year pharmacovigilance analysis. *Br J Haematol* (2019) 185(2):297–310. doi: 10.1111/bjh.15790
61. Nishimura JI, Yamamoto M, Hayashi S, Ohyashiki K, Ando K, Brodsky AL, et al. Genetic variants in C5 and poor response to eculizumab. *N Engl J Med* (2014) 370(7):632–9. doi: 10.1056/NEJMoa1311084
62. Lin Z, Schmidt CQ, Koutsogiannaki S, Ricci P, Risitano AM, Lambris JD, et al. Complement C3dg-mediated erythrophagocytosis: Implications for paroxysmal nocturnal hemoglobinuria. *Blood* (2015) 126(7):891–4. doi: 10.1182/blood-2015-02-625871
63. Rondelli T, Risitano AM, de Latour RP, Sica M, Peruzzi B, Ricci P, et al. Polymorphism of the complement receptor 1 gene correlates with the hematologic response to eculizumab in patients with paroxysmal nocturnal hemoglobinuria. *Haematologica* (2014) 99(2):262–6. doi: 10.3324/haematol.2013.090001
64. Baas I, Delvasto-Nuñez L, Ligthart, Peter Brouwer C, Folman C, Reis ES, et al. Complement C3 inhibition by compstatin Cp40 prevents intra- and extravascular hemolysis of red blood cells. *Haemotologica* (2020) 105 (57):471–3. doi: 10.3324/haematol.2019.216028
65. Mastellos DC, Yancopoulou D, Kokkinos P, Huber-Lang M, Hajishengallis G, Biglarnia AR, et al. Compstatin: A C3-targeted complement inhibitor reaching its prime for bedside intervention. *Eur J Clin Invest* (2015) 45:423–40. doi: 10.1111/eci.12419
66. Risitano AM, Marotta S, Ricci P, Marano L, Frieri C, Cacace F, et al. Anti-complement Treatment for Paroxysmal Nocturnal Hemoglobinuria: Time for proximal complement inhibition? A position paper from the SAAWP of the EBMT. *Front Immunol* (2019) 10(4):43–52. doi: 10.3389/fimmu.2019.01157
67. Haliloglu G, Maluenda J, Sayinbatur B, Aumont C, Temucin C, Tavil B, et al. Early-onset chronic axonal neuropathy, strokes, and hemolysis. *Neurology* (2015) 84:1220–4. doi: 10.1212/WNL.0000000000001391
68. Karbian N, Eshed-Eisenbach Y, Tabib A, Hoizman H, Paul Morgan B, Schueler-Furman O, et al. Molecular pathogenesis of human CD59 deficiency. *Neurol Genet* (2018) 4(6):1–9. doi: 10.1212/NXG.0000000000000280
69. Lublin DM. Cromer and DAF: role in health and disease. *Immunohematology* (2005) 21(2):39–47.
70. Hue-Roye K, Powell VI, Patel G, Lane D, Maguire M, Chung A, et al. Novel molecular basis of an Inab phenotype. *Immunohematology* (2005) 21(2):53–5.
71. Holguin MH, Martin CB, Bernshaw NJ, Parker CJ. Analysis of the effects of activation of the alternative pathway of complement on erythrocytes with an isolated deficiency of decay accelerating factor. *J Immunol* (1992) 148 (2):498–502.

72. Kurolap ARN, Eshach-Adiv O, Hershkovitz T, Paperna T, Mory A, Oz-Levi D, et al. Loss of CD55 in Eculizumab-Responsive Protein-Losing Enteropathy. *N Engl J Med* (2017) 377:87–9. doi: 10.1056/NEJMc1707173
73. Ozen A, Comrie WA, Ardy RC, Conde CD, Dalgic B, Beser ÖF, et al. CD55 deficiency, early-onset protein-losing enteropathy, and thrombosis. *N Engl J Med* (2017) 377(1):52–61. doi: 10.1056/NEJMoa1615887
74. Ozen A. CHAPLE syndrome uncovers the primary role of complement in a familial form of Waldmann's disease. *Immunol Rev* (2019) 287(1):20–32. doi: 10.1111/imr.12715
75. Shichishima T, Saitoh Y, Terasawa T, Noji H, Kai T, Maruyama Y. Complement sensitivity of erythrocytes in a patient with inherited complete deficiency of CD59 or with the Inab phenotype. *Br J Haematol* (1999) 104(2):303–6. doi: 10.1046/j.1365-2141.1999.01188.x
76. Mohandas N. Inherited hemolytic anemia: A possessive beginner's guide. *Hematology* (2018) 2018(1):377–81. doi: 10.1182/asheducation-2018.1.377
77. Wastnedge E, Waters D, Patel S, Morrison K, Goh MY, Adeloye D, et al. The global burden of sickle cell disease in children under five years of age: A systematic review and meta-analysis. *J Glob Health* (2018) 8(2):1–9. doi: 10.7189/jogh.08.021103
78. Loniewska-Lwowska A, Koza K, Mendek-Czajkowska E, Wieszczy P, Adamowicz-Salach A, Branicka K, et al. Diminished presentation of complement regulatory protein CD55 on red blood cells from patients with hereditary haemolytic anaemias. *Int J Lab Hematol* (2018) 40(2):128–35. doi: 10.1111/ijlh.12752
79. Al-Faris L, Al-Rukhayes M, Al-Humood S. Expression pattern of CD55 and CD59 on red blood cells in sickle cell disease. *Hematology* (2017) 22(2):105–13. doi: 10.1080/10245332.2016.1231988
80. Roumenina LT, Chadebech P, Bodivit G, Vieira-Martins P, Grunenwald A, Boudhabhay I, et al. Complement activation in sickle cell disease: Dependence on cell density, hemolysis and modulation by hydroxyurea therapy. *Am J Hematol* (2020) 95(5):456–64. doi: 10.1002/ajh.25742
81. De Vriese AS, Sethi S, Van Praet J, Nath KA, Fervenza FC. Kidney disease caused by dysregulation of the complement alternative pathway: An etiologic approach. *J Am Soc Nephrol* (2015) 26(12):2917–29. doi: 10.1681/ASN.2015020184
82. Jayadev R, Sherwood DR. Basement membranes. *Curr Biol* (2017) 27(6): R207–11. doi: 10.1016/j.cub.2017.02.006
83. Wong EKS, Kavanagh D. Diseases of complement dysregulation—an overview. *Semin Immunopathol* (2018) 40(1):49–64. doi: 10.1007/s00281-017-0663-8
84. Raina R, Krishnappa V, Blaha T, Kann T, Hein W, Burke L, et al. Atypical Hemolytic-Uremic Syndrome: An Update on Pathophysiology, Diagnosis, and Treatment. *Ther Apher Dial* (2019) 23(1):4–21. doi: 10.1111/1744-9987.12763
85. De Córdoba SR. aHUS: A disorder with many risk factors. *Blood* (2010) 115 (2):158–60. doi: 10.1182/blood-2009-11-252627
86. Nester CM, Barbour T, de Cordoba SR, Dragon-Durey MA, Fremeaux-Bacchi V, Goodship THJ, et al. Atypical aHUS: State of the art. *Mol Immunol [Internet]* (2015) 67(1):31–42. doi: 10.1016/j.molimm.2015.03.246
87. Arjona E, Huerta A, Goicoechea De Jorge E, Rodríguez de Córdoba S. The familial risk of developing atypical Hemolytic Uremic Syndrome. *Blood* (2020) 136(13):1558–61. doi: 10.1182/blood.2020006931
88. Urban A, Volokhina E, Felberg A, Stasiłojć G, Blom AM, Jongerius I, et al. Gain-of-function mutation in complement C2 protein identified in a patient with aHUS. *J Allergy Clin Immunol* (2020) 146(4):1–4 doi: 10.1016/j.jaci.2020.02.014
89. Moore I, Strain L, Pappworth I, Kavanagh D, Barlow PN, Herbert AP, et al. Association of factor H autoantibodies with deletions of CFHR1, CFHR3, CFHR4, and with mutations in CFH, CFI, CD46, and C3 in patients with atypical hemolytic uremic syndrome. *Blood* (2010) 115(2):379–87. doi: 10.1182/blood-2009-05-221549
90. Strobel S, Dahse H, Liu W, Hoyer PF, Oppermann M, Skerka C, et al. Brief report Anti – factor H autoantibodies block C-terminal recognition function of factor H in hemolytic uremic syndrome. *Blood* (2007) 110(5):1516–8. doi: 10.1182/blood-2007-02-071472
91. Sánchez-Corral P, Pérez-Caballero D, Huarte O, Simckes AM, Goicoechea E, López-Trascasa M, et al. Structural and functional characterization of factor H mutations associated with atypical hemolytic uremic syndrome. *Am J Hum Genet* (2002) 71(6):1285–95. doi: 10.1086/344515
92. Caprioli J, Noris M, Brioschi S, Pianetti G, Castelletti F, Bettinaglio P, et al. Genetics of HUS: The impact of MCP, CFH, and IF mutations on clinical presentation, response to treatment, and outcome. *Blood* (2006) 108 (4):1267–79. doi: 10.1182/blood-2005-10-007252
93. Bajwa R, Depalma JA, Khan T, Cheema A, Kalathil SA, Hossain MA, et al. C3 Glomerulopathy and Atypical Hemolytic Uremic Syndrome: Two Important Manifestations of Complement System Dysfunction. *Case Rep Nephrol Dial* (2018) 8(1):25–34. doi: 10.1159/000486848
94. Servais A, Noël LH, Roumenina LT, Le Quintrec M, Ngo S, Dragon-Durey MA, et al. Acquired and genetic complement abnormalities play a critical role in dense deposit disease and other C3 glomerulopathies. *Kidney Int* (2012) 82(4):454–64. doi: 10.1038/ki.2012.63
95. Chauvet S, Roumenina LT, Bruneau S, Marinozzi MC, Rybkine T, Schramm EC, et al. A familial C3GN secondary to defective C3 regulation by complement receptor 1 and complement factor H. *J Am Soc Nephrol* (2016) 27(6):1665–77. doi: 10.1681/ASN.2015040348
96. Caravaca-Fontán F, Lucientes L, Cavero T, Praga M. Update on C3 Glomerulopathy: A Complement-Mediated Disease. *Nephron* (2020) 144 (6):1–9. doi: 10.1159/000507254
97. Yeo SC, Liu X, Liew A. Complement factor H gene polymorphism rs6677604 and the risk, severity and progression of IgA nephropathy: A systematic review and meta-analysis. *Nephrology* (2018) 23(12):1096–106. doi: 10.1111/nep.13210
98. Webster AC, Nagler EV, Morton RL, Masson P. Chronic Kidney Disease. *Lancet* (2017) 389(10075):1238–52. doi: 10.1016/S0140-6736(16)32064-5
99. McClellan W, Aronoff SL, Bolton WK, Hood S, Lorber DL, Tang KL, et al. The prevalence of anemia in patients with chronic kidney disease. *Curr Med Res Opin* (2004) 20(9):1501–10. doi: 10.1185/030079904X2763
100. Al-Faris L, Al-Humood S, Behbehani F, Sallam H. Altered expression pattern of CD55 and CD59 on red blood cells in Anemia of Chronic Kidney Disease. *Med Princ Pract* (2018) 26(6):516–22. doi: 10.1159/000481823
101. Zhang G, Eddy AA. Urokinase and its receptors in chronic kidney disease. *Front Biosci* (2008) 13(14):5462–78. doi: 10.2741/3093
102. Clark SJ, McHarg S, Tilakaratna V, Brace N, Bishop PN. Bruch ' s Membrane compartmentalizes complement regulation in the eye with implications for Therapeutic Design in age-related Macular Degeneration. *Front Immunol* (2017) 8(December):1–10. doi: 10.3389/fimmu.2017.01778
103. Clark SJ, Bishop PN. The eye as a complement dysregulation hotspot. *Semin Immunopathol* (2018) 40(1):65–74. doi: 10.1007/s00281-017-0649-6
104. Geerlings MJ, de Jong EK, den Hollander AI. The complement system in age-related macular degeneration: A review of rare genetic variants and implications for personalized treatment. *Mol Immunol* (2017) 84:65–76. doi: 10.1016/j.molimm.2016.11.016
105. Toomey CB, Johnson LV, Bowes Rickman C. Complement factor H in AMD: Bridging genetic associations and pathobiology. *Prog Retin Eye Res* (2018) 62:38–57. doi: 10.1016/j.preteyeres.2017.09.001
106. Kavanagh D, Yu Y, Schramm EC, Triebwasser M, Wagner EK, Raychaudhuri S, et al. Rare genetic variants in the CFI gene are associated with advanced age-related macular degeneration and commonly result in reduced serum factor I levels. *Hum Mol Genet* (2015) 24(13):3861–70. doi: 10.1093/hmg/ddv091
107. Fritsche LG, Igl W, Bailey JNC, Grassmann F, Sengupta S, Bragg-Gresham JL, et al. A large genome-wide association study of age-related macular degeneration highlights contributions of rare and common variants. *Nat Genet* (2016) 48(2):134–43. doi: 10.1038/ng.3448
108. Hughes AE, Orr N, Esfandiary H, Diaz-Torres M, Goodship T, Chakravarthy U. A common CFH haplotype, with deletion of CFHR1 and CFHR3, is associated with lower risk of age-related macular degeneration. *Nat Genet* (2006) 38 (10):1173–7. doi: 10.1038/ng1890
109. Sánchez-Corral P, Pouw RB, López-Trascasa M, Józsi M. Self-damage caused by dysregulation of the complement alternative pathway: Relevance of the factor H protein family. *Front Immunol* (2018) 9(JUL):1–19. doi: 10.3389/fimmu.2018.01607
110. Schäfer N, Grosche A, Reinders J, Hauck SM, Pouw RB, Kuijpers TW, et al. Complement regulator FHR-3 is elevated either locally or systemically in a

selection of autoimmune diseases. *Front Immunol* (2016) 7(NOV):1–16. doi: 10.3389/fimmu.2016.00542
111. Tekin K, Inanc M, Elgin U. Monitoring and management of the patient with pseudoexfoliation syndrome: Current perspectives. *Clin Ophthalmol* (2019) 13:453–64. doi: 10.2147/OPTH.S181444
112. Botling Taube A, Konzer A, Alm A, Bergquist J. Proteomic analysis of the aqueous humour in eyes with pseudoexfoliation syndrome. *Br J Ophthalmol* (2019) 103(8):1190–4. doi: 10.1136/bjophthalmol-2017-310416
113. Zenkel M, Kruse FE, Jünemann AG, Naumann GOH, Schlötzer-Schrehardt U. Clusterin Deficiency in Eyes with Pseudoexfoliation Syndrome May Be Implicated in the Aggregation and Deposition of Pseudoexfoliative Material. *Invest Ophthalmol Vis Sci* (2006) 47(5):1982–90. doi: 10.1167/iovs.05-1580
114. Wyatt AR, Yerbury JJ, Berghofer P, Greguric I, Katsifis A, Dobson CM, et al. Clusterin facilitates in vivo clearance of extracellular misfolded proteins. *Cell Mol Life Sci* (2011) 68(23):3919–31. doi: 10.1007/s00018-011-0684-8
115. Burdon KP, Sharma S, Hewitt AW, McMellon AE, Wang JJ, Mackey DA, et al. Genetic analysis of the clusterin gene in pseudoexfoliation syndrome. *Mol Vis* (2008) 14(August):1727–36.
116. Kuot A, Hewitt AW, Griggs K, Klebe S, Mills R, Jhanji V, et al. Association of TCF4 and CLU polymorphisms with Fuchs endothelial dystrophy and implication of CLU and TGFBI proteins in the disease process. *Eur J Hum Genet* (2012) 20(6):632–8. doi: 10.1038/ejhg.2011.248
117. Cheng CY, Schache M, Ikram MK, Young TL, Guggenheim JA, Vitart V, et al. Nine loci for ocular axial length identified through genome-wide association studies, including shared loci with refractive error. *Am J Hum Genet* (2013) 93(2):264–77. doi: 10.1016/j.ajhg.2013.06.016
118. Yoshikawa M, Yamashiro K, Miyake M, Oishi M, Akagi-Kurashige Y, Kumagai K, et al. Comprehensive replication of the relationship between myopia-related genes and refractive errors in a large Japanese cohort. *Invest Ophthalmol Vis Sci* (2014) 55(11):7343–54. doi: 10.1167/iovs.14-15105
119. Long Q, Ye J, Li Y, Wang S, Jiang Y. C-reactive protein and complement components in patients with pathological myopia. *Optom Vis Sci* (2013) 90 (5):501–6. doi: 10.1097/OPX.0b013e31828daa6e
120. Mohlin C, Sandholm K, Kvanta A, Ekdahl KN, Johansson K. A model to study complement involvement in experimental retinal degeneration. *Ups J Med Sci* (2018) 123(1):28–42. doi: 10.1080/03009734.2018.1431744
121. Lyzogubov VV, Bora PS, Wu X, Horn LE, de Roque R, Rudolf XR, et al. The Complement Regulatory Protein CD46 Deficient Mouse Spontaneously Develops Dry-Type Age-Related Macular Degeneration-Like Phenotype. *Am J Pathol* (2016) 186(8):2088–2104. doi: 10.1016/j.ajpath.2016.03.021
122. Morgan BP. Complement in the pathogenesis of Alzheimer's disease. *Semin Immunopathol* (2018) 40(1):113–24. doi: 10.1007/s00281-017-0662-9
123. Lee JD, Coulthard LG, Woodruff TM. Complement dysregulation in the central nervous system during development and disease. *Semin Immunol* (2019) 45(June):1–13. doi: 10.1016/j.smim.2019.101340
124. Foster EM, Dangla-Valls A, Lovestone S, Ribe EM, Buckley NJ. Clusterin in Alzheimer's disease: Mechanisms, genetics, and lessons from other pathologies. *Front Neurosci* (2019) 13(FEB):1–27. doi: 10.3389/fnins.2019.00164
125. Yang J, Wise L, Fukuchi KI. TLR4 Cross-Talk With NLRP3 Inflammasome and Complement Signaling Pathways in Alzheimer's Disease. *Front Immunol* (2020) 11(April):1–16. doi: 10.3389/fimmu.2020.00724
126. Misra A, Charkabati SS, Gambhir IS. New genetic players in late-onset Alzheimer's disease: Findings of genome-wide association studies. *Indian J Med Res* (2018) 148):135–44. doi: 10.4103/ijmr.IJMR_473_17
127. Lambert JC, Heath S, Even G, Campion D, Sleegers K, Hiltunen M, et al. Genome-wide association study identifies variants at CLU and CR1 associated with Alzheimer's disease. *Nat Genet* (2009) 41(10):1094–9. doi: 10.1038/ng.439
128. Figueiredo Almeida JF, Ramos dos Santos L, Trancozo M, de Paula F. Updated Meta-Analysis of BIN1, CR1, MS4A6A, CLU,and ABCA7 Variants in Alzheimer's Disease. *J Mol Neurosci* (2018) 64:471–7. doi: 10.1007/s12031-018-1045-y
129. Shen N, Chen B, Jiang Y, Feng R, Liao M, Zhang L, et al. An Updated Analysis with 85,939 Samples Confirms the Association Between CR1 rs6656401 Polymorphism and Alzheimer's Disease. *Mol Neurobiol* (2015) 51(3):1017–23. doi: 10.1007/s12035-014-8761-2
130. Fonseca MI, Chu S, Pierce AL, Brubaker WD, Hauhart RE, Mastroeni D, et al. Analysis of the putative role of CR1 in Alzheimer's disease: Genetic association, expression and function. *PloS One* (2016) 11(2):1–21. doi: 10.1371/journal.pone.0149792
131. Kucukkilic E, Brookes K, Barber I, Guetta-Baranes T, Morgan K, Hollox EJ. Complement receptor 1 gene (CR1) intragenic duplication and risk of Alzheimer's disease. *Hum Genet* (2018) 137(4):305–14. doi: 10.1007/s00439-018-1883-2
132. Mahmoudi R, Feldman S, Kisserli A, Duret V, Tabary T, Bertholon LA, et al. Inherited and acquired decrease in complement receptor 1 (CR1) density on red blood cells associated with high levels of soluble CR1 in Alzheimer's disease. *Int J Mol Sci* (2018) 19(8):1–18. doi: 10.3390/ijms19082175
133. Loeffler DA, Camp DM, Conant SB. Complement activation in the Parkinson's disease substantia nigra: An immunocytochemical study. *J Neuroinflammation* (2006) 3:1–8. doi: 10.1186/1742-2094-3-29
134. Yamada T, McGeer PL, McGeer EG. Lewy bodies in Parkinson's disease are recognized by antibodies to complement proteins. *Acta Neuropathol* (1992) 84(1):100–4. doi: 10.1007/BF00427222
135. Gao J, Huang X, Park YY, Hollenbeck A, Chen H. An exploratory study on CLU, CR1 and PICALM and Parkinson disease. *PloS One* (2011) 6(8):4–8. doi: 10.1371/journal.pone.0024211
136. Van Dijk KD, Jongbloed W, Heijst JA, Teunissen CE, Groenewegen HJ, Berendse HW, et al. Cerebrospinal fluid and plasma clusterin levels in Parkinson's disease. *Parkinsonism Relat Disord* (2013) 19(12):1079–83. doi: 10.1016/j.parkreldis.2013.07.016
137. Roumenina LT, Daugan MV, Petitprez F, Sautès-Fridman C, Fridman WH. Context-dependent roles of complement in cancer. *Nat Rev Cancer* (2019) 19:698–715. doi: 10.1038/s41568-019-0210-0
138. Yu X, Rao J, Lin J, Zhang Z, Cao L, Zhang X. Tag SNPs in complement receptor-1 contribute to the susceptibility to non-small cell lung cancer. *Mol Cancer* (2014) 13(1):1–7. doi: 10.1186/1476-4598-13-56
139. Rutkowski MJ, Sughrue ME, Kane AJ, Mills SA, Parsa AT. Cancer and the complement cascade. *Mol Cancer Res* (2010) 8(11):1453–65. doi: 10.1158/1541-7786.MCR-10-0225
140. Pio R, Ajona D, Ortiz-Espinosa S, Mantovani A, Lambris JD. Complementing the cancer-immunity cycle. *Front Immunol* (2019) 10(APR):1–12. doi: 10.3389/fimmu.2019.00774
141. Ajona D, Ortiz-Espinosa S, Pio R. Complement anaphylatoxins C3a and C5a: Emerging roles in cancer progression and treatment. *Semin Cell Dev Biol* (2019) 85:153–63. doi: 10.1016/j.semcdb.2017.11.023
142. Geller A, Yan J. The role of membrane bound complement regulatory proteins in tumor development and cancer immunotherapy. *Front Immunol* (2019) 10(MAY):1–13. doi: 10.3389/fimmu.2019.01074
143. Xie YH, Chen YX, Fang JY. Comprehensive review of targeted therapy for colorectal cancer. *Signal Transduct Target Ther* (2020) 5(1):1–30. doi: 10.1038/s41392-020-0116-z
144. Nakagawa M, Mizuno M, Kawada M, Uesu T, Nasu J, Takeuchi K, et al. Polymorphic expression of decay-accelerating factor in human colorectal cancer. *J Gastroenterol Hepatol* (2001) 16:184–9. doi: 10.1046/j.1440-1746.2001.02418.x
145. Inoue H, Mizuno M, Uesu T, Ueki T, Tsuji T. Distribution of complement regulatory proteins, decay-accelerating factor, CD59/homologous restriction factor 20 and membrane cofactor protein in human colorectal adenoma and cancer. *Acta Med Okayama* (1994) 48(5):271–7. doi: 10.18926/AMO/31112
146. Shang Y, Chai N, Gu Y, Ding L, Yang Y, Zhou J, et al. Systematic immunohistochemical analysis of the expression of CD46, CD55, and CD59 in colon cancer. *Arch Pathol Lab Med* (2014) 138(7):910–9. doi: 10.5858/arpa.2013-0064-OA
147. Durrant LG, Chapman MA, Buckley DJ, Spendlove I, Robins RA, Armitage NC. Enhanced expression of the complement regulatory protein CD55 predicts a poor prognosis in colorectal cancer patients. *Cancer Immunol Immunother* (2003) 52(10):638–42. doi: 10.1007/s00262-003-0402-y
148. Mizuno M, Nakagawa M, Uesu T, Inoue H, Inaba T, Ueki T, et al. Detection of decay-accelerating factor in stool specimens of patients with colorectal cancer. *Gastroenterology* (1995) 109(3):826–31. doi: 10.1016/0016-5085(95)90390-9
149. Dho SH, Cho EH, Lee JY, Lee SY, Jung SH, Kim LK, et al. A novel therapeutic anti–CD55 monoclonal antibody inhibits the proliferation and metastasis of colorectal cancer cells. *Oncol Rep* (2019) 42(6):2686–93. doi: 10.3892/or.2019.7337

150. Kleczko EK, Kwak JW, Schenk EL, Nemenoff RA. Targeting the complement pathway as a therapeutic strategy in lung cancer. *Front Immunol* (2019) 10:1–16. doi: 10.3389/fimmu.2019.00954
151. Zhang Y, Zhang Z, Cao L, Lin J, Yang Z, Zhang X. A common CD55 rs2564978 variant is associated with the susceptibility of non-small cell lung cancer. *Oncotarget* (2017) 8(4):6216–21. doi: 10.18632/oncotarget.14053
152. Zhou J, To KKW, Dong H, Cheng ZS, Lau CCY, Poon VKM, et al. A functional variation in CD55 increases the severity of 2009 pandemic H1N1 influenza a virus infection. *J Infect Dis* (2012) 206(4):495–503. doi: 10.1093/infdis/jis378
153. Higuchi M, Endo Y, Suzuki H, Osuka F, Shio Y, Fujiu K, et al. Identification of the decay-accelerating factor CD55 as a peanut agglutinin-binding protein and its alteration in non-small cell lung cancers. *Clin Cancer Res* (2006) 12 (21):6367–72. doi: 10.1158/1078-0432.CCR-06-0836
154. Ajona D, Hsu Y-F, Corrales L, Montuenga LM, Pio R. Down-Regulation of Human Complement Factor H Sensitizes Non-Small Cell Lung Cancer Cells to Complement Attack and Reduces In Vivo Tumor Growth. *J Immunol* (2007) 178(9):5991–8. doi: 10.4049/jimmunol.178.9.5991
155. Sadallah S, Lach E, Schwarz S, Gratwohl A, Spertini O, Schifferli JA. Soluble complement receptor 1 is increased in patients with leukemia and after administration of granulocyte colony-stimulating factor. *J Leukoc Biol* (1999) 65(1):94–101. doi: 10.1002/jlb.65.1.94
156. Li JS, Jaggers J, Anderson PAW. The use of TP10, soluble complement receptor 1, in cardiopulmonary bypass. *Expert Rev Cardiovasc Ther* (2006) 4 (5):649–54. doi: 10.1586/14779072.4.5.649
157. Tomlinson S, Thurman JM. Tissue-targeted complement therapeutics. *Mol Immunol* (2018) 102:120–8. doi: 10.1016/j.molimm.2018.06.005
158. Mulligan MS, Yeh CG, Rudolph AR, Ward PA. Protective effects of soluble CR1 in complement- and neutrophil-mediated tissue injury. *J Immunol* (1992) 148(5):1479–85.
159. Singel KL, Emmons TR, Khan ANH, Mayor PC, Shen S, Wong JT, et al. Mature neutrophils suppress T cell immunity in ovarian cancer microenvironment. *JCI Insight* (2019) 4(5):1–19. doi: 10.1172/jci.insight.122311
160. Zhang R, Liu Q, Li T, Liao Q, Zhao Y. Role of the complement system in the tumor microenvironment. *Cancer Cell Int [Internet]* (2019) 19(1):1–12. doi: 10.1186/s12935-019-1027-3
161. Miranda-Filho A, Piñeros M, Znaor A, Marcos-Gragera R, Steliarova-Foucher E, Bray F. Global patterns and trends in the incidence of non-Hodgkin lymphoma. *Cancer Causes Control* (2019) 30(5):489–99. doi: 10.1007/s10552-019-01155-5
162. Charbonneau B, Maurer MJ, Fredericksen ZS, Zent CS, Link BK, Novak AJ, et al. Germline variation in complement genes and event-free survival in follicular and diffuse large B-cell lymphoma. *Am J Hematol* (2012) 87 (9):880–5. doi: 10.1002/ajh.23273
163. Rogers LM, Mott SL, Smith BJ, Link BK, Sahin D, Weiner GJ. Complement-regulatory proteins CFHR1 and CFHR3 and patient response to anti-CD20 monoclonal antibody therapy. *Clin Cancer Res* (2017) 23(4):954–61. doi: 10.1158/1078-0432.CCR-16-1275
164. Mastellos DC, Ricklin D, Lambris JD. Clinical promise of next-generation complement therapeutics. *Nat Rev Drug Discovery* (2019) 18(9):707–29. doi: 10.1038/s41573-019-0031-6
165. De Andrade LGM, Contti MM, Nga HS, Bravin AM, Takase HM, Viero RM, et al. Long-term outcomes of the Atypical Hemolytic Uremic Syndrome after kidney transplantation treated with eculizumab as first choice. *PloS One* (2017) 12(11):1–14. doi: 10.1371/journal.pone.0188155
166. Schubert J, Röth A. Update on paroxysmal nocturnal haemoglobinuria: On the long way to understand the principles of the disease. *Eur J Haematol* (2015) 94(6):464–73. doi: 10.1111/ejh.12520
167. Cavero T, Rabasco C, López A, Román E, Ávila A, Sevillano Á, et al. Eculizumab in secondary atypical haemolytic uraemic syndrome. *Nephrol Dial Transplant* (2017) 32(3):466–74. doi: 10.1093/ndt/gfw453
168. Risitano AM. Anti-Complement Treatment in Paroxysmal Nocturnal Hemoglobinuria: Where we Stand and Where we are Going. *Transl Med UniSa* (2014) 8(6):43–52. doi: 10.1517/21678707.2015.1041376
169. Holz FG, Sadda SR, Busbee B, Chew EY, Mitchell P, Tufail A, et al. Efficacy and safety of lampalizumab for geographic atrophy due to age-related macular degeneration: Chroma and spectri phase 3 randomized clinical trials. *JAMA Ophthalmol* (2018) 136(6):666–77. doi: 10.1001/jamaophthalmol.2018.1544
170. Yehoshua Z, Alexandre De Amorim Garcia Filho C, Nunes RP, Gregori G, Penha FM, Moshfeghi AA, et al. Systemic complement inhibition with eculizumab for geographic atrophy in age-related macular degeneration: The COMPLETE study. *Ophthalmology* (2014) 121(3):693–701. doi: 10.1016/j.ophtha.2013.09.044
171. Perego F, Wu MA, Valerieva A, Caccia S, Suffritti C, Zanichelli A, et al. Current and emerging biologics for the treatment of hereditary angioedema. *Expert Opin Biol Ther* (2019) 19(6):517–26. doi: 10.1080/14712598.2019.1595581
172. Schröder-Braunstein J, Kirschfink M. Complement deficiencies and dysregulation: Pathophysiological consequences, modern analysis, and clinical management. *Mol Immunol* (2019) 114(August):299–311. doi: 10.1016/j.molimm.2019.08.002
173. Emmens RW, Wouters D, Zeerleder S, van Ham SM, Niessen HWM, Krijnen PAJ. On the value of therapeutic interventions targeting the complement system in acute myocardial infarction. *Transl Res* (2017) 182:103–22. doi: 10.1016/j.trsl.2016.10.005
174. Koles K, van Berkel PHC, Pieper FR, Nuijens JH, Mannesse MLM, Vliegenthart JFG, et al. N- and O-glycans of recombinant human C1 inhibitor expressed in the milk of transgenic rabbits. *Glycobiology* (2004) 14(1):51–64. doi: 10.1093/glycob/cwh010
175. Wouters D, Wagenaar-Bos I, Van Ham M, Zeerleder S. C1 inhibitor: Just a serine protease inhibitor? New and old considerations on therapeutic applications of C1 inhibitor. *Expert Opin Biol Ther* (2008) 8(8):1225–40. doi: 10.1517/14712598.8.8.1225
176. Caliezi C, Wuillemin WA, Zeerleder S, Redondo M, Eisele B, Hack CE. C1-esterase inhibitor: An anti-inflammatory agent and its potential use in the treatment of diseases other than hereditary angioedema. *Pharmacol Rev* (2000) 52(1):91–112.
177. Wouters D, Stephan F, Strengers P, de Haas M, Brouwer C, Hagenbeek A, et al. C1-esterase inhibitor concentrate rescues erythrocytes from complement-mediated destruction in autoimmune hemolytic anemia. *Blood* (2013) 121(7):1242–4. doi: 10.1182/blood-2012-11-467209
178. Jordan SC, Choi J, Aubert O, Haas M, Loupy A, Huang E, et al. A phase I/II, double-blind, placebo-controlled study assessing safety and efficacy of C1 esterase inhibitor for prevention of delayed graft function in deceased donor kidney transplant recipients. *Am J Transplant* (2018) 18(12):2955–64. doi: 10.1111/ajt.14767
179. Pandey S, Vyas GN. Adverse Effects of Plasma Transfusion. *Transfusion* (2012) 52:1–23. doi: 10.1111/j.1537-2995.2012.03663.x
180. Kasanmoentalib ES, Valls Serón M, Engelen-Lee JY, Tanck MW, Pouw RB, Van Mierlo G, et al. Complement factor H contributes to mortality in humans and mice with bacterial meningitis. *J Neuroinflammation* (2019) 16 (1):1–14. doi: 10.1186/s12974-019-1675-1
181. Fakhouri F, De Jorge EG, Brune F, Azam P, Cook HT, Pickering MC. Treatment with human complement factor H rapidly reverses renal complement deposition in factor H-deficient mice. *Kidney Int* (2010) 78 (3):279–86. doi: 10.1038/ki.2010.132
182. Pickering MC, Cook HT, Warren J, Bygrave AE, Moss J, Walport MJ, et al. Uncontrolled C3 activation causes membranoproliferative glomerulonephritis in mice deficient in complement factor h. *Nat Genet* (2002) 31(4):424–8. doi: 10.1038/ng912
183. Feng S, Liang X, Cruz MA, Vu H, Zhou Z, Pemmaraju N, et al. The Interaction between Factor H and Von Willebrand Factor. *PloS One* (2013) 8 (8):1–15. doi: 10.1371/journal.pone.0073715
184. Sharma AK, Pangburn MK. Biologically active recombinant human complement factor H: synthesis and secretion by the baculovirus system. *Gene* (1994) 143(2):301–2. doi: 10.1016/0378-1119(94)90116-3
185. Michelfelder S, Parsons J, Bohlender LL, Hoernstein SNW, Niederkrüger H, Busch A, et al. Moss-produced, glycosylation-optimized human Factor H for therapeutic application in complement disorders. *J Am Soc Nephrol* (2017) 28(5):1462–74. doi: 10.1681/ASN.2015070745
186. Büttner-Mainik A, Parsons J, Jérôme H, Hartmann A, Lamer S, Schaaf A, et al. Production of biologically active recombinant human factor H in Physcomitrella. *Plant Biotechnol J* (2011) 9(3):373–83. doi: 10.1111/j.1467-7652.2010.00552.x

187. Top O, Parsons J, Bohlender LL, Michelfelder S, Kopp P, Busch-Steenberg C, et al. Recombinant production of MFHR1, a novel synthetic multitarget complement inhibitor, in moss bioreactors. *Front Plant Sci* (2019) 10 (March):1–14. doi: 10.3389/fpls.2019.00260
188. Sugita Y, Ito K, Shiozuka K, Suzuki H, Gushima H, Tomita M, et al. Recombinant soluble CD59 inhibits reactive haemolysis with complement. *Immunology* (1994) 82(1):34–41.
189. Christiansen D, Milland J, Thorley BR, McKenzie IFC, Loveland BE. A functional analysis of recombinant soluble CD46 in vivo and a comparison with recombinant soluble forms of CD55 and CD35 in vitro. *Eur J Immunol* (1996) 26(3):578–85. doi: 10.1002/eji.1830260312
190. Moran P, Beasley H, Gorrell A, Martin E, Gribling P, Fuchs H, et al. Human recombinant soluble decay accelerating factor inhibits complement activation in vitro and in vivo. *J Immunol* (1992) 149(5):1736–43.
191. Smith GP, Smith RAG. Membrane-targeted complement inhibitors. *Mol Immunol* (2001) 38(2–3):249–55. doi: 10.1016/S0161-5890(01)00047-5
192. Schmid RA, Hillinger S, Hamacher J, Stammberger U. TP20 is superior to TP10 in reducing ischemia/reperfusion injury in rat lung grafts. *Transplant Proc* (2001) 33(1–2):948–9. doi: 10.1016/S0041-1345(00)02279-X
193. Sellier-Leclerc AL, Fremeaux-Bacchi V, Dragon-Durey MA, Macher MA, Niaudet P, Guest G, et al. Differential impact of complement mutations on clinical characteristics in atypical hemolytic uremic syndrome. *J Am Soc Nephrol* (2007) 18(8):2392–400. doi: 10.1681/ASN.2006080811
194. Ricklin D, Mastellos DC, Reis ES, Lambris JD. The renaissance of complement therapeutics. *Physiol Behav* (2018) 14(1):1–47. doi: 10.1038/nrneph.2017.156
195. Harder MJ, Anliker M, Höchsmann B, Simmet T, Huber-Lang M, Schrezenmeier H, et al. Comparative Analysis of Novel Complement-Targeted Inhibitors, MiniFH, and the Natural Regulators Factor H and Factor H–like Protein 1 Reveal Functional Determinants of Complement Regulation. *J Immunol* (2016) 196(2):866–76. doi: 10.4049/jimmunol.1501919
196. Schmidt CQ, Bai H, Lin Z, Risitano AM, Barlow PN, Ricklin D, et al. Rational Engineering of a Minimized Immune Inhibitor with Unique Triple-Targeting Properties. *J Immunol* (2013) 190(11):5712–21. doi: 10.4049/jimmunol.1203548
197. Schmidt CQ, Harder MJ, Nichols EM, Hebecker M, Anliker M, Höchsmann B, et al. Selectivity of C3-opsonin targeted complement inhibitors: A distinct advantage in the protection of erythrocytes from paroxysmal nocturnal hemoglobinuria patients. *Immunobiology* (2016) 221(4):503–11. doi: 10.1016/j.imbio.2015.12.009
198. Yang Y, Denton H, Davies OR, Smith-Jackson K, Kerr H, Herbert AP, et al. An engineered complement factor H construct for treatment of C3 glomerulopathy. *J Am Soc Nephrol* (2018) 29(6):1649–61. doi: 10.1681/ASN.2017091006
199. Souza DG, Esser D, Bradford R, Vieira AT, Teixeira MM. APT070 (Mirococept), a membrane-localised complement inhibitor, inhibits inflammatory responses that follow intestinal ischaemia and reperfusion injury. *Br J Pharmacol* (2005) 145(8):1027–34. doi: 10.1038/sj.bjp.0706286
200. Patel H, Smith RAG, Sacks SH, Zhou W. Therapeutic strategy with a membrane-localizing complement regulator to increase the number of usable donor organs after prolonged cold storage. *J Am Soc Nephrol* (2006) 17(4):1102–11. doi: 10.1681/ASN.2005101116
201. Kassimatis T, Qasem A, Douiri A, Ryan EG, Rebollo-Mesa I, Nichols LL, et al. A double-blind randomised controlled investigation into the efficacy of Mirococept (APT070) for preventing ischaemia reperfusion injury in the kidney allograft (EMPIRIKAL): Study protocol for a randomised controlled trial. *Trials* (2017) 18(1):1–11. doi: 10.1186/s13063-017-1972-x
202. Drage M. *An investigation into the treatment of the donor kidney to see if this improves the recovery of the kidney after transplantation.* ISCRTN Registry. doi: 10.1186/ISRCTN49958194
203. Fridkis-Hareli M, Storek M, Mazsaroff I, Risitano AM, Lundberg AS, Horvath CJ, et al. Design and development of TT30, a novel C3d-targeted C3/C5 convertase inhibitor for treatment of human complement alternative pathway-mediated diseases. *Blood* (2011) 118(17):4705–13. doi: 10.1182/blood-2011-06-359646
204. Dobó J, Kocsis A, Gál P. Be on target: Strategies of targeting alternative and lectin pathway components in complement-mediated diseases. *Front Immunol* (2018) 9(AUG):1–22. doi: 10.3389/fimmu.2018.01851
205. Pérez-Alós L, Bayarri-Olmos R, Skjoedt MO, Garred P. Combining MAP-1:CD35 or MAP-1:CD55 fusion proteins with pattern-recognition molecules as novel targeted modulators of the complement cascade. *FASEB J* (2019) 33 (11):12723–34. doi: 10.1096/fj.201901643R
206. Takasumi M, Omori T, Machida T, Ishida Y, Hayashi M, Suzuki T, et al. A novel complement inhibitor sMAP-FH targeting both the lectin and alternative complement pathways. *FASEB J* (2020) 34(5):1–15. doi: 10.1096/fj.201902475R
207. Panwar HS, Ojha H, Ghosh P, Barage SH, Raut S, Sahu A. Molecular engineering of an efficient four-domain DAF-MCP chimera reveals the presence of functional modularity in RCA proteins. *PNAS* (2019) 116 (20):9953–8. doi: 10.1073/pnas.1818573116
208. Song C, Xu Z, Miao J, Xu J, Wu X, Zhang F, et al. Protective effect of scFv-DAF fusion protein on the complement attack to acetylcholine receptor: A possible option for treatment of myasthenia gravis. *Muscle Nerve* (2012) 45 (5):668–75. doi: 10.1002/mus.23247
209. Kusner LL, Satija N, Cheng G, Kaminski HJ. Targeting therapy to the neuromuscular junction: Proof of concept. *Muscle Nerve* (2014) 49(5):749–56. doi: 10.1002/mus.24057
210. Katschke KJ, Helmy KY, Steffek M, Xi H, Yin JP, Lee WP, et al. A novel inhibitor of the alternative pathway of complement reverses inflammation and bone destruction in experimental arthritis. *J Exp Med* (2007) 204 (6):1319–25. doi: 10.1084/jem.20070432
211. Helmy KY, Katschke KJ, Gorgani NN, Kljavin NM, Elliott JM, Diehl L, et al. CRIg: A macrophage complement receptor required for phagocytosis of circulating pathogens. *Cell* (2006) 124(5):915–27. doi: 10.1016/j.cell.2005.12.039
212. Chen M, Muckersie E, Luo C, Forrester JV, Xu H. Inhibition of the alternative pathway of complement activation reduces inflammation in experimental autoimmune uveoretinitis. *Eur J Immunol* (2010) 40 (10):2870–81. doi: 10.1002/eji.201040323
213. Wang X, Van Lookeren Campagne M, Katschke KJ, Gullipalli D, Miwa T, Ueda Y, et al. Prevention of Fatal C3 Glomerulopathy by Recombinant Complement Receptor of the Ig Superfamily. *J Am Soc Nephrol* (2018) 29 (8):2053–9. doi: 10.1681/ASN.2018030270
214. Shaughnessy J, Vu DM, Punjabi R, Serra-Pladevall J, De Oliveira RB, Granoff DM, et al. Fusion protein comprising factor H domains 6 and 7 and human IgG1 Fc as an antibacterial immunotherapeutic. *Clin Vaccine Immunol* (2014) 21(10):1452–9. doi: 10.1128/CVI.00444-14
215. Blom AM, Magda M, Kohl L, Shaughnessy J, Lambris JD, Ram S, et al. Factor H–IgG Chimeric Proteins as a Therapeutic Approach against the Gram-Positive Bacterial Pathogen Streptococcus pyogenes. *J Immunol* (2017) 199 (11):3828–39. doi: 10.4049/jimmunol.1700426
216. Wong SM, Shaughnessy J, Ram S, Akerley BJ. Defining the binding region in factor H to develop a therapeutic factor H-Fc fusion protein against non-typeable Haemophilus influenzae. *Front Cell Infect Microbiol* (2016) 6 (APR):1–10. doi: 10.3389/fcimb.2016.00040
217. Pouw RB, Brouwer MC, de Gast M, van Beek AE, van den Heuvel LP, Schmidt CQ, et al. Potentiation of complement regulator factor H protects human endothelial cells from complement attack in aHUS sera. *Blood Adv* (2019) 3(4):621–32. doi: 10.1182/bloodadvances.2018025692
218. Dekkers G, Brouwer M, Jeremiasse J, Kamp A, Biggs RM, Van G. Unravelling the effect of a potentiating anti-Factor H antibody on atypical hemolytic uremic syndrome associated factor H variants. *J Immunol* (2020) 205(9):1–9. doi: 10.1101/2020.04.08.026906
219. Zell S, Geis N, Rutz R, Schultz S, Giese T, Kirschfink M. Down-regulation of CD55 and CD46 expression by anti-sense phosphorothioate oligonucleotides (S-ODNs) sensitizes tumour cells to complement attack. *Clin Exp Immunol* (2007) 150(3):576–84. doi: 10.1111/j.1365-2249.2007.03507.x
220. Kourtzelis I, Rafail S. The dual role of complement in cancer and its implication in anti-tumor therapy. *Ann Transl Med* (2016) 4(14):1–14. doi: 10.21037/atm.2016.06.26
221. Zhao W-P, Zhu B, Duan Y-Z, Chen Z-T. Neutralization of complement regulatory proteins CD55 and CD59 augments therapeutic effect of herceptin against lung carcinoma cells WEI-PENG. *Oncol Rep* (2009) 21:1405–11. doi: 10.3892/or_00000368
222. Dho SH, Kim SY, Chung C, Cho EH, Lee SY, Kim JY, et al. Development of a radionuclide-labeled monoclonal anti-CD55 antibody with theranostic

potential in pleural metastatic lung cancer. *Sci Rep* (2018) 8(1):1–12. doi: 10.1038/s41598-018-27355-8

223. Gelderman KA, Blok VT, Fleuren GJ, Gorter A. The inhibitory effect of CD46, CD55, and CD59 on complement activation after immunotherapeutic treatment of cervical carcinoma cells with monoclonal antibodies or bispecific monoclonal antibodies. *Lab Investig* (2002) 82(4):483–93. doi: 10.1038/labinvest.3780441
224. Gelderman KA, Kuppen PJK, Okada N, Fleuren GJ, Gorter A. Tumor-specific inhibition of membrane-bound complement regulatory protein Crry with bispecific monoclonal antibodies prevents tumor outgrowth in a rat colorectal cancer lung metastases model. *Cancer Res* (2004) 64(12):4366–72. doi: 10.1158/0008-5472.CAN-03-2131
225. Macor P, Tripodo C, Zorzet S, Piovan E, Bossi F, Marzari R, et al. In vivo targeting of human neutralizing antibodies against CD55 and CD59 to lymphoma cells increases the antitumor activity of rituximab. *Cancer Res* (2007) 67(21):10556–63. doi: 10.1158/0008-5472.CAN-07-1811
226. Bresin E, Rurali E, Caprioli J, Sanchez-Corral P, Fremeaux-Bacchi V, De Cordoba SR, et al. Combined complement gene mutations in atypical hemolytic uremic syndrome influence clinical phenotype. *J Am Soc Nephrol* (2013) 24(3):475–86. doi: 10.1681/ASN.2012090884

20

Complement Activation in Kidneys of Patients with COVID-19

Frederick Pfister[1†], Eva Vonbrunn[1†], Tajana Ries[1], Hans-Martin Jäck[2], Klaus Überla[3], Günter Lochnit[4], Ahmed Sheriff[5], Martin Herrmann[6], Maike Büttner-Herold[1], Kerstin Amann[1] and Christoph Daniel[1]*

[1] Department of Nephropathology, Institute of Pathology, Friedrich-Alexander-University (FAU) Erlangen-Nürnberg, Erlangen, Germany, [2] Nikolaus-Fiebinger-Center FAU, Department of Medicine 3, Division of Molecular Immunology, Friedrich-Alexander-University (FAU) Erlangen-Nürnberg, Erlangen, Germany, [3] Department of Virology, Friedrich-Alexander-University (FAU) Erlangen-Nürnberg, Erlangen, Germany, [4] Department of Biochemistry, Division Protein Analystics, Justus-Liebig-University Giessen, Giessen, Germany, [5] Pentracor GmbH, Henningsdorf, Germany, [6] Department of Medicine 3, Institute for Rheumatology and Immunology, Friedrich-Alexander-University (FAU) Erlangen-Nürnberg, Erlangen, Germany

***Correspondence:**
Christoph Daniel
Christoph.Daniel@uk-erlangen.de

[†]These authors have contributed equally to this work

Most patients who became critically ill following infection with COVID-19 develop severe acute respiratory syndrome (SARS) attributed to a maladaptive or inadequate immune response. The complement system is an important component of the innate immune system that is involved in the opsonization of viruses but also in triggering further immune cell responses. Complement activation was seen in plasma adsorber material that clogged during the treatment of critically ill patients with COVID-19. Apart from the lung, the kidney is the second most common organ affected by COVID-19. Using immunohistochemistry for complement factors C1q, MASP-2, C3c, C3d, C4d, and C5b-9 we investigated the involvement of the complement system in six kidney biopsies with acute kidney failure in different clinical settings and three kidneys from autopsy material of patients with COVID-19. Renal tissue was analyzed for signs of renal injury by detection of thrombus formation using CD61, endothelial cell rarefaction using the marker E-26 transformation specific-related gene (ERG-) and proliferation using proliferating cell nuclear antigen (PCNA)-staining. SARS-CoV-2 was detected by *in situ* hybridization and immunohistochemistry. Biopsies from patients with hemolytic uremic syndrome (HUS, n = 5), severe acute tubular injury (ATI, n = 7), zero biopsies with disseminated intravascular coagulation (DIC, n = 7) and 1 year protocol biopsies from renal transplants (Ctrl, n = 7) served as controls. In the material clogging plasma adsorbers used for extracorporeal therapy of patients with COVID-19 C3 was the dominant protein but collectin 11 and MASP-2 were also identified. SARS-CoV-2 was sporadically present in varying numbers in some biopsies from patients with COVID-19. The highest frequency of CD61-positive platelets was found in peritubular capillaries and arteries of COVID-19 infected renal specimens as compared to all controls. Apart from COVID-19 specimens, MASP-2 was detected in glomeruli with DIC and ATI. In contrast, the classical pathway (i.e. C1q) was hardly seen in COVID-19 biopsies. Both C3 cleavage products C3c and C3d were strongly detected in renal arteries but also occurs in glomerular capillaries of COVID-19 biopsies, while tubular C3d was stronger than C3c in biopsies from COVID-19 patients. The membrane attack complex C5b-9, demonstrating terminal pathway activation, was predominantly deposited in COVID-19 biopsies in peritubular capillaries, renal arterioles, and tubular basement membrane with similar or even higher frequency compared to controls. In conclusion, various complement pathways were activated in COVID-19 kidneys, the lectin pathway mainly in peritubular capillaries and in part the classical pathway in renal arteries whereas the alternative pathway seem to be crucial for tubular complement activation. Therefore, activation of the complement system might be involved in the worsening of renal injury. Complement inhibition might thus be a promising treatment option to prevent deregulated activation and subsequent collateral tissue injury.

Keywords: complement—immunological term, COVID-19, kidney, endothelial injury, lectin pathway activation

INTRODUCTION

Patients who became critically ill due to SARS-Cov2 virus infection developed severe acute respiratory distress syndrome (ARDS). ARDS is induced by damage of lung alveoli by endothelial injury followed by a maladaptive immune response (1). Tissue damage is not restricted to the respiratory tract since patients with severe COVID-19 often developed multiorgan failure including cardiac and acute kidney injury (2, 3). In a consecutive study of 701 patients with COVID-19 hospitalized in Wuhan, 44% and 27% had proteinuria and hematuria on admission, respectively (4). Furthermore, kidney disease in COVID-19 patients was associated with in-hospital mortality (3). While some reports suggested a direct viral infection of the kidney with infection of glomerular (5) and tubular cells (6–8) other studies support indirect pathomechanisms (9–11). Histopathological findings in postmortem renal biopsies (8, 10, 11) or native and allograft kidney biopsies (9) reported a wide spectrum of glomerular and tubular injury. However, by far the most common renal complication is acute kidney injury (AKI) (8–11). Additionally, scarce focal kidney fibrin thrombi occur (11). The pathophysiology of COVID-19–induced kidney damage is not well understood, but is primarily a result of the host immune response driving hypercytokinemia and aggressive inflammation (12, 13). The cytokine storm that causes lung injury associated with infections is reportedly driven by factors of the complement system (14), which as part of the innate immune system plays an important role in defense against infections. Complement opsonizes viruses or bacteria, activates and attracts leukocytes and lyses bacteria and cells (15). The complement system can be activated by three different pathways, (i) the classical pathway, activated by any structure that is recognized by C1q (16), (ii) the lectin pathway, activated when mannan-binding lectin-associated serine protease 2 (MASP-2) complexes with mannose-binding lectin (MBL), ficolins, or collectin-11 bound to saccharide patterns expressed on bacteria or cells (17, 18) and (iii) the alternative pathway, activated through spontaneous hydrolysis of C3 (19). All complement activation pathways form C3 convertases, which finally initiate the formation of the C5 convertase, which leads to the assembly of C5b-9, the terminal membrane attack complex. In addition, cleavage products C3a and C5a serve as anaphylatoxins that activate and attract leukocytes (15). Since complement activation could be detected in plasma (20), lung and skin (21) from COVID-19 patients and seems to be involved in promoting inflammatory processes that lead to tissue damage in COVID-19 patients we here investigated complement activation in six renal biopsies and three postmortem kidneys from patients with COVID-19. Complement involvement was compared to renal biopsies of acute tubular injury (ATI), known kidney diseases with distinct endothelial cell injury including hemolytic uremic syndrome (HUS) and disseminated intravascular coagulation (DIC) and a control group of 1 year protocol biopsies from stable renal transplants (Ctrl).

MATERIALS AND METHODS

Analysis of Plasma Adsorber–Bound Proteins

Plasma adsorbers (Pentracor CRP, Pentracor, Henningsdorf, Germany) that clogged during the treatment of critically ill COVID-19 patients were analyzed to study proteins involved in this plasma reaction. A sample of 0.5 ml agarose (plasma adsorber material) was washed with 25 ml of 0.9% NaCl solution to remove unbound proteins. After that, 0.5 ml of 2 mg/ml DNase I (Roche, in 10 mM Tris HCl, 2.5 mM $MgCl_2$ and 0.5 mM $CaCl_2$, pH 7.6) was added and the mixture was incubated for 30 min at 37°C on a tilt shaker. The DNase I and released proteins were eluted with 5 ml PBS, boiled for 15 min in reducing SDS-buffer (10% SDS in 250 mM Tris pH 6.8 supplemented with 2.83 M mercaptoethanol) and then separated by gradient SDS polyacrylamide gel electrophoresis (4–20% Acrylamid). Bands of interest were excised from gels and the proteins were digested with trypsin (10 ng/μl sequencing grade Promega, Mannheim). Tryptic peptides were eluted from the gel slices with 1% trifluoric acid.

Matrix-Assisted Laser-Desorption Ionization Time-of-Flight Mass Spectrometry (MALDI-TOF-MS) and Protein Identification

MALDI-TOF-MS was performed on an Ultraflex TOF/TOF mass spectrometer (Bruker Daltonics, Bremen) equipped with a nitrogen laser and a LIFT-MS/MS facility. The instrument was operated in the positive-ion reflectron mode using 2.5-dihydroxybenzoic acid and methylendiphosphonic acid as matrix. Sum spectra consisting of 200–400 single spectra were acquired. For data processing and instrument control the Compass 1.4 software package consisting of FlexControl 4.4, FlexAnalysis 3.4 4, Sequence Editor and BioTools 3.2 and ProteinScape 3.1. were used. External calibration was performed with a peptide standard (Bruker Daltonics).

Proteins were identified by MASCOT peptide mass fingerprint search (http://www.matrixscience.com) using the Uniprot Human database (version 20200226, 210438 sequence entries; $p<0.05$). For the search, a mass tolerance of 75 ppm was allowed and oxidation of methionine as the variable modification was used.

Human Renal Tissue Specimens

To evaluate the relevance of complement in mediation of renal pathological changes during COVID-19 we used six formalin-fixed paraffin-embedded (FFPE) kidney biopsies of patients with COVID-19 and renal insufficiency in different clinical settings (four transplant kidneys, one ANCA-associated vasculitis, one multiple organ dysfunction syndrome) and three FFPE autopsy kidneys of patients who died with multiple organ dysfunction syndrome following SARS-CoV-2 infection. Kidney biopsies of patients with hemolytic uremic syndrome (HUS, n = 5), severe acute tubular injury due to septic shock (ATI n = 7), zero-biopsies with disseminated intravascular coagulation (DIC, n = 7) and 1 year protocol biopsies from stable renal transplants (Ctl; n = 7) served as controls. All tissue samples were collected from the archive of the Department of Nephropathology, Friedrich-Alexander-University Erlangen-Nuremberg and analysis was approved by the local Ethics committee (reference number 4415). Patient characteristics of the investigated cases with COVID-19 are described in **Table 1**.

In Situ Hybridization

In situ hybridization, for detection of SARS-CoV-2 RNA in FFPE tissue, was performed using a V nCoV2019-S probe (848561; ACD, Hayward, CA, USA), specific for the S gene encoding the spike protein from SARS-CoV-2, and the RNAscope 2.5 HD RED Kit (ACD). Tissue sections of 4 µm thickness were deparaffinized in xylene, dehydrated in ethanol and blocked with peroxidase. Slides were boiled in kit-provided antigen retrieval buffer at 95°C for 15 min and digested afterwards with protease at 40°C for 30 min. The target probe were hybridized with kidney sections in the HybEZ hybridization oven (ACD) at 40°C for 2 h. Pre-amplification and amplification steps were conducted using kit-provided reagents according to the manufacturer's recommendations. For signal detection sections were incubated with Fast Red substrate for 10 min at room temperature followed by counterstaining with hematoxylin, drying at 60°C for 15 min and mounting with Eco Mount (ACD). The same procedure was used for *in situ* hybridization with the Hs-COLEC11 probe (542431; ACD) for the detection of human collectin 11 mRNA.

Immunohistochemistry

For immunohistochemical stainings formalin-fixed paraffin-embedded (FFPE) kidney biopsies were cut into 2 µm sections, deparaffinized and rehydrated. Antigen retrieval was performed using pronase E (Sigma Aldrich, Taufkirchen, Germany) digestion for 30 min at 37°C (C1q, C3c, C5b-9) or cooking in target retrieval solution pH 6 (DAKO Deutschland GmbH, Hamburg, Germany) for 2.5 min (C3d, C4d, MASP-2, CD61, COVID-19 spike protein). Endogenous peroxidase was blocked with 3% H_2O_2 and unspecific antigens with Avidin-Biotin (Vector laboratories, Burlingame, CA, USA) and normal goat or horse serum in blotto (1:5). The following primary antibodies were diluted in 50 mM Tris pH 7,4 and incubated over-night at 4°C or for 1 h at room temperature: C1q, a rabbit polyclonal antibody against human C1q (A0136; DAKO Deutschland GmbH); C3c, a rabbit polyclonal antibody against human C3c (A0062; DAKO Deutschland GmbH); C3d, a rabbit monoclonal antibody against human C3d (ab136916; Abcam, Cambridge, UK); C5b-9, a mouse monoclonal antibody against human C5b-9 (M0777; DAKO Deutschland GmbH); MASP-2, a rabbit polyclonal antibody against human Mannan-binding lectin serine peptidase 2 (HPA029313; Sigma Aldrich); CD61 a mouse monoclonal antibody against human platelet glycoprotein IIIa (M0753; DAKO Deutschland GmbH), C4d, a rabbit polyclonal antibody against human C4d (BI-RC4D;

TABLE 1 | Clinical, laboratory, and histopathological findings in patients with COVID-19 infection.

Pt	Age	Sex	Biopsy indication	Comorbidities/ circumstances	SARS-CoV-2 infection	PU	Serumcreatinine [mg/dl]	Bx diagnosis
1	40	M	AKI, PU, HU, ANCA positivity	HTN	Current	1 g/g	3,1	ANCA-asso. Crescentic GN, ATN
2	76	M	MODS, AKI	DM	Current	++	7,5	ATN
3	69	M	AKI, ESKD, RTx 2007	DM, HTN, acute enteritis	Current	0,7 g/g	2,1	ATN
4	52	F	AKI, progress PU, ESKD, RTx 2011	DM, HTN	Current	1,5 g/g	1,5	ATN
5	70	M	AKI, ESKD, RTx	Bacterial pneumonia	Current	++	1,4	ATN, infect-asso.GN, cellular borderline changes
6	35	M	AKI, progress PU, ESKD, RTx 2019	–	Current	1,5 g/g	2,1	ATN, recurrent FSGS
7	41	F	ARDS, MODS, AKI, post-mortem	Pregnancy (32gw)	Current	Nd	Nd	ATN
8	64	M	ARDS, MODS, AKI, post-mortem	HTN	Current	Nd	Nd	ATN
9	71	M	ARDS, MODS, AKI, LE, post-mortem	HTN	Current	Nd	Nd	ATN

Pt, patient; M, male; F, female; PU, proteinuria measured as g proteinuria/g creatinine or dipstick; HU, hematuria; AKI, acute kidney insufficiency; ESKD, end-stage kidney disease; RTx, renal transplantation; ARDS, acute respiratory distress syndrome; MODS, multiple organ dysfunction syndrome; HTN, hypertension; DM, diabetes mellitus; ATN, acute tubular necrosis; FSGS, focal-segmental glomerulosclerosis; ANCA, anti-neutrophilic cytoplasmatic antibody; GN, glomerulonephritis; Nd, unknown.

Biomedica, Vienna, Austria) and SARS-CoV-2 spike protein, a mouse monoclonal antibody against SARS-CoV-2 spike protein (clone 224.2, kindly provided by M.-H. Jäck, Department of Molecular Immunology, FAU Erlangen-Nürnberg). After washing with 50 mM Tris pH 7.4, sections were incubated with biotinylated secondary goat anti-rabbit IgG (BA-1000; Vector laboratories) or horse anti-mouse IgG (BA-2001, Vector laboratories). Detection of bound antibodies was conducted using ABC-Kit and DAB-Impact as a substrate (both from Vector laboratories), while nuclei were counter stained with hematoxylin. For negative controls primary antibody was substituted by antibody dilution buffer (50 mM Tris pH 7,4) (**Supplemental Figure 3**). An overview with representative stainings of all cases is shown in **Supplemental Figure 2**.

Immunofluorescence Double Staining

For evaluation of endothelial cell injury and proliferative activity we performed immunofluorescence double staining on rehydrated FFPE kidney sections using a rabbit anti-human E26-transformation- specific related gene (ERG) antibody for detection of endothelial cells (diluted 1:100 in 50 mM Tris pH 7,4; EP111, Cell Marque, Rocklin, CA, USA) and a mouse anti-human proliferating cell nuclear antigen (PCNA, M0879, diluted 1:1000 in 50 mM Tris pH 7.4; DAKO Deutschland GmbH, Hamburg Germany). After dewaxing, sections were incubated with primary antibodies over-night at 4°C followed by washing with 50 mM Tris pH 7.4 supplemented with 0.05% Tween 20. A donkey anti-rabbit IgG Alexa Fluor 568 and a donkey anti-mouse IgG Alexa633 (both from Thermo Fisher Scientific, Waltham, MA, USA) were used as secondary antibodies diluted 1:200 in 50 mM Tris pH 7.4 and incubated at room temperature for 30 min. After subsequent washing, cell nuclei were stained with DAPI (diluted 0.2 µg/ml in distilled water) for 5 min, followed by rinsing in Tris buffer. Finally, sections were covered with Mowiol mounting medium (Calbiochem, La Jolla, USA) and analyzed using laser scanning confocal microscopy (LSM Zeiss 710) and quantification of fluorescence positive area by Zen software (Zeiss GmbH, Jena, Germany).

Semi-Quantitative Evaluation of Complement and CD61 in Renal Biopsies

Complement staining in renal biopsies was graded in different vascular compartments of the kidney (i.e. in the glomeruli, peritubular capillaries and arteries), using a semi-quantitative immunohistochemical staining score (score 0, 1 or 2), which describes the distribution and intensity of staining signal in the micro- and macrovascular structures. In detail for CD61, score 0 was defined as no positive thrombocytes within vascular lumina, score 1 was defined as single/scattered positive thrombocytes in vascular lumina and score 2 was defined as presence of intravascular thrombocyte aggregates of any size. For the components of the complement system (C1q, C3c, C3d, C4dC5b-9, MASP-2) score 0 was defined as no specific granular reactivity along endothelial cell surfaces in the different vascular compartments or tubular basement membrane, score 1 was defined as minimal reactivity in single glomeruli and peritubular capillaries and mild reactivity along endothelial cells or in the intima of arteries and focal reactivity along the tubular basement membrane and score 2 was defined as reactivity in > 10% to 20% of glomeruli and peritubular capillaries and moderate reactivity in the majority (>50%) of arteries and diffuse clear reactivity along tubular basement membranes.

Transient Expression of SARS-CoV-2 Spike Protein

Cells producing membrane-anchored CoV-2 spike protein cells were established by co-transfecting HEK 293T with the PEI method with a GFP reporter plasmid and a pCG1-based expression vector for the spike protein of SARS-CoV-2 (position 21580 – 25400 from accession no. NC_045512).

Generation of Anti-SARS-CoV-2 Spike Protein Ab

The monoclonal IgG2c antibody against the CoV-2 spike protein was isolated from a hybridoma line that was established by the conventional hybridoma technology from spleen cells of Trianni mice that were immunized with DNA-encoding CoV-2 spike protein and purified CoV-2 spike protein. The Trianni mouse line (Patent US 2013/0219535 A1) carried the complete repertoire of human variable region gene segments of immunoglobulin (Ig) heavy (HC) and L chains (LC).

Statistical Analyses

After testing for normal distribution of values using Kolmogorov-Smirnov test, data were analyzed using Kruskal-Wallis test with Dunn's Multiple Comparison test as *post hoc* test for comparison of multiple groups. In all tests $p<0.05$ was accepted as statistically significant. Statistical analyses were performed using GraphPad Prism 8 for Windows software (version 8.3, GraphPad software Inc., San Diego, CA, USA).

RESULTS

Complement C3 Was the Main Component in Clotted Plasma Adsorber From Patients With COVID-19

When seriously ill patients with COVID-19 in our clinic were connected to plasma absorption columns for therapeutic purposes, we observed that these columns quickly clogged. From more than 90 patients treated with CRP apheresis with various diseases (including severe myocardial infarction (STEMI), cardiogenic shock, after bypass surgery, severe COVID-19, acute pancreatitis, sepsis, SIRS after failed bypass surgery) the massive clogging of the columns only occurred in patients with severe COVID-19. In patients with heart attack much smaller clots were observed on the sieve filters but not on the adsorber material. To identify the proteins that are involved in this clot-forming reaction of the plasma, the proteins were detached from the adsorber material and sieve filters by treatment with DNase1 and separated by electrophoresis.

Individual bands were digested with trypsin and finally examined by MALDI-TOF (**Figure 1A**). First, we analyzed the most prominent bands of an electrophoretic separation in an unbiased manner for the major peptides and detected C3 and C3 fragments with a sequence coverage of 52% (**Figure 1B**). Next, we analyzed the candidate peptides of mannose-binding protein-associated serine protease 2 (MASP-2) and collectin 11 involved in complement activation *via* the lectin pathway and detected both molecules (MASP-2; sequence coverage 12%) and collectin 11 (sequence coverage 33%) (**Figure 1B**). MASP-2. In contrast, the investigation of the clots from treatment of heart attack patients showed haptoglobin as main component and only little C3a (data not shown). This finding might indicate an important role of complement in the pathogenesis of COVID-19 disease and encouraged us to investigate complement activation in the kidneys of COVID-19 patients in more detail.

Histopathology, Proliferative Activity, and Loss of Endothelial Cells in Kidneys From Patients With COVID-19

In this study, six kidney biopsies of patients with COVID-19 infection (four transplant kidneys, 1 ANCA-associated vasculitis, one multiple organ dysfunction syndrome) and three autopsy kidneys of patients who died with multiple organ dysfunction syndrome following COVID-19 infection were analyzed (**Table 1**). In all tissue samples a moderate to severe acute tubular injury (ATI) with tubular dilatation and vacuolization of swollen tubular epithelial cells was found (**Figure 2A**) and in one of the postmortem tissue samples isolated glomerular microthrombi were present (**Figure 2B**). In addition, an infect-associated glomerulonephritis (most likely related to a bacterial pneumonia the patient developed secondary to the COVID-19) was diagnosed in one proteinuric transplant patient (patient 5), accompanied by acute T-cell mediated borderline-rejection. Another proteinuric transplant patient suffered from recurrence of podocytopathy with focal-segmental glomerulosclerosis in the transplanted kidney and in the biopsy of patient 1 an ANCA-associated crescentic glomerulonephritis was diagnosed. SARS-CoV-2 was sporadically detected by *in situ* hybridization in renal tubules and endothelial cells in six of nine kidney specimens of patients with COVID-19 (**Figure 2C**). However, renal infection with COVID-19 could be confirmed in only one case by immunohistochemistry with an antibody directed against the SARS-CoV-2 spike protein (**Figure 2D**), indicating at least low renal virus load. In contrast, this antibody sensitively recognized paraffin embedded HEK293T cells transfected with SARS-CoV-2 spike protein (**Figure 2E**). To further assess renal damage in patients with COVID-19, we examined proliferating cell nuclear antigen (PCNA) as a marker of increased repair and the expression of the endothelial cell marker ERG in COVID-19 kidney biopsies and compared these to biopsies of kidney diseases characterized by tubular or endothelial damage. Compared to biopsies with hemolytic uremic syndrome (HUS) the kidneys of patients with COVID-19 (COV) showed significantly lower proliferative activity measured as PCNA positive area, which was comparably low to those of biopsies with acute tubular injury (ATI), disseminated intravascular coagulation (DIC) and in 1 year protocol biopsies that served as controls (Ctrl) (**Figures 3A, C–G**, green staining). Capillarization of COVID-19 biopsies, measured as ERG-positive area, was less 50% and 40% than in Ctrl and HUS (**Figures 3B, C, E, G**, red staining). Only DIC showed higher endothelial cell loss while endothelial cell loss in ATI was comparable to COV (**Figures 3B, D, F**).

Thrombus-Forming CD61-Positive Platelets Were Frequently Detected in Kidneys From Patients With COVID-19

First, we investigated CD61-positive platelets in COVID-19 renal biopsies, which are involved in thrombus formation and detected glomerular CD61-positive platelets in 8/9 of the COVID-19 cases (**Figures 4A, B**). Glomerular CD61-positive platelets were comparable in Ctrl and COVID-19, and decreased compared to DIC and HUS glomeruli but ATI had the lowest number of CD61-positive platelets (**Figure 3A**). In peritubular capillaries and renal arteries, CD61-positive platelets counts were higher in COVID-19 biopsies as compared to DIC, HUS and ATI and Ctrl (**Figures 4C–F**). The overall score for CD61, summarizing the scores of all three vascular beds, was highest in COVID-19 compared to all controls (**Table 2**).

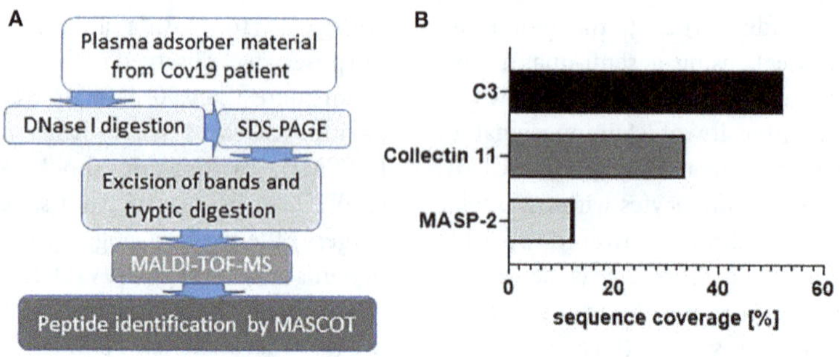

FIGURE 1 | Involvement of complement components in COVID-19. Workflow for the analysis of clotted material isolated from plasma adsorber material collected from treated COVID-19 patient **(A)**. Coverage rates of complement factors C3, collectin 11, and mannose-binding protein-associated serine protease 2 (MASP-2) analyzed by MALDI-TOF **(B)**.

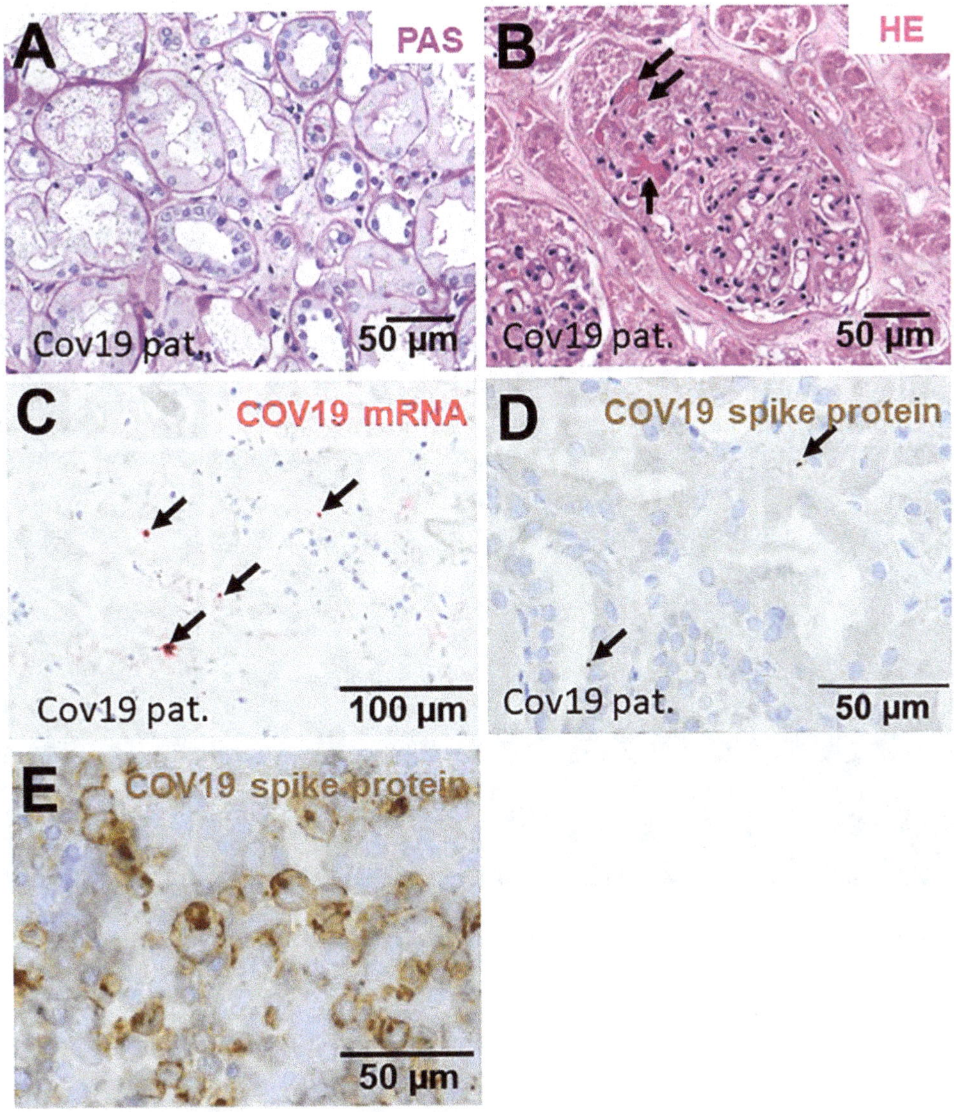

FIGURE 2 | Renal injury in kidney biopsies from patients infected with SARS-CoV-2. Representative pictures of a PAS-stained COVID-19 renal biopsy showing acute tubular injury with swollen and vacuolized cells **(A)** and glomerular microthrombi in HE-stained section (**B**, arrows). In situ hybridization for SARS-CoV-2 mRNA showed few positive signals in tubular and endothelial localization (**C**, pink signals marked by arrows). Immunohistochemistry for SARS-CoV-3 spike protein detected sporadic positive signals in renal biopsies from patients with COVID-19 (**D**, brown signals marked by arrows). As positive control, we employed HEK293T cells transfected with a plasmid expressing SARS-CoV-2 spike protein, fixed with formalin, embedded in paraffin followed by staining of sections by immunohistochemistry using anti-SARS-CoV-2 spike antibody (**E**, brown staining).

Marked Complement Activation Occurs in Kidney Vascular Beds of Patients With COVID-19

As first complement factor, we detected the glomerular deposition of MASP-2, a serine protease, that complexes with the lectin pathway initiators (MBL, ficolins, and collectins) and becomes activated upon binding to the lectin ligand and found it in 2/9 of the COVID-19 biopsies. Compared to COVID-19 glomerular MASP-2 expression was higher in DIC, comparable in Ctrl, slightly lower in ATI and did not occur at all in HUS (**Figures 5A, B**). Additionally, in peritubular capillaries and renal arteries, MASP-2 was detected in only 22% 2/9 of cases from patients with COVID-19 respectively, but could otherwise only be detected in renal arteries of HUS and in peritubular capillaries in HUS and ATI groups and not at all in the Ctrl biopsies (**Figures 5C–F**). Next, we studied the renal deposition of C1q, which is part of the classical pathway (**Figure 6**). We rarely detected C1q in glomerular and peritubular capillaries in a single COVID-19 biopsy (1/9), which was comparable to Ctrl. In HUS and DIC renal biopsies it was present in the glomeruli of all

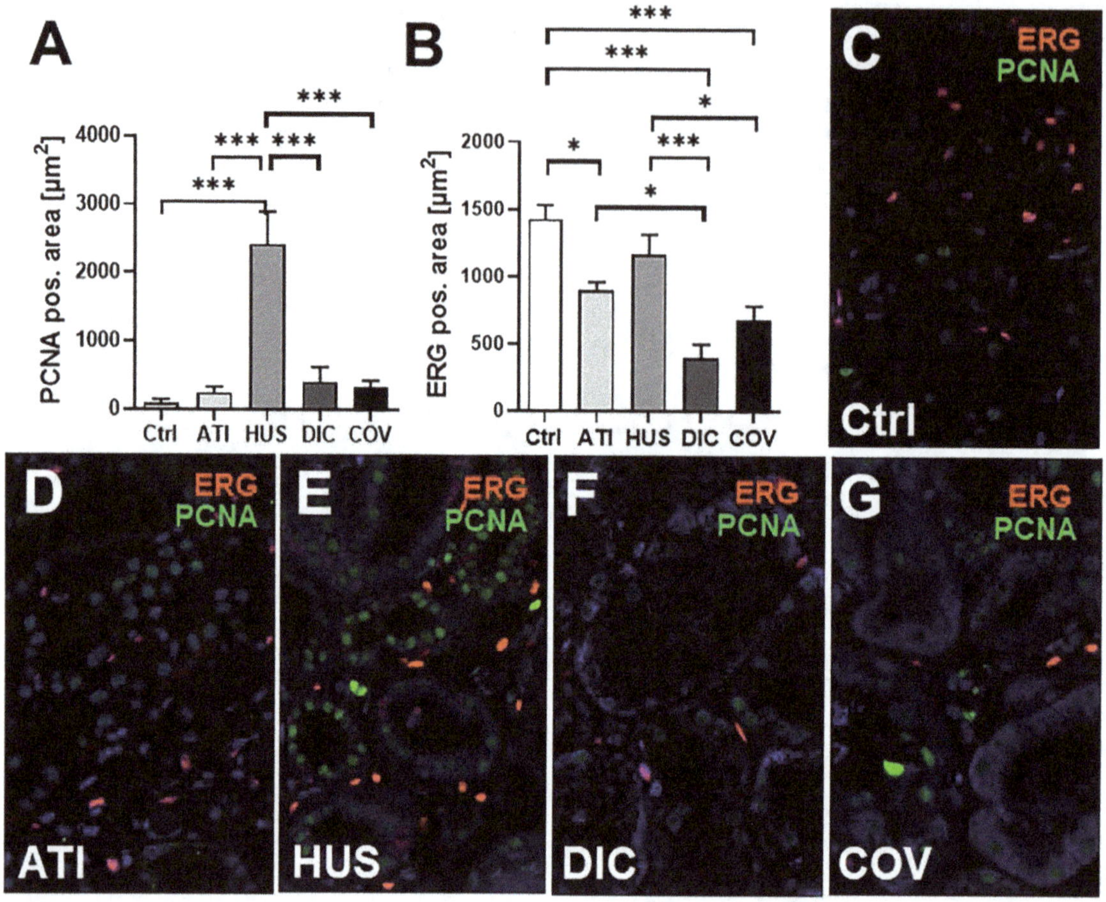

FIGURE 3 | Endothelial rarefaction and proliferative activity in kidney biopsies from patients infected with SARS-CoV-2. Renal proliferation, as assessed by PCNA-staining **(A)** and ERG-positive endothelial cells **(B)** were evaluated by immunofluorescence staining analyzed by confocal microscopy and quantification by ZEN-software in COVID-19 biopsies (COV, n = 7) compared to renal control biopsies taken 1 year after transplantation (Ctrl, n=7), biopsies with acute tubular injury (ATI, n = 7), hemolytic uremic syndrome (HUS, n = 5) and disseminated intravascular coagulation (DIC, n = 7). Representative pictures of immunofluorescence double staining showing PCNA (green staining) and ERG (red staining) double staining were shown in biopsies of Ctrl **(C)**, ATI **(D)**, HUS **(E)**, DIC **(F)**, and COV **(G)**.
*$p < 0.05$; ***$p < 0.001$.

biopsies and peritubular capillaries in 40% to 60% of the biopsies (**Figures 6A–D**). In COVID-19, C1q deposition in the renal arteries was seen in 4/9 of biopsies (**Figures 6E, F**) and even more commonly in HUS and DIC (**Figure 6E**). In Ctrl C1q deposition was slightly lower compared to COVID-19 while renal biopsies of patients with ATI showed no C1q deposition at all (**Figures 6A, C, E**). Next, we analyzed fragments of C3 that are formed by all complement pathways: C3c, a stable activation fragment and C3d an activation fragment that is able to covalently bind to surfaces. The stable C3 fragment C3c was detectable in the glomeruli of 4/9 of the COVID-19 biopsies, while glomerular C3c signals were comparable in ATI and more frequent and stronger in HUS and DIC and lower in Ctrl (**Figures 7A, B**). In peritubular capillaries, C3c was visible in 2/9 of COVID-19 biopsies, one of them at high intensity, and was thus comparable in frequency to ATI and HUS (**Figures 7C, D**). Only in DIC peritubular C3c was present in 6/7 of biopsies but also occurred in 4/7 Ctrl biopsies (**Figure 7C**). In renal arteries, the deposition of C3c was common in all groups and showed less intensity in Ctrl while other groups frequently showed intense staining (**Figures 7E, F**). C3d,. was detectable in the glomeruli of 8/9 of COVID-19 biopsies, while glomerular C3d signals were lower in ATI and completely lacking in Ctrl (**Figures 8A, B**). In contrast, more frequent glomerular C3d deposition was detected in HUS and DIC (**Figures 8A, B**). In peritubular capillaries, C3d was negative in all investigated groups (**Figures 8C, D**). In renal arteries, the deposition of C3d was common in all groups but strongest staining was observed in COVID-19 (**Figures 8E, F**). Interestingly, the complement split product C4d, that was commonly used to assess whether antibodies are participating in antibody-mediated rejection of renal transplants, was not detected in any of the kidney samples tested; neither in biopsies of COVID-19 patients nor in the controls (**Supplemental Figure 3**, **Table 2**). Finally, we studied C5b-9 deposition in renal specimens, the membrane attack complex formed in the terminal complement pathway (**Figure 9**). While

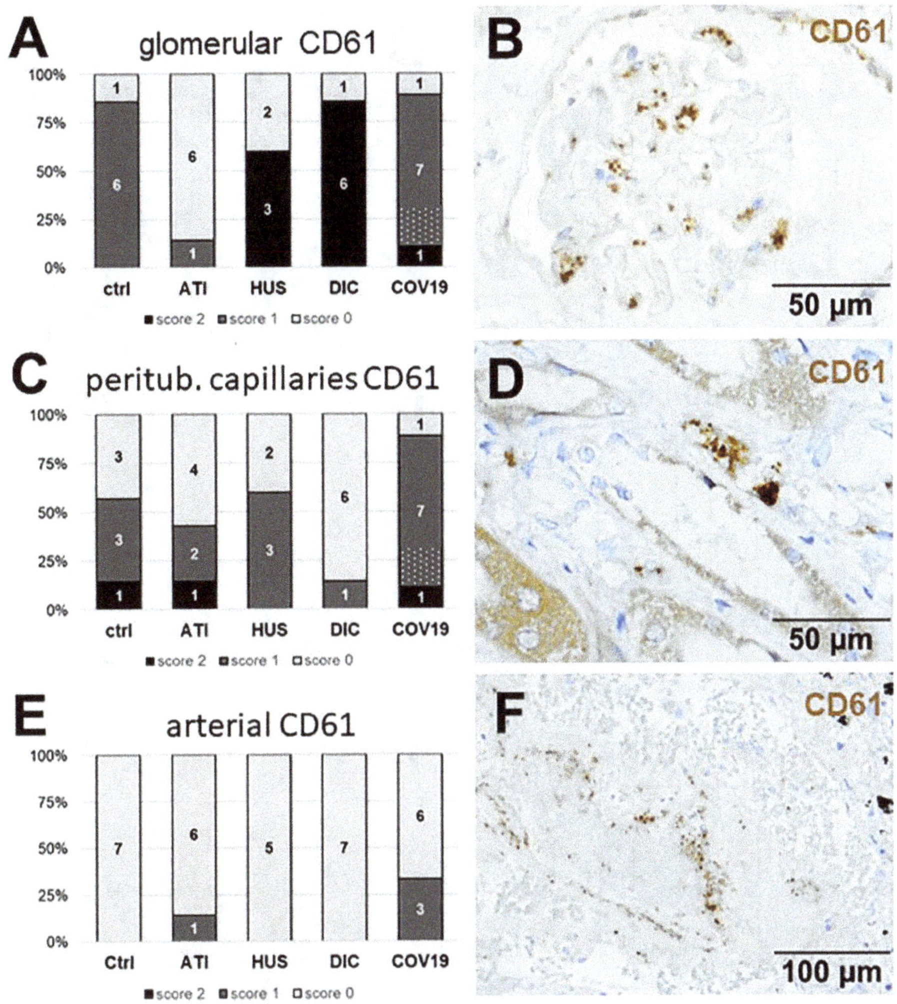

FIGURE 4 | Frequency and localization of CD61-positive platelets in renal biopsies with COVID-19 compared to Ctrl, ATI, HUS, and DIC. Frequency and amount of CD61-positive platelets was analyzed in glomerular capillaries **(A)**, peritubular capillaries **(C)** and renal arteries **(E)** in renal control biopsies taken 1 year after transplantation (Ctrl, n = 7), biopsies with acute tubular injury (ATI, n = 7), hemolytic uremic syndrome (HUS, n = 5), disseminated intravascular coagulation (DIC, n = 7), and COVID-19 (COVID-19, n = 9) using immunohistochemistry and semi-quantitative scoring. The proportion of CD61-positive stained cases that belongs to cases with comorbidities with known involvement of complement activation is marked by hatching in the bars representing the COVID-19 cohort. Representative pictures of COVID-19 biopsies positive for CD61 were shown for glomerular (**B**, brown staining), peritubular (**D**, brown staining), and arterial localization (**F**, brown staining).

TABLE 2 | Overview of renal complement deposition in patients with COVID-19 compared to Ctrl, ATI, HUS and DIC.

	Ctrl	ATI	HUS	DIC	COVID-19
CD61	0.52	0.29	0.6	0.61	0.78
MASP-2	0.07	0.07	0.1	0.2	0.22
C1q	0.14	0	0.8	0.79	0.19
C3c	0.54	0.89	1	1.25	0.75
C3d	0.39	0.48	0.55	0.61	0.89
C4d	0	0	0	0	0
C5b-9	0.5	0.43	0.65	0.93	1

The mean values of all semi-quantitative compartment-specific scores were summarized and displayed on a heat map.
Ctrl, 1 year renal transplant protocol biopsies; ATI, acute tubular injury; HUS, hemolytic uremic syndrome; DIC, disseminated intravascular coagulation.

C5b-9 was lacking in Ctrl and low in the glomeruli of ATI, it was deposited in four of nine COVID-19 cases, sometimes heavily (**Figures 9A, B**). The most intense deposition of C5b-9 was observed in DIC, while in HUS 3/5 of biopsies were also positive but showed only weak glomerular staining (**Figure 9A**). In contrast, peritubular C5b-9 was most common in COVID-19 (**Figures 9C, D**); in comparison Ctrl and DIC cases showed comparatively less C5b-9 and HUS showed less positive staining (**Figure 9C**). Comparable arterial C5b-9 deposits with light to intense staining were observed in COVID-19 and DIC, while in HUS arterial C5b-9 was similarly frequent but showed less intense staining (**Figure 9E**). Similar to most other complement components in this study, C5b-9 in renal arteries was lowest in ATI (**Figure 8E**) while Ctrl showed positive

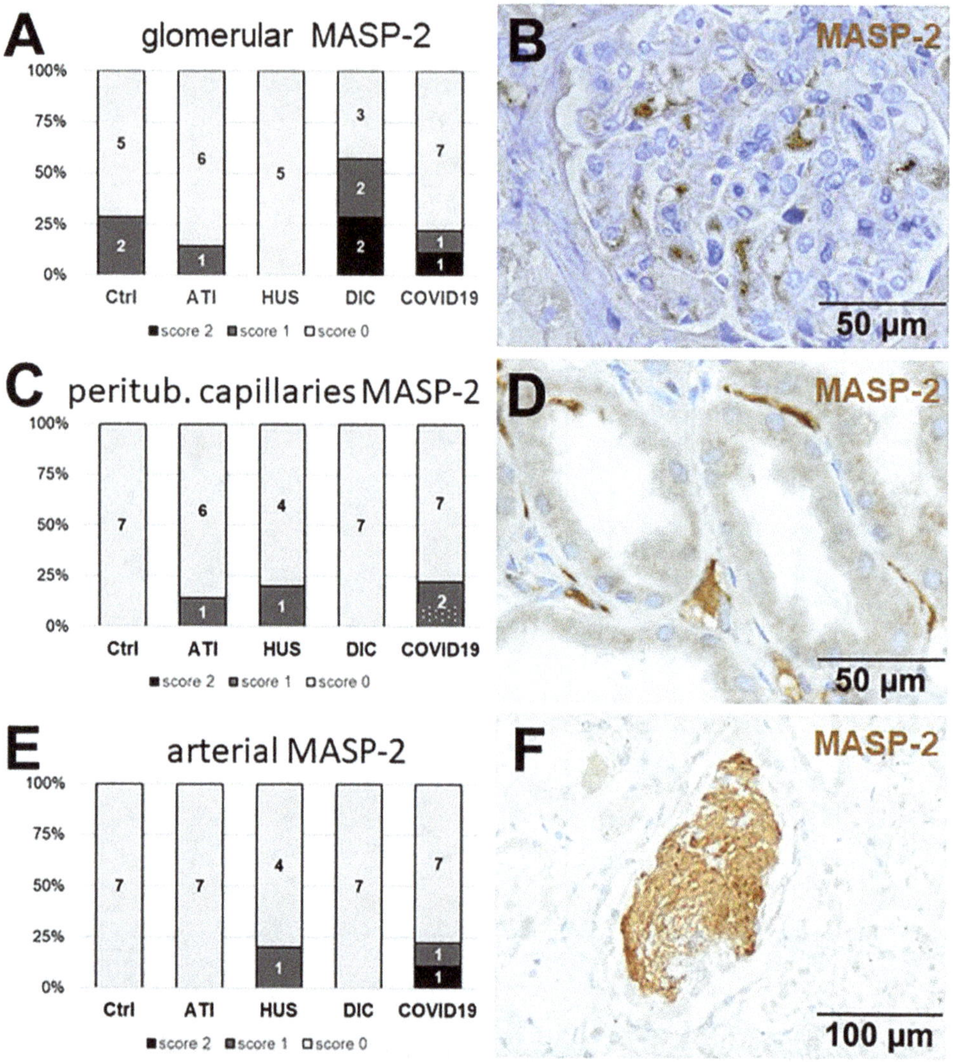

FIGURE 5 | Frequency and vascular localization of MASP-2 deposition in renal biopsies with COVID-19 compared to Ctrl, ATI, HUS, and DIC. Frequency and amount of mannose-binding protein-associated serine protease 2 (MASP-2) deposition was analyzed in glomerular capillaries **(A)**, peritubular capillaries **(C)** and renal arteries **(E)** in renal control biopsies taken 1 year after transplantation (Ctrl, n = 7), biopsies with acute tubular injury (ATI, n = 7), hemolytic uremic syndrome (HUS, n = 5), disseminated intravascular coagulation (DIC, n = 7), and COVID-19 (COVID-19, n = 9) using immunohistochemistry and semi-quantitative scoring. The proportion of MASP-2–positive stained cases that belongs to cases with comorbidities with known involvement of complement activation is marked by hatched bars representing the COVID-19 cohort. Representative pictures of COVID-19 biopsies positive for MASP-2 were shown for glomerular (**B**, brown staining), peritubular (**D**, brown staining) and arterial localization (**F**, brown staining).

staining in all cases but with less intensity (**Figure 9E**). In summary, COVID-19 leads to endothelial cell damage in the kidney with the accumulation of platelets and significant activation of the complement system (summarized in **Table 2**), which might at least in part occur *via* the lectin pathway.

Tubular Complement Activation Was Highest in Kidneys of Patients With COVID-19 and Restricted to C3c, C3d and C5b-9

Since we observed tubular injury in all biopsies from patients with COVID-19, we next investigated complement deposition in the tubular compartment and detected complement deposition along the tubular basement membranes (**Figures 10B, D, F**). No tubular deposition could be detected for MASP-2 and C1q in our cohort (data not shown). Tubular C3c, was detected in 5/9 biopsies from COVID-19 patients, while tubular C3c deposition in HUS was comparable and more frequent in ATI and DIC (**Figure 10A**). In contrast, tubular C3d was detectable in all COVID-19 biopsies and showed the most frequent and intense staining compared to all other groups (**Figure 10C**). Interestingly, the C3d staining was strongest in kidneys from patients who died due to severe COVID-19 infection, indicating that complement mediated tubular damage is might be dependent on the severity of the COVID-19 disease. Tubular

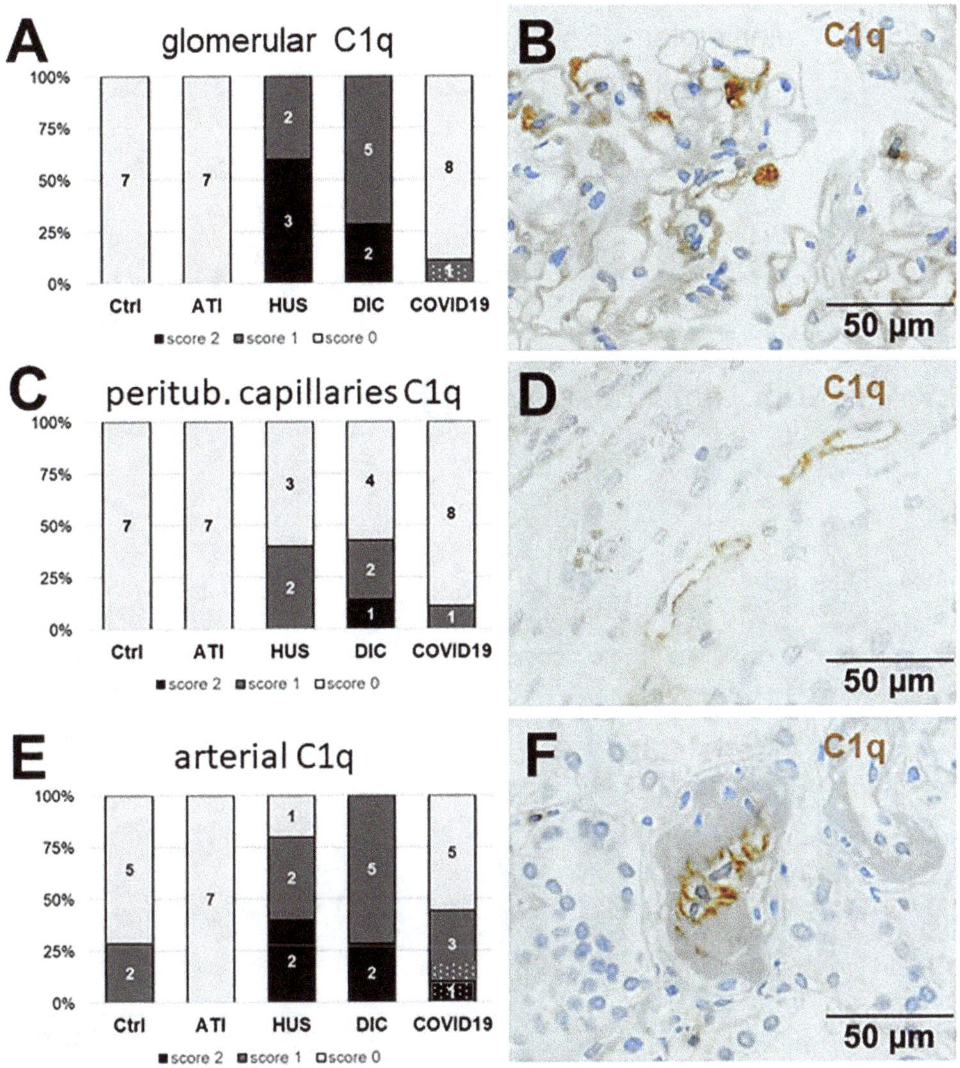

FIGURE 6 | Frequency and vascular localization of C1q deposition in renal biopsies with COVID-19 compared to Ctrl, ATI, HUS, and DIC. Frequency and amount of C1q deposition were analyzed in glomerular capillaries **(A)**, peritubular capillaries **(C)**, and renal arteries **(E)** in renal control biopsies taken 1 year after transplantation (Ctrl, n = 7), biopsies with acute tubular injury (ATI, n = 7), hemolytic uremic syndrome (HUS, n = 5), disseminated intravascular coagulation (DIC, n = 7) and COVID-19 (COVID-19, n = 9) using immunohistochemistry and semi-quantitative scoring. The proportion of C1q-positive stained cases that belongs to cases with comorbidities with known involvement of complement activation is marked by hatched bars representing the COVID-19 cohort. Representative pictures of COVID-19 biopsies positive for C1q were shown for glomerular (**B**, brown staining), peritubular (**D**, brown staining) and arterial localization (**F**, brown staining).

C5b-9 deposits could also be detected in 7/9 biopsies of patients with COVID-19 and again showed the highest intensity compared to the other groups (**Figure 10E**).

In summary, when the compartment-specific scores for all stainings were added up to a total score for the respective factor, biopsies of COVID-19 patients contained the highest number of CD61-positive platelets compared to the other groups (**Table 2**). This parallels with the deposition of C3d, C5b-9 and on a lower level with the deposition of MASP-2 (**Table 2**). C1q deposition in biopsies from patients with COVID-19 was comparable with Ctrl and even higher in HUS and DIC (**Table 2**), indicating that in COVID-19 renal complement was not activated *via* the classical but by the lectin or alternative pathway.

DISCUSSION

Complement factors were major components that clogged CRP adsorber columns during the treatment of critically ill patients with COVID-19 prompting further studies on a role of complement in COVID-19 infection. C5b-9 and the complement cleavage product and anaphylatoxin C5a were increased in the plasma of patients with moderate and severe disease compared to healthy controls (20). Furthermore, lung epithelial cells infected with SARS-CoV-2 highly expressed the complement factors C1r, C1s, C3 and factor B (22). Studies by immunohistology on complement-mediated microvascular damage showed deposits of MASP-2, C4d, and C5b-9 in the

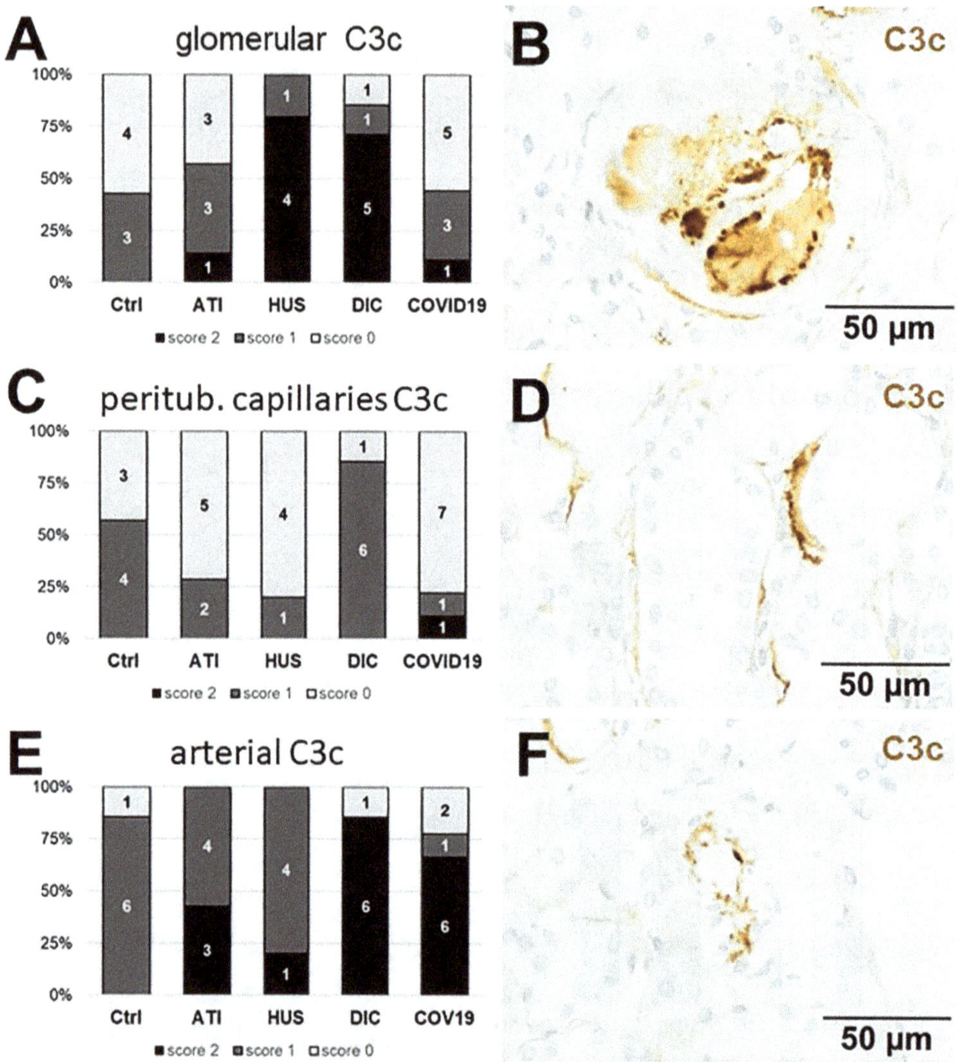

FIGURE 7 | Frequency and vascular localization of C3c deposition in renal biopsies with COVID-19 compared to Ctrl, ATI, HUS and DIC. Frequency and amount of C3c deposition were analyzed in glomerular capillaries **(A)**, peritubular capillaries **(C)**, and renal arteries **(E)** in renal control biopsies taken 1 year after transplantation (Ctrl, n = 7), biopsies with acute tubular injury (ATI, n = 7), hemolytic uremic syndrome (HUS, n = 5), disseminated intravascular coagulation (DIC, n = 7) and COVID-19 (COVID-19, n = 9) using immunohistochemistry and semi-quantitative scoring. The proportion of C3d-positive stained cases that belongs to cases with comorbidities with known involvement of complement activation is marked by hatched bars representing the COVID-19 cohort. Representative pictures of COVID-19 biopsies positive for C3c were shown for glomerular (**B**, brown staining), peritubular (**D**, brown staining) and arterial localization (**F**, brown staining).

lungs and skins of severely ill patients (21). In a preprint study Gao et al. demonstrated, that the SARS-CoV-2 nucleocapsid protein bound to MASP-2 and activated complement; blockade of this interaction improved the survival of mice with COVID-19 nucleocapsid potentiated LPS-induced pneumonia (23). In our study in kidney biopsies from patients with COVID-19, we for the first time detected enhanced renal complement deposition in vascular beds and tubuli supporting the idea that the complement system is a potential mediator of COVID-19–induced kidney injury. The observed kidney damage in COVID-19 biopsies was primarily acute kidney injury (AKI) with mild to severe tubular injury and in rare cases glomerular thrombi. This is consistent with the observations of other histopathological studies examining kidneys of the patients with COVID-19 and identifying AKI in 37% to 98% of all examined cases (9–11). Interestingly, especially the tubular deposition of C3d was highest in biopsies from patients with COVID-19 and seem to be dependent on the severity of the disease, supporting the role of complement as a mediator of tubular damage. In addition, we investigated endothelial cell loss in COVID-19 biopsies. The endothelium plays an important role in the pathogenesis of COVID-19–mediated tissue damage, both as an effector contributing to inflammation and thrombosis, and as a target organ, whose dysfunction may contribute to poor outcome (24). In an autopsy study from patients who died of COVID-19, pulmonary vessels showed widespread thrombosis,

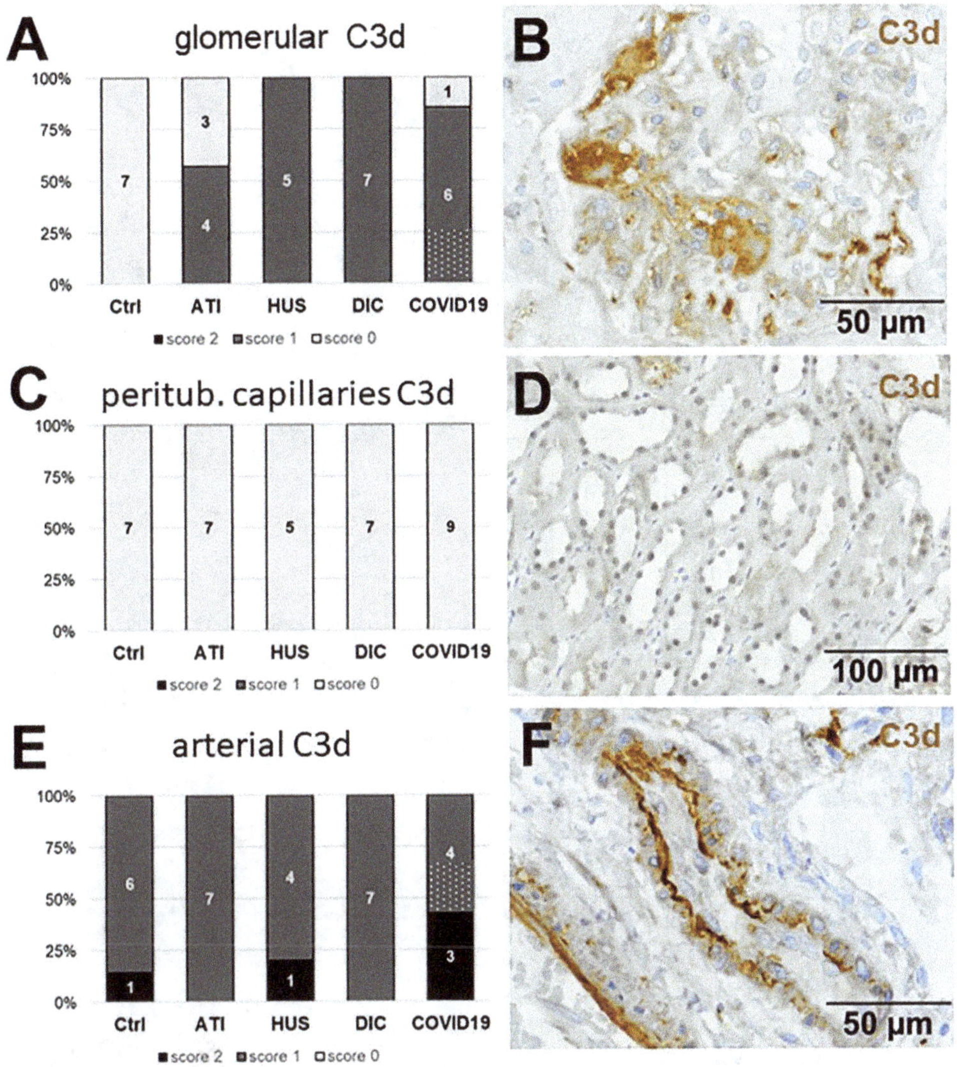

FIGURE 8 | Frequency and vascular localization of C3d deposition in renal biopsies with COVID-19 compared to Ctrl, ATI, HUS, and DIC. Frequency and amount of C3d deposition were analyzed in glomerular capillaries **(A)**, peritubular capillaries **(C)** and renal arteries **(E)** in renal control biopsies taken 1 year after transplantation (Ctrl, n = 7), biopsies with acute tubular injury (ATI, n = 7), hemolytic uremic syndrome (HUS, n = 5), disseminated intravascular coagulation (DIC, n = 7) and COVID-19 (COVID-19, n = 9) using immunohistochemistry and semi-quantitative scoring. The proportion of C3d-positive stained cases that belongs to cases with comorbidities with known involvement of complement activation is marked by hatched bars representing the COVID-19 cohort. Representative pictures of COVID-19 biopsies positive for C3d were shown for glomerular (**B**, brown staining), peritubular (**D**, brown staining) and arterial localization (**F**, brown staining).

capillary microthrombi and increased neovascularization (25). In renal biopsies we observed a reduction of the endothelial cell marker ERG, similar to the endothelial damage in ATI, but less pronounced than in DIC. Renal capillarization was highest in HUS, indicating that the endothelial cell damage already started to be repaired by high proliferative activity. In contrast to reports in the lung (25), microthrombi and endothelial proliferation were rare in COVID-19 renal biopsies. However, CD61-positive platelets in peritubular capillaries were highest in COVID-19 biopsies compared to all other groups. In comparison with other renal diseases with distinct endothelial cell injury, like HUS or DIC, we demonstrate similar complement activation in COVID-19 renal biopsies with some differences in the involved pathways.

The lectin pathway can be activated by sugar residues bound to pattern recognition molecules followed by activation of MASP-2 complexes with collectin 11. In ischemic kidneys, collectin 11 recognized an abnormal L-fucose pattern on tubular cells and consequently activated the lectin pathway (26). Interestingly, in tubuli from COVID-19 biopsies we observed a higher collectin 11 mRNA expression compared to 1 year biopsies, HUS and ATI controls (**Supplemental Figure 1**) and MASP-2 deposition in some of the COVID-19 cases, indicating that activation of the lectin pathway in COVID-19 was not restricted to lung or skin (21). Activation of the classical pathway can be mediated for example by natural IgM antibodies that recognize viral antigens or neo-antigens exposed on damaged host tissues (27). C1q, the

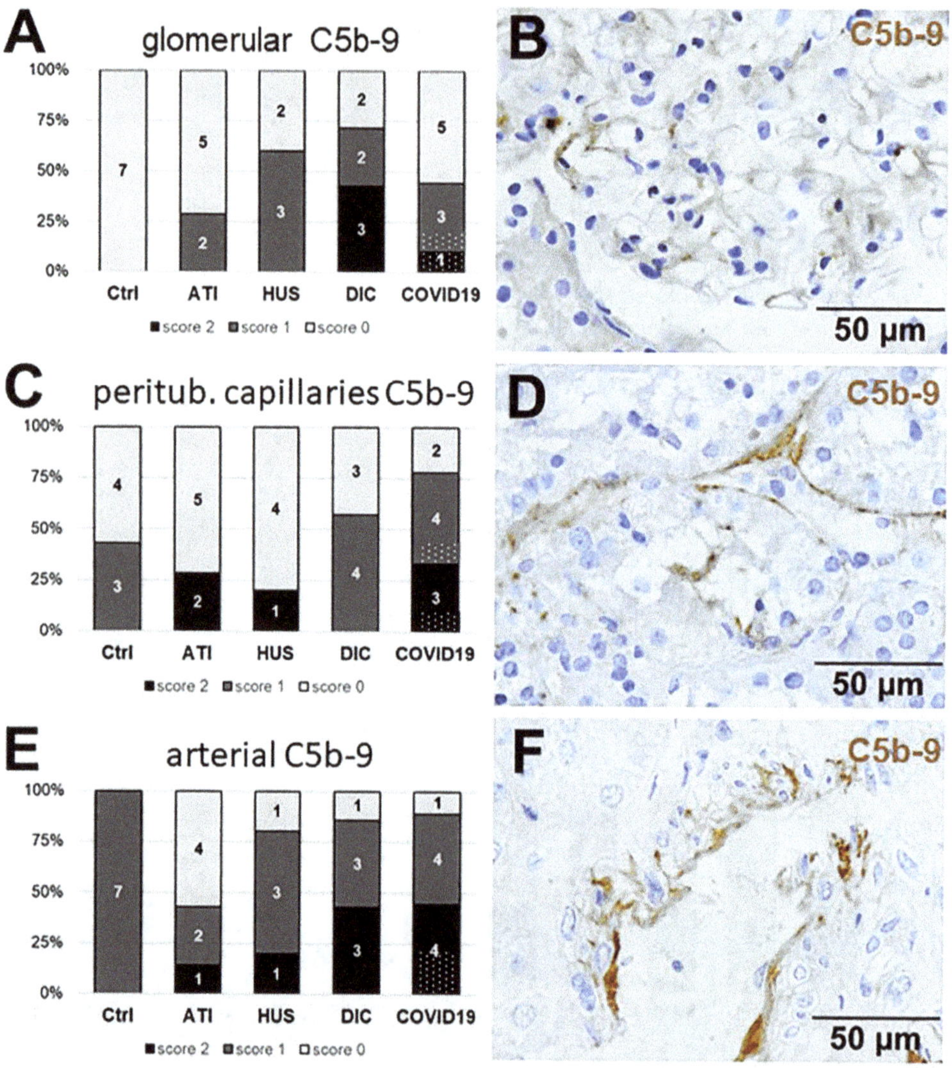

FIGURE 9 | Frequency and vascular localization of C5b-9 deposition in renal biopsies with COVID-19 compared to Ctrl, ATI, HUS, and DIC. Frequency and amount of C5b-9 deposition were analyzed in glomerular capillaries **(A)**, peritubular capillaries **(C)** and renal arteries **(E)** in renal control biopsies taken 1 year after transplantation (Ctrl, n = 7), biopsies with acute tubular injury (ATI, n = 7), hemolytic uremic syndrome (HUS, n = 5), disseminated intravascular coagulation (DIC, n = 7) and COVID-19 (COVID-19, n = 9) using immunohistochemistry and semi-quantitative scoring. The proportion of C5b-9–positive stained cases that belongs to cases with comorbidities with known involvement of complement activation is marked by hatched bars representing the COVID-19 cohort. Representative pictures of COVID-19 biopsies positive for C5b-9 were shown for glomerular (**B**, brown staining), peritubular (**D**, brown staining) and arterial localization (**F**, brown staining).

starter of the classical pathway, was more frequently detected in COVID-19 as compared to ATI but, nevertheless, rarely detected in glomeruli and peritubular capillaries compared to HUS and DIC cases. However, the highest C1q deposition in COVID-19 biopsies was seen in renal arteries. C3 cleavage products occur in all three complement activation pathways and were detected as the stable cleavage product C3c and C3d, which can bind covalently to cell surfaces. Interestingly, deposition of these C3 cleavage products were not similarly deposited in the renal biopsies. C3d was highest in biopsies from patients with COVID-19, C3c was also increased compared to controls but even higher in HUS and DIC. Differences in staining patterns are may be due to the specificity of the used antibodies. While the anti-C3c antibody also recognize C3 the anti-C3d do not detect intact C3. C5b-9, as a marker of the terminal complement cascade, was strongly and similarly detectable in glomerular capillaries and even more strongly deposited in the peritubular capillaries than in HUS and DIC biopsies. Significant C5b-9 deposition was also described in lung and skin biopsies from patients with COVID-19 (21).

In summary, in our study complement activation in COVID-19 was not restricted to a specific activation pathway. Complement was reportedly activated by all three known pathways during COVID-19 infection (28). It is conceivable that complement activation can occur both through direct interaction with the SARS-CoV-2 virus or indirectly by

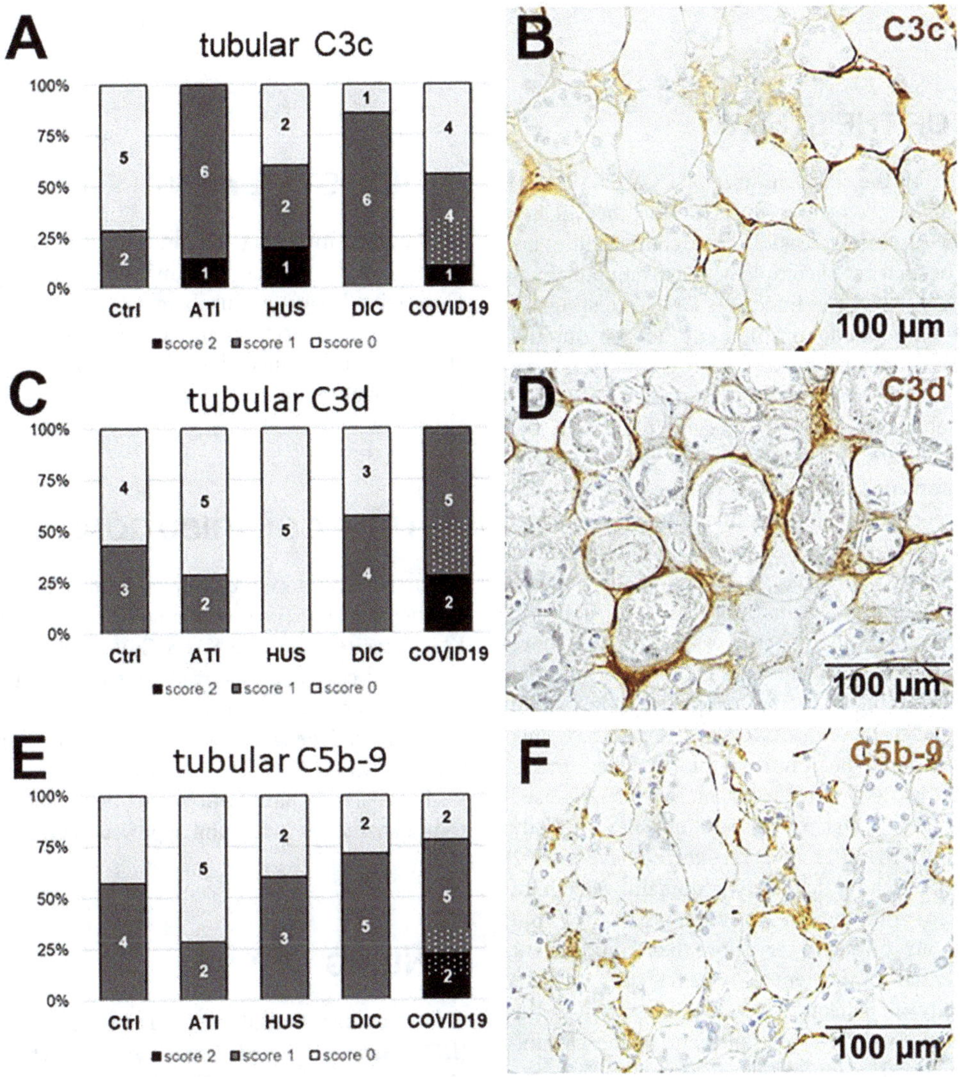

FIGURE 10 | Frequency and tubular localization of C3c, C3d, and C5b-9 deposition in renal biopsies with COVID-19 compared to Ctrl, ATI, HUS and DIC. Frequency and amount of tubular C3c **(A)**, C3d **(C)**, and C5b-9 **(E)** deposition were analyzed in renal control biopsies taken 1 year after transplantation (Ctrl, n = 7), biopsies with acute tubular injury (ATI, n = 7), hemolytic uremic syndrome (HUS, n = 5), disseminated intravascular coagulation (DIC, n = 7), and COVID-19 (COVID-19, n = 9) using immunohistochemistry and semi-quantitative scoring. The proportion of complement-positive stained cases that belongs to cases with comorbidities with known involvement of complement activation is marked by hatched bars representing the COVID-19 cohort. Representative pictures of COVID-19 biopsies positive for tubular C3c (**B**, brown staining), C3d (**D**, brown staining), and C5b-9 (**F**, brown staining) were shown.

tissue damage and dying cells. Presumably, the complement activation in kidneys of COVID-19 patients observed in our study was rather indirect, since we could hardly detect viruses by in-situ hybridization and even fewer pathogens by immunohistochemistry so that we cannot exclude that these are unspecific background signals. This goes inline with findings of other groups, which have also not found robust signals of SARS-CoV-2 in the kidneys (9–11). In contrast, in other studies SARS-CoV-2 was detected in the kidney (5, 7, 8), so that we cannot exclude the possibility that SARS-CoV-2 was present in the kidney at an earlier time interval before biopsy was taken and that complement was activated directly by the virus. Our own and data of other groups showed that complement activation might be an important pathomechanism of tissue damage in COVID-19 opening the possibility of treatment with complement inhibitors. Anecdotal reports of the successful treatment of seriously ill patients with COVID-19 employing the C5 inhibitor Eculizumab (29) or the C3 inhibitor AMY-101 (30) have already been published. Clinical studies with complement inhibitors in patients with COVID-19 will show the efficiency of this treatment. Several clinical trials are currently ongoing to investigate the protective effects of purified/recombinant complement regulators (e.g. C1-esterase inhibitor) or complement inhibitors directed against MASP-2, C3, C5, or the C5a receptor on COVID-19 outcomes ranging from changes in oxygenation to mortality (31)(https://www.trialsitenews.com/category/masp-2/).

LIMITATION OF THE STUDY

Our study is limited by the small number of COVID-19 renal biopsies and the different co-morbidities of the investigated patients with kidney disease. At least 3 of the comorbidities are also known for the occurrence of complement activation, namely ANCA-associated GN, FSGS and infectious GN. To distinguish between COVID-19–related complement activation and complement activation that might be related to the diagnosed renal disease, the proportion of positively stained cases that belongs to the 3 above mentioned cases is marked in the figures by hatching. Indeed, we frequently but not necessarily always detected complement deposition outline biopsies with these diseases. However, the percentage of complement-positive cases in COVID-19 with known potential complement involvement represented on average 30.2% of all positive COVID-19 cases. Although we cannot rule out that the observed complement deposition in the cases with the above mentioned kidney diseases was due to this comorbidity and not to the COVID-19 infection, the renal complement deposition was by far not limited to these cases. Renal thrombi were only found in one investigated post-mortem biopsy, therefore it remains unclear if thrombi only occur in severely diseased kidneys or during peri-mortal processes. Since the antibody used for detection of MASP-2 also recognize the MASP-2 splice variant MAp19, lacking the catalytic domain, we cannot distinguish between complement activating MASP-2 and Map19. Although our initial observation that complement factors are an essential component of plasma clots in CRP adsorbers in critically ill patients with COVID-19 led to the studies in the kidney, the role of complement in the clotting process remains open and needs further investigation.

In conclusion, we observed marked complement deposition in kidneys of patients with COVID-19 similar to other known renal diseases with a distinct endothelial injury. Complement deposition could be also detected on tubular basement membranes in biopsies from patients with COVID-19. Therefore, we speculate that complement is, most likely involved in vascular and tubular kidney damage in COVID-19. Specific complement inhibition might thus be a promising treatment option to prevent deregulated complement activation and subsequent collateral tissue injury. Further studies with larger biopsy numbers are necessary to elucidate the involvement of the complement system in COVID-19–induced renal damage.

ETHICS STATEMENT

The studies involving human participants were reviewed and approved by Ethics Committee of Friedrich-Alexander-University Erlangen-Nürnberg (Reference No. 4415). Written informed consent for participation was not required for this study in accordance with the national legislation and the institutional requirements.

AUTHOR CONTRIBUTIONS

EV and FP conducted experiments, analyzed data, and wrote the manuscript. TR carried out immunohistological staining. H-MJ and KÜ generated the anti-SARS-CoV-2 spike antibody, supplied transfected cells, and proofread the paper. GL performed MALDI-TOF. AS isolated proteins from plasma adsorber material. MH conceived and designed the plasma adsorber analysis and revised the manuscript. KA, MB-H, and CD conceived and designed the study, analyzed data, and wrote the manuscript. All authors contributed to the article and approved the submitted version.

FUNDING

This study was funded by the Deutsche Forschungsgemeinschaft (DFG, German Research Foundation), project number 387509280, SFB 1350 and supported by the DEFEAT Pandemics autopsy platform of the Federal Ministry of Education and Research (BMBF).

ACKNOWLEDGMENTS

The technical assistance of E. Roth, S. Söllner, Lisa Stelzer, Britta Hähnel, and M. Reutelshöfer is gratefully acknowledged.

REFERENCES

1. Guan WJ, Ni ZY, Hu Y, Liang WH, Ou CQ, He JX, et al. Clinical Characteristics of Coronavirus Disease 2019 in China. *N Engl J Med* (2020) 382(18):1708–20. doi: 10.1056/NEJMoa2002032
2. Gupta A, Madhavan MV, Sehgal K, Nair N, Mahajan S, Sehrawat TS, et al. Extrapulmonary manifestations of COVID-19. *Nat Med* (2020) 26(7):1017–32. doi: 10.1038/s41591-020-0968-3
3. Chen YT, Shao SC, Hsu CK, Wu IW, Hung MJ, Chen YC. Incidence of acute kidney injury in COVID-19 infection: a systematic review and

meta-analysis. *Crit Care* (2020) 24(1):346. doi: 10.1186/s13054-020-03009-y
4. Cheng Y, Luo R, Wang K, Zhang M, Wang Z, Dong L, et al. Kidney disease is associated with in-hospital death of patients with COVID-19. *Kidney Int* (2020) 97(5):829–38. doi: 10.1016/j.kint.2020.03.005
5. Puelles VG, Lütgehetmann M, Lindenmeyer MT, Sperhake JP, Wong MN, Allweiss L, et al. Multiorgan and Renal Tropism of SARS-CoV-2. *N Engl J Med* (2020) 383(6) :590–2. doi: 10.1056/NEJMc2011400
6. Soleimani M. Acute Kidney Injury in SARS-CoV-2 Infection: Direct Effect of Virus on Kidney Proximal Tubule Cells. *Int J Mol Sci* (2020) 21(9):1–6. doi: 10.3390/ijms21093275
7. Farkash EA, Wilson AM, Jentzen JM. Ultrastructural Evidence for Direct Renal Infection with SARS-CoV-2. *J Am Soc Nephrol* (2020) 31(8):1683–7. doi: 10.1681/asn.2020040432
8. Su H, Yang M, Wan C, Yi LX, Tang F, Zhu HY, et al. Renal histopathological analysis of 26 postmortem findings of patients with COVID-19 in China. *Kidney Int* (2020) 98(1):219–27. doi: 10.1016/j.kint.2020.04.003
9. Kudose S, Batal I, Santoriello D, Xu K, Barasch J, Peleg Y, et al. Kidney Biopsy Findings in Patients with COVID-19. *J Am Soc Nephrol* (2020) 31(9):1959–68. doi: 10.1681/asn.2020060802
10. Golmai P, Larsen CP, DeVita MV, Wahl SJ, Weins A, Rennke HG, et al. Histopathologic and Ultrastructural Findings in Postmortem Kidney Biopsy Material in 12 Patients with AKI and COVID-19. *J Am Soc Nephrol* (2020) 31 (9):1944–7. doi: 10.1681/asn.2020050683
11. Santoriello D, Khairallah P, Bomback AS, Xu K, Kudose S, Batal I, et al. Postmortem Kidney Pathology Findings in Patients with COVID-19. *J Am Soc Nephrol* (2020) 31(9):2158–67. doi: 10.1681/asn.2020050744
12. Chen G, Wu D, Guo W, Cao Y, Huang D, Wang H, et al. Clinical and immunological features of severe and moderate coronavirus disease 2019. *J Clin Invest* (2020) 130(5):2620–9. doi: 10.1172/jci137244
13. Leppkes M, Knopf J, Naschberger E, Lindemann A, Singh J, Herrmann I, et al. Vascular occlusion by neutrophil extracellular traps in COVID-19. *EBioMedicine* (2020) 58:102925. doi: 10.1016/j.ebiom.2020.102925
14. Wang R, Xiao H, Guo R, Li Y, Shen B. The role of C5a in acute lung injury induced by highly pathogenic viral infections. *Emerg Microbes Infect* (2015) 4 (5):e28. doi: 10.1038/emi.2015.28
15. Noris M, Remuzzi G. Overview of complement activation and regulation. *Semin Nephrol* (2013) 33(6):479–92. doi: 10.1016/j.semnephrol.2013.08.001
16. Kojouharova M, Reid K, Gadjeva M. New insights into the molecular mechanisms of classical complement activation. *Mol Immunol* (2010) 47 (13):2154–60. doi: 10.1016/j.molimm.2010.05.011
17. Farrar CA, Zhou W, Sacks SH. Role of the lectin complement pathway in kidney transplantation. *Immunobiology* (2016) 221(10):1068–72. doi: 10.1016/j.imbio.2016.05.004
18. Dobo J, Pal G, Cervenak L, Gal P. The emerging roles of mannose-binding lectin-associated serine proteases (MASPs) in the lectin pathway of complement and beyond. *Immunol Rev* (2016) 274(1):98–111. doi: 10.1111/imr.12460
19. Pangburn MK, Schreiber RD, Muller-Eberhard HJ. Formation of the initial C3 convertase of the alternative complement pathway. Acquisition of C3b-like activities by spontaneous hydrolysis of the putative thioester in native C3. *J Exp Med* (1981) 154(3):856–67. doi: 10.1084/jem.154.3.856
20. Cugno M, Meroni PL, Gualtierotti R, Griffini S, Grovetti E, Torri A, et al. Complement activation in patients with COVID-19: A novel therapeutic target. *J Allergy Clin Immunol* (2020) 146(1):215–7. doi: 10.1016/j.jaci.2020.05.006
21. Magro C, Mulvey JJ, Berlin D, Nuovo G, Salvatore S, Harp J, et al. Complement associated microvascular injury and thrombosis in the pathogenesis of severe COVID-19 infection: a report of five cases. *Transl Res* (2020) 220:1–13. doi: 10.1016/j.trsl.2020.04.007
22. Yan B, Freiwald T, Chauss D, Wang L, West E, Bibby J, et al. SARS-CoV2 drives JAK1/2-dependent local and systemic complement hyper-activation. *Res Sq* (2020). doi: 10.21203/rs.3.rs-33390/v1
23. Gao T, Hu M, Zhang X, Li H, Zhu L, Liu H, et al. Highly pathogenic coronavirus N protein aggravates lung injury by MASP-2-mediated complement over-activation. *medRxiv* (2020). doi: 10.1101/2020.03.29.2004196
24. Evans PC, Ed Rainger G, Mason JC, Guzik TJ, Osto E, Stamataki Z, et al. Endothelial dysfunction in COVID-19: a position paper of the ESC Working Group for Atherosclerosis and Vascular Biology, and the ESC Council of Basic Cardiovascular Science. *Cardiovasc Res* (2020) 116(14) :2177–84. doi: 10.1093/cvr/cvaa230
25. Ackermann M, Verleden SE, Kuehnel M, Haverich A, Welte T, Laenger F, et al. Pulmonary Vascular Endothelialitis, Thrombosis, and Angiogenesis in Covid-19. *N Engl J Med* (2020) 383(2):120–8. doi: 10.1056/NEJMoa2015432
26. Farrar CA, Tran D, Li K, Wu W, Peng Q, Schwaeble W, et al. Collectin-11 detects stress-induced L-fucose pattern to trigger renal epithelial injury. *J Clin Invest* (2016) 126(5):1911–25. doi: 10.1172/jci83000
27. Zhang M, Carroll MC. Natural IgM-mediated innate autoimmunity: a new target for early intervention of ischemia-reperfusion injury. *Expert Opin Biol Ther* (2007) 7(10):1575–82. doi: 10.1517/14712598.7.10.1575
28. Song WC, FitzGerald GA. COVID-19, microangiopathy, hemostatic activation, and complement. *J Clin Invest* (2020) 130(8):3950–3. doi: 10.1172/jci140183
29. Diurno F, Numis FG, Porta G, Cirillo F, Maddaluno S, Ragozzino A, et al. Eculizumab treatment in patients with COVID-19: preliminary results from real life ASL Napoli 2 Nord experience. *Eur Rev Med Pharmacol Sci* (2020) 24 (7):4040–7. doi: 10.26355/eurrev_202004_20875
30. Mastaglio S, Ruggeri A, Risitano AM, Angelillo P, Yancopoulou D, Mastellos DC, et al. The first case of COVID-19 treated with the complement C3 inhibitor AMY-101. *Clin Immunol* (2020) 215:108450. doi: 10.1016/j.clim.2020.108450
31. Conigliaro P, Triggianese P, Perricone C, Chimenti MS, Perricone R. COVID-19: disCOVering the role of complement system. *Clin Exp Rheumatol* (2020) 38(4):587–91. doi: 10.1016/j.autrev.2020.102590

Permissions

All chapters in this book were first published by Frontiers; hereby published with permission under the Creative Commons Attribution License or equivalent. Every chapter published in this book has been scrutinized by our experts. Their significance has been extensively debated. The topics covered herein carry significant findings which will fuel the growth of the discipline. They may even be implemented as practical applications or may be referred to as a beginning point for another development.

The contributors of this book come from diverse backgrounds, making this book a truly international effort. This book will bring forth new frontiers with its revolutionizing research information and detailed analysis of the nascent developments around the world.

We would like to thank all the contributing authors for lending their expertise to make the book truly unique. They have played a crucial role in the development of this book. Without their invaluable contributions this book wouldn't have been possible. They have made vital efforts to compile up to date information on the varied aspects of this subject to make this book a valuable addition to the collection of many professionals and students.

This book was conceptualized with the vision of imparting up-to-date information and advanced data in this field. To ensure the same, a matchless editorial board was set up. Every individual on the board went through rigorous rounds of assessment to prove their worth. After which they invested a large part of their time researching and compiling the most relevant data for our readers.

The editorial board has been involved in producing this book since its inception. They have spent rigorous hours researching and exploring the diverse topics which have resulted in the successful publishing of this book. They have passed on their knowledge of decades through this book. To expedite this challenging task, the publisher supported the team at every step. A small team of assistant editors was also appointed to further simplify the editing procedure and attain best results for the readers.

Apart from the editorial board, the designing team has also invested a significant amount of their time in understanding the subject and creating the most relevant covers. They scrutinized every image to scout for the most suitable representation of the subject and create an appropriate cover for the book.

The publishing team has been an ardent support to the editorial, designing and production team. Their endless efforts to recruit the best for this project, has resulted in the accomplishment of this book. They are a veteran in the field of academics and their pool of knowledge is as vast as their experience in printing. Their expertise and guidance has proved useful at every step. Their uncompromising quality standards have made this book an exceptional effort. Their encouragement from time to time has been an inspiration for everyone.

The publisher and the editorial board hope that this book will prove to be a valuable piece of knowledge for researchers, students, practitioners and scholars across the globe.

List of Contributors

Yanyan Liu, Kun Wang, Yueqiang Li, Ying Zhang, Chunxiu Zhang, Haotian Wei, Ran Luo, Shuwang Ge and Gang Xu
Division of Internal Medicine, Department of Nephrology, Tongji Hospital, Tongji Medical College, Huazhong University of Science and Technology, Wuhan, China

Xinjun Liang
Hubei Cancer Hospital, Tongji Medical College, Huazhong University of Science and Technology, Wuhan, China

Felix Poppelaars, Mariana Gaya da Costa, Casper F. M. Franssen, Willem J. van Son, Stefan P. Berger, and Marc A. Seelen
Division of Nephrology, Department of Internal Medicine, University of Groningen, University Medical Center Groningen, Groningen, Netherlands
Nephrology and Infectious Diseases Research and Development Group, University of Porto, Porto, Portugal

Bernardo Faria
Department of Internal Medicine, Division of Nephrology, University Medical Center Groningen, Groningen, Netherlands
Nephrology and Infectious Diseases Research and Development Group, University of Porto, Porto, Portugal
Nephrology and Infecciology Group, INEB/I3S, University of Porto, Porto, Portugal
Department of Nephrology, Hopsital Braga, Braga, Portugal

V. Michael Holers and Nirmal K. Banda
Division of Rheumatology, Department of Medicine, University of Colorado Anschutz Medical Campus, Aurora, CO, United States

Jenny Giang and Jeffrey Damman
Department of Pathology, Erasmus Medical Center Rotterdam, Rotterdam, Netherlands

Martijn B. A. van Doorn and Errol P. Prens
Department of Dermatology, Erasmus Medical Center Rotterdam, Rotterdam, Netherlands

Christopher L. Nauser, Mark C. Howard, Giorgia Fanelli, Conrad A. Farrar and Steven Sacks
MRC Centre for Transplantation, School of Immunology and Microbial Sciences, King's College London, Guy's and St.Thomas' NHS Foundation Trust, London, United Kingdom

Robert Rissmann
Center for Human Drug Research, Leiden, Netherlands

Giuseppe Castellano, Rossana Franzin, Alessandra Stasi, Chiara Divella, Paola Pontrelli and Loreto Gesualdo
Nephrology, Dialysis and Transplantation Unit, Department of Emergency and Organ Transplantation, University of Bari Aldo Moro, Bari, Italy

Fabio Sallustio
Nephrology, Dialysis and Transplantation Unit, Department of Emergency and Organ Transplantation, University of Bari Aldo Moro, Bari, Italy
Department of Basic Medical Sciences, Neuroscience and Sense Organs, University of Bari Aldo Moro, Bari, Italy

Giuseppe Lucarelli and Michele Battaglia
Urology, Andrology and Renal Transplantation Unit, Department of Emergency and Organ Transplantation, University of Bari Aldo Moro, Bari, Italy

Francesco Staffieri and Antonio Crovace
Veterinary Surgery Unit, Department of Emergency and Organ Transplantation, University of Bari Aldo Moro, Bari, Italy

Giovanni Stallone and Giuseppe Grandaliano
Nephrology, Dialysis and Transplantation Unit, Department of Medical and Surgical Sciences, University of Foggia, Foggia, Italy

Gregor Sommer
Clinic of Radiology and Nuclear Medicine, University Hospital Basel, Basel, Switzerland

Günter Lochnit
Department of Biochemistry, Division Protein Analystics, Justus-Liebig-University Giessen, Giessen, Germany

Solmaz Assa
Department of Cardiology, University of Groningen, University Medical Center Groningen, Groningen, Netherlands

Mohamed R. Daha
Division of Nephrology, Department of Internal Medicine, University of Groningen, University Medical Center Groningen, Groningen, Netherlands
Department of Nephrology, University of Leiden, Leiden University Medical Center, Leiden, Netherlands

José Osmar Medina Pestana
Nephrology Division, Federal University of São Paulo, São Paulo, Brazil

Anne Troldborg and Kristian Stengaard-Pedersen
Department of Rheumatology, Aarhus University Hospital, Aarhus, Denmark
Institute of Clinical Medicine, Aarhus University, Aarhus, Denmark

Bent Deleuran
Department of Rheumatology, Aarhus University Hospital, Aarhus, Denmark
Department of Biomedicine, Aarhus University, Aarhus, Denmark

Lisbeth Jensen, Steffen Thiel and Jens Christian Jensenius
Department of Biomedicine, Aarhus University, Aarhus, Denmark

Anneza Panagiotou
Division of Internal Medicine, University Hospital Basel, Basel, Switzerland

Marten Trendelenburg and Michael Osthoff
Division of Internal Medicine, University Hospital Basel, Basel, Switzerland
Department of Biomedicine, University Hospital Basel, University of Basel, Basel, Switzerland

Karin Ekholt
Department of Immunology, Oslo University Hospital, Rikshospitalet, Oslo, Norway
University of Oslo, Oslo, Norway

Hilde L. Orrem, Søren E. Pischke and Andreas Barratt-Due
Department of Immunology, Oslo University Hospital, Rikshospitalet, Oslo, Norway
University of Oslo, Oslo, Norway
Division of Emergencies and Critical Care, Department of Anesthesiology, Oslo University Hospital, Rikshospitalet, Oslo, Norway

Per H. Nilsson
Department of Immunology, Oslo University Hospital, Rikshospitalet, Oslo, Norway
University of Oslo, Oslo, Norway
KG Jebsen Inflammation Research Centre, University of Oslo, Oslo, Norway
Linnaeus Centre for Biomaterials Chemistry, Linnaeus University, Kalmar, Sweden

Ola Kleveland and Rune Wiseth
Clinic of Cardiology, St. Olavs Hospital, Trondheim, Norway
Department of Circulation and Medical Imaging, Faculty of Medicine and Health Sciences, Norwegian University of Science and Technology, Trondheim, Norway

Ida Gregersen
Research Institute of Internal Medicine, Oslo University Hospital, Rikshospitalet, Oslo, Norway
Faculty of Medicine, University of Oslo, Oslo, Norway

Arne Yndestad, Bente Halvorsen and Thor Ueland
KG Jebsen Inflammation Research Centre, University of Oslo, Oslo, Norway
Research Institute of Internal Medicine, Oslo University Hospital, Rikshospitalet, Oslo, Norway
Faculty of Medicine, University of Oslo, Oslo, Norway
KG Jebsen Center for Cardiac Research, University of Oslo, Oslo, Norway
Center for Heart Failure Research, Oslo University Hospital, Oslo, Norway

Jan K. Damås and Terje Espevik
Centre of Molecular Inflammation Research, Department of Clinical and Molecular Medicine, Norwegian University of Science and Technology, Trondheim, Norway

Bjørn Bendz
Department of Cardiology, Oslo University Hospital, Rikshospitalet, Oslo, Norway

Lars Gullestad
KG Jebsen Center for Cardiac Research, University of Oslo, Oslo, Norway
Center for Heart Failure Research, Oslo University Hospital, Oslo, Norway
Department of Cardiology, Oslo University Hospital, Rikshospitalet, Oslo, Norway

Geir Ø. Andersen
Center for Heart Failure Research, Oslo University Hospital, Oslo, Norway
Center for Clinical Heart Research, Oslo University Hospital, Ullevål, Oslo, Norway
Department of Cardiology, Oslo University Hospital, Ullevål, Oslo, Norway

Pål Aukrust
KG Jebsen Inflammation Research Centre, University of Oslo, Oslo, Norway
Research Institute of Internal Medicine, Oslo University Hospital, Rikshospitalet, Oslo, Norway
Faculty of Medicine, University of Oslo, Oslo, Norway
Section of Clinical Immunology and Infectious Diseases, Oslo University Hospital, Oslo, Norway

Tom E. Mollnes
Department of Immunology, Oslo University Hospital, Rikshospitalet, Oslo, Norway
University of Oslo, Oslo, Norway
KG Jebsen Inflammation Research Centre, University of Oslo, Oslo, Norway
Centre of Molecular Inflammation Research, Department of Clinical and Molecular Medicine, Norwegian University of Science and Technology, Trondheim, Norway
Research Laboratory, Nordland Hospital, Bodø, Norway
K.G. Jebsen TREC, University of Tromsø, Tromsø, Norway

Romain Paule
INSERM, UMR_S 1138, Centre de Recherche des Cordeliers, Paris, France

Florian Delguste and Eric Boulanger
INSERM, UMR 995, Lille, France

Olivia May
INSERM, UMR_S 1138, Centre de Recherche des Cordeliers, Paris, France
INSERM, UMR 995, Lille, France
University of Lille, CHU Lille, Nephrology Department, Lille, France

Marc Hazzan and Marie Frimat
INSERM, UMR 995, Lille, France
University of Lille, CHU Lille, Nephrology Department, Lille, France

Nicolas S. Merle, Tania Robe-Rybkine, Jordan D. Dimitrov and Lubka T. Roumenina
INSERM, UMR_S 1138, Centre de Recherche des Cordeliers, Paris, France
Sorbonne Universités, UPMC Univ Paris 06, Paris, France
Université Paris Descartes, Sorbonne Paris Cité, Paris, France

Cloé Payet
INSERM, UMR_S 1138, Centre de Recherche des Cordeliers, Paris, France
Sorbonne Universités, UPMC Univ Paris 06, Paris, France

Juliette Leon
INSERM, UMR_S 1138, Centre de Recherche des Cordeliers, Paris, France
Université Paris Descartes, Sorbonne Paris Cité, Paris, France

Viviane Gnemmi
University of Lille, INSERM, CHU Lille, Department of Pathology, UMR-S 1172 - Jean-Pierre Aubert Research Center, Lille, France

Anne Grunenwald
INSERM, UMR_S 1138, Centre de Recherche des Cordeliers, Paris, France
University of Lille, CHU Lille, Nephrology Department, Lille, France
University of Lille, INSERM, CHU Lille, Department of Pathology, UMR-S 1172 - Jean-Pierre Aubert Research Center, Lille, France

Simon C. Satchell
Bristol Renal, University of Bristol, Bristol, United Kingdom

Peter W. Mathieson
University Lodge, University of Hong Kong, Hong Kong, Hong Kong

Veronique Fremeaux-Bacchi
INSERM, UMR_S 1138, Centre de Recherche des Cordeliers, Paris, France
Assistance Publique - Hôpitaux de Paris, Service d'Immunologie Biologique, Hôpital Européen Georges Pompidou, Paris, France

Frida C. Mohlin and Anna M. Blom
Department of Translational Medicine, Lund University, Malmö, Sweden

Piet Gros
Crystal and Structural Chemistry, Bijvoet Center for Biomolecular Research, Department of Chemistry, Utrecht University, Utrecht, Netherlands

Eric Mercier and Jean-Christophe Raymond Gris
Laboratory of Hematology, University Hospital, Nimes, France

Sandra Jeremias Catarino, Fabiana Antunes Andrade and Iara Jose Messias-Reason
Molecular Immunopathology Laboratory, Department of Medical Pathology, Clinical Hospital, Federal University of Paraná, Curitiba, Brazil

Angelica Beate Winter Boldt
Molecular Immunopathology Laboratory, Department of Medical Pathology, Clinical Hospital, Federal University of Paraná, Curitiba, Brazil
Human Molecular Genetics Laboratory, Department of Genetics, Federal University of Paraná, Curitiba, Brazil

Luiza Guilherme
Heart Institute (InCor), School of Medicine, University of São Paulo, São Paulo, Brazil

Shinjini Chakraborty, Ebru Karasu and Markus Huber-Lang
Institute of Clinical and Experimental Trauma-Immunology, University Hospital of Ulm, Ulm, Germany

Anouk G. van Mourik
Sanquin Research, Department of Immunopathology, and Landsteiner Laboratory, Amsterdam University Medical Centre, Amsterdam Infection and Immunity Institute, Amsterdam, Netherlands

Esther C. W. de Boer and Ilse Jongerius
Sanquin Research, Department of Immunopathology, and Landsteiner Laboratory, Amsterdam University Medical Centre, Amsterdam Infection and Immunity Institute, Amsterdam, Netherlands
Department of Pediatric Immunology, Rheumatology, and Infectious Diseases, Emma Children's Hospital, Amsterdam University Medical Centre, Amsterdam, Netherlands

Frederick Pfister, Eva Vonbrunn, Tajana Ries, Maike Büttner-Herold, Kerstin Amann and Christoph Daniel
Department of Nephropathology, Institute of Pathology, Friedrich-Alexander-University (FAU) Erlangen-Nürnberg, Erlangen, Germany

Hans-Martin Jäck
Nikolaus-Fiebinger-Center FAU, Department of Medicine 3, Division of Molecular Immunology, Friedrich-Alexander-University (FAU) Erlangen-Nürnberg, Erlangen, Germany

Klaus Überla
Department of Virology, Friedrich-Alexander-University (FAU) Erlangen-Nürnberg, Erlangen, Germany

Ahmed Sheriff
Pentracor GmbH, Henningsdorf, Germany

Martin Herrmann
Department of Medicine 3, Institute for Rheumatology and Immunology, Friedrich-Alexander-University (FAU) Erlangen-Nürnberg, Erlangen, Germany

Index

www.ingramcontent.com/pod-product-compliance
Lightning Source LLC
LaVergne TN
LVHW082149200926
848484LV00008B/2129